Surgical Anatomy and Technique

Lee J. Skandalakis
Editor

Surgical Anatomy and Technique

A Pocket Manual

Fifth Edition

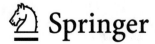 Springer

Editor
Lee J. Skandalakis
Department of Surgery
Piedmont Hospital
Atlanta, GA, USA

ISBN 978-3-030-51312-2   ISBN 978-3-030-51313-9   (eBook)
https://doi.org/10.1007/978-3-030-51313-9

This Springer imprint is published by the registered company Springer Nature Switzerland AG
The registered company address is: Gewerbestrasse 11, 6330 Cham, Switzerland

As always, my father's presence is felt. I can feel him breathing down my back saying his mantra "study, study, study." So again I dedicate this book to my father.

Preface to the Fifth Edition

It is not the critic who counts; not the man who points out how the strong man stumbles, or where the doer of deeds could have done them better. The credit belongs to the man who is actually in the arena, whose face is marred by dust and sweat and blood; who strives valiantly; who errs, who comes short again and again, because there is no effort without error and shortcoming; but who does actually strive to do the deeds; who knows great enthusiasms, the great devotions; who spends himself in a worthy cause; who at the best knows in the end the triumph of high achievement, and who at the worst, if he fails, at least fails while daring greatly, so that his place shall never be with those cold and timid souls who neither know victory nor defeat.
Theodore Roosevelt
Paris, April 23, 1910

The fifth edition of *Surgical Anatomy and Technique: A Pocket Manual* underwent a major revision with new color illustrations and chapters. Color illustrations make it much easier for the student young and old to follow the technique and better appreciate the anatomy. In the chapter on the abdominal wall and hernias, operating room strategies have been updated again and techniques of historical interest only have been removed. These new illustrations have made the transversus abdominus release technique much easier to follow. I would like to thank my friends at Emory who made tremendous contributions to this fifth edition. Major revisions were done on the stomach and extrahepatic biliary tract by Drs Jaja and Patel and the pancreas by Drs Ramonel and Patel. Dr Elwood made major revisions and updates to the chapter on the duodenum. Dr Marty T. Sellers enhanced the liver chapter which he had revised in the fourth edition.

Dr Feldman of Piedmont Hospital made major revision to the longest chapter in this book, Colon and Anorectum. Piedmont Hospital vascular surgeons Ross, Untzeitig, Chahwala, and Craddock made major revisions as well as a new chapter on ablative techniques for venous disease. Dr Hoadley from Northside Hospital contributed a new chapter on sports hernia. Dr John G. Seiler updated his chapter on carpal tunnel. Dr Procter updated his chapter on bariatric surgery adding technique for the duodenal switch. Dr Roger Eduardo revised the chapters on the small bowel and appendix. Dr C Dan Smith updated the chapters on the esophagus and diaphragm adding the new and novel LINX procedure for reflux.

Dr Feigelson, my old partner whom I sorely miss (not dead, just gone!), revised the chapters on the breast and adrenals. Dr Mullins made sure that treatment of melanoma of the skin was current and lastly Drs Shah and Muhletaler provided a new chapter on the kidney and ureter. Yes, general surgeons should know their way around those structures!

We have tried again to present what are considered to be basic surgical techniques. However, as I have stated before, what used to be advanced laparoscopic skills have been downgraded to basic laparoscopic skills.

Though the senior and principal author (JES) passed away in 2009, he continues to influence this and future editions of this text. He is sorely missed.

Atlanta, GA, USA   Lee J. Skandalakis

Acknowledgments

For some reason it seems that every subsequent edition of this book gets harder to write. We try to cut outdated material and revise to what is currently being taught and done. This project started about 2 years ago so by the time it gets into your hands it may be dated. Unfortunately, that is the case with every surgical text written. Nevertheless, I want to thank all of the surgeons who contributed and made this a much better edition than the previous. So again, I thank the people at Springer including Richard Hruska, Senior Editor of Clinical Medicine, for making this possible. More than halfway into this I had told Richard that I felt we needed to make the transition to colored illustrations. He gladly complied and we have a much better text for it.

In previous editions I had two editorial assistants helping me. This time I had one doing the work of two. Connie Walsh, Developmental Editor for Springer, did a fantastic job of dealing with all the surgeons, reading over the chapters and revisions, and making sure everything was just right. Thank you for your hard work and perseverance.

Finally, I would like to thank Dr Panagiotis G. Skandalakis for his great ideas for this book and the wonderful illustrations that kick-started this entire endeavor many years ago.

Contents

Contributors

Veer Chahwala, MD, RPVI Vascular and Endovascular Surgery, Piedmont Atlanta Vein Center, Piedmont Atlanta Hospital, Atlanta, GA, USA

Garnet Roy Craddock Jr, MD, RPVI, FACS Southern Vein Care, The Piedmont Clinic, Piedmont Newnan Hospital, Newnan, GA, USA

Roger Eduardo, MD Department of Surgery, Beltline Bariatric and Surgical Group, Atlanta, GA, USA

David R. Elwood, MD Division of General and Gastrointestinal Surgery, Department of Surgery, Emory University, Atlanta, GA, USA

Bruce J. Feigelson, MD, FACS Department of General Surgery, Colorado Permanente Medical Group, Denver, CO, USA

Evan N. Feldman, MD ATL Colorectal Surgery, P.C, Atlanta, GA, USA

M. Fred Muhletaler, MD, FACS Robotic and Minimally Invasive Surgery, Department of Surgery, Palms West Hospital and Palm Beach Urology, Wellington, FL, USA

Jeffrey S. Hoadley, MD Department of Surgery, North Atlanta Surgical Associates, Atlanta, GA, USA

Mohammad Raheel Jajja, MD Department of Surgery, Winship Cancer Institute, Emory University, Atlanta, GA, USA

John David Mullins, MD, FACS Department of Surgery, Piedmont Hospital, Atlanta, GA, USA

Shatul Parikh, MD Northwest Thyroid and Parathyroid Center, Northwest ENT and Allergy Center, Atlanta, GA, USA

Snehal Patel, MD Department of Surgery, Emory University, Atlanta, GA, USA

Charles D. Procter Jr, MD, FACS, FASMBS Department of Surgery, Piedmont Atlanta Hospital, Atlanta, GA, USA

Kimberly M. Ramonell, MD Department of General Surgery, Emory University, Atlanta, GA, USA

Charles B. Ross, MD, RPVI, FACS Vascular and Endovascular Services, Piedmont Heart Institute, Piedmont Atlanta Vein Center, Piedmont Atlanta Hospital, Atlanta, GA, USA

John Gray Seiler III, MD Department of Orthopaedic Surgery, Emory University, Atlanta, GA, USA

Piedmont Hospital, Atlanta, GA, USA

Marty T. Sellers, MD, MPH Department of Surgery, Emory University, Atlanta, GA, USA

Nikhil L. Shah, DO, MPH Minimally Invasive, Minimal Access & Robotic Surgery, Department of Surgery, Piedmont Health Care, Atlanta, GA, USA

Lee J. Skandalakis, MD, FACS Department of Surgery, Piedmont Hospital, Atlanta, GA, USA

C. Daniel Smith, MD Esophageal Institute of Atlanta, Atlanta, GA, USA

Ramon A. Suarez, MD, FACOG Department of Gynecology and Obstetrics, Emory University School of Medicine, Atlanta, GA, USA

Gynecology – Obstetrics, Piedmont Hospital, Atlanta, GA, USA

Andrew Walter Unzeitig, MD Department of Vascular Surgery, Piedmont Atlanta Hospital, Atlanta, GA, USA

Skin, Scalp, and Nail

1

John David Mullins and Lee J. Skandalakis

Anatomy

Skin and Subcutaneous Tissue (Fig. 1.1)

Incisions are necessary but need to be undertaken with respect to the potential complications or long-term effects. Some general considerations can often minimize problems.

The scalpel direction in almost all cases is best performed as a perpendicular division of the tissue through all the dermal layers to the underlying subcutaneous tissue. A "skiving" or angled incision will have more of a tendency to be problematic in healing or scar formation with residual deformity.

An incision that is in proximity to a scar or additional incision should be done with caution. The poor vascular supply between parallel incisions should be considered.

Likewise, converging incisions can create an area of poor vascularization at the apex.

The skin is the largest organ of the body and is composed of two primary layers: the epidermis (superficial) and the dermis (under the epidermis). The thickness of the skin varies from 0.5 to 3.0 mm. There are some references to a hypodermis or adjacent subcutaneous tissue which, although not part of the skin as such, does contain some deeper appendages. In some references this is considered a third layer.

The epidermis is avascular and is composed of stratified squamous epithelium. It has a thickness of 0.04–0.4 mm. The palms of the hands and the soles of the feet are thicker than the skin of other areas of the human body, such as the eyelids. Melanocytes are found in the epidermis.

J. D. Mullins (✉) · L. J. Skandalakis
Department of Surgery, Piedmont Hospital, Atlanta, GA, USA

© Springer Nature Switzerland AG 2021
L. J. Skandalakis (ed.), *Surgical Anatomy and Technique*,
https://doi.org/10.1007/978-3-030-51313-9_1

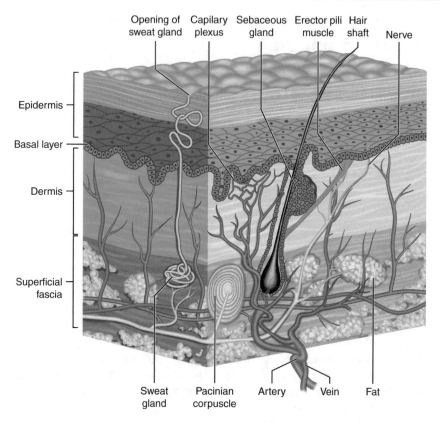

Fig. 1.1 Structures of the skin

The dermis has a thickness of 0.5–2.5 mm and contains smooth muscles and sebaceous and sweat glands. Various mechanoreceptors are found in the dermis. Hair roots are located in the dermis and may extend into the subcutaneous tissue or hypodermis.

Vascular System

There are two arterial plexuses: one close to the subcutaneous fat (subdermal) and the second in the subpapillary area. Venous return is accomplished by a subpapillary plexus to a deep plexus and then to the superficial veins. A lymphatic plexus is situated in the dermis, which drains into the subcutaneous tissue. The lymphatic drainage into anatomic basins of lymph node collections is an important subject to become acquainted.

Nervous System

For innervation of the skin, there is a rich sensory and sympathetic supply.

Remember
- The epidermis is avascular.
- The dermis is tough, strong, and very vascular.
- The superficial fascia is the subcutaneous tissue that blends with the reticular layer of the dermis.
- The principal blood vessels of the skin lie in subdermal areas.
- The basement membrane is the lowest layer of the epidermis.
- The papillary dermis is the upper (superficial) layer of the dermis, just below the basement membrane.
- The reticular dermis is the lower (deep) layer of the dermis, just above the fat.

Scalp

The following mnemonic device will serve as an aid in remembering the structure of the scalp (see also Fig. 1.2).

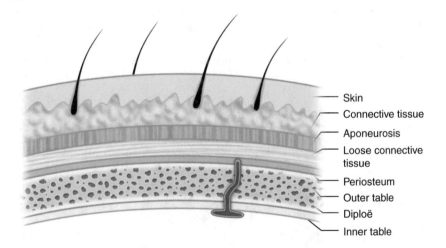

Skin
Connective tissue
Aponeurosis
Loose connective tissue
Periosteum
Outer table
Diploë
Inner table

Fig. 1.2 Structures of the scalp

	Layers	Description	Observations
S	Skin	Hair, sebaceous glands	
C	Connective close subcutaneous tissue	Superficial layer avascular deep layer vascular (internal and external carotid lymphatic network). Nerves are present (cervical, trigeminal)	Bleeding due to gap and nonvascular contraction
A	Aponeurosis epicranial, galea	Aponeurosis of the occipitofrontalis muscle	Sensation present
L	Loose connective tissue	Emissary veins	Dangerous zone = extracranial and intracranial infections
P	Pericranium–periosteum		No sensation. Heavy fixation at the suture lines, so infection is limited

Vascular System

Arterial Supply

The arteries of the scalp are branches of the internal and external carotid arteries. The internal carotid in this area becomes the supratrochlear and supraorbital arteries (Fig. 1.3), both of which are terminal branches of the ophthalmic artery. The external carotid becomes a large occipital artery and two small arteries: the superficial temporal and the posterior auricular (see Fig. 1.3). Abundant anastomosis takes place among all these arteries. All are superficial to the epicranial aponeurosis.

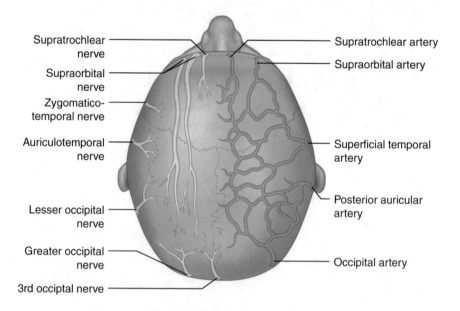

Fig. 1.3 Arterial blood supply shown on *right*. Nerve distribution shown on *left*. Veins are not shown, but follow the arteries

Venous Drainage
Veins follow the arteries.

Lymphatic Drainage
The lymphatic network of the scalp is located at the deep layer of the dense connective subcutaneous tissue just above the aponeurosis (between the connective tissue and aponeurosis). The complex network has frequent anastomoses. The three principal zones are the frontal, parietal, and occipital.

Note
- The blood supply of the scalp is rich. Arteries are anastomosed very freely.
- The arteries and veins travel together in a longitudinal fashion.
- A transverse incision or laceration will produce a gap. Dangerous bleeding will take place from both vascular ends due to nonretraction of the arteries by the close, dense, connective layer.
- Always repair the aponeurotic galea to avoid hematoma under it.
- With elective cases (excision of sebaceous cysts, etc.), whenever possible, make a longitudinal incision.
- Drain infections of the scalp and face promptly. Use antibiotics to prevent intracranial infections via the emissary veins.
- After cleansing the partially avulsed scalp, replace it and débride the wound; then suture with nonabsorbable sutures.
- Use pressure dressing as required. Sutures may be removed in 3–10 days.
- Be sure about the diagnosis. A very common sebaceous cyst could be an epidermoid cyst of the skull involving the outer or inner table, or both, with extension to the cerebral cortex. In such a case, call for a neurosurgeon. The best diagnostic procedure is an AP and lateral film of the skull to rule out bony involvement
- Because the skin, connective tissue, and aponeurosis are so firmly interconnected, for practical purposes, they form one layer: the surgical zone of the scalp.

Nerves (Figs. 1.3 and 1.4)
The following nerves innervate the scalp (their origins are in parentheses):
- Lesser occipital (second and third ventral nerves)
- Greater occipital (second and third dorsal nerves)
- Auriculotemporal (mandibular nerve)
- Zygomaticotemporal and zygomaticofacial (zygomatic [maxillary] nerve)
- Supraorbital (ophthalmic nerve)
- Supratrochlear (ophthalmic nerve)

Nail

The anatomy of the nail may be appreciated from Figs. 1.5 and 1.6.

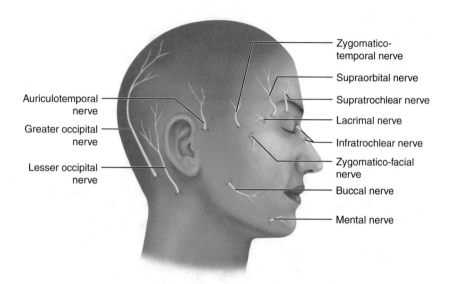

Fig. 1.4 Sensory Nerves of the scalp and face

Fig. 1.5 Structures of the nail

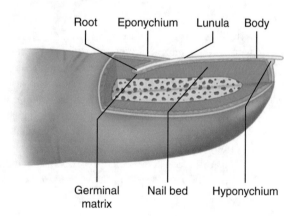

Fig. 1.6 Nail bed

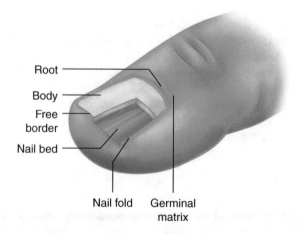

Technique

Benign Skin Lesions (Figs. 1.7, 1.8, and 1.9)

Benign skin lesions fall into several groups. Cystic lesions include epidermal inclusion cysts, sebaceous cysts, pilonidal cysts, and ganglia. Another group includes warts, keratoses, keloids, hemangiomatas, arteriovenous malformations, glomus tumors, and capillary malformations.

A third group includes decubitus ulcers, hidradenitis suppurativa, and burns. Junctional, compound, and intradermal nevi and malignant lentigos compose another group.

- **Step 1.** For a cyst, make an elliptical incision. An infected sebaceous cyst may best be treated in 2 stages. The first will be to incise and drain the contents until the inflammatory response has resolved. A loose pack or drain may be placed until this can be achieved. Closure of an infected wound will likely require a subsequent drainage procedure. For a noncystic lesion, be sure to include approximately 2.0 mm of tissue beyond the lesion when making the elliptical incision.

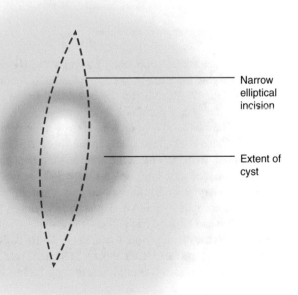

Narrow elliptical incision

Extent of cyst

Fig. 1.7 Incision for cyst removal

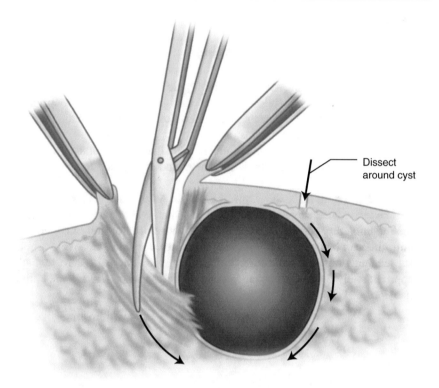

Dissect
around cyst

Fig. 1.8 Dissection to subcutaneous tissue

- **Step 2.** Place the incision along Langer's lines (Kraissl's) and perpendicular to the underlying muscles, but seldom parallel to the underlying muscle fibers.
- **Step 3.** Dissect down to the subcutaneous tissue but not to the fascia. Avoid breaking the cyst, if possible.
- **Step 4.** Handle the specimen with care by not crushing the skin or the lesion.
- **Step 5.** Close in two layers only in the absence of infection. Undermine the skin as required. Remember that the dermis is the strongest layer. For the dermis, use absorbable synthetic interrupted suture 3–0 (undyed Vicryl); for the epidermis, use 5–0 Vicryl subcuticular continuous and reinforce with Steri-strips or skin glue. It is acceptable to use 6–0 interrupted nylon sutures very close to the edges of the skin and close to each other.
- **Step 6.** Remove interrupted sutures in 8–10 days and again reinforce with Steri-strips, especially if the wound is located close to a joint. For most cases, a nylon epidermal continuous suture may be left in for 2 weeks without any problems.

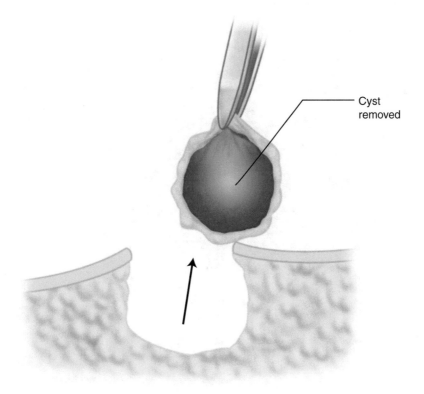

Cyst removed

Fig. 1.9 Excision of cyst

Malignant Skin Lesions (Figs. 1.10 and 1.11)

Malignant skin lesions include melanoma, basal cell carcinoma, squamous cell carcinoma, sweat gland carcinoma, fibrosarcoma, hemangiopericytoma, Kaposi's sarcoma, and dermatofibrosarcoma protuberans.

When removing the lesion, 1.0 cm of healthy skin around it must also be removed, as well as the subcutaneous layer.

Remember
- Send specimen to the lab for frozen section of the lesion and margins. Not recommended for melanoma. Many labs prefer permanent fixation for histologic diagnosis.
- Prior to surgery explain to the patient about scarring, recurrence, margins, etc.
- If the case involves a large facial lesion, obtain the advice of a plastic surgeon.

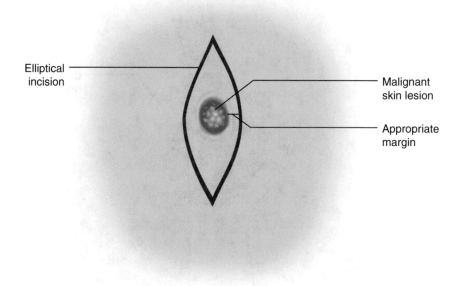

Fig. 1.10 Incision for removal of malignant skin lesion

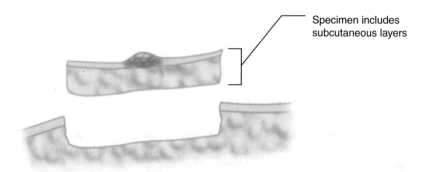

Fig. 1.11 Resection of malignant skin lesion

Melanoma

The Clark classification has fallen out of favor due to the levels varying based on location on the body. This led to less of a correlation of metastasis compared to the Breslow classification.

Staging of Malignant Melanoma (After Clark)

Level I. Malignant cells are found above the basement membrane.

Level II. Malignant cells infiltrate into the papillary dermis.

Level III. Malignant cells fill the papillary layer and extend to the junction of the papillary and reticular layers but do not enter the reticular layer.

Level IV.   Malignant cells extend into the reticular layer of the dermis.
Level V.   Malignant cells extend into the subcutaneous tissue.

Tumor Thickness (After Breslow)
Level I.   Tumor thickness less than 0.76 mm
Level II.   Tumor thickness 0.76–1.5 mm
Level III. Tumor thickness 1.51–2.25 mm
Level IV.   Tumor thickness 2.26–3 mm
Level V.   Tumor thickness greater than 3 mm

> **Remember**
> - Perform a sentinel lymph node biopsy, and, if positive, follow up with a complete lymph node dissection. Management with consultation of an oncologist is always encouraged if possible. Amputate a digit if melanoma is present. Be sure to consider the size, depth, and topography of the defect.
> - For all pigmented nevi, ask for a second opinion. Remember that the depth of invasion is critical and full-thickness biopsy will be necessary for determination.

Margins

Tumor thickness	Margins
In situ lesions	0.5–1.0 cm
≤ 1.0 mm	1.0 cm
1.01–2.0 mm	1.0–2.0 cm
≥2.01	2.0 cm

Lesion Thickness and Regional Lymph Node Staging
For Breslow's levels 1 and 5, very few lymphadenectomies are performed. The philosophy is that with a level 1 lesion, the chance of metastasis is remote; hence, a lymph node dissection is not warranted. The level 5 lesion is so advanced that a lymph node dissection will not alter the outcome. For intermediate levels 2–4, lymphadenectomy can be therapeutic. In recent large studies the breakpoint for indicated sentinel lymph node biopsy is 0.86 mm thickness for the melanoma. A sentinel lymph node biopsy is done first and, if positive, is followed by a complete lymphadenectomy. If there are palpable lymph nodes, then a radical lymphadenectomy is performed.

Sentinel Lymph Node Biopsy

- **Step 1.** Radiologist have localized sentinel lymph node preoperatively by injecting radioisotope and blue dye around the lesion (on breast: around nipple).
- **Step 2.** In the operating room, an incision is made over the area with the highest radioactivity count.

- **Step 3.** Dissect down to lymph node.
- **Step 4.** Using Geiger counter device as well as looking for the blue lymph node, identify and remove the sentinel lymph node.
- **Step 5.** If frozen section of sentinel lymph node is found to be positive, consider proceeding to a full lymph node dissection if staging information has been completed and indication has been confirmed.

Excision of Malignant Lesion (Melanoma, Squamous Cell Epithelioma)

The procedure is similar to that for a benign lesion. For melanoma, make a wide excision depending upon the thickness of the lesion as reported by the pathologist. Scalp melanomas metastasize, and sentinel lymph node biopsy may be performed, regardless of depth: if radical neck surgery is done for frontal lesions, include the superficial lobe of the parotid; for temporal and occipital lesions, include the post-auricular and occipital nodes. When a posterior scalp melanoma is present, a posterior neck dissection may be performed. See details on malignant skin lesions earlier in this chapter.

For squamous cell epitheliomas, wide excision is the procedure of choice. If the bone is involved, plastic and neurosurgical procedures should follow.

Skin Grafts

Free skin grafts include split-thickness grafts, postage-stamp grafts (a type of split-thickness graft), full-thickness grafts, and pinch grafts (not described here due to space limitations). Another classification, pedicle grafts, also is not described because a general surgeon who lacks the proper training to perform pedicle grafts should refer such cases to a plastic surgeon.

Split-Thickness Graft (Epidermis Plus Partial Dermis)

Definition: Large pieces of skin including part of the dermis but leaving deeper dermal elements to allow healing of the donor site.

Indications: Non-infected area that has adequate granulation to support a split-thickness graft. It is not uncommon for the initial role of the surgeon is to prepare the recipient site. Negative pressure wound therapy as well as topical wound care therapies have been advanced in the past few years to facilitate a proper "wound bed."

Contraindications: Infection, exposed bone without periosteum, exposed cartilage without perichondrium, and exposed tendon without sheath. Coverage over a joint is often discouraged due to the reduced elasticity of a healed split-thickness graft. Consider a full-thickness graft in this setting. Radiated tissue is considered a relative contraindication for grafting with a significant failure rate.

Donor Area: Consider the size of the graft to be harvested. Also consider the need for the donor site to heal without trauma or disruptive motion. The lateral thighs are often used as donor sites as occlusive dressings can be maintained without the problems of restrictive positioning.

Complications: Infection, failure to take, contractures and donor site failure to heal.

The progression or conversion of a split-thickness donor site to a full-thickness wound should be a complication to keep in mind and avoid by all means.

- **Step 1.** Prepare both areas. Prepare the donor site first as this is the "clean" site and must not be contaminated. Skin of the donor area must be kept taut by applying hand or board pressure. The motion of the dermatome may be facilitated by application of oil or saline.
- **Step 2.** Remove estimated skin. We use a Zimmer dermatome set at a thickness of 0.026 cm for harvesting of skin. In most cases, we mesh the skin using a 1.5:1 mesh ratio.
- **Step 3.** Place the graft over the receiving area.
- **Step 4.** Suture or staple the graft to the skin. If the graft was not meshed, perforate it for drainage.
- **Step 5.** Dress using Xeroform gauze covered by moist 4 × 4 s or cotton balls. Then cover with roll gauze of appropriate size circumferentially. A tie-over bolster may be used to prevent shifting of the graft.
- **Step 6.** Change dressing in 3 days.
- Alternative procedure: Place a wound VAC white gauze over the graft. Change in 5–7 days.

Full-Thickness Graft (Fig. 1.12)

Definition: The skin in toto, but not the subcutaneous tissue.

Indications: Facial defects, fresh wounds, covering of defects after removal of large benign or malignant tumors. Coverage over joints or tissues requiring flexibility such as "web" sites.

Contraindications: Infections. Poor recipient site vascularity or granulation tissue. The full-thickness grafts require better vascularity in general.

Donor Area: The full-thickness graft will require closure of the defect or a possible lengthy course for healing by secondary intention. Previous incisions may

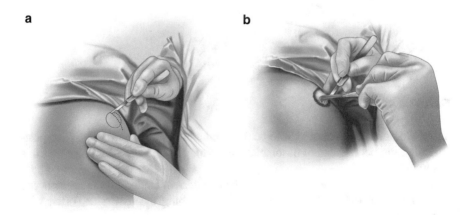

Fig. 1.12 How to prepare a "full-thickness skin graft". The first step is skin excision (**a**, **b**)... can be anywhere anatomically. Then placement of the hemostats (**c**), inversion of the skin over a fingertip (**d**), and then tangential thinning with surgical scissors (**e**)

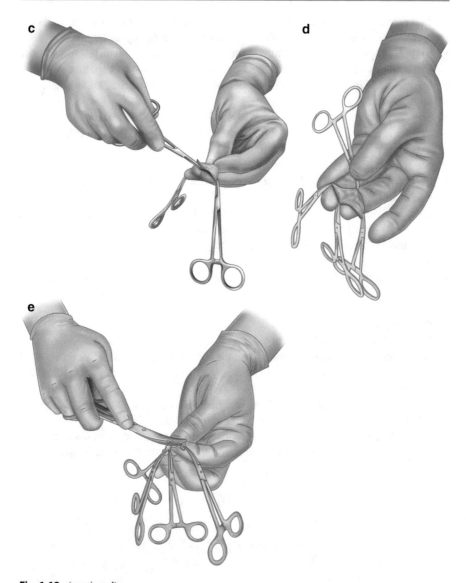

Fig. 1.12 (continued)

allow additional ellipses of skin to be removed and re-closed primarily. Also post-auricular, supraclavicular, or nasolabial tissues may be considered if color match is desired.

Technique: Excise the skin sharply to be transferred. Undermine as necessary to close the donor defect. Prepare the graft by thinning the underside, often with curved iris or Mayo scissors.

Fenestration may be needed to prevent accumulation of fluid beneath the graft. Fixation of the graft is the same as with the split graft although a longer period of time may be required before dressing removal and inspection.

Scalp Surgery

Excision of Benign Lesion
- **Step 1. Consider cutting** hair with scissors, but shaving has shown to be unnecessary.
- **Step 2.** Make longitudinal or elliptical incision, removing an elliptical piece of skin to include the lesion if dermal, overlying the cystic lesion if in the subcutaneous tissue.
- **Step 3.** Elevate limited flaps in the subcutaneous plane if necessary.
- **Step 4.** Obtain hemostasis if identifiable blood vessels, but compression against the underlying bone may be effective.
- **Step 5.** Remove cyst.
- **Step 6.** Close skin with a continuous suture to compress the wound edges. Alternatively, staples can provide a hemostatic closure.

Biopsy of Temporal Artery
Temporal artery biopsy is used to diagnose patients with symptoms such as fever, weight loss, or malaise and more specifically headaches, loss of visual acuity, diplopia, and temporal artery tenderness.

Step 1. Shave hair at the point of maximal pulsation at the preauricular area or above the zygomatic process.

Step 2. Make a longitudinal incision (Fig. 1.13).

Step 3. Carefully incise the aponeurosis (Fig. 1.14).

Step 4. After proximal and distal ligation with 2–0 silk, remove arterial segment at least 2 cm long (Fig. 1.15).

Step 5. Close in layers.

Remember
- The temporal artery is closely associated with the auriculotemporal nerve, which is behind it, and with the superficial temporal vein, which is also behind it, medially or laterally.
- In front of the ear, the temporal artery is subcutaneous. The temporal and zygomatic branches of the facial nerve emerge several centimeters anterior to the tragus but should be considered in danger of injury if the biopsy site is misplaced.
- Perform biopsy above the zygomatic process.

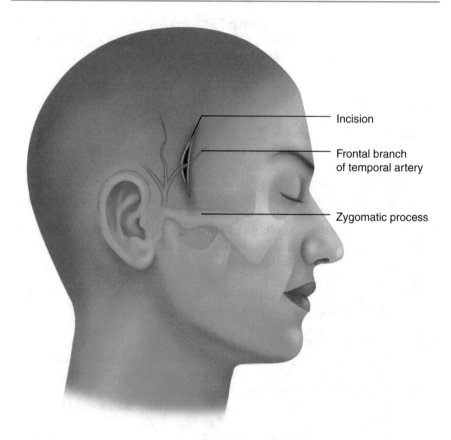

Incision

Frontal branch
of temporal artery

Zygomatic process

Fig. 1.13 Anatomical landmarks for temporal artery biopsy

Fig. 1.14 Incision for
temporal artery biopsy

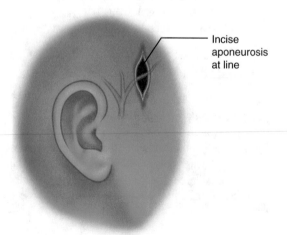

Incise
aponeurosis
at line

Fig. 1.15 Removal of
arterial segment

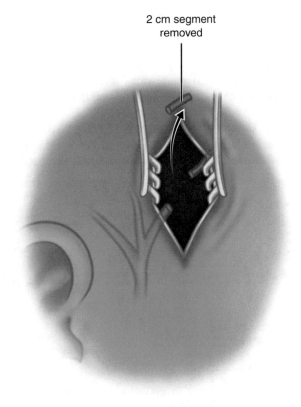

Ingrown Toenail

Definition: Inflammatory process with or without abscess formation secondary to
embedment of the lateral or medial edge of the nail into the nail fold.

Conservative Treatment
Good hygiene requires that the nail be cut in transverse, straight fashion without any
trimming of the edges (the square nail-cutting technique). Carefully elevate the
embedded edge and insert a piece of cotton between the infected nail fold and the
nail. Repeat the procedure until the ingrown nail edge grows above and distal to the
nail fold.

Total Excision (Avulsion) of Nail
- **Step 1.** Prepare distal half of foot.
- **Step 2.** Use double rubber band around the proximal phalanx for avascular field.
  Inject lidocaine, 1–2% without epinephrine, at the lateral and medial aspect of
  the second phalanx.
- **Step 3.** Insert a straight hemostat under the nail at the area of the inflammatory
  process until the edge of the instrument reaches the lunula.

- **Step 4.** Roll instrument and nail toward the opposite side for the avulsion of the nail.
- **Step 5.** Occasionally a small fragment of nail remains in situ and should be removed.
- **Step 6.** Excise all granulation tissue.
- **Step 7.** Cover area with antibiotic ointment and apply sterile dressing.

Partial Excision of Nail and Matrix (Figs. 1.16, 1.17, and 1.18)
Proceed as in total excision; except in step 4, remove only the involved side of the nail. Remove all granulation tissue, necrotic skin, matrix, and periosteum.

> **Remember**
> - The removal of the matrix in the designated area should be complete. Use curette as required. If in doubt, make a small vertical incision at the area for better exposure of the lateral nail and matrix to aid complete removal of these entities.

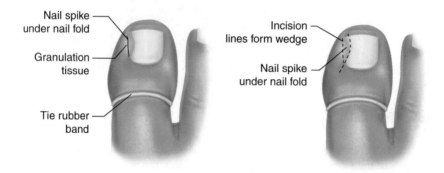

Fig. 1.16 Preparation of nail, showing incision lines

Fig. 1.17 Avulsion

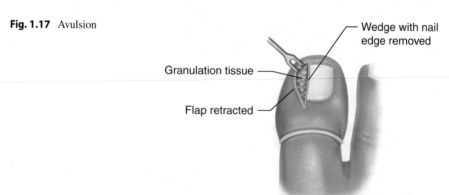

Fig. 1.18 Removal of
granulation tissue

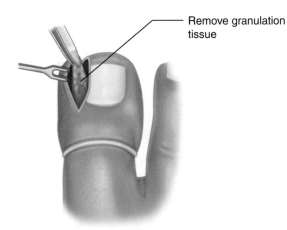

Remove granulation
tissue

Radical Excision of Nail and Matrix

Follow the total excision procedure described above, and then continue with
steps 4a–4d:

- **Step 4a.** Make vertical incisions medially and laterally.
- **Step 4b.** Elevate flaps for exposure of the matrix.
- **Step 4c.** Remove matrix in toto with knife and, as required, with curette.
- **Step 4d.** Loosely approximate the skin.

   Note: This procedure is done only if there is no evidence of inflammatory
process.

Neck

2

Lee J. Skandalakis and Shatul Parikh

Anatomy

Anterior Cervical Triangle (Fig. 2.1)

The boundaries are:
- Lateral: sternocleidomastoid muscle
- Superior: inferior border of the mandible
- Medial: anterior midline of the neck

This large triangle may be subdivided into four more triangles: submandibular, submental, carotid, and muscular.

Submandibular Triangle

The submandibular triangle is demarcated above by the inferior border of the mandible and below by the anterior and posterior bellies of the digastric muscle.

The largest structure in the triangle is the submandibular salivary gland. A number of vessels, nerves, and muscles also are found in the triangle.

For the surgeon, the contents of the triangle are best described in four layers, or surgical planes, starting from the skin. It must be noted that severe inflammation of the submandibular gland can destroy all traces of normal anatomy. When this occurs, identifying the essential nerves becomes a great challenge.

L. J. Skandalakis
Department of Surgery, Piedmont Hospital, Atlanta, GA, USA

S. Parikh (✉)
Northwest Thyroid and Parathyroid Center, Northwest ENT and Allergy Center, Atlanta, GA, USA
e-mail: sparikh@nw-ent.com

© Springer Nature Switzerland AG 2021
L. J. Skandalakis (ed.), *Surgical Anatomy and Technique*,
https://doi.org/10.1007/978-3-030-51313-9_2

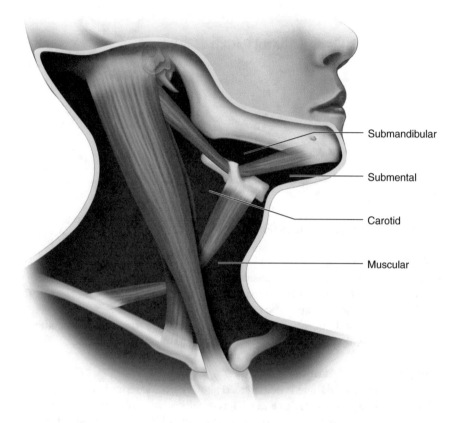

Fig. 2.1 The subdivision of the anterior triangle of the neck

Roof of the Submandibular Triangle

The roof—the first surgical plane—is composed of skin, superficial fascia enclosing platysma muscle and fat, and the mandibular and cervical branches of the facial nerve (VII) (Fig. 2.2).

It is important to remember that (1) the skin should be incised 4–5 cm below the mandibular angle; (2) the platysma and fat compose the superficial fascia, and (3) the cervical branch of the facial nerve (VII) lies just below the angle, superficial to the facial artery (Fig. 2.3).

The mandibular (or marginal mandibular) nerve passes approximately 3 cm below the angle of the mandible to supply the muscles of the corner of the mouth and lower lip.

The cervical branch of the facial nerve divides to form descending and anterior branches. The descending branch innervates the platysma and communicates with

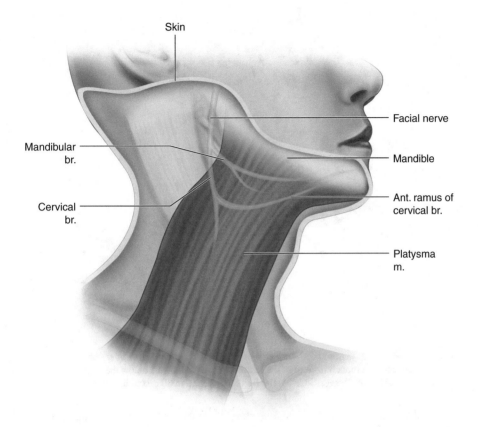

Skin

Facial nerve

Mandibular br.

Mandible

Cervical br.

Ant. ramus of cervical br.

Platysma m.

Fig. 2.2 The roof of the submandibular triangle (the first surgical plane). The platysma lies over the mandibular and cervical branches of the facial nerve

the anterior cutaneous nerve of the neck. The anterior branch—the ramus colli mandibularis—crosses the mandible superficial to the facial artery and vein and joins the mandibular branch to contribute to the innervation of the muscles of the lower lip.

Injury to the mandibular branch results in severe drooling at the corner of the mouth. It also causes an asymmetry in lower lip function that can identified when the patient smiles or purses their lips. Injury to the anterior cervical branch produces minimal side effects.

The distance between these two nerves and the lower border of the mandible is shown in Fig. 2.3.

Contents of the Submandibular Triangle

The structures of the second surgical plane, from superficial to deep, are the anterior and posterior facial vein, part of the facial (external maxillary) artery, the submental branch of the facial artery, the superficial layer of the submaxillary fascia (deep

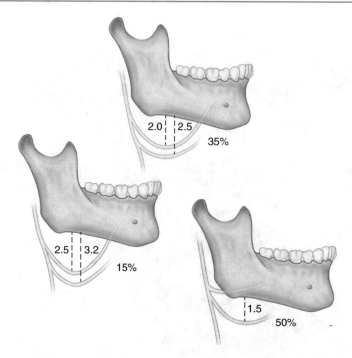

Fig. 2.3 The neural "hammocks" formed by the mandibular branch (*upper*) and the anterior ramus of the cervical branch (*lower*) of the facial nerve. The distance below the mandible is given in centimeters, and *percentages* indicate the frequency found in 80 dissections of these nerves

cervical fascia), the lymph nodes, the deep layer of the submaxillary fascia (deep cervical fascia), and the hypoglossal nerve (XII) (Fig. 2.4).

It is necessary to remember that the facial artery pierces the stylomandibular ligament. Therefore, it must be ligated before it is cut to prevent bleeding after retraction. Also, it is important to remember that the lymph nodes lie within the envelope of the submandibular fascia in close relationship with the gland. Differentiation between gland and lymph node may be difficult.

The anterior and posterior facial veins cross the triangle in front of the submandibular gland and unite close to the angle of the mandible to form the common facial vein, which empties into the internal jugular vein near the greater cornu of the hyoid bone. It is wise to identify, isolate, clamp, and ligate both of these veins.

The facial artery—a branch of the external carotid artery—enters the submandibular triangle under the posterior belly of the digastric muscle and under the stylohyoid muscle. At its entrance into the triangle, it is under the submandibular gland. After crossing the gland posteriorly, the artery passes over the mandible, lying always under the platysma. It can be ligated easily.

Floor of the Submandibular Triangle

The structures of the third surgical plane, from superficial to deep, include the mylohyoid muscle with its nerve, the hyoglossus muscle, the middle constrictor muscle covering the lower part of the superior constrictor, and part of the styloglossus muscle (Fig. 2.5).

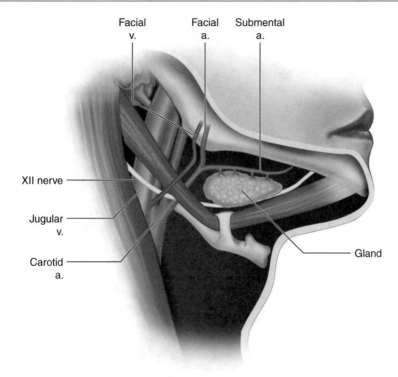

Fig. 2.4 The contents of the submandibular triangle (the second surgical plane). Exposure of the superficial portion of the submandibular gland

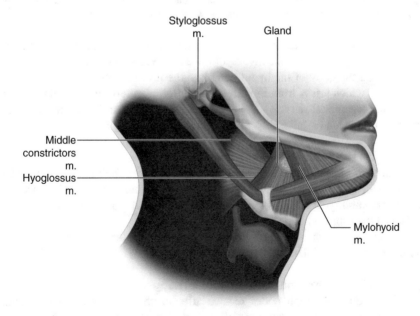

Fig. 2.5 The floor of the submandibular triangle (the third surgical plane). Exposure of mylohyoid and hyoglossus muscles

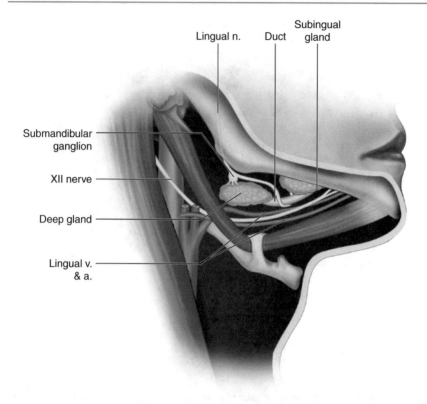

Fig. 2.6 The basement of the submandibular triangle (the fourth surgical plane). Exposure of the deep portion of the submandibular gland, the lingual nerve, and the hypoglossal (XII) nerve

The mylohyoid muscles are considered to form a true diaphragm of the floor of the mouth. They arise from the mylohyoid line of the inner surface of the mandible and insert on the body of the hyoid bone into the median raphe. The nerve to the mylohyoid, which arises from the inferior alveolar branch of the mandibular division of the trigeminal nerve (V), lies on the inferior surface of the muscle. The superior surface is in relationship with the lingual and hypoglossal nerves.

Basement of the Submandibular Triangle
The structures of the fourth surgical plane, or basement of the triangle, include the deep portion of the submandibular gland, the submandibular (Wharton's) duct, lingual nerve, sublingual artery, sublingual vein, sublingual gland, hypoglossal nerve (XII), and the submandibular ganglion (Fig. 2.6).

The submandibular duct lies below the lingual nerve (except where the nerve passes under it) and above the hypoglossal nerve.

Lymphatic Drainage of the Submandibular Triangle
The submandibular lymph nodes receive afferent channels from the submental nodes, oral cavity, and anterior parts of the face. Efferent channels drain primarily

into the jugulodigastric, jugulocarotid, and jugulo-omohyoid nodes of the chain accompanying the internal jugular vein (deep cervical chain). A few channels pass by way of the subparotid nodes to the spinal accessory chain.

Submental Triangle (See Fig. 2.1)

The boundaries of this triangle are:
- Lateral: anterior belly of digastric muscle
- Inferior: hyoid bone
- Medial: midline
- Floor: mylohyoid muscle
- Roof: skin and superficial fascia

The lymph nodes of the submental triangle receive lymph from the skin of the chin, the lower lip, the floor of the mouth, and the tip of the tongue. They send lymph to the submandibular and jugular chains of nodes.

Carotid Triangle (See Fig. 2.1)

The boundaries are:
- Posterior: sternocleidomastoid muscle
- Anterior: anterior belly of omohyoid muscle
- Superior: posterior belly of digastric muscle
- Floor: hyoglossus muscle, inferior constrictor of pharynx, thyrohyoid muscle, longus capitis muscle, and middle constrictor of pharynx
- Roof: investing layer of deep cervical fascia

Contents of the carotid triangle: bifurcation of carotid artery; internal carotid artery (no branches in the neck); external carotid artery branches, e.g., superficial temporal artery, internal maxillary artery, occipital artery, ascending pharyngeal artery, sternocleidomastoid artery, lingual artery (occasionally) , and external maxillary artery (occasionally); jugular vein tributaries, e.g., superior thyroid vein, occipital vein, common facial vein, and pharyngeal vein; and vagus nerve, spinal accessory nerve, hypoglossal nerve, ansa hypoglossi, and sympathetic nerves (partially).

Lymph is received by the jugulodigastric, jugulocarotid, and jugulo-omohyoid nodes and by the nodes along the internal jugular vein from submandibular and submental nodes, deep parotid nodes, and posterior deep cervical nodes. Lymph passes to the supraclavicular nodes.

Muscular Triangle (Fig. 2.1)

The boundaries are:
- Superior lateral: anterior belly of omohyoid muscle
- Inferior lateral: sternocleidomastoid muscle
- Medial: midline of the neck
- Floor: prevertebral fascia and prevertebral muscles; sternohyoid and sternothyroid muscles
- Roof: investing layer of deep fascia; strap, sternohyoid, and cricothyroid muscles
- Contents of the muscular triangle include: thyroid and parathyroid glands, trachea, esophagus, and sympathetic nerve trunk.

Remember that occasionally the strap muscles must be cut to facilitate thyroid surgery. They should be cut across the upper third of their length to avoid sacrificing their nerve supply.

Posterior Cervical Triangle (Fig. 2.7)

The posterior cervical triangle is sometimes considered to be two triangles—occipital and subclavian—divided by the posterior belly of the omohyoid muscle or, perhaps, by the spinal accessory nerve (see Fig. 2.7); we will treat it as one.

The boundaries of the posterior triangle are:
- Anterior: sternocleidomastoid muscle
- Posterior: anterior border of trapezius muscle
- Inferior: clavicle
- Floor: prevertebral fascia and muscles, splenius capitis muscle, levator scapulae muscle, and three scalene muscles
- Roof: superficial investing layer of the deep cervical fascia

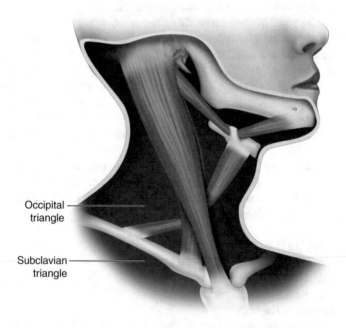

Occipital triangle

Subclavian triangle

Fig. 2.7 The posterior triangle of the neck. The triangle may be divided into two smaller triangles by the omohyoid muscle

Contents of the posterior cervical triangle include subclavian artery, subclavian vein, cervical nerves, brachial plexus, phrenic nerve, accessory phrenic nerve, spinal accessory nerve, and lymph nodes.

The superficial occipital lymph nodes receive lymph from the occipital region of the scalp and the back of the neck. The efferent vessels pass to the deep occipital lymph node (usually only one), which drains into the deep cervical nodes along the spinal accessory nerve.

Fasciae of the Neck

Our classification of the rather complicated fascial planes of the neck follows the work of several investigators. It consists of the superficial fascia and three layers that compose the deep fascia.

Superficial Fascia
The superficial fascia lies beneath the skin and is composed of loose connective tissue, fat, the platysma muscle, and small unnamed nerves and blood vessels (Fig. 2.8). The surgeon should remember that the cutaneous nerves of the neck and the anterior and external jugular veins are between the platysma and the deep cervical fascia. If these veins are to be cut, they must first be ligated. Because of their attachment to the platysma above and the fascia below, they do not retract; bleeding from them may be serious. For all practical purposes, there is no space between this layer and the deep fascia.

Deep Fascia

Investing, Anterior, or Superficial Layer (Figs. 2.9 and 2.10)
This layer envelops two muscles (the trapezius and the sternocleidomastoid) and two glands (the parotid and the submaxillary) and forms two spaces (the supraclavicular and the suprasternal). It forms the roof of the anterior and posterior cervical triangles and the midline raphe of the strap muscles.

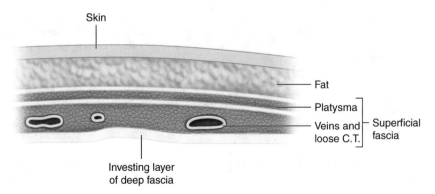

Fig. 2.8   The superficial fascia of the neck lies between the skin and the investing layer of the deep cervical fascia

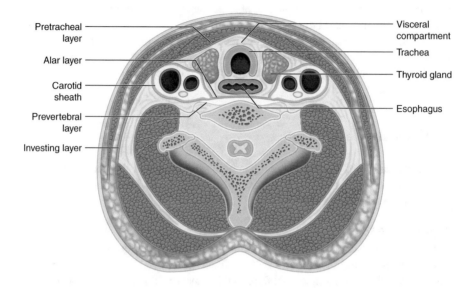

Fig. 2.9 Diagrammatic cross section through the neck below the hyoid bone showing the layers of the deep cervical fascia and the structures that they envelop

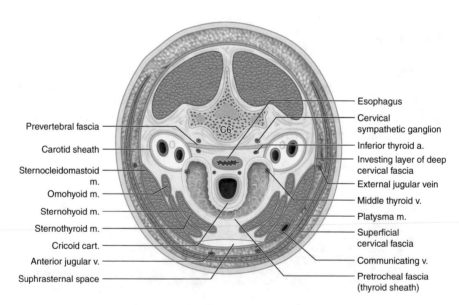

Fig. 2.10 Diagrammatic cross section of the neck through the thyroid gland at the level of the sixth cervical vertebra showing the fascial planes, muscles, and vessels that may be encountered in an incision for thyroidectomy

Pretracheal or Middle Layer
The middle layer of the deep fascia splits into an anterior portion that envelops the strap muscles and a posterior layer that envelops the thyroid gland, forming the false capsule of the gland.

Prevertebral, Posterior, or Deep Layer
This layer lies in front of the prevertebral muscles. It covers the cervical spine muscles, including the scalene muscles and vertebral column anteriorly. The fascia divides to form a space in front of the vertebral bodies, the anterior layer being the alar fascia and the posterior layer retaining the designation of prevertebral fascia.

Carotid Sheath
Beneath the sternocleidomastoid muscle, all the layers of the deep fascia contribute to a fascial tube, the carotid sheath. Within this tube lie the common carotid artery, internal jugular vein, vagus nerve, and deep cervical lymph nodes.

Buccopharyngeal Fascia
This layer covers the lateral and posterior surfaces of the pharynx and binds the pharynx to the alar layer of the prevertebral fascia.

Axillary Fascia
This fascia takes its origin from the prevertebral fascia. It is discussed in Chap. 3.

Spaces of the Neck

There are many spaces in the neck defined by the fasciae, but for the general surgeon, the visceral compartment is the most important; be very familiar with its boundaries and contents.

The boundaries of the visceral compartment of the neck are:
- Anterior: pretracheal fascia
- Posterior: prevertebral fascia
- Lateral: carotid sheath
- Superior: hyoid bone and thyroid cartilage
- Posteroinferior: posterior mediastinum
- Anteroinferior: bifurcation of the trachea at the level of the fifth thoracic vertebra

Contents of the spaces of the neck include part of esophagus, larynx, trachea, thyroid gland, and parathyroid glands.

Lymphatics of the Neck/Right and Left Thoracic Ducts

The overall anatomy of the lymphatics of the head and neck may be appreciated from Table 2.1 and Fig. 2.11.

Table 2.1 Lymph nodes and the lymphatic drainage of the head and neck

Location		Lymphatics	
		From	To
Superior horizontal chain:			
Submental nodes	Submental triangle	Skin of chin, lip, floor of mouth, tip of tongue	Submandibular nodes or jugular chain
Submandibular nodes	Submandibular triangle	Submental nodes, oral cavity, face, except forehead and part of lower lip	Intermediate jugular nodes, deep posterior cervical nodes
Preauricular (parotid) nodes	In front of tragus	Lateral surface of pinna, side of scalp	Deep cervical nodes
Postauricular (mastoid) nodes	Mastoid process	Temporal scalp, medial surface of pinna, external auditory meatus	Deep cervical nodes
Occipital node	Between mastoid process and external occipital protuberance	Back of scalp	Deep cervical nodes
Vertical chain:			
Posterior cervical (posterior triangle) nodes		Subparotid nodes, jugular chain, occipital, and mastoid area	Supraclavicular and deep cervical nodes
Superficial	Along external jugular vein		
Deep	Along spinal accessory nerve		
Intermediate (jugular) nodes		All other nodes of the neck	Lymphatic trunks to left and right thoracic ducts
Jugulocarotid (subparotid) nodes	Angle of mandible, near parotid nodes		
Jugulodigastric (subdigastric) nodes	Junction of common facial and internal jugular veins	Palatine tonsils, base of tongue	
Jugulocarotid (bifurcation) nodes	Bifurcation of common carotid artery close to carotid body	Tongue, except tip, oropharynx, hypopharynx, larynx	
Jugulo-omohyoid (omohyoid) nodes	Crossing of omohyoid and internal jugular vein	Tip of tongue	
Anterior (visceral) nodes			
Parapharyngeal nodes	Lateral and posterior wall of pharynx	Deep face and esophagus	Intermediate nodes

(continued)

Table 2.1 (continued)

Paralaryngeal nodes	Lateral wall of larynx	Larynx and thyroid gland	Deep cervical nodes
Paratracheal nodes	Lateral wall of trachea	Thyroid gland, trachea, esophagus	Deep cervical and mediastinal nodes
Prelaryngeal (Delphian) nodes	Cricothyroid ligament	Thyroid gland, pharynx	Deep cervical nodes
Pretracheal nodes	Anterior wall of trachea below isthmus of thyroid gland	Thyroid gland, trachea, esophagus	Deep cervical and mediastinal nodes
Inferior horizontal chain:			
Supraclavicular and scalene nodes	Subclavian triangle	Axilla, thorax, vertical chain	Jugular or subclavian trunks to right lymphatic duct and thoracic duct

By permission of JE Skandalakis, SW Gray, and JR Rowe. *Anatomical Complications in General Surgery*. New York: McGraw-Hill, 1983

Fig. 2.11 The lymph nodes of the neck. *SH* superior horizontal chain, *IH* inferior horizontal chain, *PV* posterior vertical chain, *IV* intermediate vertical chain, *AV* anterior vertical chain

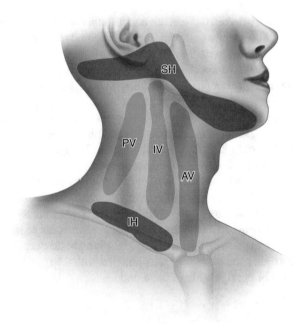

The thoracic duct originates from the cisterna chyli and terminates in the left subclavian vein (Fig. 2.12). It is approximately 38–45 cm long. The duct begins at about the level of the second lumbar vertebra from the cisterna chyli or, if the cisterna is absent (about 50% of cases), from the junction of the right and left lumbar lymphatic trunks and the intestinal lymph trunk. It ascends to the right of the midline on the anterior surface of the bodies of the thoracic vertebrae. It crosses the

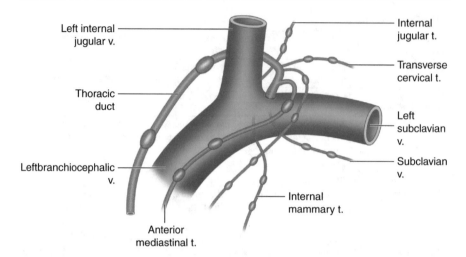

Left internal jugular v.

Internal jugular t.

Transverse cervical t.

Thoracic duct

Left subclavian v.

Leftbranchiocephalic v.

Subclavian v.

Internal mammary t.

Anterior mediastinal t.

Fig. 2.12 The thoracic duct and main left lymphatic trunks. Trunks are variable and may enter the veins with the thoracic duct or separately

midline between the seventh and fifth thoracic vertebrae to lie on the left side, to the left of the esophageal wall. It passes behind the great vessels at the level of the seventh cervical vertebra and descends slightly to enter the left subclavian vein (see Fig. 2.12). The duct may have multiple entrances to the vein, and one or more of the contributing lymphatic trunks may enter the subclavian or the jugular vein independently. It may be ligated with impunity, but improper ligation can result in a chyle leak which can be a very difficult postoperative complication to manage.

The thoracic duct collects lymph from the entire body below the diaphragm, as well as from the left side of the thorax. Lymph nodes may be present at the caudal end, but there are none along its upward course. Injury to the duct in supraclavicular lymph node dissections results in copious lymphorrhea. Ligation is the answer.

The right lymphatic duct is a variable structure about 1 cm long formed by the right jugular, transverse cervical, internal mammary, and mediastinal lymphatic trunks (Fig. 2.13). If these trunks enter the veins separately, there is no right lymphatic duct. When present, the right lymphatic duct enters the superior surface of the right subclavian vein at its junction with the right internal jugular vein and drains most of the right side of the thorax.

Anatomy of the Thyroid Gland

The thyroid gland consists typically of two lobes, a connecting isthmus, and an ascending pyramidal lobe. One lobe, usually the right, may be smaller than the other (7% of cases) or completely absent (1.7%). The isthmus is absent in about 10% of thyroid glands, and the pyramidal lobe is absent in about 50% (Fig. 2.14). A minute epithelial tube or fibrous cord—the thyroglossal duct—almost always extends between the thyroid gland and the foramen cecum of the tongue.

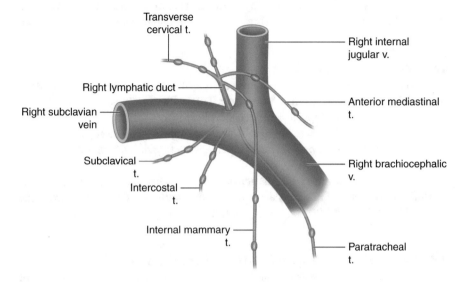

Fig. 2.13 The right lymphatic duct is formed by the junction of several lymphatic trunks. If they enter the veins separately, there may be no right lymphatic duct

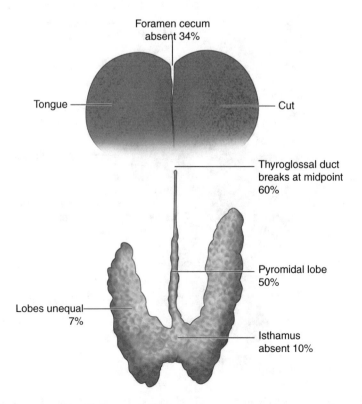

Fig. 2.14 Normal vestiges of thyroid gland development. None are of clinical significance, but their presence may be of concern to the surgeon

The thyroid gland normally extends from the level of the fifth cervical vertebra to that of the first thoracic vertebra. It may lie higher (lingual thyroid), but rarely lower.

Capsule of the Thyroid Gland

The thyroid gland has a connective tissue capsule which is continuous with the septa and which makes up the stroma of the organ. This is the *true* capsule of the thyroid.

External to the true capsule is a well-developed (to a lesser or greater degree) layer of fascia derived from the pretracheal fascia. This is the *false* capsule, *perithyroid sheath*, or *surgical capsule*. The false capsule, or fascia, is not removed with the gland at thyroidectomy.

The superior parathyroid glands normally lie between the true capsule of the thyroid and the fascial false capsule. The inferior parathyroids may be between the true and the false capsules, within the thyroid parenchyma, or lying on the outer surface of the fascia.

Arterial Supply of the Thyroid and Parathyroid Glands

Two paired arteries, the superior and inferior thyroid arteries, and an inconstant midline vessel—the thyroid ima artery—supply the thyroid (Fig. 2.15).

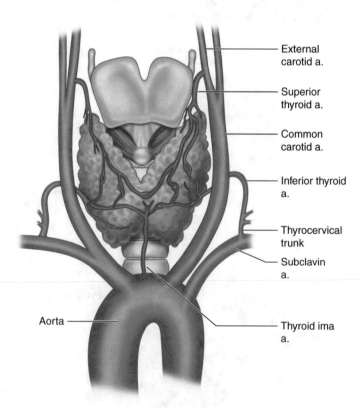

External
carotid a.

Superior
thyroid a.

Common
carotid a.

Inferior thyroid
a.

Thyrocervical
trunk

Subclavin
a.

Aorta

Thyroid ima
a.

Fig. 2.15 The arterial supply to the thyroid gland. The thyroid ima artery is only occasionally present

The superior thyroid artery arises from the external carotid artery just above, at, or just below the bifurcation of the common carotid artery. It passes downward and anteriorly to reach the superior pole of the thyroid gland. Along part of its course, the artery parallels the external branch of the superior laryngeal nerve. At the superior pole the artery divides into anterior and posterior branches. From the posterior branch, a small parathyroid artery passes to the superior parathyroid gland.

The inferior thyroid artery usually arises from the thyrocervical trunk or from the subclavian artery. It ascends behind the carotid artery and the internal jugular vein, passing medially and posteriorly on the anterior surface of the longus colli muscle. After piercing the prevertebral fascia, the artery divides into two or more branches as it crosses the ascending recurrent laryngeal nerve. The nerve may pass anterior or posterior to the artery or between its branches (Fig. 2.16). The lowest branch sends

Fig. 2.16 Relations at the crossing of the recurrent laryngeal nerve and the inferior thyroid artery. (**a–c**) Common variations. Their frequencies are given in Table 2.2. (**d**) A non-recurrent nerve is not related to the inferior thyroid artery. (**e**) The nerve loops beneath the artery

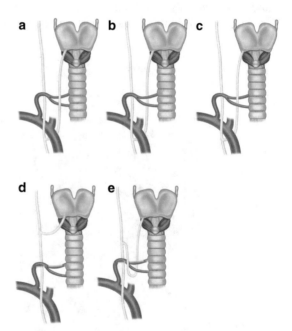

Table 2.2 Recurrent laryngeal nerve vulnerability

Cause of vulnerability	Percent encountered
Lateral and anterior location	1.5–3.0
Tunneling through thyroid tissue	2.5–15.0
Fascial fixation	2.0–3.0
Arterial fixation	5.0–12.5
Close proximity to inferior thyroid vein	1.5–2.0+

Data from Chang-Chien Y. Surgical anatomy and vulnerability of the recurrent laryngeal nerve. *Int Surg* 1980; 65:23

a twig to the inferior parathyroid gland. On the right, the inferior thyroid artery is absent in about 2% of individuals. On the left, it is absent in about 5%. The artery is occasionally double.

The arteria thyroidea ima is unpaired and inconstant. It arises from the brachiocephalic artery, the right common carotid artery, or the aortic arch. Its position anterior to the trachea makes it important for tracheostomy.

Venous Drainage

The veins of the thyroid gland form a plexus of vessels lying in the substance and on the surface of the gland. The plexus is drained by three pairs of veins (Fig. 2.17):
- The superior thyroid vein accompanies the superior thyroid artery.
- The middle thyroid vein arises on the lateral surface of the gland at about two-thirds of its anteroposterior extent. No artery accompanies it. This vein may be absent; occasionally it is double.
- The inferior thyroid vein is the largest and most variable of the thyroid veins.

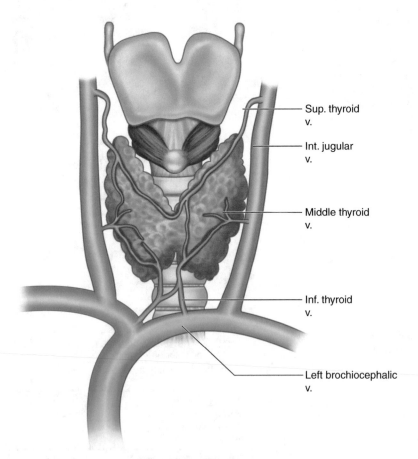

Fig. 2.17 The venous drainage of the thyroid gland. The inferior thyroid veins are quite variable

Recurrent Laryngeal Nerves (Figs. 2.16 and 2.18)

The right recurrent laryngeal nerve branches from the vagus as it crosses anterior to the right subclavian artery, loops around the artery from posterior to anterior, crosses

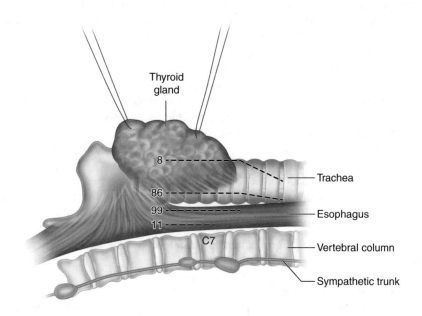

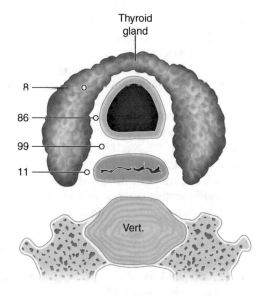

Fig. 2.18 The course of the recurrent laryngeal nerve at the level of the thyroid gland in 102 cadavers. In about one-half of the cases, the nerve lay in the groove between the trachea and the esophagus. (*Top*) Lateral view. (*Bottom*) Cross-sectional view

behind the right common carotid, and ascends in or near the tracheoesophageal groove. It passes posterior to the right lobe of the thyroid gland to enter the larynx behind the cricothyroid articulation and the inferior cornu of the thyroid cartilage.

The left recurrent laryngeal nerve arises where the vagus nerve crosses the aortic arch, just distal to the origin of the left subclavian artery from the aortic arch. It loops under the ligamentum arteriosum and the aorta and ascends in the same manner as the right nerve. Both nerves cross the inferior thyroid arteries near the lower border of the middle third of the gland.

In about 1% of patients, the right recurrent nerve arises normally from the vagus but passes medially almost directly from its origin to the larynx without looping under the subclavian artery. In these cases, the right subclavian artery arises from the descending aorta and passes to the right behind the esophagus. This anomaly is asymptomatic, and the thyroid surgeon will rarely be aware of it prior to operation. Even less common is a non-recurrent left nerve in the presence of a right aortic arch and a retroesophageal left subclavian artery.

In the lower third of its course, the recurrent laryngeal nerve ascends behind the pretracheal fascia at a slight angle to the tracheoesophageal groove. In the middle third of its course, the nerve may lie in the groove or within the substance of the thyroid gland.

The vulnerability of the recurrent laryngeal nerve may be appreciated from Table 2.2.

Exposure of the Laryngeal Nerves

The recurrent laryngeal nerve forms the medial border of a triangle bounded superiorly by the inferior thyroid artery and laterally by the carotid artery. The nerve can be identified where it enters the larynx just posterior to the inferior cornu of the thyroid cartilage. If the nerve is not found, a non-recurrent nerve should be suspected, especially on the right.

In the lower portion of its course, the nerve can be palpated as a tight strand over the tracheal surface. There is more connective tissue between the nerve and the trachea on the right than on the left. Visual identification, with avoidance of traction, compression, or stripping the connective tissue, is all that is necessary.

The superior laryngeal nerve arises from the vagus nerve just inferior to its lower sensory ganglion just outside the jugular foramen of the skull. The nerve passes inferiorly, medial to the carotid artery. At the level of the superior cornu of the hyoid bone, it divides into a large, sensory, internal laryngeal branch, and a smaller, motor, external laryngeal branch, serving the cricothyroid muscle and the cricopharyngeus. The point of division is usually within the bifurcation of the common carotid artery (Fig. 2.19).

The internal laryngeal branch is rarely identified by the surgeon (Fig. 2.20).

The external laryngeal branch, together with the superior thyroid vein and artery, passes under the sternothyroid muscles, posterior and medial to the vessels. The nerve then passes beneath the lower border of the thyrohyoid muscle to continue inferiorly to innervate the cricothyroid muscle.

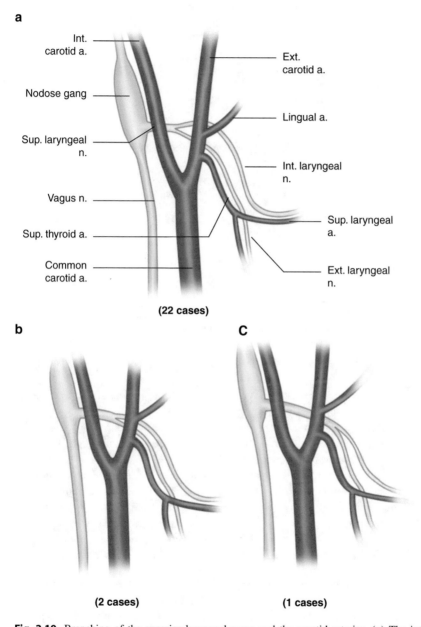

Fig. 2.19 Branching of the superior laryngeal nerve and the carotid arteries. (**a**) The internal branch crosses the external carotid artery above the origin of the lingual artery. (**b**) The internal branch crosses below the origin of the lingual artery. (**c**) The nerve divides medial to the external carotid artery

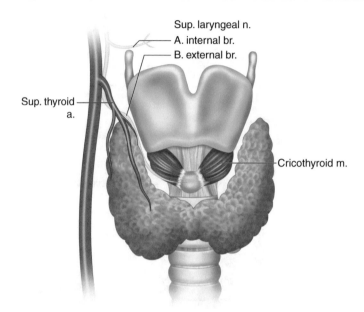

Sup. laryngeal n.
A. internal br.
B. external br.

Sup. thyroid a.

Cricothyroid m.

Fig. 2.20 Relations of the internal and external branches of the superior laryngeal nerve to the superior thyroid artery and the upper pole of the thyroid gland

Remember
- The results of injury to the recurrent laryngeal nerve and the external branch of the superior laryngeal nerve are as follows:
  - *Unilateral recurrent nerve injury.* The affected vocal cord is paramedian owing to adduction by the cricothyroid muscle. Voice is preserved but often breathy with poor cough.
  - *Unilateral recurrent and superior laryngeal nerve injury.* The affected cord is in an intermediate position, resulting in hoarseness and inability to cough. The affected cord will move toward the midline with time. Voice improves, but improvement is followed by narrowing of the airway.

Postoperative hoarseness is not always the result of operative injury to laryngeal nerves. From 1% to 2% of patients have a paralyzed vocal cord prior to thyroid operations. Researchers at the Mayo Clinic examined 202 cases of vocal cord paralysis, of which 153 (76%) followed thyroidectomy, 36 (18%) were of various known etiologies, and 13 (6%) were of idiopathic origin. We strongly advise the general surgeon to perform a mirror laryngoscopy or flexible nasolaryngoscopy prior to thyroidectomy.

We believe that the patient should be told that in spite of all precautions, there is a possibility of some vocal disability following thyroidectomy.

A sympathetic ganglion can be confused with a lymph node and removed when the surgeon operates for metastatic papillary carcinoma of the thyroid. In one of our patients, the inferior cervical and first thoracic ganglia were fused to form a node-like structure that was removed. The surgeon must identify any apparent lymph node related to the vertebral artery and fixed in front of the transverse process of the seventh cervical vertebra.

Injury to the cervical sympathetic nerve results in Horner's syndrome: (1) constriction of the pupil, (2) partial ptosis of the upper eyelid, (3) apparent enophthalmos, (4) dilatation of the retinal vessels, and (5) flushing and drying of the facial skin on the affected side.

Persistent Remnants of the Thyroglossal Duct

The foramen cecum of the tongue and the pyramidal lobe of the thyroid gland are normal remnants of the thyroglossal duct. Between these structures is a very small epithelial tube, usually broken in several places. Occasionally these epithelial fragments hypertrophy, secrete fluid, and form cysts. Drainage or aspiration of these cysts is futile and often results in formation of a fistula, that usually becomes infected.

All fragments of the duct, the foramen cecum, and the midportion of the hyoid bone should be removed (Sistrunk procedure). Recurrence of the cyst is the result of failure to remove the entire duct or the central portion of the hyoid bone.

Anatomy of the Parathyroid Glands

The parathyroid glands are usually found on the posterior surface of the thyroid gland, each with its own capsule of connective tissue. They are occasionally included in the thyroid capsule, or one of them may even follow a blood vessel deep into a sulcus of the thyroid.

Extreme locations are very rare, although glands have been found as high as the bifurcation of the carotid artery and as low as the mediastinum. In practice, the surgeon should start at the point at which the inferior thyroid artery enters the thyroid gland. The superior parathyroid glands will *probably* lie about 1 in. above it, and the inferior parathyroid glands will *probably* lie 1/2 in. below it. If the inferior gland is not found, it is more likely to be lower than higher.

It is not uncommon to have more or fewer than four parathyroid glands.

Blood Supply

The inferior thyroid artery is responsible in most cases for the blood supply of both the upper and lower parathyroid glands (see material on arterial supply of thyroid and parathyroid glands).

Anatomy of the Trachea

The trachea, together with the esophagus and thyroid gland, lies in the visceral compartment of the neck. The anterior wall of the compartment is composed of sternothyroid and sternohyoid muscles. It is covered anteriorly by the investing layer of the deep cervical fascia and posteriorly by the prevertebral fascia (Fig. 2.9). The trachea begins at the level of the sixth cervical vertebra. Its bifurcation is at the level of the sixth thoracic vertebra in the erect position, or the fourth to fifth thoracic vertebrae when supine.

Vascular System
The chief sources of arterial blood to the trachea are the inferior thyroid arteries. At the bifurcation, these descending branches anastomose with ascending branches of the bronchial arteries.

Small tracheal veins join the laryngeal vein or empty directly into the left inferior thyroid vein.

The pretracheal and paratracheal lymph nodes receive the lymphatic vessels from the trachea.

Nervous System
The trachealis muscle and the tracheal mucosa receive fibers from the vagus nerve, recurrent laryngeal nerves, and sympathetic trunks. Small autonomic ganglia are numerous in the tracheal wall.

Anatomic Landmarks
The usual site of a tracheostomy is between the second and fourth or third and fifth tracheal rings. Several structures are encountered. The platysma lies in the superficial fascia and is absent in the midline. The anterior jugular veins may lie close to the midline; more importantly, they may be united by a jugular venous arch at the level of the seventh to eighth tracheal rings in the suprasternal space of Burns.

The investing layer of deep cervical fascia is encountered when the superficial fascia is reflected. Deep to the investing fascia are the sternohyoid and sternothyroid muscles. These muscles lie between the investing layer and the pretracheal fascia on either side of the midline.

Within the visceral compartment under the pretracheal fascia, the isthmus of the thyroid gland will be found, except that in 10% it is absent. A thyroid ima artery is possible, as well as a suspensory ligament of the thyroid and a levator thyroid muscle in, or close to, the midline.

Parotid Gland (Fig. 2.21)

Relations of the Parotid Gland
The parotid gland lies beneath the skin in front of and below the ear. It is contained within the investing layer of the deep fascia of the neck, called locally the parotid fascia, and the gland can be felt only under pathological conditions.

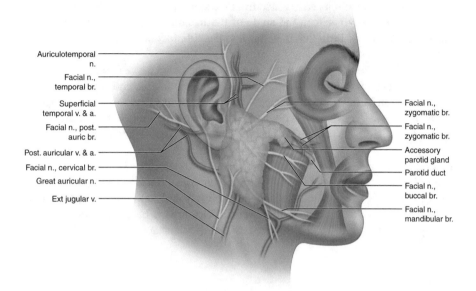

Fig. 2.21 Relations of the parotid gland to the facial nerve and its branches

The boundaries are:
- Anterior: masseter muscle, ramus of mandible, and medial pterygoid muscle
- Posterior: mastoid process, sternocleidomastoid muscle, and posterior belly of the digastric muscle and facial nerve
- Superior: external auditory meatus, and temporomandibular joint
- Inferior: sternocleidomastoid muscle and posterior belly of digastric muscle
- Lateral: investing layer of deep cervical fascia, skin, and platysma muscle
- Medial: investing layer of deep cervical fascia, styloid process, internal jugular vein, internal carotid artery, and pharyngeal wall

From the anterolateral edge of the gland, the parotid duct (Stensen's) passes lateral to the masseter muscle and turns medial at the anterior margin of the muscle. The duct pierces the buccinator muscle and enters the oral cavity at the level of the upper second molar tooth.

Structures Traversing the Parotid Gland

Facial Nerve

There is a superficial lobe and a deep lobe of the gland; the branches of the facial nerve run between them. In contrast, some anatomists visualize the gland as essentially unilobular, with the branches of the facial nerve enmeshed within the gland tissue with no cleavage plane between nerve and gland. The view that one may accept does not change the actual surgical procedure.

The main trunk of the facial nerve enters the posterior surface of the parotid gland about 1 cm from its emergence from the skull through the stylomastoid foramen, about midway between the angle of the mandible and the cartilaginous ear canal (Fig. 2.21). At birth the child has no mastoid process; the stylomastoid foramen is subcutaneous.

About 1 cm from its entrance into the gland, the facial nerve typically divides to form five branches: temporal, zygomatic, buccal, mandibular, and cervical. In most individuals, an initial bifurcation called the pes anserinus forms an upper temporofacial and a lower cervicofacial division, but six major patterns of branching, based on a series of simple to complex arrangements, have been distinguished.

Arteries

The external carotid artery enters the inferior surface of the gland and divides at the level of the neck of the mandible into the maxillary and superficial temporal arteries. The latter gives rise to the transverse facial artery. Each of these branches emerges separately from the superior or anterior surface of the parotid gland (Fig. 2.22).

Veins

The superficial temporal vein enters the superior surface of the parotid gland. It receives the maxillary vein to become the retromandibular vein. Still within the gland, the retromandibular vein divides. The posterior branch joins the posterior auricular vein to form the external jugular vein. The anterior branch emerges from the gland to join with the facial vein, thereby forming the common facial vein, a tributary to the internal jugular (Fig. 2.23).

Remember, the facial nerve is superficial, the artery is deep, and the retromandibular vein lies between them.

Fig. 2.22 Relations of the parotid gland to branches of the external carotid artery

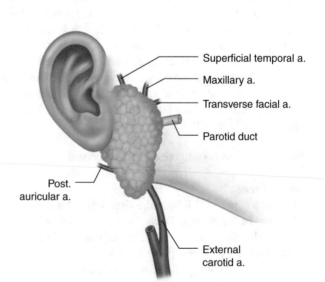

Superficial temporal a.

Maxillary a.

Transverse facial a.

Parotid duct

Post. auricular a.

External carotid a.

Fig. 2.23 Relations of the parotid gland to tributaries of the external and internal jugular veins

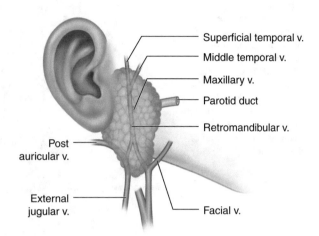

Superficial temporal v.

Middle temporal v.

Maxillary v.

Parotid duct

Retromandibular v.

Post auricular v.

External jugular v.

Facial v.

Lymphatics

The preauricular lymph nodes in the superficial fascia drain the temporal area of the scalp, upper face, lateral portions of the eyelids, and the anterior pinna. Parotid nodes within the gland drain the gland itself, as well as the nasopharynx, nose, palate, middle ear, and external auditory meatus. These nodes, in turn, send lymph to the subparotid nodes and eventually to the nodes of the internal jugular vein and spinal accessory chains (Table 2.1).

Great Auricular Nerve

The great auricular nerve reaches the posterior border of the sternocleidomastoid muscle and, on the surface of the parotid gland, follows the course of the external jugular vein. It is often sacrificed at parotidectomy. Injury to this nerve results in numbness in the preauricular region, lower auricle, and the lobe of the ear, but it disappears after 4–6 months.

Auriculotemporal Nerve

The auriculotemporal nerve, a branch of the mandibular division of the trigeminal cranial nerve, traverses the upper part of the parotid gland and emerges with the superficial temporal blood vessels from the superior surface of the gland. Within the gland, the auriculotemporal nerve communicates with the facial nerve.

Usually, the order of the structures from the tragus anteriorly is the following: auriculotemporal nerve, superficial temporal artery and vein, and temporal branch of the facial nerve. The auriculotemporal nerve carries sensory fibers from the trigeminal nerve and motor (secretory) fibers from the glossopharyngeal nerve.

Injury to the auriculotemporal nerve produces Frey's syndrome, in which the skin anterior to the ear sweats during eating ("gustatory sweating").

Fig. 2.24 Lateral view of the structures in the left carotid sheath at the base of the skull. The posterior belly of the digastric is shown in dotted outline. The hypoglossal nerve (not shown) hooks around the vagus and appears between the artery and the vein below the lower border of the digastric

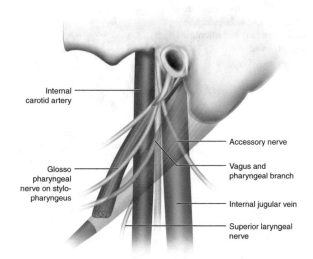

Parotid Bed

Complete removal of the parotid gland reveals the following structures (the acronym VANS may be helpful in remembering them):

- One **V**ein: internal jugular
- Two **A**rteries: external and internal carotid
- Four **N**erves: glossopharyngeal (IX), vagus (X), spinal accessory (XI), and hypoglossal (XII) (Fig. 2.24)
- Four anatomic entities starting with **S**: styloid process, and styloglossus, stylopharyngeus, and stylohyoid muscles

Identification of the Facial Nerve

The main trunk of the facial nerve is within a triangle bounded by the mastoid process, the external auditory meatus, and the angle of the mandible. The lower tip of the mastoid process is palpated, and a fingertip is placed on the lateral surface pointing forward. The trunk of the facial nerve will be found deep and anterior to the center of the fingertip.

Remember
- The stem of the nerve lies between the parotid gland and its fascia, deep in front of the mastoid, and medially at the midpoint between the mandibular angle and the cartilaginous ear canal. The stylomastoid foramen and the facial nerve are subcutaneous.

The facial nerve and its branches are in danger during parotidectomy. The facial trunk is large enough for anastomosis of the cut ends, should this be necessary.

Branchial Cleft Sinuses and Cysts

Anatomy of Branchial Remnants

Fistulas

Fistulas are patent duct-like structures that have both external and internal orifices. Cervicoaural fistulas extend from the skin at the angle of the jaw and may open into the external auditory canal. These fistulas lie anterior to the facial nerve. They are remnants of the ventral portion of the first branchial cleft (Fig. 2.25).

Lateral cervical fistulas almost always arise from the ventral portion of the second branchial cleft and pouch. They originate on the lower third of the neck on the anterior border of the sternocleidomastoid muscle. The path is upward through the platysma muscle and deep fascia. Above the hyoid bone the track turns medially to pass beneath the stylohyoid and the posterior belly of the digastric muscle, in front of the hypoglossal nerve, and between the external and internal carotid arteries. It enters the pharynx on the anterior surface of the upper half of the posterior pillar of the fauces (Fig. 2.26a). It may open into the supratonsillar fossa or even into the tonsil itself.

Sinuses

External sinuses are blindly ending spaces that extend inward from openings in the skin. *Internal sinuses* are blindly ending spaces that extend outward from openings in the pharynx.

External sinuses usually arise at the anterior border of the sternocleidomastoid muscle and end in a cystic dilatation (Fig. 2.26b). Internal sinuses are usually asymptomatic and hence undetected.

Fig. 2.25 Congenital cervicoaural fistula or cyst. This is a persistent remnant of the ventral portion of the first branchial cleft. The tract may or may not open into the external auditory canal

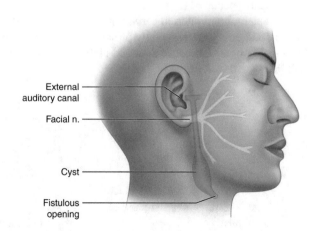

External auditory canal

Facial n.

Cyst

Fistulous opening

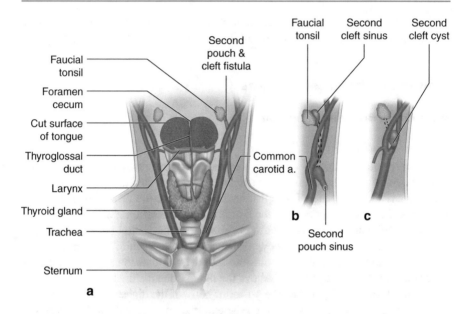

Fig. 2.26 Track of a second-pouch and second-cleft fistula passing from the tonsillar fossa of the palatine (faucial) tonsils to the neck. (**a**) Complete fistula. (**b**) External (cervical) and internal (pharyngeal) sinuses. (**c**) Cyst of branchial cleft origin lying in the carotid notch

Cysts

Cysts are spherical or elongated spaces lying in the track of a branchial pouch or cleft and have no communication with the pharynx or skin.

Superficial cysts lie at the edge of the sternocleidomastoid muscle. Deeper cysts lie on the jugular vein or in the bifurcation of the carotid artery (Fig. 2.26c). These are of branchial cleft origin and are lined with stratified squamous epithelium. Cysts on the pharyngeal wall deep to the carotid arteries are usually of branchial cleft origin. They are lined with ciliated epithelium unless inflammatory or pressure changes have occurred (Fig. 2.27).

The external and internal carotid arteries just above the bifurcation of the common carotid artery are especially prone to injury while performing excision of the branchial remnants, because a second-cleft cyst or the path of a second-cleft fistula will lie in the crotch of the bifurcation.

Remember
- A first-cleft sinus or cyst passes over or under the facial nerve below and anterior to the ear. The cyst may displace the nerve either upward or downward. While removing the cyst, the surgeon must be careful to protect the nerve.
- Several nerves will be found above the pathway of a second-cleft or second-pouch branchial fistula:
  - Mandibular and cervical branches of the facial nerve
  - Spinal accessory nerve, which may be injured when trying to free a cyst or fistulous tract from the sternocleidomastoid muscle

Fig. 2.27 Incomplete closure of the second branchial cleft or pouch may leave cysts. Type I, superficial, at the border of the sternocleidomastoid muscle. Type II, between the muscle and the jugular vein. Type III, in the bifurcation of the carotid artery. Type IV, in the pharyngeal wall. Types I, II, and III are of second-cleft origin; Type IV is from the second pouch. *M* sternocleidomastoid muscle, *V* jugular vein, *A* carotid artery

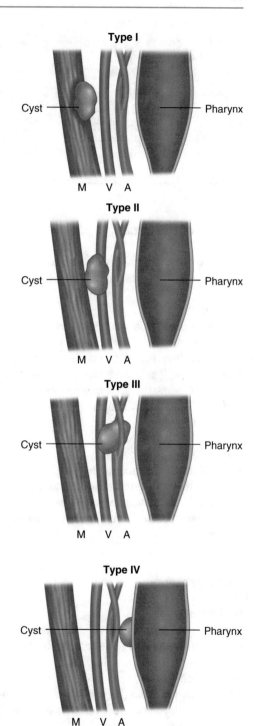

- Descendens hypoglossi—superior root of the ansa cervicalis—which may be cut with impunity
- Hypoglossal nerve (the fistula crosses the nerve above the bifurcation of the common carotid artery)
- Superior laryngeal nerves
- Vagus nerve, which lies parallel to the carotid artery. (The fistula crosses the nerve near the level of the carotid bifurcation.)

Technique

Masses of the Neck

Diagnosis of nonthyroid neck masses follows a well-marked pathway. With a little rounding of the figures, an easily remembered rule is apparent:

Rule of 80
- 80% of nonthyroid neck masses are neoplastic.
- 80% of neoplastic neck masses are in males.
- 80% of neoplastic neck masses are malignant.
- 80% of malignant neck masses are metastatic.
- 80% of metastatic neck masses are from primary sites above the clavicle.

In addition, the probable diagnosis may be based on the average duration of the patient's symptoms:

Rule of 7
- Mass from inflammation has existed for 7 days.
- Mass from a neoplasm has existed for 7 months.
- Mass from a congenital defect has existed for 7 years.

However, acquired immune deficiency syndrome (AIDS) perhaps changes these rules a little.

Parotidectomy

Indications
The most common indications for removal of the parotid gland are tumors and chronic obstruction of Stensons duct by calculi.

Technique
Position the head and prepare the skin as in thyroid surgery but uncover the lateral angle of the eye and the labial commissure. Sterilize the external auditory canal. Use intravenous antibiotic of choice.

Nerve Monitoring

EMG monitoring the facial nerve during parotidectomy is now standard of care. Numerous devices exist to allow the surgeon to safely monitor the nerve passively and actively during surgery.

- **Step 1.** *Incision*: Inverted T or modified Y (Figs. 2.28 and 2.29).

Inverted T: Make a vertical preauricular incision about 3 mm in front of the ear with downward curved extension at the posterior angle of the mandible. Make a

Fig. 2.28 Modified Y incision

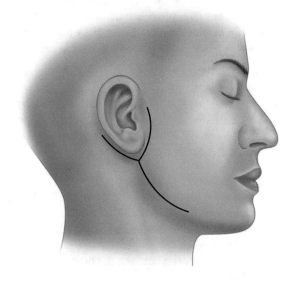

Fig. 2.29 Inverted T-incision

Inverted T

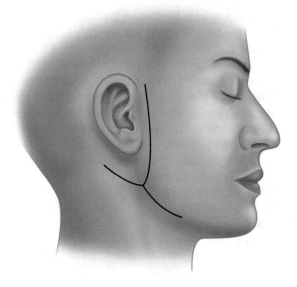

transverse curved incision 3 cm below the mandible with posterior extension close to the mastoid.

Modified Y: Make vertical pre- and postauricular incisions that unite approximately at the angle of the mandible, forming a Y which again meets a transverse incision 3 cm below the mandible.

Make a deep incision into the superficial cervical fascia (anteriorly, fat and platysma; posteriorly, fat only).

• **Step 2.** Formation of flaps (Fig. 2.30).

Carefully elevate skin and fat using knife, scissors, and blunt dissection upward, medially, laterally, downward, and posteriorly.

For the upper flap, provide traction upward and medially on the dissected skin, and laterally toward the external auditory canal. Form the lower flap by dissection of the skin downward and posteriorly toward the mastoid process.

Remember
• Sacrifice the great auricular nerve and the posterior facial vein. Both are very close to and topographicoanatomically situated in the vicinity of the lower flap and the lower parotid border.

• **Step 3.** Facial nerve identification (Fig. 2.31)
  (a) Place the distal phalanx of the left index finger on the mastoid, pointing to the eye of the patient.
  (b) Carefully incise the parotid fascia and further mobilize the superficial part of the parotid.
  (c) Insert a hemostat between the mastoid and the gland and bluntly spread the gland medially.
  (d) The stem of the nerve will always be found at a depth of less than 0.5 cm. If there is any doubt whether the nerve has been identified, use electrical stimulation.
  (e) Exert upward traction on the superficial lobe and, with a curved hemostat, begin dissection over the nerve.
  (f) Identify all five branches.
• **Step 4.** Resection of the superficial lobe (Fig. 2.32).

With gentle traction of the gland and further anterior nerve dissection toward the periphery of the gland, totally mobilize and resect the superficial lobe. As the dissection is carried toward the ends of the branches of the facial nerve, Stensen's duct will be encountered and should be ligated and divided.

Step 5. Resection of the deep lobe (Fig. 2.33).

The following anatomical entities should be kept in mind:
• Pterygoid venous plexus
• External carotid artery
• Maxillary nerve
• Superficial temporal nerve
• Posterior facial vein

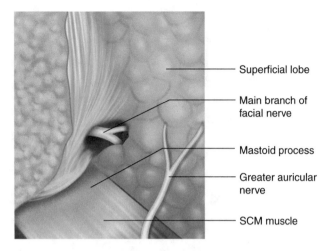

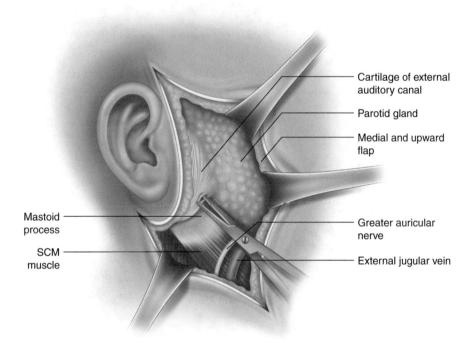

Fig. 2.30 Parotid gland exposure. *Inset*: Facial nerve and greater auricular nerve

Pterygoid venous plexus bleeding may be stopped by compression. Do not go deep: remember VANS (see "Parotid Bed" earlier in this chapter). Remove the deep lobe carefully, working under the facial nerve by the piecemeal dissection technique. Obtain good hemostasis.

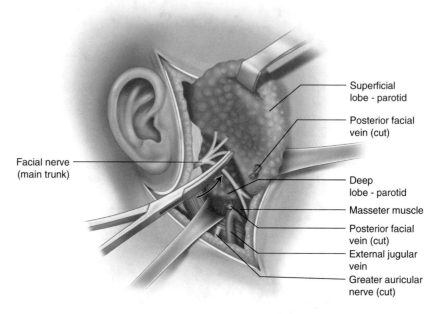

Fig. 2.31 Facial nerve identification

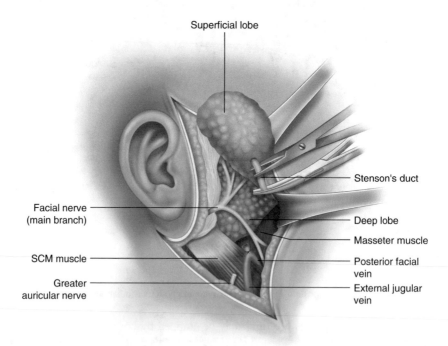

Fig. 2.32 Resection of the superficial lobe

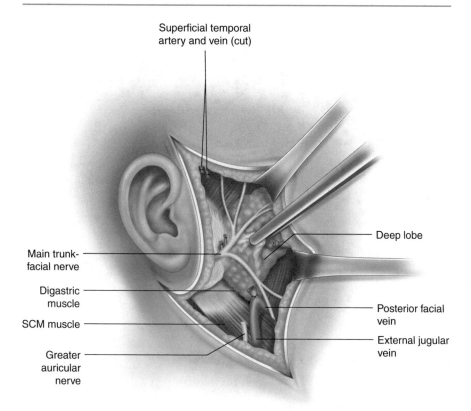

Fig. 2.33 Resection of the deep lobe

Radical Parotidectomy (Fig. 2.34)

Excise the parotid in toto, as well as the facial nerve and the regional lymph nodes; also, if necessary, perform ipsilateral radical neck dissection.

Autologous graft microanastomosis should be considered for reconstruction of the facial nerve. The greater and lesser occipital nerves can serve as donors.

> **Remember**
> - Try to save zygomatic marginal branches if possible. If not, use microanastomosis end to end.

Insert a Jackson–Pratt drain through a lower stab wound. To close the wound, use interrupted 3–0 Vicryl for platysma and fat and interrupted 6–0 nylon for skin.

Resection of Submaxillary Gland (Figs. 2.1, 2.2, 2.3, 2.4, 2.5, and 2.6)

Position and Preparation: As in parotidectomy. The upper half of the face should be covered, but the labial commissure should be uncovered.

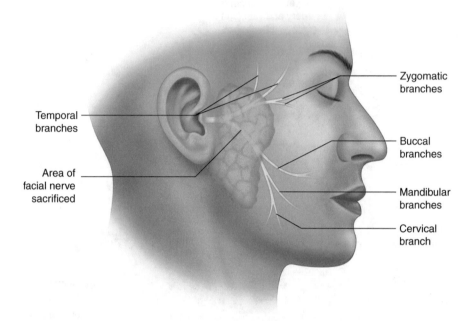

Fig. 2.34 Typical positions of the branches of the facial nerve

Fig. 2.35 Incision of the superficial fascia

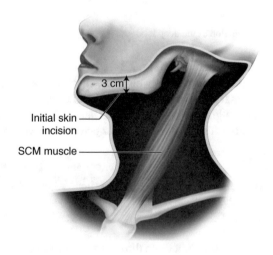

Incision: Make a transverse incision 3 cm below the lower border of the mandible. Incise the superficial fascia from the anterior border of the sternocleidomastoid muscle (SCM) to 2–3 cm from the midline (Fig. 2.35).

Remember
- The two branches of the facial nerve (mandibular and cervical) are under the platysma and the deep fascia of the submaxillary gland. Identify and protect them. Apply retractors carefully.

Surgical Field in View
- Superior: inferior border of mandible
- Inferior: digastric and stylohyoid muscles
- Medial: mylohyoid muscle
- Lateral: sternocleidomastoid muscle
- Center: deep cervical fascia covering the gland

The common facial vein, its anterior tributary, or its posterior tributary is now in view close to the sternocleidomastoid muscle. Continue to observe the marginal branch of the facial nerve, which is superficial to the facial vessels (occasionally at a lower level).

Remember
- There are lymph nodes outside the capsule close to the vessels. With benign disease, removal of these is not necessary.

Step 1. Ligate the facial vessels (Fig. 2.36).
Step 2. With curved hemostat, separate inferiorly the gland from the digastric muscle (Fig. 2.37).

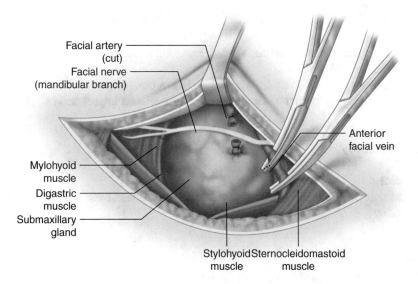

Fig. 2.36 Exposure of common facial artery, vein, and nerve

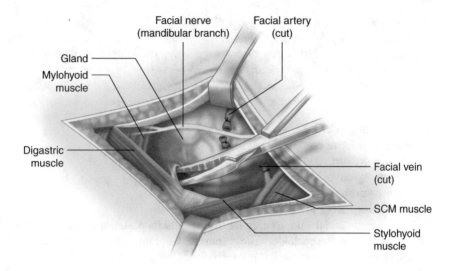

Fig. 2.37 Exposure of the gland

Remember
- The hypoglossal nerve is located very close to the digastric tendon and is accompanied by the lingual vein and deeper, by the external maxillary artery. Both vessels should be ligated carefully. Elevate the mylohyoid muscle to expose the deep part of the submaxillary gland. Separate the gland slowly. Just under the gland and cephalad to it, the following anatomical entities are in view: lingual nerve, chorda tympani, submaxillary ganglion, and Wharton's duct.

- **Step 3.** Ligate and cut Wharton's duct. Protect the lingual nerve (Fig. 2.38). Continue blunt dissection.
- **Step 4.** Insert Jackson–Pratt drain and close in layers.
  Caution: Avoid injury to the mandibular, hypoglossal, and lingual nerves.

Thyroidectomy

Indications
Indeterminate thyroid masses, cancer, goiters, Graves' disease, toxic adenomas and toxic goiters.

Technique
Step 1. Position
  (a) Put the patient in semi-Fowler position.
  (b) Patient's neck should be hyperextended.

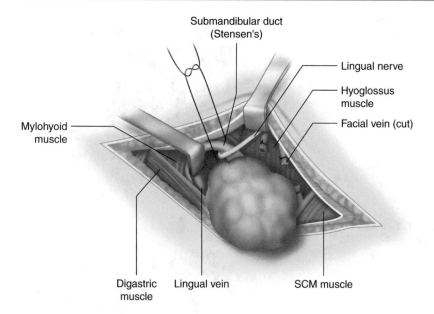

Fig. 2.38 Blunt dissection

Fig. 2.39 Location for incision

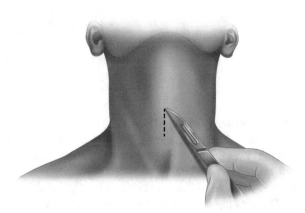

(c) Place small pillow at the area of the upper thoracic spine, beneath the shoulders.

(d) Place a doughnut support under the head.

Step 2. Preparation of skin

(a) Use Betadine or any other solution of the surgeon's choice.

(b) Be sure the chin and long axis of the body are aligned at the midline.

(c) Palpate or ultrasound the thyroid gland and use a marking pen to denote a 3–5 cm incision overlying the gland

Step 3. Incise the mark of the incision, carrying out the incision through the superficial fascia (subcutaneous fat and platysma). Establish good hemostasis by electrocoagulation (Figs. 2.39 and 2.40)

Fig. 2.40 Incision through
superficial fascia

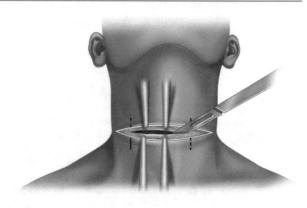

Fig. 2.41 Elevation
of flaps

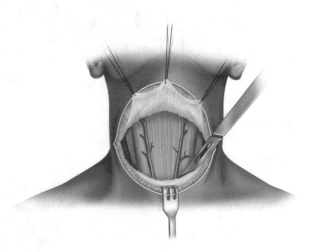

Step 4. Formation of flaps (Fig. 2.41)

By blunt dissection, elevate the upper flap to the notch of the thyroid cartilage
and the lower flap to the jugular (sternal) notch. Use Mahorner's, Murphy's, or other
self-retaining retractors.

Step 5. Opening of the deep fascia (Figs. 2.42 and 2.43)

The opening is accomplished by a longitudinal midline incision along the raphe
of the strap muscles, which is actually the deep fascia. This can be performed using
the electrocautery pencil.

Step 6. Elevation of the strap muscles (Figs. 2.44, 2.45, and 2.46)

The sternohyoid muscles are easily elevated, but the thyrohyoid and sternothyroid muscles are attached to the false thyroid capsule and should be separated carefully to avoid injuring the gland and causing bleeding. In extremely rare cases, when
the thyroid gland is markedly enlarged, section of the strap muscles becomes necessary. Divide them at the proximal (upper) one-third to avoid paralysis due to injury
of the ansa hypoglossi (C_1, C_2, C_3, and XII).

Fig. 2.42 Raphe of
strap muscles

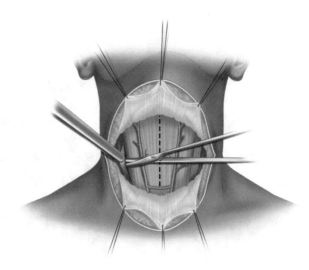

Fig. 2.43 Incising
strap muscles

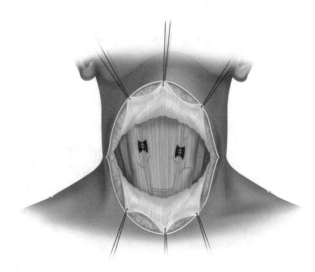

The sternohyoid muscles are the most superficial, and the sternothyroid and thyrohyoid are underneath. For practical purposes, the thyrohyoid is an upward continuation of the sternothyroid.

Step 7. Exposure and mobilization of the gland

With all strap muscles elevated and retracted, the index finger of the surgeon is gently inserted between the thyroid and the muscles (Fig. 2.45). A lateral elevation is also taking place, occasionally using all the fingers except the thumb. It not only breaks the remaining muscular or pathological attachments but enables the surgeon to appreciate the gross pathology of the gland in toto. Occasionally the strap muscles should be divided (Figs. 2.46 and 2.47).

Fig. 2.44 Sternohyoid
muscles

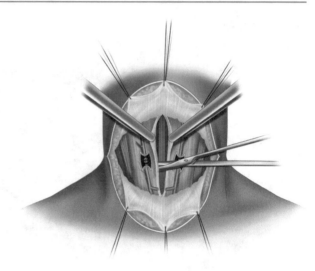

Fig. 2.45 Breaking of
attachments

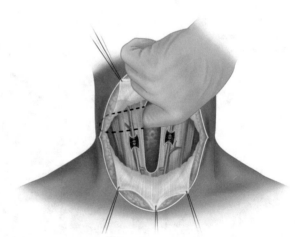

Fig. 2.46 Separation and
division

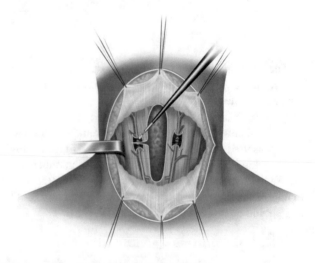

Fig. 2.47 Lateral elevation

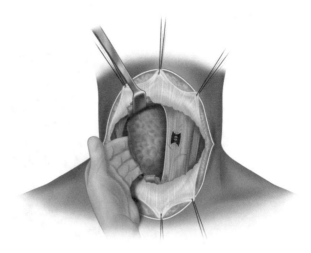

Fig. 2.48 Exposure

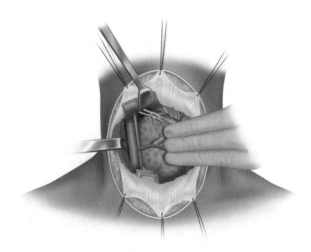

The anatomy of the normal and the abnormal must be studied carefully regarding size, extension, consistency, and fixation of the gland. Is a pyramidal lobe present? How thick is the isthmus? Are a Delphian node and other lymph nodes present? If so, excision of the Delphian node and perhaps one or two of the other palpable lymph nodes is in order. Frozen section should follow.

Step 8. Total lobectomy (Figs. 2.48, 2.49, and 2.50)

    (a) Retract the lobe medially and anteriorly by clamps.

    (b) Ligate the middle thyroid vein by LigaSure or Harmonic scalpel.

    (c) Identify the recurrent laryngeal nerve by blunt dissection into the tracheo-esophageal groove.

    (d) Identify and protect the parathyroids. Minimize manipulation of the parathyroid glands

Fig. 2.49 Retraction

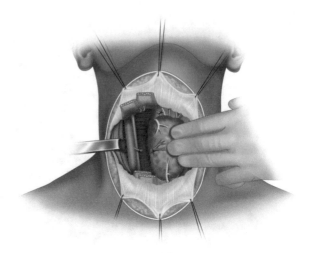

Fig. 2.50 Ligation

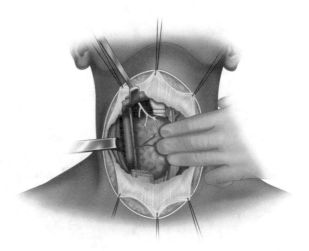

(e) Ligate the inferior thyroid artery. Superior and inferior pole vessels may also be divided with the LigaSure or Harmonic scalpel.

(f) Ligate the lower pole vessels.

(g) Carefully ligate the upper pole. Perform en masse ligation, thereby ligating the superior thyroid artery, or, if possible, prepare the artery above the pole and ligate. This ligation should be performed close to the thyroid gland to minimize injury to the superior laryngeal nerve.

(h) Dissect the lobe from the trachea by dividing the gland between straight mosquitoes. With bipolar cautery, Berry's ligament, the attachment of the isthmus to the thyroid, can be transected. Alternatively, the Harmonic Scalpel can be used with the same effect.

(i) If the pyramidal lobe is present, ligate its most distal part, and remove it together with the lobe.

(j) Ligate the isthmus if present.
(k) Obtain meticulous hemostasis. Using bipolar cautery with care to protect the recurrent nerve and parathyroidectomy.
(l) If a total thyroidectomy is necessary, the contralateral lobe should be resected in the same fashion and the gland sent en bloc for permanent pathology.
(m) Frozen section is rarely used for diagnostic purposes.

Parathyroidectomy

Indications
Patients with primary hyperparathyroidism (PHPT), with kidney stones, bone fractures. For asymptomatic PHPT with elevated serum calcium, osteoporosis, vertebral fractures kidney stones, elevated urine calcium, age <50, neurocognitive disorders such as difficulty concentrating, sleep disturbances, depression, consider surgery.

Technique
Step 1. The following steps are a strategy for finding abnormal parathyroid locations.
(a) Perform preoperative CT angiogram (CTA) to identify parathyroid adenoma.
(b) Explore the superior surface of the thyroid gland. Ligate the middle thyroid veins, retract the lobe medially and anteriorly, and expose the recurrent laryngeal nerve.
(c) Dissect the superior anterior mediastinum as far as possible, with special attention to the thymus or its remnant behind the manubrium.
(d) Explore the region above the upper pole of the thyroid gland as far as the hyoid bone.
(e) Explore the retroesophageal, retropharyngeal, and retrosternal spaces.
(f) Perform subtotal thyroidectomy.
(g) Confirm removal of parathyroid adenoma via intraoperative parathyroid monitoring.
(h) Further explore the mediastinum at a second operation. This should be done only after the pathology report on thymus and thyroid tissue has been received and no parathyroid tissue is reported.

Remember
- The best anatomical landmark is the inferior thyroid artery.
- The most useful instrument for palpation is the distal phalanx of the index finger.

Step 2. In the patient with a localized gland identified by preoperative imaging including ultrasound, sestamibi, and CT scan, the incision is made directly over the gland between the sternocleidomastoid muscle and the strap muscles. In a patient with hyperplasia, remove 2–3½ glands. The remaining ½ gland can be left in situ or implanted into the sternocleidomastoid muscle. In any case, cryopreserve a parathyroid for reimplantation in case the patient becomes hypoparathyroid. When a patient is explored for a suspected adenoma, the healthy glands will be smaller than normal. If a parathyroid adenoma has been identified by imaging, it is not necessary to identify all the glands. After removal of the enlarged gland, there should be at least an 80% reduction in the PTH level. The reduction should be at least 80% and into normal or below normal range. If the PTH level does not show a significant decrease, then the presence of a second and possibly a third adenoma should be investigated. Always send adenomas for frozen section. If the gland is determined to be malignant, which is incredibly rare the surrounding tissue should be removed.

Step 3. Reconstruction.

Insert a Penrose or a Jackson–Pratt drain if necessary. Close the midline and the superficial fascia, approximating the marked points and avoiding dog-ears. Closure of the skin is up to the surgeon: use subcuticular sutures with Steri-strips or Dermabond. Remember to check the patient's voice for normal vocal function as soon as the endotracheal tube has been removed.

Thyroid Reoperation

- **Step 1.** Carefully read the patient's previous operating report.
- **Step 2.** Inspect vocal cords.
- **Step 3.** Incise through the previous scar, but add 1–2 cm on each side laterally.
- **Step 4.** Make flaps as in thyroidectomy.
- **Step 5.** Identify the sternocleidomastoid muscle; incise, dissect, and elevate its medial border.
- **Step 6.** Carefully elevate the strap muscles.
- **Step 7.** There are two ways to re-explore the thyroid: from the periphery (this anatomically intact area has less scar tissue) to the center and from the midline/isthmic area to the periphery.
  (a) From the periphery to the center
- Most likely, the virgin area after thyroid surgery is the area corresponding to the medial border of the sternocleidomastoid. The best anatomical landmark is the proximal part of the inferior thyroid artery, since the distal was probably ligated. Any white, thin, cordlike structure should be protected, since this is probably the recurrent laryngeal nerve. If in doubt, stop the dissection in this area, and try to find the nerve at the cricothyroid area above or at the supraclavicular area below. The most virgin area is just above the clavicle, and the least virgin (if total lobectomy was performed previously) is the cricothyroid area. The parathyroids will be found above and below the inferior thyroid artery. The remnants of the thyroid glands will be found in the tracheoesophageal groove or in the area of the upper thyroid pole.
  (b) From the midline/isthmic area to the periphery.

The anatomical area to be explored with this procedure is the tracheoesophageal groove, in the hope that the recurrent laryngeal nerve is somewhere in the vicinity. Small curved mosquito or Mixter clamps may be used for elevation of the thyroid remnants, location of the nerve, and location of the parathyroids.

If re-exploration is performed for malignant disease, then a modified radical neck dissection is in order. In the modified procedure the sternocleidomastoid muscle and the internal jugular vein are preserved. The recurrent nerve also should be saved; it should be sacrificed only if it is fixed to the tumor.

Parathyroid Reoperation

- **Step 1.** Read about normal and abnormal locations of parathyroids.
- **Step 2.** Carefully read the patient's previous operating report and pay special attention to:
  - (a) Number of parathyroids removed.
  - (b) Sites (right or left).
  - (c) Together with the radiologist, study all possible results of techniques for localization (ultrasonography, CTA, MRI, sestamibi scan, selective venous catheterization with parathyroid hormone immunoassay evaluation, digital subtraction angiography).
- **Step 3.** Reexplore the neck as in thyroidectomy.
- **Step 4.** Locate and mark the inferior thyroid artery.
- **Step 5.** Protect the recurrent laryngeal nerve.
- **Step 6.** Palpate the "certain" location and all possible locations of parathyroid glands, such as tracheoesophageal groove, retropharyngeal, retroesophageal, retrocarotid, anterior mediastinum (thymus), posterior mediastinum, middle mediastinum (pericardium) within the carotid sheath, suprathyroid, infrathyroid, intrathyroid, and posterior triangle.
- **Step 7.** Remove the tumor. A patient diagnosed with hyperplasia probably has one gland or only 1/2 of the fourth gland (if the patient has only four glands) with hyperplastic or adenomatous changes. Perform a total parathyroidectomy and transplant multiple pieces (1 mm in diameter) of the adenoma or the hyperplastic gland into the biceps muscle, being sure to mark the location. If there is an adenoma that was not found previously, remove it. If the frozen section is determined to be malignant, the surrounding tissue should be removed.

Thyroglossal Duct Cystectomy (Fig. 2.51)

Position and prepare as for thyroidectomy.
- **Step 1.** Make a transverse incision over the cyst. Incise the superficial fascia (fat and platysma) and mark the skin at the midline to facilitate good closure. Formation of flaps: the upward elevation reaches the hyoid bone and extends cephalad 1–2 cm. Elevate the lower flap almost to the isthmus of the thyroid

Fig. 2.51 Various locations of thyroglossal duct cysts. (**a**) In front of the foramen cecum. (**b**) At the foramen cecum. (**c**) Above the hyoid bone. (**d**) Below the hyoid bone. (**e**) In the region of the thyroid gland. (**f**) At the suprasternal notch. About 50% of the cysts are located at (**d**), below the hyoid bone

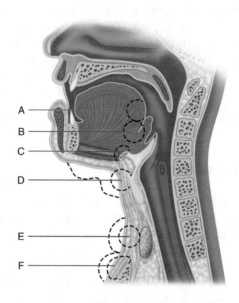

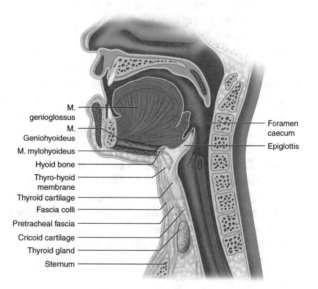

gland. One self-retaining retractor is enough to keep the field open. Open the deep fascia in a longitudinal fashion.

- **Step 2.** Dissect the cyst and isolate it with a small hemostat and plastic scissors (Fig. 2.52). The involved anatomical entities depend upon the location of the cyst (Fig. 2.53): suprahyoid (rare), hyoid (common), and infrahyoid or suprasternal (rare). (Knowledge of the embryology plays a great role here.)

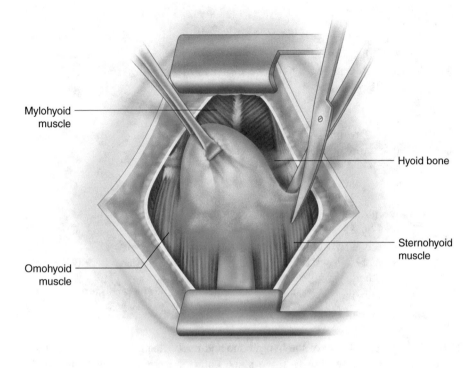

Fig. 2.52 Dissection of cyst

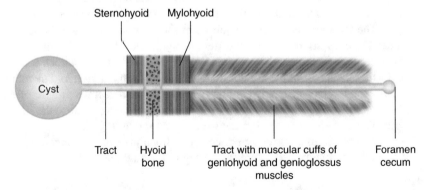

Fig. 2.53 Diagrammatic presentation of tract

Remember

- The embryologic path of descent of the thyroid gland (from the foramen cecum to the manubrium sterni).
- The thyroglossal duct (a midline cordlike formation) travels, in most cases, through the hyoid bone.
- The anatomical entities involved in most of the cases are:
  - Foramen cecum
  - Thyroid membrane
  - Mylohyoid muscle
  - Geniohyoid muscle
  - Genioglossus muscle
  - Sternohyoid muscle
  - Anterior belly of digastric muscle
- The mylohyoid is fixed to the hyoid bone above; the sternohyoid is fixed to the hyoid bone below.
- Occasionally, the anterior belly of the digastric muscle may partially cover the hyoid bone laterally.
- The geniohyoid is between the thyroid membrane and the mylohyoid.

Step 3. Take special care of the hyoid bone and tract. Clean the central part of the hyoid bone, but be sure to leave some cuffs of sternohyoid and mylohyoid attached to the bone, as well as some cuffs of the underlying geniohyoid and genioglossus attached to the cephalad tract (Fig. 2.54). Insert a curved hemostat under the central part of the hyoid bone. With heavy scissors or small bone cutter, cut the bone on both sides. Continue upward dissection bilaterally to the midline where the tract is located. The thyrohyoid membrane is now exposed (Fig. 2.55).

Step 4. The foramen cecum also requires special attention. The anesthesiologist's index finger is inserted into the patient's mouth, elevating the foramen cecum. With continuous cephalad dissection, the surgeon reaches the foramen cecum by palpating the finger of the anesthesiologist just under the thyrohyoid membrane. Excise the foramen cecum in continuity and close the defect with figure-of-eight 4–0 chromic catgut or any other absorbable suture. Drainage is up to the surgeon. Establish good hemostasis. Irrigate with normal saline (Fig. 2.56).

Step 5. Reconstruction. Perform midline approximation of the mylohyoid and sternohyoid with interrupted sutures as for thyroid operation.

Note

- In the case of a sinus without cyst, follow the same steps.

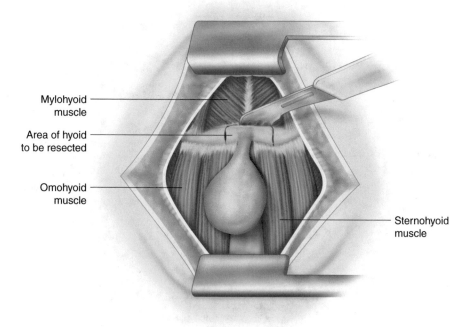

Fig. 2.54 Preparation of surgical field

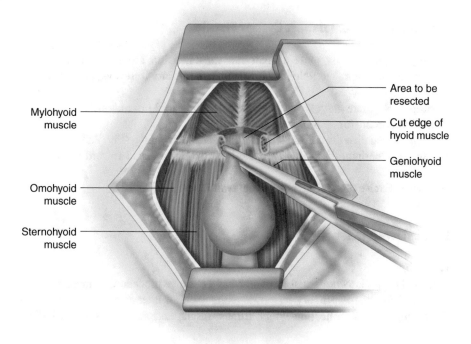

Fig. 2.55 Resection

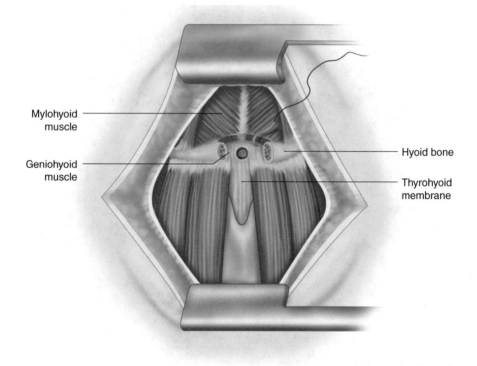

Mylohyoid muscle

Geniohyoid muscle

Hyoid bone

Thyrohyoid membrane

Fig. 2.56 Closure of defect

Excision of Branchial Cleft Cyst or Fistula

- **Step 1.** Above a cyst, make a small transverse incision; around a sinus, make an elliptical incision. Multiple incisions will be necessary if the cyst or sinus is low (Fig. 2.57).
- **Step 2.** Separate and elevate the sternocleidomastoid muscle, always using the medial border (Fig. 2.58).
- **Step 3.** Visualize the carotid sheath and hypoglossal nerve (Fig. 2.59).
- **Step 4.** Continue dissection of the cyst or sinus cephalad toward the pharyngeal wall.
- **Step 5.** Excise the minute pharyngeal wall if pathology exists.

Radical Neck Dissection

Overview

A radical neck dissection must be planned as a curative procedure. It involves complete excision of the primary lesion, together with all nonessential structures and their lymph nodes, collecting lymph trunks, fascia, and fat. The bed of a radical

Fig. 2.57 Location of
incision

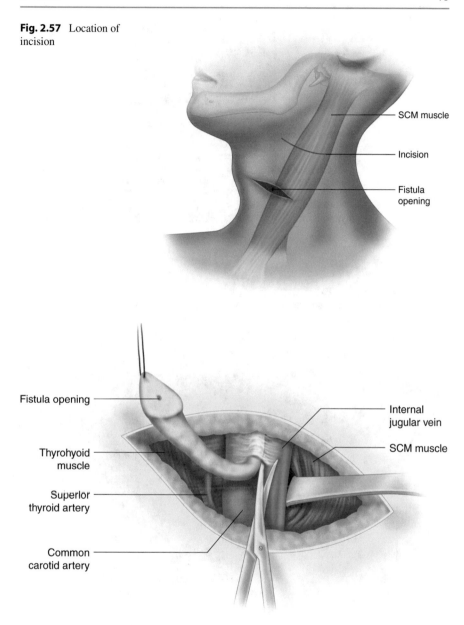

SCM muscle

Incision

Fistula
opening

Fistula opening

Thyrohyoid
muscle

Superior
thyroid artery

Common
carotid artery

Internal
jugular vein

SCM muscle

Fig. 2.58 Exposure of fistulous tract

neck dissection is bounded superiorly by the inferior border of the mandible, inferiorly by the clavicle, posteriorly by the anterior border of the trapezius muscle, and anteriorly by the midline.

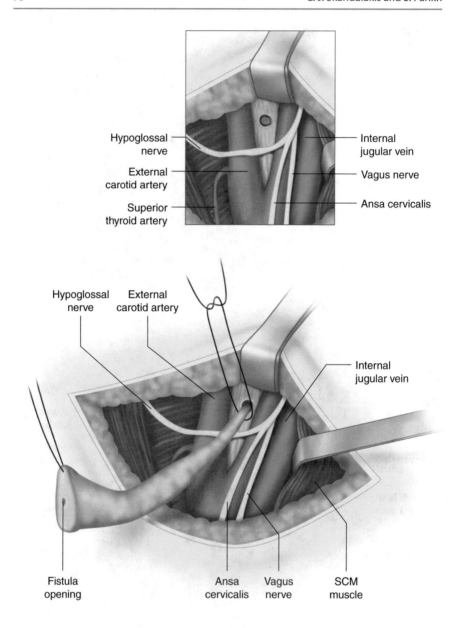

Fig. 2.59 Excision of fistula. Inset: structures of surgical field

Lymphatic tissue must be removed as completely as possible. Nonlymphatic tissue falls into three categories: (1) structures that can be sacrificed with impunity; (2) structures whose sacrifice is controversial, especially for cosmetic reasons; and (3) structures that must be preserved unless directly invaded by cancer. Structures in these categories are listed in Table 2.3.

Table 2.3 Synopsis of radical neck procedures

Structures	May be sacrificed	Controversial	Must be preserved[a]
Organs	Submaxillary gland, lower pole of parotid gland	None	Thyroid gland, parathyroid glands
Muscles	Omohyoid, sternocleidomastoid	Platysma, digastric, stylohyoid	All other muscles
Vessels	External jugular vein, facial artery and vein, superior thyroid artery, lingual artery	Internal jugular vein	External carotid artery, internal carotid artery, subclavian artery and vein, thoracic duct
Nerves	Anterior cutaneous C_2–C_3, supraclavicular C_3–C_4, ansa hypoglossi, great auricular nerve	Spinal accessory nerve	Mandibular branch of facial nerve, superior laryngeal nerve, recurrent laryngeal nerve, facial nerve, lingual nerve, hypoglossal nerve, phrenic nerve, vagus nerve, cervical sympathetic nerve, carotid sinus nerves, brachial plexus, nerves to rhomboid and serratus muscles

[a]Unless invaded by cancer. (By permission of JE Skandalakis, SW Gray, and JR Rowe. *Anatomical Complications in General Surgery*. New York: McGraw-Hill, 1983)

Anatomical Elements

Superficial Cervical Fascia
The anterior cutaneous nerves and the supraclavicular nerves must be sacrificed. The platysma muscle should be preserved.

Deep Cervical Fascia
The deep cervical fascia must be removed as completely as possible since lymph nodes and lymphatic vessels are largely distributed in the connective tissue between the layers of the fascia. The carotid sheath and the internal jugular vein also should be sacrificed.

Anterior Triangle
- Submental triangle: Remove the entire contents.
- Submandibular triangle: Remove the submaxillary gland and lymph nodes.
- Carotid triangle: Remove the internal jugular vein. High ligation of the vein is facilitated by removal of the lower pole of the parotid gland. The great auricular nerve and all superficial branches of the cervical nerves should be cut. All lymph nodes along the internal jugular vein must be removed. The final result is shown in Fig. 2.60.

Posterior Triangle
Remove all tissue above the spinal accessory nerve without injury to the nerve. With blunt dissection, free the nerve from the underlying tissue. Ligate the external jugular vein close to the subclavian vein and transect the sternocleidomastoid and omohyoid muscles.

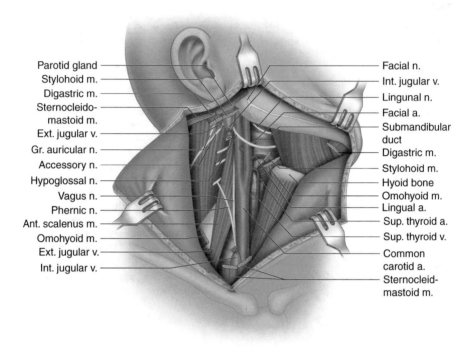

Parotid gland — Facial n.
Stylohoid m. — Int. jugular v.
Digastric m. — Lingunal n.
Sternocleido- — Facial a.
  mastoid m. — Submandibular
Ext. jugular v. —   duct
Gr. auricular n. — Digastric m.
Accessory n. — Stylohoid m.
Hypoglossal n. — Hyoid bone
Vagus n. — Omohyoid m.
Phernic n. — Lingual a.
Ant. scalenus m. — Sup. thyroid a.
Omohyoid m. — Sup. thyroid v.
Ext. jugular v. — Common
Int. jugular v. —   carotid a.
— Sternocleid-
  mastoid m.

Fig. 2.60 The completed radical dissection of the neck. Remaining structures may be removed if they are involved in malignant growth

The area beneath the spinal accessory nerve is the "danger zone" of Beahrs. It contains a number of structures that must be saved if possible: the nerves to rhomboid and serratus muscles, the brachial plexus, the subclavian artery and vein with the anterior scalene muscle between, and the phrenic nerve. The object of dissection in this area is to remove completely the transverse cervical (inferior horizontal) and spinal accessory chains of lymph nodes (see Fig. 2.11).

Deep to the sternocleidomastoid muscle and posterolateral to the internal jugular vein, the thoracic duct on the left and the right lymphatic duct on the right lie in a mass of areolar connective tissue. They should be preserved if possible; if they have been injured, ligate.

Between the jugular vein and the carotid artery lies the ansa cervicalis, which innervates the strap muscles of the neck. This nerve is on or in the carotid sheath medial to the internal jugular vein. It may be cut with impunity.

Procedure

Position and prepare as in parotidectomy.

• **Step 1.** Incision (Figs. 2.61, 2.62, and 2.63).

Make a T-incision with the horizontal part extending from the midline to the submastoid area approximately 3 cm below the inferior border of the mandible and

Fig. 2.61 T-incision

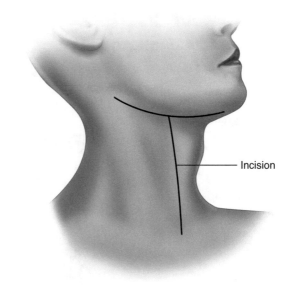

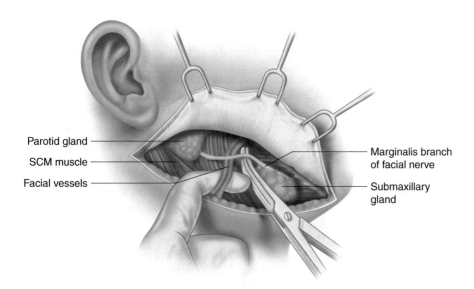

Parotid gland

SCM muscle

Facial vessels

Marginalis branch
of facial nerve

Submaxillary
gland

Fig. 2.62 Development of upper flap

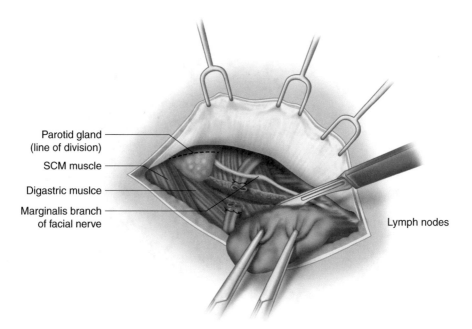

Parotid gland
(line of division)
SCM muscle
Digastric muslce
Marginalis branch
of facial nerve

Lymph nodes

Fig. 2.63 Dissection of submental and submandibular triangles

the vertical part extending from the midpoint of the horizontal down to 1 cm above the clavicle. Alternative incisions are the H type, the I type, or one shaped like an H lying on its side (lazy H).

The upper flap of the horizontal part. Incise the superficial fascia (fat and platysma) by deepening the skin incision and elevate the upper flap. The anterior facial vessels are located at the upper part of the flap snaking in front of the mandible. The mandibular and cervical branches of the facial nerves are located superficially to these vessels. Protect both nerves, especially the marginal branch, by careful dissection and isolation. If necessary, the cervical branch may be cut. Elevate the anterior facial vessels, then clamp, divide, and ligate them.

Detach the deep cervical fascia from the mandible and push it downward bluntly, including the submental area and the submaxillary gland, fat, and lymph nodes. Occasionally, the lower pole of the parotid is removed below the disappearing point of the marginal branch. Then, in this procedure, the contents of the submental and submandibular triangles are dissected as well as the lower pole of the parotid.

Vertical incision and formation of flaps. To form flaps, deepen the existing skin incision. Prepare the anterior neck triangle, and elevate the anterior flap to the midline and the posterior flap to the anterior border of the trapezius muscle. The sternocleidomastoid muscle is essentially in the middle of the surgical field.

- **Step 2.** Exploration of the posterior triangle (Fig. 2.64).
  The following anatomical entities should be identified:
- Spinal accessory nerve

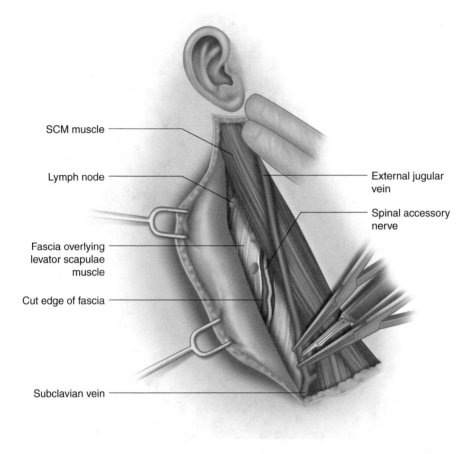

Fig. 2.64 Contents of posterior triangle

- External jugular vein
- Cervical nerves (not shown)
- Brachial plexus (between anterior and middle scalene) (not shown)
- Phrenic nerve (resting on the anterior scalene) (not shown)

All but the spinal accessory nerve are under the "carpet" (the splitting of the deep fascia) of the floor of the posterior triangle.

Carefully ligate the external jugular vein close to the subclavian vein while protecting the other four entities listed above. The upper part of the posterior triangle is cleaned by blunt dissection, pushing fibrofatty tissue, and lymph nodes cephalad.

- **Step 3.** After elevating and protecting the anatomical entities of the carotid sheath, carefully transect the clavicular and sternal insertions of the sternocleidomastoid muscle.

The next step is a low division of the omohyoid behind the sternocleidomastoid muscle. Continue cleaning the floor of the posterior triangle (Figs. 2.65 and 2.66).

Fig. 2.65 Transection of
omohyoid muscle

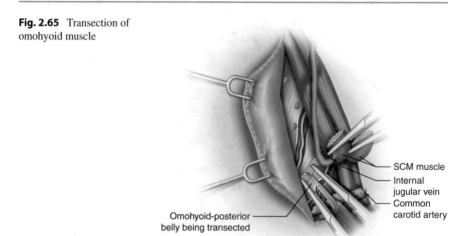

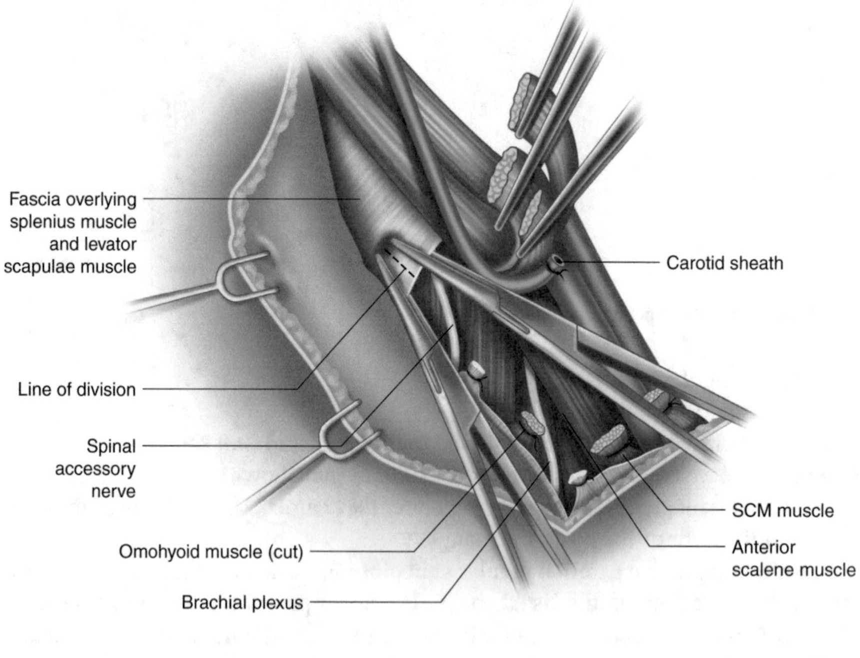

Fig. 2.66 Exploration of overlying fascia

Fig. 2.67 Removal of
carotid sheath

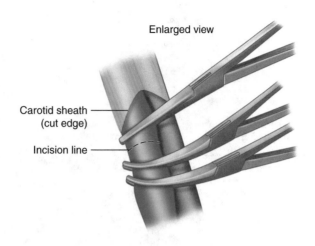

Enlarged view

Carotid sheath —
(cut edge)

Incision line —

Step 4. Open the anterior wall of the carotid sheath, ligate the internal jugular vein close to the clavicle, and remove the sheath together with the vein and all fibro-fatty tissue in the vicinity. Protect the phrenic nerve and ligate the transverse scapular and transverse cervical arteries and the right or left thoracic ducts as required. Proceeding upward, remember the posterior belly of the digastric muscle is an excellent anatomical landmark. Just underneath are internal and external carotid arteries; the internal jugular vein, which should be ligated; cranial nerves (X, XI, XII); and the sympathetic chain (Fig. 2.67).

Step 5. Working now at the anterior triangle, avoid cutting the external branch of the superior laryngeal nerve. Ligate the branches of the external carotid artery. Protect and save the hypoglossal nerve. Continue to work on both the submental and the submandibular triangles. Ligate the submaxillary duct, but protect and save its fellow traveler, the lingual nerve. Spare the submaxillary ganglion. Establish good hemostasis (Fig. 2.68).

Step 6. Remove the specimen en bloc (Fig. 2.69). Figure 2.60 shows the surgical field after removal of the specimen.

Note
- Under certain circumstances, such as thyroid cancer, a modified radical neck dissection or central neck dissection may be more appropriate than the radical dissection.

In the beautiful book, *An Atlas of the Surgical Techniques of Oliver H. Beahrs* (Beahrs OH, Kiernan PD, Hubert JP Jr. Philadelphia: Saunders, 1985), Dr. Beahrs gives an excellent description of the technique of radical neck dissection, one of the most complicated surgeries of the human body. We strongly advise the reader to consult his book, as well as an article in *Surgical Clinics of North America* 1977;57(4):663–700, Philadelphia: Saunders.

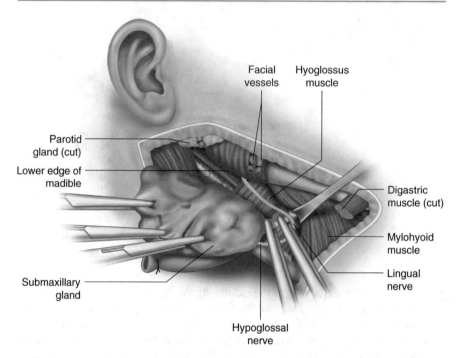

Fig. 2.68 Dissection of anterior triangle

Tracheostomy

Step 1. Position: semi-Fowler; hyperextension of the neck; small pillow at the area of the upper thoracic spine beneath the shoulders; doughnut support under the head.

Step 2. Preparation of skin: use Betadine or any other solution of surgeon's choice. Be sure that chin and long axis of the body are aligned at the midline.

Mark the location of the incision with 2–0 silk, two fingerbreadths above the sternal notch.

With a knife, mark very superficially the middle and edges of the previously marked location of the incision.

Use of an endotracheal tube is a wise step.

Step 3. In children, make a vertical incision to avoid injury of the arteries and veins located under the anterior border of the sternocleidomastoid muscle.

In adults, use vertical or transverse incision and proceed as in thyroid surgery (Fig. 2.70).

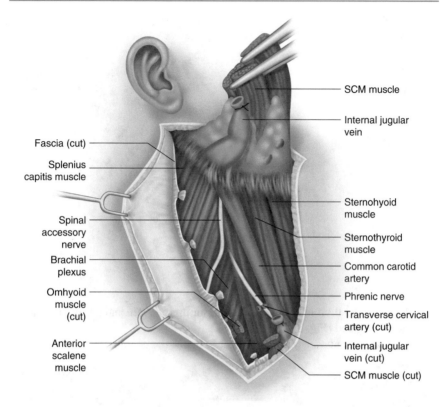

Fig. 2.69 Specimen removal

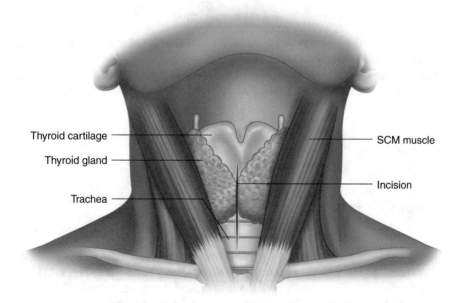

Fig. 2.70 Incision for tracheostomy

Fig. 2.71 Thyroid isthmus

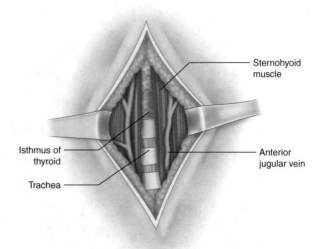

Step 4. Locate the thyroid isthmus. The inferior thyroid vein and thyroid ima artery should be ligated (Fig. 2.71).

Step 5. Clean the anterior wall of the trachea below the isthmus.

> **Remember**
> • Dissection too deep toward the superior mediastinum will injure the jugular venous arch, and dissection too lateral will injure the vessels of the carotid sheath. The thyroid isthmus should be retracted or cut between clamps for more tracheal room.

Step 6. Immobilize and elevate the anterior tracheal wall using a hook at the lower border of the cricoid cartilage.

Step 7. Make a vertical incision through the second or third tracheal ring or form a window at the anterior tracheal wall by removing the anterior central segment of the two rings (Fig. 2.72).

> **Remember**
> • Be careful when you incise the trachea. The posterior wall of the trachea is not protected, so injury to the esophagus is an obvious risk.
> • Protect the cricoid cartilage and first tracheal ring to avoid postoperative tracheal stenosis.

Step 8. Spread the tracheal opening with a tracheal spreader. Insert a Hardy–Shiley tracheostomy tube as the endotracheal tube is slowly backed out (Fig. 2.73).

Step 9. With umbilical tape, secure the tube around the patient's neck. Pack iodoform in the subcutaneous tissue around the tracheostomy tube.

Fig. 2.72 Incising trachea

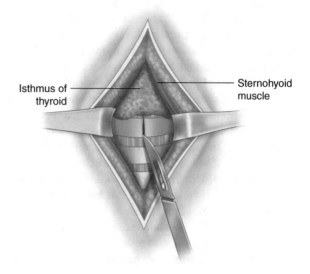

Isthmus of thyroid

Sternohyoid muscle

Fig. 2.73 Tracheal opening

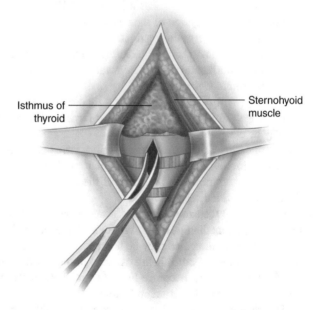

Isthmus of thyroid

Sternohyoid muscle

Anatomical Complications

Nerve Injuries

Nerves at risk during thyroidectomy and parathyroidectomy include the recurrent laryngeal nerves, the external branches of the superior laryngeal nerves, and the cervical sympathetic nerve trunks. In a series of 217 thyroid operations, Holt et al. found nine laryngeal nerve injuries, four of them permanent. In the same series, there were three injuries to superior laryngeal nerves; one was permanent.

Most recurrent laryngeal nerve injuries occur "just below that point to where the nerve passed under the lower fibers of the inferior constrictor muscle to become intralaryngeal." The usual cause is a hemostatic stitch. Another source of injury is mass ligation of the vessels of the lower pole of the thyroid. Such ligation may include a recurrent nerve which is more anterior than usual. The nerve should be identified before ligating the inferior thyroid vein.

Sites of possible nerve injury in thyroidectomy are as follows:

1. External branch of the superior laryngeal nerve during ligation of the superior thyroid vascular pedicle.
2. Recurrent laryngeal nerve as it traverses the ligament of Berry during total lobectomy. The recurrent nerve usually courses posterior to the "adherent zone" (ligament of Berry); however, in 25% of cases, it passes through it. The nerve traverses the thyroid itself at this level in 10% of patients. By retraction on the lobe, the recurrent nerve can be pulled forward into the operative field and be injured. In addition, traction can injure the nerve.
3. Recurrent laryngeal nerve during ligation of the inferior thyroid artery. It is important to ligate branches of the artery while keeping the nerve under direct vision.
4. Recurrent laryngeal nerve during ligation of the inferior thyroid veins. The nerve is anterolateral to the trachea in about 10% of cases and may be caught and divided during ligation of the veins.
5. Non-recurrent nerve during ligation of the inferior thyroid artery. A non-recurrent nerve may be mistaken for the inferior thyroid artery and ligated, because it takes a parallel horizontal course from the cervical vagus to the larynx. Fortunately, this anatomic variant is rare.
6. Cervical sympathetic trunk during ligation of the inferior thyroid artery. If the inferior thyroid artery is ligated too far lateral, the cervical sympathetic trunk may be caught in the tie.

Specific causes of recurrent nerve injury have been detailed by Chang. Separation of the inferior thyroid artery from the recurrent laryngeal nerve requires care. Where the nerve passes between branches of the artery, the individual branches must be ligated and divided separately.

Injury to the recurrent laryngeal nerve usually is complete. The vocal cord then takes up a paramedian position. When only one side is involved, the airway is adequate. However, the voice may be hoarse until one cord compensates by adducting over to the opposite cord. If the external branch of the superior laryngeal nerve is also injured, the cord becomes flaccid as well as paralyzed. This may cause noisy breathing on both inspiration and expiration.

The recurrent laryngeal nerve carries both adductor and abductor fibers. The abductor fibers are more superficial and more vulnerable to injury. The abductors may be preferentially damaged by traction, cautery, and other procedures. Such incomplete bilateral damage to the recurrent laryngeal nerves is more dangerous and more potentially life-threatening than is bilateral complete injury, since damage to abductor fibers results in unopposed function of adductor fibers, which draw the cords toward the midline, narrowing the glottic opening to a slit and resulting in severe respiratory distress, which may necessitate emergent tracheostomy.

Injury to the external branch of the superior laryngeal nerve results in dysfunction of the cricothyroid muscle, with ensuing hoarseness. The voice is usually "breathy" and aspiration of liquids is a frequent complication. Bilateral damage to both external branches results in flaccid vocal cords and extreme weakness of the voice on phonation. The superior thyroid artery should not be clamped above the upper pole of the thyroid because the external laryngeal nerve may be injured. The branches of the artery should be divided individually.

Postoperative hoarseness is not always the result of operative injury to laryngeal nerves. One percent to 2% of patients have a paralyzed vocal cord prior to thyroid resection. Based on several large series, it is recommended that the patient be informed that, despite all precautions, there is a possibility (1–2%) of some vocal disability following thyroidectomy or parathyroidectomy.

A sympathetic ganglion may be confused with a lymph node and removed when the surgeon operates for metastatic papillary carcinoma of the thyroid. Injury to the cervical sympathetic nerve results in Homer's syndrome (constriction of the pupil, ptosis of the upper eyelid, apparent enophthalmos, and dilation of retinal vessels).

Hypoparathyroidism

With total thyroidectomy, transient hypocalcemia may occur in 5–10% of patients. The incidence of permanent hypoparathyroidism is less than 1% in patients operated on by experienced surgeons, especially with preservation or autotransplantation of resected tissue from a normal parathyroid gland. The surgeon performing thyroidectomy should be familiar with the technique of parathyroid fragment autografting. It is important to recognize arterial or venous compromise to a parathyroid and autograft its fragments rather than assuming that it is viable in situ. With careful dissection, most normal parathyroids can be spared in situ; but in 5–10% pf thyroidectomies at least one parathyroid will require autografting, usually because its arterial supply is intimate to the thyroid capsule. If a parathyroid is not found during thyroidectomy, the surface of the resected thyroid specimen should be inspected.

Vascular Injuries

Thyroid arteries must be ligated carefully with double or suture ligature of the superior and inferior thyroid arteries. The superior thyroid artery tends to retract. The middle thyroid vein is short and easily torn and, if divided accidentally, will retract, making hemostasis difficult. With too much traction of the thyroid gland, the vein becomes flattened and bloodless, making it difficult to recognize. The tear is often at the junction of the middle thyroid vein with the jugular vein. The thoracic duct is rarely injured in thyroidectomy, although it may be injured during neck dissection. The duct may be ligated with impunity.

Organ Injuries

The pleurae are injured rarely, except in cases such as a huge goiter extending into the mediastinum. Both anteriorly and posteriorly, the two pleurae approach the midline and hence each other. Intrathoracic goiter may descend into the anterior or posterior mediastinum, bringing the thyroid gland close to the pleurae.

The trachea and esophagus may be injured in the presence of thyroiditis, calcified adenoma, or malignancy. The true capsule of the thyroid, the pretracheal fascia, the trachea, and the esophagus maybe fixed to one another, and vigorous attempts at separation may perforate the trachea. Tracheal perforation may require immediate tracheostomy but usually can be repaired primarily with absorbable suture, after advancing the cuff of endotracheal tube below the perforation. Facial nerve injury is related to tumor location and the experience of the operator. Temporary nerve paresis, especially of the marginal mandibular and temporal branches, is not uncommon. When removing the gland, care must be taken to not apply too much traction on the specimen. Hematoma and infection are extremely rare if proper surgical technique is used.

Frey's syndrome is localized sweating and flushing during the mastication of food. This common disorder occurs in 35–60% of patients after parotidectomy with facial nerve dissection. The syndrome usually is noted several months after surgery, with varying degrees of severity. It may result from aberrant regeneration of nerve fibers from postganglionic secretomotor parasympathetic innervation to the parotid gland occurring through the severed axon sheaths of the postganglionic sympathetic fibers that supply the sweat glands of the skin. The majority of affected patients do not seek treatment.

Bleeding from the thyroid or great vessels may occur. The innominate artery or right common carotid artery may cross the trachea above the sternal notch, so care must be taken during an emergency tracheostomy. Midline dissection prevents injury to the esophagus and recurrent laryngeal nerves.

False passage of the tracheostomy tube may result in a pneumothorax or pneumomediastinum. Improper tube placement may result in perforation of the lateral or posterior tracheal wall. Postoperative complications include erosion into a major vessel or the esophagus. Long-term tracheal intubation may result in tracheal stenosis.

Breast

3

Bruce J. Feigelson

Anatomy

General Description of the Breast

The adult female breast is located within the superficial fascia of the anterior chest wall. The base of the breast extends from the second rib superiorly to the sixth or seventh rib inferiorly and from the sternal border medially to the midaxillary line laterally. Two-thirds of the base of the breast lies anterior to the pectoralis major muscle; the remainder lies anterior to the serratus anterior muscle. A small part may lie over the aponeurosis of the external oblique muscle.

In about 95% of women, there is a prolongation of the upper lateral quadrant toward the axilla. This tail (of Spence) of breast tissue enters a hiatus (of Langer) in the deep fascia of the medial axillary wall. This is the only breast tissue found normally beneath the deep fascia.

Deep Fascia

The deep pectoral fascia envelops the pectoralis major muscle, and the clavipectoral fascia envelops the pectoralis minor and part of the subclavius muscles. The axillary fascia lying across the base of the axillary pyramidal space is an extension of the pectoralis major fascia and continues as the fascia of the latissimus dorsi. It forms the dome of the axilla (Fig. 3.1a). Where the axillary vessels and nerves to the arm pass through the fascia, they take with them a tubular fascial sleeve, the axillary sheath.

B. J. Feigelson (✉)
Department of General Surgery, Colorado Permanente Medical Group, Denver, CO, USA
e-mail: Bruce.X.Feigelson@kp.org

© Springer Nature Switzerland AG 2021
L. J. Skandalakis (ed.), *Surgical Anatomy and Technique*,
https://doi.org/10.1007/978-3-030-51313-9_3

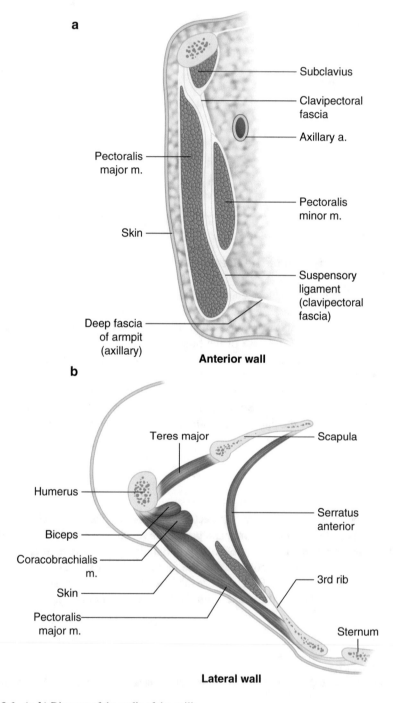

Fig. 3.1 (**a**, **b**) Diagram of the walls of the axilla

The clavipectoral fascia (Fig. 3.1a) can be thought of as consisting of five parts:

- The attachment to the clavicle and the envelope of the subclavius muscle
- That part between the subclavius and pectoralis minor muscles, referred to by some as "the costocoracoid membrane"
- The thickened lateral band between the first rib and the coracoid process, the costocoracoid ligament
- The pectoralis minor envelope
- The suspensory ligament of the axilla attaching to the axillary fascia

Axilla

The axilla is shaped like a pyramid with an apex, a base, and four walls. The apex is a triangular space bordered by the clavicle, the upper border of the scapula, and the first rib. The base consists of the axillary fascia beneath the skin of the axillary fossa. The anterior wall is composed of three muscles—the pectoralis major, the pectoralis minor, and the subclavius—and the clavipectoral fascia, which envelops the muscles and fills the spaces between them. The posterior wall is formed by the scapula and three muscles: the subscapularis, the latissimus dorsi, and the teres major. The medial wall consists of the lateral chest wall, with the second to sixth ribs, and the serratus anterior muscle. The lateral wall is the narrowest of the walls, being formed by the bicipital groove of the humerus (Fig. 3.1b).

The axilla contains lymph nodes (about which more will be said); the axillary sheath, which covers blood vessels and nerves; and the tendons of the long and short heads of the biceps brachii muscle and the coracobrachialis muscle (Fig. 3.2).

Muscles and Nerves

The muscles and nerves with which the surgeon must be familiar are listed in Table 3.1.

Morphology of the Breast

Each breast is composed of between 15 and 20 lobes, some larger than others, within the superficial fascia, which is loosely connected with the deep fascia. Between the superficial and deep fasciae is the retromammary (submammary) space, which is rich in lymphatics (Fig. 3.3).

Each lobe has a duct terminating at the nipple. These lobes, together with their ducts, are anatomical but not surgical units. A breast biopsy is not a lobectomy; in the latter, parts of one or more lobes are removed.

In the fat-free area under the areola, the dilated portions of the lactiferous ducts (the lactiferous sinuses) are the only sites of actual milk storage. Intraductal papillomas may develop here.

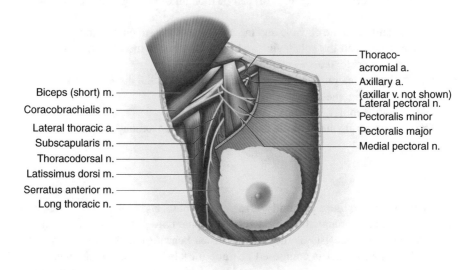

Fig. 3.2 Topography of the axilla. Anterior view

The suspensory ligaments of Cooper form a network of strong connective tissue fibers passing between the lobes of parenchyma and connecting the dermis of the skin with the deep layer of the superficial fascia. Occasionally the superficial fascia is fixed to the skin in such a way that ideal subcutaneous total mastectomy is impossible.

With malignant invasion, portions of the ligaments of Cooper may contract, producing a characteristic fixation and retraction or dimpling of the skin. This must not be confused with the retraction called *peau d'orange* secondary to lymphatic obstruction.

Vascular System of the Breast

Arterial Supply
The breast is supplied with blood from three sources, with considerable variation (Figs. 3.2 and 3.4).

Internal Thoracic Artery
The internal thoracic (or internal mammary) artery is a branch of the subclavian artery that parallels the lateral border of the sternum behind the internal intercostal muscles.

Table 3.1 Muscles and nerves involved in mastectomy

Muscle	Origin	Insertion	Nerve supply	Comments
Pectoralis major	Medial half of clavicle, lateral half of sternum, second to sixth costal cartilages, aponeurosis of external oblique muscle	Greater tubercle of humerus	Lateral anterior thoracic nerve	Clavicular portion of pectoralis forms upper extent of radical mastectomy; lateral border forms medial boundary of modified radical mastectomy; both nerves should be preserved in modified radical procedure
Pectoralis minor	Second to fifth ribs	Coracoid process of scapula	Medial anterior thoracic nerve	
Deltoid	Lateral half of clavicle, lateral border of acromion process, spine of scapula	Deltoid tuberosity of humerus	Axillary nerve	
Serratus anterior (three parts)	1. First and second ribs	Costal surface of scapula at superior angle	Long thoracic nerve	Injury produces "winged scapula"
	2. Second to fourth ribs	Vertebral border of scapula		
	3. Fourth to eighth ribs	Costal surface of scapula at inferior angle		
Latissimus dorsi	Back, to crest of ilium	Crest of lesser tubercle and inter-tubercular groove of humerus	Thoracodorsal nerve	Anterior border forms lateral extent of radical mastectomy; injury results in weakness of rotation and abduction of arm
Subclavius	Junction of first rib and its cartilage	Groove of lower surface of clavicle	Subclavian nerve	
Subscapularis	Costal surface of scapula	Lesser tubercle of humerus	Subscapular nerve	Subscapular nerve should be spared
External oblique aponeurosis	External oblique muscle	Rectus sheath and linea alba, crest of ilium		Remember the interdigitation with serratus anterior and pectoralis muscles
Rectus abdominis	Ventral surface of fifth to seventh costal cartilages and xiphoid process	Crest and superior ramus of pubis	Branches of seventh to 12th thoracic nerves	Rectus sheath is lower limit of radical mastectomy

By permission of JE Skandalakis, SW Gray, and JR Rowe. *Anatomical Complications in General Surgery*. New York: McGraw-Hill, 1983

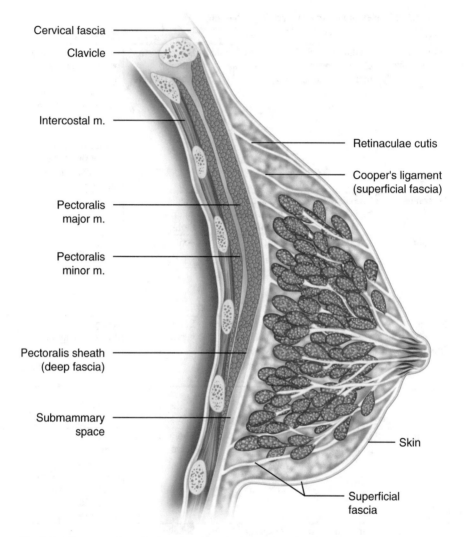

Fig. 3.3 Diagrammatic sagittal section through the non-lactating female breast and anterior thoracic wall

Branches of the Axillary Artery

Four branches of the axillary artery may supply the breast. They are, in order of appearance, (1) the supreme thoracic branch, (2) the pectoral branches of the thoracoacromial artery, (3) the lateral thoracic arteries, and (4) unnamed mammary branches.

Intercostal Arteries

The lateral half of the breast may also receive branches of the third, fourth, and fifth intercostal arteries.

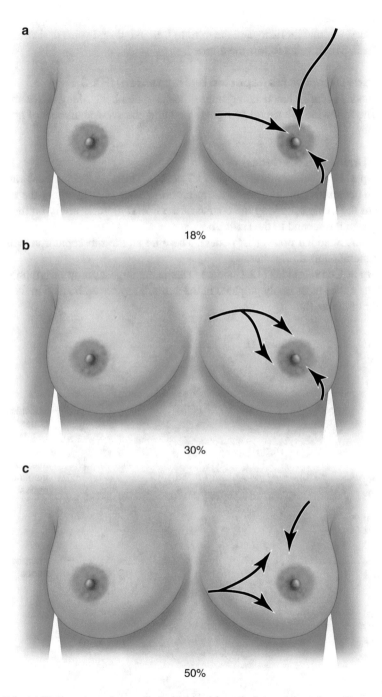

Fig. 3.4 (a) The breast may be supplied with blood from the internal thoracic, axillary, and intercostal arteries in 18% of individuals. (b) In 30%, the contribution from the axillary artery is negligible. (c) In 50%, the intercostal arteries contribute little or no blood to the breast. In the remaining 2%, other variations may be found

Venous Drainage

The axillary, internal thoracic, and the third to fifth intercostal veins drain the mammary gland. These veins follow the arteries.

Lymphatic Drainage (as Reported by Haagensen) (Fig. 3.5)

Lymph nodes occur in inconstant groups of varying numbers. Many nodes are very small. The following is a useful grouping, including the average number of nodes in each group.

Axillary Drainage (35.3 Nodes)

- **Group 1**. External mammary nodes (1.7 nodes). These lie along the lateral edge of the pectoralis minor, deep to the pectoralis major muscle, along the medial side of the axilla following the course of the lateral thoracic artery on the chest wall from the second to the sixth rib.
- **Group 2**. Scapular nodes (5.8 nodes). These lie on the subscapular vessels and their thoracodorsal branches.
- **Group 3**. Central nodes (12.1 nodes). This is the largest group of lymph nodes and the nodes most easily palpated in the axilla. They are embedded in fat in the center of the axilla.

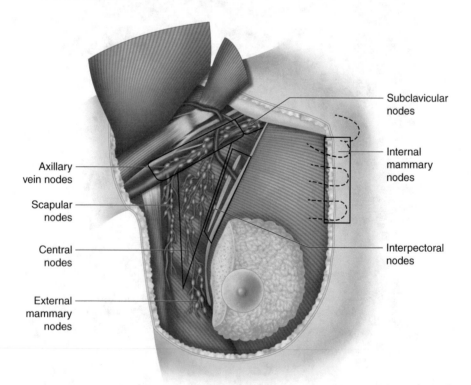

Fig. 3.5 Lymph nodes of the breast and axilla. Classification of Haagensen and coworkers

- **Group 4**. Interpectoral nodes (Rotter's nodes) (1.4 nodes). These lie between the pectoralis major and minor muscles. Often there is a single node. They are the smallest group of the axillary nodes and will not be found unless the pectoralis major is removed.
- **Group 5**. Axillary vein nodes (10.7 nodes). This is the second largest group of lymph nodes in the axilla. They lie on the caudal and ventral surfaces of the lateral part of the axillary vein.
- **Group 6**. Subclavicular nodes (3.5 nodes). These lie on the caudal and ventral surfaces of the medial part of the axillary vein. Haagensen and coworkers consider them to be inaccessible unless the pectoralis minor muscle is sacrificed.

Internal Thoracic (Mammary) Drainage (8.5 Nodes)
The nodes, about four or five on each side, are small and are usually in the fat and connective tissue of the intercostal spaces. The internal thoracic trunks empty into the thoracic duct or the right lymphatic duct. This route to the venous system is shorter than the axillary route.

The presence of regional lymph nodes is an important prognostic indicator and suggests systemic disease. Performing a sentinel lymph node biopsy can spare the patient an unnecessary axillary dissection. If a sentinel node is positive, the resultant axillary dissection is not—in most surgeons' view—a curative procedure but one that controls local disease. In many patients, positive axillary nodes mandate chemotherapy, although indications for chemotherapy are continuously evolving.

Surgical Anatomy of Mastectomy

Anatomy of the Axillary Triangular Bed of Modified Radical Mastectomy
The medial side of the surgical field is the upward and medially retracted axillary margin of the pectoralis major muscle. The lateral side is the medial border of the latissimus dorsi muscle, and the superior side is the axillary vein. The floor of the triangular bed is formed by the serratus anterior and the subscapularis muscles. This results in a smaller triangle than would be used for a radical mastectomy but one that is adequate for good dissection (Fig. 3.6).

After the breast and the underlying fascia are removed, a good dissection consists of (1) removing remnants of the pectoralis major fascia at its axillary border, (2) entering the axilla by incising and stripping the axillary fascia, (3) further stripping the fascia of the pectoralis minor (lower clavipectoral fascia), (4) exposing the axillary vein, (5) downward dissection of axillary fat and lymph nodes after ligating tributaries of the axillary vein from the thoracic wall, and (6) continuing the dissection downward, partially removing the fascia of the serratus anterior, the subscapularis, and the medial border of the latissimus dorsi muscles.

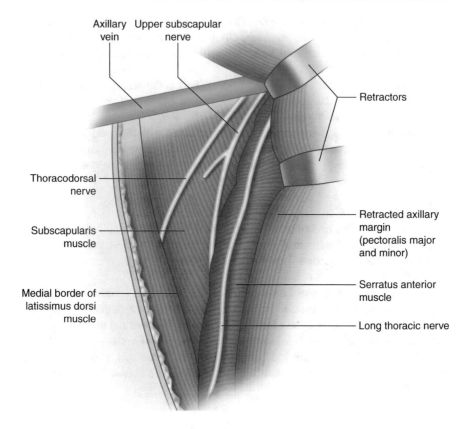

Fig. 3.6 The triangular bed of a modified radical mastectomy. The pectoralis muscles are retracted, rather than removed

Remember
- The *thoracodorsal nerve* lies on the subscapularis muscle and innervates the latissimus dorsi muscle (Fig. 3.6). If it is cut, internal rotation and abduction will be weakened, although there is no deformity. The nerve and its associated vessels can be found near the medial border of the latissimus dorsi about 5 cm above a plane passing through the third sternochondral junction. Once located, the neurovascular bundle should be marked with an umbilical tape. If there is obvious involvement of lymph nodes around the nerve, it must be sacrificed.

- The *long thoracic nerve* innervates the serratus anterior muscle and lies on it (Fig. 3.6). Division of the nerve results in the "winged scapula" deformity. Unless actually invaded by cancer, this nerve should be spared. The landmark for locating the nerve is the point at which the axillary vein passes over the second rib. Careful dissection of this area will reveal the nerve descending on the second rib posterior to the axillary vein.
- The *medial anterior thoracic nerve* is superficial to the axillary vein and lateral to the pectoralis minor muscle. The *lateral anterior thoracic nerve*, which is the nerve supply of the clavicular as well as of the sternal portions of the pectoralis major muscle, also is superficial to the axillary vein and lies at the medial edge of the pectoralis minor.
- If branches of one or both anterior thoracic nerves are injured, the result will be atrophy of the pectoralis major and minor muscles. If the few lymph nodes of the interpectoral group are involved and are fixed to the nerves, these nerves should be sacrificed.

Technique

Breast Biopsy/Lumpectomy

- By definition, these operations remove as much breast tissue as required to achieve the desired goal (tissue diagnosis or definitive surgical management of cancer) and leave as much breast tissue as possible, whether this is for benign, malignant, or unknown pathology.
- For benign lesions or lesions still being evaluated for possible malignancy, a more focal excision can be performed.
- Proven malignancy requires a larger excision in order to obtain disease free margins.
- Applicable for both palpable and nonpalpable lesions. Nonpalpable lesions require breast imaging assistance for localization and removal. Needle localization, placed the day of surgery, or implanted identifiable markers (RF reflector, implantable magnet, or radioactive seed may be placed prior to the day of surgery), may be employed.
- Appropriate incision placement is critical for both successful excision and for optimal cosmesis.
- If combined with axillary surgery (either Sentinel Node Biopsy or Axillary node dissection), I usually utilize a separate incision unless the breast lesion is high in the UOQ.

- **Step 1.** Using the location of the area of concern, decide on placement of the incision. If an implanted devise has been deployed, locating this prior to making an incision is critical. Try to avoid the upper inner quadrant if possible for cosmetic considerations. Wire entry site, if used, is also an important consideration for incision choice. Useful incisions include periareolar (Fig. 3.7) or along Langer's lines. I draw all incisions and place perpendicular cross marks as this facilitates proper skin alignment during closure.

- **Step 2.** Raise skin flaps to approach the lesion (Fig. 3.8). Reviewing breast imaging intraoperatively allows understanding of location of the area of concern, assessment of anterior and posterior margins, how thin/thick flaps can be, and if posterior pectoralis fascia requires resection.
- **Step 3.** Excise the lesion with a margin of normal breast tissue. For patients with nonpalpable lesions located with one of the localization techniques, intraoperative post-excision imaging should be performed to ensure successful removal of the area of concern, marking clip, and the localization device. The specimen should be appropriately marked for tissue orientation to assist the pathologist with communicating the final margins. Sutures, clips, or tags may be used. It is

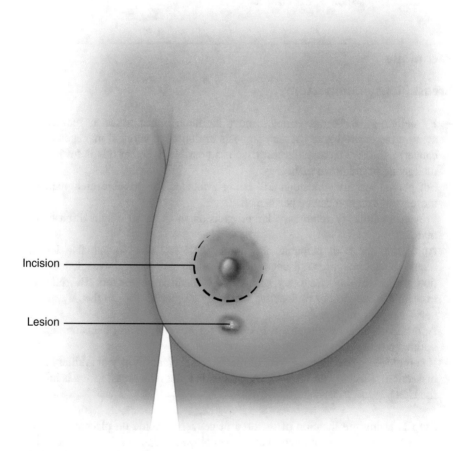

Fig. 3.7 Periareolar incision for lower central lesion

critical that these orienting designations are properly placed and communicated to the OR team handling the specimen and ultimately to the pathologist in order to have an accurate margin report on the final pathology.

- **Step 4.** We mark lumpectomy cavities with clips to assist the radiation oncology team with identification of the tumor site if boost radiation is utilized. Implantable marking devices are commercially available as well.
- **Step 5.** Establish hemostasis with electrocautery. Inject local anesthesia liberally for post-op pain control. Consider approximating the mammary tissue with 2–0 Vicryl, using oncoplastic techniques. Some surgeons prefer not to approximate the breast defect, reasoning that if hemostasis is good, in time the formed seroma will form fibrous tissue, and no or minimal skin depression will result. We prefer to place a few superficial sutures only for smaller resections and then approximate the edges of the incision, leaving the cavity alone, with occasional use of level 1 oncoplastic closure strategies. Use subcutaneous interrupted sutures with 3–0 Vicryl and close the skin with running

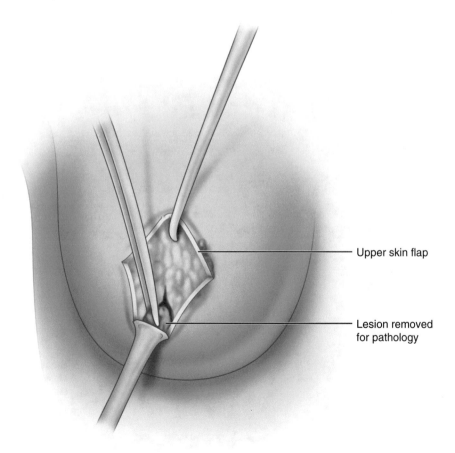

Upper skin flap

Lesion removed for pathology

Fig. 3.8 Creation of flaps

4–0 Monocryl subcuticular sutures (Fig. 3.9). We cover the wound(s) with surgical glue.
- **Step 6.** I recommend a supportive bra for the first 1–2 weeks post-op. An ice bag intermittently to the breast for 24 h may be used.

Simple Mastectomy/Modified Radical Mastectomy

– Removal of 99% + of breast tissue, but not 100%. Skin flaps should be of appropriate thickness for viability, yet leaving as little breast tissue as possible. I wear a headlight during surgery for optimal visualization and to allow transillumination of the flap, so my assistant can continuously monitor flap thickness. I frequently palpate the flaps to monitor flap thickness.
– Multiple variations of mastectomy exist, including traditional (removal of nipple areolar complex plus surrounding ellipse of skin), skin sparing (taking only the nipple areolar complex), and nipple sparing (leave all skin and utilize a single linear incision either lateral radial or inframammary). Multiple mastectomy incision options exist as well, based on the patient breast anatomy, ptosis, weight, and tumor location.

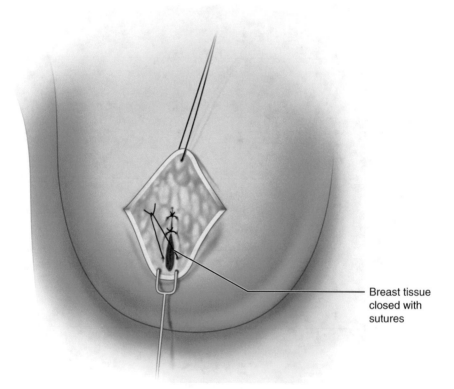

Breast tissue closed with sutures

Fig. 3.9 Suturing the defect

– Long wide strokes with the energy source help making the flaps even and smooth. Use of a suction tip electrocautery devise will maximize smoke evacuation during dissection.
– Unless performing nipple sparing mastectomy, any needed axillary surgery can be performed through this incision. For nipple sparing mastectomy, I often will make a separate axillary incision.

• **Step 1.** Prior to incision, mark the contour of the breast to determine its edges, especially when the patient is obese. This minimizes unnecessary dissection (Fig. 3.10). Frequently I will do this in the pre-op area with the patient upright.
• **Step 2.** An obliquely oriented elliptical incision of some variety is created. Use electrocautery for the formation of the superior and inferior flaps. The superior flap should be taken to the clavicle or well above the superior margin of the breast which is sometimes easily seen. The inferior flap should be taken down to the inframammary fold (Fig. 3.11). Medial margin of dissection is the lateral portion of the sternum and, laterally, the latissimus muscle. Carry these dissections until you reach chest wall or pectoralis muscle. Reaching these boundaries as the flaps are created will facilitate removal of the breast from the chest as it establishes the resection margins.

If mastectomy combined with axillary dissection continue to step 3
If mastectomy combined with Axillary Sentinel Node Biopsy skip steps 5–9
If no axillary component, skip to step 9

• **Step 3.** As the breast is separated from the overlying flaps laterally and the axilla is approached, the clavipectoral fascia is encountered. When this is opened, there is access to the axilla (Fig. 3.12). Protect the pectoralis major and minor. Rarely, however, the pectoralis minor may be cut for a more complete axillary dissection (Fig. 3.13).
• **Step 4.** If performing an axillary sentinel node biopsy at time of mastectomy, I usually perform the SLNB after creating my flaps but prior to removing the breast from the pectoralis. Please refer to the previously described sentinel node technique (Chap. 1).

Briefly, interrogate the axilla with the radioactivity detecting probe, look for blue dye, and remove involved nodes. Consider sending for frozen section, based on your individual algorithm for immediate axillary lymph node dissection. I have moved away from routine frozen section for sentinel nodes, as there are now multiple axillary algorithms for positive nodes based on size of axillary metastasis, number of positive nodes, and extent of extranodal extension. An axillary drain is only used for axillary dissections.

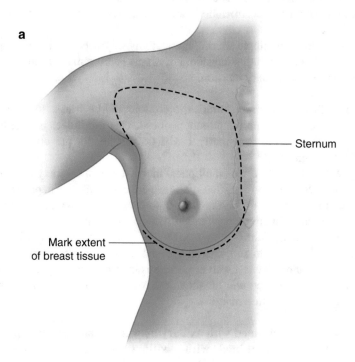

Sternum

Mark extent of breast tissue

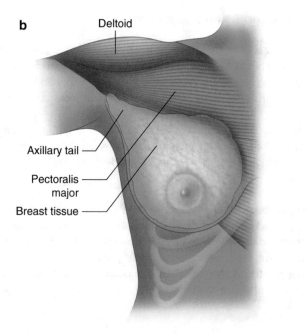

Deltoid

Axillary tail

Pectoralis major

Breast tissue

Fig. 3.10 (a) Breast contour. (b) Underlying structures

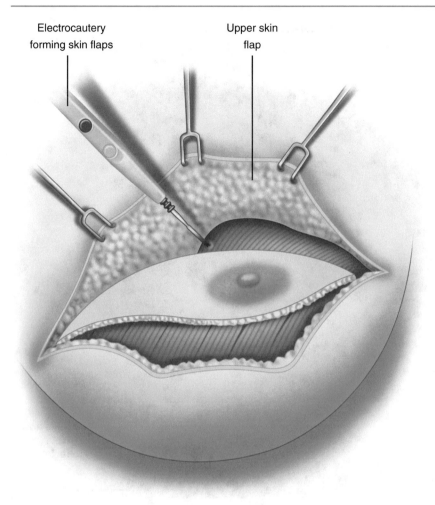

Fig. 3.11 Flap formation

- **Step 5.** After opening the clavipectoral fascia, use finger dissection and occasional cautery to dissect along the lateral chest wall, looking for the long thoracic nerve. The patient should NOT be paralyzed, so this nerve can be stimulated intraoperatively to assist with identification. This nerve is usually quite posterior.
- **Step 6.** Sweep the mobilized portion of the axillary contents laterally and inferiorly to locate the axillary vein (Fig. 3.14). Follow the vein laterally to identify the vascular tributaries, which come of the inferior margin of the axillary vessels. With 3–0 or 4–0 Vicryl, or other vessel sealing devise, ligate all tributaries toward the breast and axilla.
- **Step 7.** Using a hemostat, gently sweep the axillary contents of fat and lymph nodes inferiorly, retracting inferiorly and in continuity (Fig. 3.15). Send all removed contents/pieces to pathology as occasionally additional nodal tissue

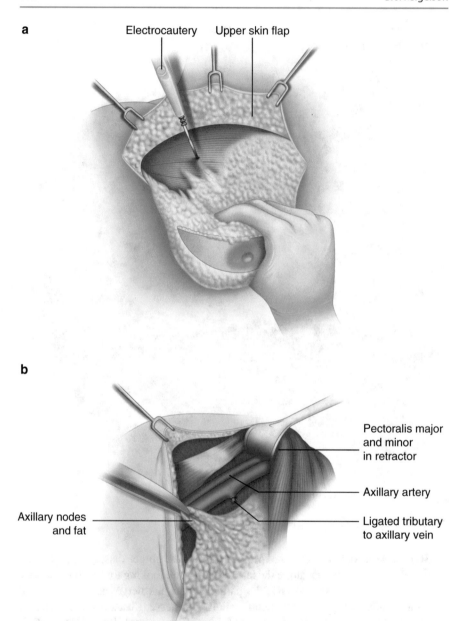

Fig. 3.12 (**a**) Axilla is exposed. (**b**) Structures of the axillary region

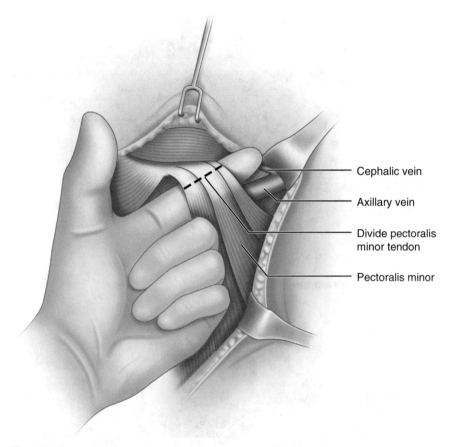

Fig. 3.13 Pectoralis minor

will be separated from the main body of axillary contents. I use vessel sealing devise to divide all lymphatic and most vessels.

- **Step 8.** Five nerves* CAN be identified and protected if possible (Figs. 3.2 and 3.16):
  - (a) Long thoracic, where the axillary vein passes over the second rib
  - (b) Thoracodorsal, at the medial border of the latissimus dorsi
  - (c) Medial anterior thoracic (pectoral), superficial to the axillary vein and lateral to the pectoralis minor muscle
  - (d) Lateral anterior thoracic (pectoral), at the medial edge of the pectoralis minor and superficial to the axillary vein
  - (e) Subscapular, at the vicinity of the subscapular artery and vein

*In practice, I only typically identify the long thoracic and thoracodorsal nerves.

As you sweep the contents inferiorly, and as your dissection extends further posteriorly, begin to look for the thoracodorsal nerve. This is usually associated with an

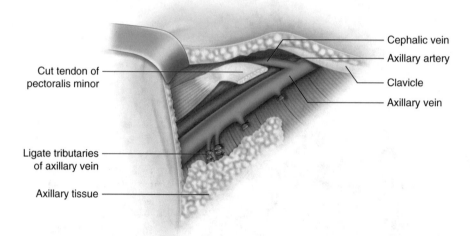

Cut tendon of
pectoralis minor

Cephalic vein

Axillary artery

Clavicle

Axillary vein

Ligate tributaries
of axillary vein

Axillary tissue

Fig. 3.14 Axillary vein and artery

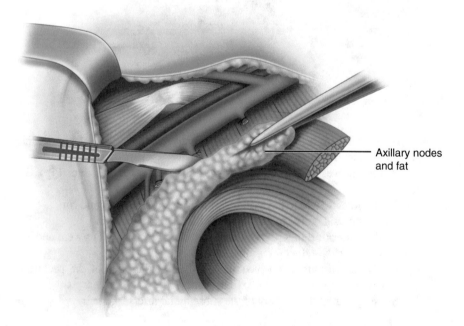

Axillary nodes
and fat

Fig. 3.15 Evacuation of axillary contents

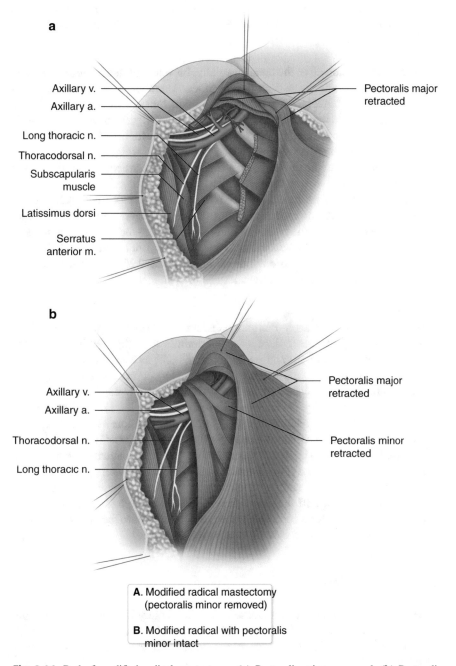

a

Axillary v.

Axillary a.

Long thoracic n.

Thoracodorsal n.

Subscapularis
muscle

Latissimus dorsi

Serratus
anterior m.

Pectoralis major
retracted

b

Axillary v.

Axillary a.

Thoracodorsal n.

Long thoracic n.

Pectoralis major
retracted

Pectoralis minor
retracted

A. Modified radical mastectomy
(pectoralis minor removed)

B. Modified radical with pectoralis
minor intact

Fig. 3.16 Bed of modified radical mastectomy. (**a**) Pectoralis minor removed. (**b**) Pectoralis major and minor are retracted

accompanying artery and vein, is in the posterior aspect of the axilla, and is about 2 cm lateral to the long thoracic nerve. Stimulate with a hemostat to confirm its identity.

- **Step 9.** Begin removal of the breast medially. Elevate it off the pectoralis muscle, taking the pectoralis fascia with the specimen. There are many arterial perforators entering the medial breast that will require ligation with 2–0 Vicryl. The vessel sealing device can be used in lieu of suture ligations. Pectoralis fascia MUST be removed with the breast. Tag the specimen for proper orientation.
  - If reconstruction is considered, it may be helpful to weigh the specimen (and document this in the operative note if delayed reconstruction) as it may assist the plastic surgeon with reconstruction.
- **Step 10.** Consider a rib block. I perform a 4 level nerve block with 0.25% bupivacaine, for the 2/3/4 or 3/4/5 ribs. I place 5 cc at each level, followed by another 10 cc between the pectoralis major and minor. I place the needle very tangentially to avoid creating a pneumothorax and aspirate prior to injecting. Volume of local used should be based on patient weight (1 cc 0.25% bupivacaine/kg). I always communicate this with the anesthesiologist.

Closing

- **Step 11.** Place one Jackson–Pratt drain under the inferior skin flap. If an axillary dissection was performed, place a second drain in the axilla. While a "Y" connector is pictured (Fig. 3.17), I prefer separate bulbs as each drain output is followed, managed, and removed independently. On rare occasion, for very large breast patients, I will place 2 drains under the mastectomy flaps.
- **Step 12.** I prefer to align the incision with temporary staples. Frequently a medial or lateral "dog ear" is addressed while aligning the incision with staples. There are many described techniques to address the lateral "dog ear" problem, but not reviewed in this text. This is a frequent problem in obese patients. I then replace the staples with 3–0 Vicryl deep dermal sutures, and final skin closure with 4–0 Monocryl subcuticular suture. Final dressing is surgical glue. I do cover the wound/chest with a fluff dressing and a surgical bra. We traditionally admitted our mastectomy patients for overnight observation but have recently offered outpatient mastectomies on a case by case basis.

Axillary Dissection

Make an incision through a skin crease along the axillary hair line and extending close to the lateral margin of the pectoralis muscle. The patient must not be paralyzed in order to stimulate the motor nerves (long thoracic and thoracodorsal) during the dissection.

Follow steps 6–9 above.

Close in layers of absorbable suture over a single 10 mm flat or 15 mm round closed suction drain.

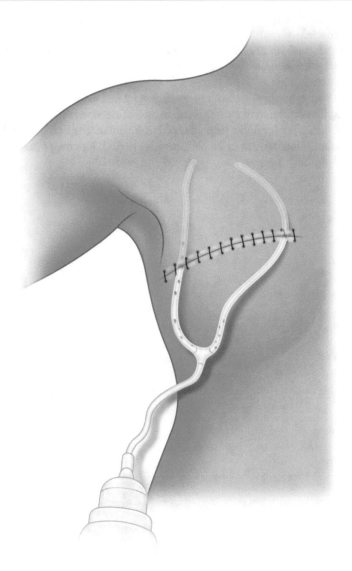

Fig. 3.17 Placement of drains

Anatomical Complications

- Injury to long thoracic nerve resulting in winged scapula.
- Extensive resection of brachial lymphatic vessels resulting in increased risk for arm lymphedema.
- Injury to the thoracodorsal nerve, weakening the latissimus dorsi muscle leading to decreased ability for adduction.

- Injury to the medial pectoral nerves resulting in partial atrophy of the pectoralis major muscle.
- Total division of the intercostobrachial nerve resulting in numbness and dysesthesia under the arm.
- Flap necrosis.
- Axillary web syndrome: an axillary syndrome related to extensive lymphovascular disruption during axillary lymph node or sentinel node dissection. Occurs in some women who develop a palpable cord of subcutaneous tissue from the axilla down to the ipsilateral arm in the postoperative period. This may often be relieved by early physical therapy.

Abdominal Wall and Hernias

4

Lee J. Skandalakis

Anatomy

General Description of the Anterior Abdominal Wall

The anterior abdominal wall can be thought of as having two parts: anterolateral and midline. The *anterolateral portion* is composed of the external oblique, internal oblique, and transversus abdominis muscles (often referred to as "the three flat muscles of the anterior abdominal wall"). These muscles are arranged such that their fibers are roughly parallel as they approach their insertion on the rectus sheath.

The *midline (middle) portion* is composed of the rectus abdominis and pyramidal muscles. The rectus muscle is enclosed in a stout sheath formed by the bilaminar aponeuroses of the three flat muscles, which divide and pass anteriorly and posteriorly around it. The sheath attaches medially to the linea alba (Fig. 4.1), which is formed by decussation. In 10–20% of the subjects, the pyramidal muscle is absent on one or both sides, but when present its insertion into the linea alba is a landmark for an accurate midline incision.

The following array shows some comparisons between the structures of the upper three-quarters of the midline portion of the abdominal wall and the lower one-quarter:

Upper midline	Lower midline
Linea alba well developed	Linea alba poorly developed
Right and left recti well separated	Right and left recti close together
Anterior and posterior layers of rectus sheath present	Only anterior layer of rectus sheath present
Aponeurosis of external oblique weak or absent	Aponeurosis of external oblique strong and well developed

L. J. Skandalakis (✉)
Department of Surgery, Piedmont Hospital, Atlanta, GA, USA

© Springer Nature Switzerland AG 2021
L. J. Skandalakis (ed.), *Surgical Anatomy and Technique*,
https://doi.org/10.1007/978-3-030-51313-9_4

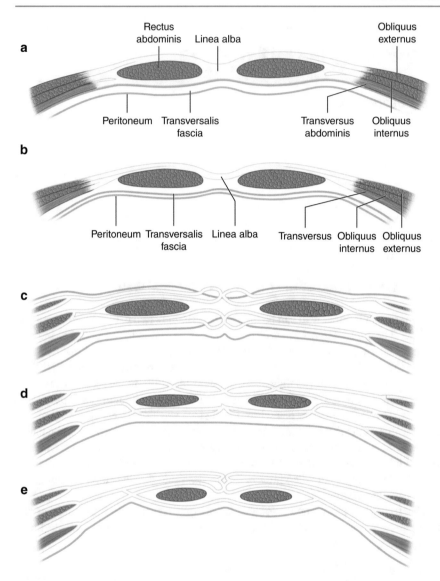

Fig. 4.1 (**a**) Transverse sections through the anterior abdominal wall, traditional view: immediately above the umbilicus. (**b**) Below the arcuate line. (**c–e**) Schematic transverse sections through the ventral abdominal wall showing bilaminar aponeuroses, external oblique, internal oblique, transversus abdominis, and sites of linear decussation that compacted from linea alba

In the lower one-quarter of the abdominal wall, the aponeuroses of the internal oblique and transversus abdominis muscles pass anterior to the rectus muscle, which is bounded posteriorly by the transversalis fascia only (Fig. 4.1). The dividing line is the linea semicircularis of Douglas, which marks the level at which the rectus sheath loses its posterior wall. The line is well marked if the change is abrupt but less definite if the change is gradual.

Umbilical Region

The variations of the anatomy of the umbilical region may be appreciated from the drawing presenting the relations of the umbilical ring to the linea alba, round ligament, urachus (median umbilical ligament), and umbilical fascia (Fig. 4.2).

Figures 4.3 and 4.4 present variations of the umbilical fascia in relation to several anatomical entities. Note that in Fig. 4.4a, the fascia covers the umbilical ring in toto.

Layers of the Lower Anterior Body Wall

In the inguinal region, the layers of the abdominal wall are:

- Skin.
- Subcutaneous fasciae (Camper and Scarpa) containing fat (superficial fascia).
- Innominate fascia (Gallaudet). It is not always recognized as a distinct entity. Its absence is of no surgical importance. It is responsible for the formation of the external spermatic fascia.
- External oblique aponeurosis, including the inguinal, lacunar, and reflected inguinal ligaments.
- Spermatic cord.
- Transversus abdominis muscle and aponeurosis, internal oblique muscle, falx inguinalis (Henle), and the conjoined tendon (when present).
- Anterior lamina of transversalis fascia.
- Posterior lamina of transversalis fascia.
- Preperitoneal connective tissue with fat.
- Peritoneum.

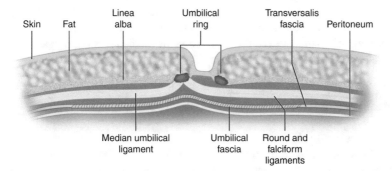

Fig. 4.2 Diagrammatic sagittal section through a normal umbilicus showing the relation of the umbilical ring to the linea alba, the round ligament, the urachus, and the umbilical and transversalis fasciae. Note the absence of subcutaneous fat over the umbilical ring

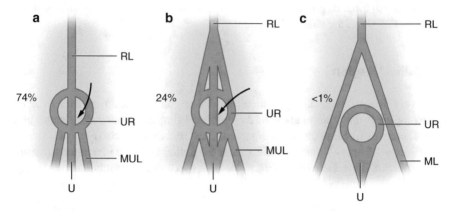

Fig. 4.3 Variations in the disposition of the umbilical ligaments as seen from the posterior (peritoneal) surface of the body wall. *Arrows* indicate (**a**) usual relations (74%) of the umbilical ring (UR), the round ligament (RL), the urachus (U), and the medial umbilical ligaments (MUL). The round ligament crosses the umbilical ring to insert on its inferior margin. (**b**) Less common configuration (24%). The round ligament splits and is attached to the superior margin of the umbilical ring. (**c**) Rare configuration (less than 1%). The round ligament branches before reaching the umbilical ring. Each branch continues with the medial umbilical ligament without attaching to the umbilical ring

Fossae of the Lower Anterior Abdominal Wall (Fig. 4.5)

The inner (posterior) surface of the anterior body wall above the inguinal ligament and below the umbilicus is divided into three shallow fossae on either side of a low ridge formed in the midline by the median umbilical ligament, the obliterated urachus. Each of these fossae is a potential site for a hernia. From lateral to medial, these fossae are:

- The *lateral fossa*, bounded medially by the inferior epigastric arteries. It contains the internal inguinal ring, the site of indirect inguinal hernia.
- The *medial fossa*, between the inferior epigastric artery and the medial umbilical ligament (remnant of the umbilical artery). It is the site of direct inguinal hernia.
- The *supravesical fossa*, between the medial and the median umbilical ligaments. It is the site of external supravesical hernia.

Anatomical Entities of the Groin

Superficial Fascia (Fig. 4.6)
This fascia (described here only for the male) is divided into a superficial part (Camper) and a deep part (Scarpa). The superficial part extends upward on the abdominal wall and downward over the penis, scrotum, perineum, thigh, and buttocks. The deep part extends from the abdominal wall to the penis (Buck's fascia), the scrotum (dartos), and the perineum (Colles' fascia).

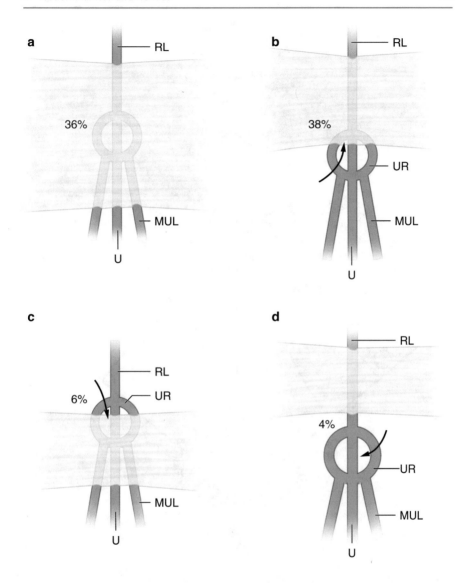

Fig. 4.4 Variations in the presence and form of the insertion of the umbilical fascia as seen from the posterior (peritoneal) surface of the body wall. (**a**) The thickened transversalis fascia forms the umbilical fascia covering the umbilical ring (36%). *Arrows* indicate (**b**) the umbilical fascia covers only the superior portion of the umbilical ring (38%); (**c**) the umbilical fascia covers only the inferior portion of the umbilical ring (6%); (**d**) though present, the umbilical fascia does not underlie the umbilical ring (4%). (No figure: fascia is entirely absent in 16%)

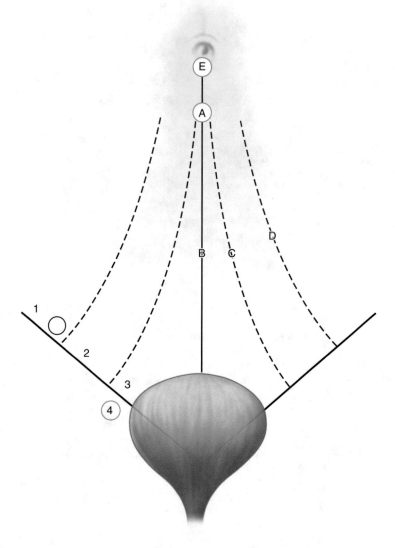

Fig. 4.5 Diagram of the fossae of the anterior abdominal wall and their relation to the sites of groin hernias: (**a**) umbilicus, (**b**) median umbilical ligament (obliterated urachus), (**c**) medial umbilical ligament (obliterated umbilical arteries), (**d**) lateral umbilical ligament containing inferior (deep) epigastric arteries, and (**e**) falciform ligament. Sites of possible hernias: (**1**) lateral fossa (indirect inguinal hernia), (**2**) medial fossa (direct inguinal hernia), (**3**) supravesical fossa (supravesical hernia), and (**4**) femoral ring (femoral hernia)

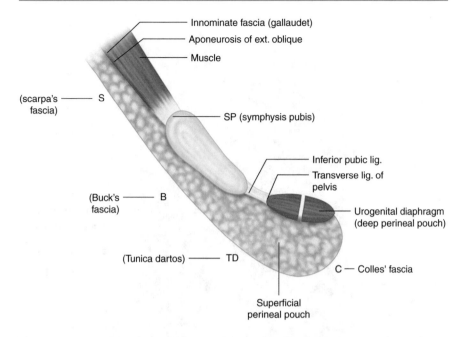

Fig. 4.6 Diagram of the relations of the superficial fasciae of the inguinal area showing the formation of the superficial perineal pouch

Usually two spaces are formed: the superficial perineal cleft and the superficial perineal pouch. The cleft is situated between Colles' fascia and the muscle fascia that covers the muscles of the superficial perineal pouch. The pouch is defined by the perineal membrane, the external perineal fascia (Gallaudet), and the ischiopubic rami.

Aponeurosis of the External Oblique Muscle (Fig. 4.6)

Below the arcuate line (Douglas), the aponeurosis of the external oblique muscle joins with the aponeuroses of the internal oblique and transversus abdominis muscles to form the anterior layer of the rectus sheath. This aponeurosis forms or contributes to three anatomical entities in the inguinal canal:

- Inguinal ligament (Poupart)
- Lacunar ligament (Gimbernat)
- Reflected inguinal ligament (Colles)

(Included sometimes is the pectineal ligament (Cooper), which is also formed from tendinous fibers of the internal oblique, transversus, and pectineus muscles.)

Inguinal Ligament (Poupart) (Fig. 4.7)

This is the thickened lower part of the external oblique aponeurosis from the anterior superior iliac spine laterally to the superior ramus of the pubic tubercle. The middle one-third has a free edge. The lateral two-third is attached strongly to the underlying iliopsoas fascia.

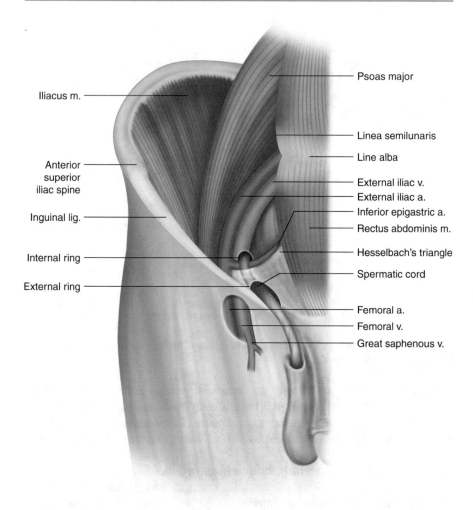

Fig. 4.7 Hesselbach triangle, site of direct inguinal hernia. Medial border of triangle is related to the lateral border of the rectus abdominis, site of supravesical hernia

Lacunar Ligament (Gimbernat) (Fig. 4.8)

This is the most inferior portion of the inguinal ligament and is formed from external oblique tendon fibers arising at the anterior superior iliac spine. Its fibers recurve through an angle of less than 45° before attaching to the pectineal ligament. Occasionally it forms the medial border of the femoral canal.

Pectineal Ligament (Cooper) (Fig. 4.8)

This is a thick, strong tendinous band formed principally by tendinous fibers of the lacunar ligament and aponeurotic fibers of the internal oblique, transversus abdominis, and pectineus muscles and, with variation, the inguinal falx. It is

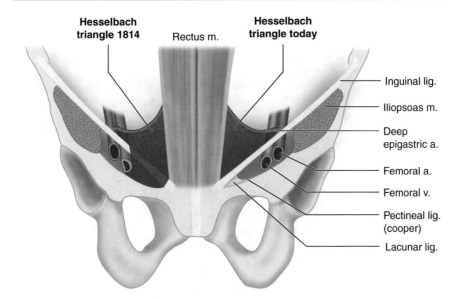

Fig. 4.8 *Left*: triangle described by Hesselbach (1814). *Right*: the slightly smaller triangle accepted today

fixed to the periosteum of the superior pubic ramus and, laterally, the periosteum of the ilium. The tendinous fibers are lined internally by transversalis fascia.

Conjoined Area (Fig. 4.9)

By definition, this is the fusion of fibers of the internal oblique aponeurosis with similar fibers from the aponeurosis of the transversus abdominis muscle, just as they insert on the pubic tubercle, the pectineal ligament, and the superior ramus of the pubis.

The above configuration is rarely encountered; published data suggest that it will be found in 5% of individuals or fewer. We have proposed the term *conjoined area*. This has obvious practical application to the region containing the falx inguinalis (Henle ligament), the transversus abdominis aponeurosis, the inferomedial fibers of the internal oblique muscle or aponeurosis, the reflected inguinal ligament, and the lateral border of the rectus sheath.

Arch of the Transversus Abdominis

The inferior portion of the transversus abdominis, the transversus arch, becomes increasingly less muscular and more aponeurotic as it approaches the rectus sheath. Close to the internal ring, it is covered by the much more muscular arch of the internal oblique muscle. Remember that in the inguinal canal region, the internal oblique is muscular. The transversus abdominis is aponeurotic.

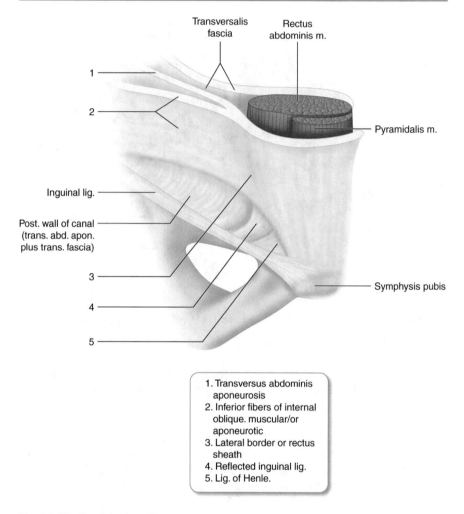

Fig. 4.9 The "conjoined area"

Falx Inguinalis (Henle Ligament) (Fig. 4.9)

Henle ligament is the lateral, vertical expansion of the rectus sheath that inserts on the pecten of the pubis. It is present in 30–50% of individuals and is fused with the transversus abdominis aponeurosis and transversalis fascia.

Interfoveolar Ligament (Hesselbach)

This is not a true ligament. It is a thickening of the transversalis fascia at the medial side of the internal ring. It lies anterior to the inferior epigastric vessels.

Reflected Inguinal Ligament (Colles') (Fig. 4.9)

This is formed by aponeurotic fibers from the inferior crus of the external ring that extend to the linea alba.

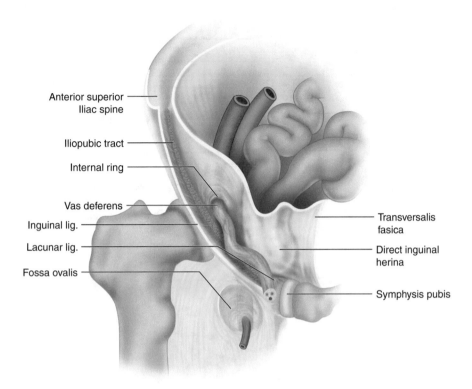

Fig. 4.10 Site of direct inguinal hernia. Note the internal ring and the iliopubic tract

Iliopubic Tract (Fig. 4.10)

This is an aponeurotic band extending from the iliopectineal arch to the superior ramus of the pubis. It forms part of the deep musculoaponeurotic layer together with the transversus abdominis muscle and aponeurosis and the transversalis fascia.

The tract passes medially, contributing to the inferior border of the internal ring. It crosses the femoral vessels to form the anterior margin of the femoral sheath, together with the transversalis fascia. The tract curves around the medial surface of the femoral sheath to attach to the pectineal ligament. It can be confused with the inguinal ligament.

Transversalis Fascia (Fig. 4.11)

Although the name transversalis fascia may be restricted to the internal fascia lining the transversus abdominis muscle, it is often applied to the entire connective tissue sheath lining the abdominal cavity. In the latter sense, it is a fascial layer covering the muscles, aponeuroses, ligaments, and bones. In the inguinal area, the transversalis fascia is bilaminar, enveloping the inferior epigastric vessels.

Related to the transversalis fascia is the space of Bogros, which is, for all practical purposes, a lateral extension of the retropubic space of Retzius. It is located just beneath the posterior lamina of the transversalis fascia out in front of the peritoneum (Fig. 4.11). The space of Bogros is used for the location of prostheses during the repair of inguinal hernias.

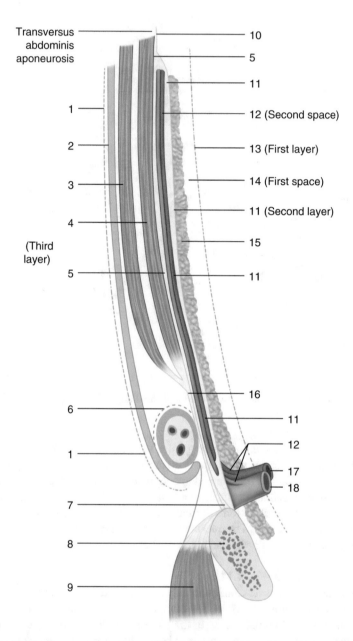

Fig. 4.11 Highly diagrammatic representation of the layers and spaces of the inguinal area and the space of Bogros: **(1)** innominate fascia; **(2)** external oblique aponeurosis; **(3)** internal oblique muscle; **(4)** transversus abdominis muscle and its aponeurosis; **(5)** transversalis fascia anterior; **(6)** external spermatic fascia; **(7)** Cooper ligament; **(8)** pubic bone; **(9)** pectineus muscle; **(10)** transversalis fascia; **(11)** transversalis fascia posterior lamina; **(12)** vessels; **(13)** peritoneum; **(14)** home (space) of the prosthesis, space of Bogros; **(15)** preperitoneal fat; **(16)** transversus abdominis aponeurosis and anterior lamina of transversalis fascia; **(17)** femoral artery; and **(18)** femoral vein

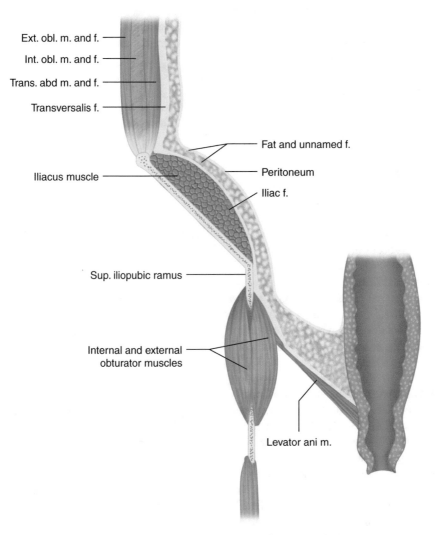

Fig. 4.12 Diagram of the normal relations of the transversalis fascia in the lateral and lower parts of the abdominal wall

Figure 4.12 shows normal relations of the transversalis fascia in the lateral and lower parts of the abdominal wall.

Iliopectineal Arch

This is a medial thickening of the iliopsoas fascia deep to the inguinal ligament. The surgeon does not directly use this arch, but it is important as the junction of a number of structures of the groin. These structures are:

- The insertion of fibers of the external oblique aponeurosis.
- The insertion of fibers of the inguinal ligament.

- The origin of part of the internal oblique muscle.
- The origin of part of the transversus abdominis muscle.
- Part of the lateral attachment of the iliopubic tract. It contributes also to the lateral wall of the femoral sheath.

Hesselbach Triangle (Fig. 4.8)
As described by Hesselbach in 1814, the base of the triangle was formed by the pubic pecten and the pectineal ligament. The boundaries of this triangle as usually described today are:

- Superolateral: the inferior (deep) epigastric vessels
- Medial: the rectus sheath (lateral border)
- Inferior (or, the base): the inguinal ligament

This is smaller than that described by Hesselbach in 1814. Most direct inguinal hernias occur in this area.

Inguinal Canal
The inguinal canal is an oblique passage through the abdominal wall that contains the spermatic cord or the round ligament of the uterus; embryologically, however, the canal develops before the descent of these entities. The inguinal canal has two openings, the deep and the superficial rings, an anterior and posterior wall, and a roof and a floor.

Boundaries of the Inguinal Canal
The anterior wall of the canal is formed by the aponeurosis of the external oblique. The external oblique muscle caudally ends in a thickening, the inguinal ligament (Poupart ligament), which extends from the anterior superior iliac spine laterally to the superior ramus of the pubis. This ligament is not cord-like, but the lower edge of the external oblique aponeurosis.

The posterior wall is given by the fascia transversalis and the transversus abdominis aponeurosis. The roof of the canal is formed by the arched fibers of the lower edge of the internal oblique muscle and by the transversus abdominis muscle and aponeurosis. The internal oblique and the transversalis muscle attach to the lateral two-thirds or one-half of the inguinal ligament and then arch over the spermatic cord to reach the pubic tubercle (and also the pectinate line). Close to the deep ring, the arch of the internal oblique muscle is more muscular, while that of the transversus more aponeurotic. Sometimes the lower fibers of these muscles fuse to be inserted together to the pubic tubercle and thus form the so-called conjoint tendon. A true fusion is, however, rare (5%), and maybe the term "conjoined area" should be more exact to describe this mass of aponeuroses inserting together to the tubercle. Many times the "conjoined tendon" has been confused with the falx inguinalis (ligament of Henle), which is the lateral, vertical expansion of the rectus sheath that inserts on the pectin of the pubis (present in 30% to 50%) and fuses with the transversus abdominis aponeurosis. The floor of the inguinal canal is formed by the shelving lower border of the inguinal ligament and the lacunar ligament (Gimbernat ligament). The lacunar ligament is in fact the extension of the inguinal ligament backward and laterally to attach to the pectineal line and form a triangular ligament with apex the pubic tubercle. Occasionally, it forms the medial border of the femoral canal. A lateral periosteal extension of the lacunar ligament along the pectineal line forms the pectineal ligament (Cooper ligament). According to O'Rahilly, the pectineal ligament provides a firm anchor for the attachment of muscular, tendinous, and fascial layers of the groin and thereof is used in the surgical repair of inguinal hernia.

Beneath the inguinal ligament is found a collagenous band, the iliopubic tract, extending from close to anterior inferior iliac spine to the pubic tubercle (Fig. 4.13). It is said to be a thickening of the transversalis fascia below the inguinal ligament, or a band between the transversalis fascia and the ligament, or even to disappear when the transversalis fascia is freed from the adjacent preperitoneal tissue (McVay and Anson). It arches over the femoral vessels and contributes to the medial margin

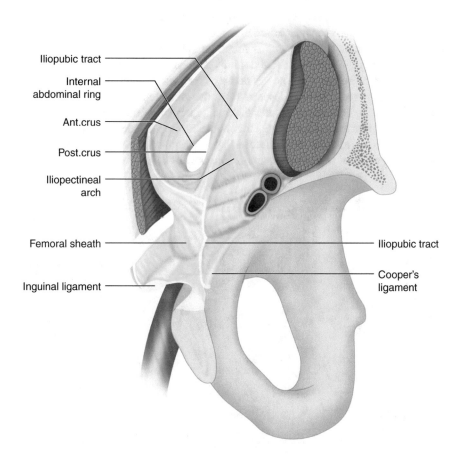

Fig. 4.13 Ligamentous attachments of the deep inguinal region

of the femoral canal. In any case, the iliopubic tract is found in a deeper layer and should not be confused with the inguinal ligament.

Beneath the inguinal ligament is found a collagenous band, the iliopubic tract, extending from close to anterior inferior iliac spine to the pubic tubercle (Fig. 4.12). It is said to be a thickening of the transversalis fascia below the inguinal ligament, or a band between the transversalis fascia and the ligament, or even to disappear when the transversalis fascia is freed from the adjacent preperitoneal tissue (McVay and Anson). It arches over the femoral vessels and contributes to the medial margin of the femoral canal. In any case, the iliopubic tract is found in a deeper layer and should not be confused with the inguinal ligament.

The Deep (Internal) Inguinal Ring

The deep inguinal ring is an opening of the transversalis fascia. It resembles a funnel directed downward and medially. There is no opening of the transversalis aponeurosis for the passage of the spermatic cord—it courses under the arch of the transversus abdominis muscle (and aponeurosis). The iliopubic tract lies under the deep ring and is said to reinforce it (or contribute to it, according to others). These relations are evident when the peritoneum is removed and the deep ring is seen from within the abdomen: the deep ring is found laterally to the inferior epigastric vessels, delineated by the transverse abdominis arch superolaterally and the iliopubic tract coursing inferolaterally. The vas deferens courses from the pelvis and is found medially; the gonadal vessels descend from the abdomen and are found laterally. Between the two, descending resides the genital branch of the genitofemoral nerve (Fig. 4.14). After the internal ring, this nerve is not included in the part of the spermatic cord surrounded by the internal spermatic fascia (given from the internal oblique) but external to it, in companion with the cremasteric vessels.

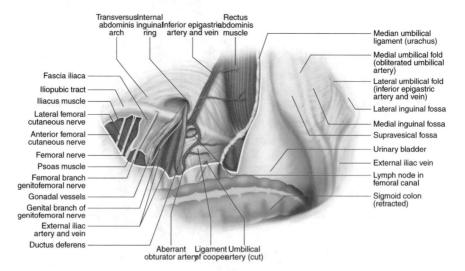

Fig. 4.14 Panoramic extraperitoneal view of the anatomical entities of the inguinal area

The Secondary Internal Inguinal Ring (Fig. 4.15)

The secondary internal inguinal ring was first noted by Lytle in 1945 and later defined correctly in 1975 by Fowler. Dr. Mirilas has brought this ring back in focus (see Mirilas et al. *J Am Col Surg* 2008). The secondary internal inguinal ring arises from the membranous layer of the extraperitoneal fascia located immediately deep to the transversalis fascia. In males, the vas deferens hooks around the inferomedial lip of the secondary internal inguinal ring in order to enter the inguinal canal. The gonadal vessels, which lie lateral to the vas deferens in the extraperitoneal fat and deep to the membranous layer, also traverse the secondary internal inguinal ring in order to become incorporated in the cord. This is readily appreciated when viewing

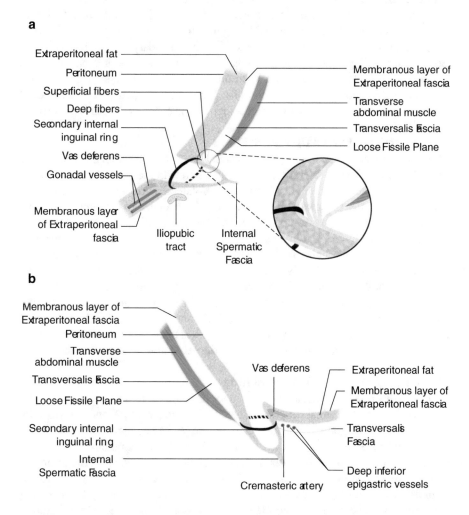

Fig. 4.15 Diagrammatic representation of a parasagittal (**a**) and horizontal (**b**) section of the anterior abdominal wall through the area of the secondary internal inguinal ring. The term "loose fissile plane" stands for the areolar extraperitoneal tissue

the deep ring from a preperitoneal exposure and is sometimes mistaken for the transversalis fascia during anterior exposure of the groin.

As said above, the membranous layer of the extraperitoneal fascia divides the extraperitoneal space into a parietal and a visceral plane. The parietal plane, between the transversalis fascia and the membranous layer of the extraperitoneal fascia, contains the deep inferior epigastric vessels, the cremasteric vessels, and the genital branch of the genitofemoral nerve. The visceral plane, between the membranous layer of the extraperitoneal fascia and the peritoneum, contains the median and medial umbilical ligaments, the vas deferens/round ligament, the gonadal vessels, and the ureter. This plane is equivalent to the space of Retzius, defined between the peritoneum and the "posterior lamina of the transversalis fascia"; here redefined as membranous layer of the extraperitoneal tissue. The secondary internal inguinal ring has important applications to surgery of the inguinal canal. During the repair of an indirect inguinal hernia, the correct site of sac ligation lies at the level of the secondary internal inguinal ring. Either using the inguinal or the preperitoneal open approach, the internal spermatic fascia should be incised to allow for exposure of the secondary internal ring. At this level, the membranous layer is incised in its thicker area, the peritoneum is detached from the cord structures, and a truly high ligation or inversion of the sac is performed.

The Superficial (External) Inguinal Ring

The superficial ring is an opening in the aponeurosis of the external oblique muscle found 2.5 cm above and laterally to the pubic tubercle in the adult. Although called "ring," it is somehow triangular, with a superolateral border (superior crus), an inferomedial border (inferior crus), and an open base related to the pubic crest. The superior crus is formed by the aponeurosis of the external oblique. The inferior crus is largely formed by the inguinal ligament, which also inserts in the pubic tubercle. Usually, there are superficial transverse fibers superior at the beginning of the diversion of the crura. Superficially to these, there is a fascia that continues from the aponeurosis of the external oblique muscle on to the spermatic cord; this is the outer investing fascia of the muscle that gives the external spermatic fascia extending between the crura of the ring (thereof also called "intercrural" fascia). After removal of the superficial fascia, the thin intercrural fascia is opened during surgical dissection, and the thick aponeurotic semicircle of the external ring is easily found.

The Secondary External Inguinal Ring

In dissections done by Mirilas the secondary inguinal ring was rediscovered. The secondary external inguinal ring, discovered by McGregor (1929) and described by Martin (1984)—forgotten thereafter (see Mirilas & Mentessidou, *Hernia* 2013). The secondary external inguinal ring arises from the membranous layer of the superficial fascia of the anterior abdominal wall below the classic superficial ring. It is tube-like arrangement of Scarpa fascia, which constitutes the entrance into the scrotum. An examining finger can be easily inserted in the secondary external ring at the root of the scrotum and follows the spermatic cord until the external inguinal ring. A similar ring-like arrangement of Scarpa fascia has been also noted around the round ligament in female cadavers.

The secondary external inguinal ring is implicated in several disorders of the inguinoscrotal area. Adhesive obstruction, underdevelopment, or congenital absence of the secondary external ring has been considered responsible for some cases of incomplete testicular descent or testicular ectopy. The secondary external ring usually constitutes an anatomical obstacle for hernia sacs to enter the scrotum. In the case that a hernia passes the secondary external ring, the hernia becomes scrotal.

The contents of the inguinal canal for males and females are as follows.

Male

The spermatic cord contains a matrix of connective tissue continuous with the preperitoneal connective tissue. The cord consists of:

- Ductus deferens
- Three arteries: the internal spermatic (testicular), deferential, and external spermatic (cremasteric)
- One venous plexus (pampiniform)
- Genital branch of the genitofemoral nerve
- Ilioinguinal nerve
- Sympathetic fibers from the hypogastric plexus
- Three layers of fascia: the external spermatic fascia, a continuation of the innominate fascia; the middle, cremasteric layer, continuous with the internal oblique muscle fibers and muscle fascia; and the internal spermatic fascia, an extension of the transversalis fascia

Female

- Round ligament of the uterus
- Genital branch of the genitofemoral nerve
- Cremasteric vessels
- Ilioinguinal nerve
- Coverings as described for the male, although usually less distinct

Fruchaud viewed hernias not by their clinical presentation but rather by their origin within the groin, in an area he termed the myopectineal orifice (Fig. 4.16). This area is bounded superiorly by the arch of the internal oblique muscle and transversus abdominis muscle, laterally by the iliopsoas muscle, medially by the lateral border of the rectus muscle and its anterior lamina, and inferiorly by the pubic pecten. The inguinal ligament spans and divides this framework.

Surgical Ellipse (Fig. 4.17)

With the patient in the supine position, the surgeon is dealing with the following anatomical areas and entities of the inguinal region, which are incorporated into an elliptical area: floor of the inguinal canal, superior medial edge (above), inferior lateral edge (below), medial apex, and lateral apex.

The *floor* (posterior wall) of the ellipse is formed by the transversus abdominis aponeurosis and the transversalis fascia. If the posterior wall is intact, its integrity

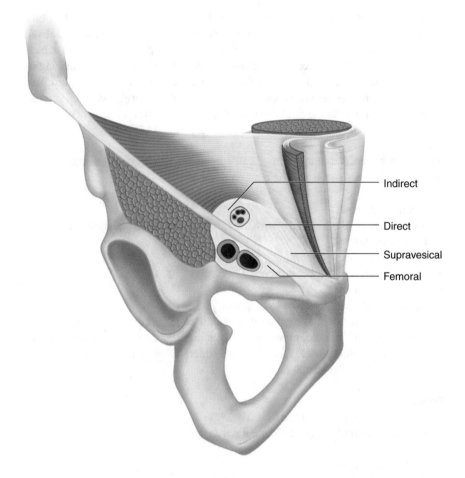

Fig. 4.16 Anterior view of Fruchaud's myopectineal orifice

prevents herniation; none of the four types of inguinal hernia (indirect, direct, external supravesical, femoral) will develop.

The *superior medial* (*upper*) *edge* of the ellipse is formed by the conjoined area and the arch (internal oblique muscle and transversus abdominis muscle with their aponeuroses).

The *inferior lateral* (*lower*) *edge* is formed by the inguinal ligament, iliopubic tract, femoral sheath, and Cooper ligament. The iliopubic tract, femoral sheath, Cooper ligament, and occasionally the inguinal ligament are used for repair.

The *medial apex*—close to the symphysis pubis—is formed by Gimbernat ligament below and the conjoined area above.

The *lateral apex*—at the internal ring—is formed by the arch (internal oblique and transversus abdominis muscles and aponeuroses), transversalis fascia and crura, iliopubic tract, femoral sheath, and inguinal ligament.

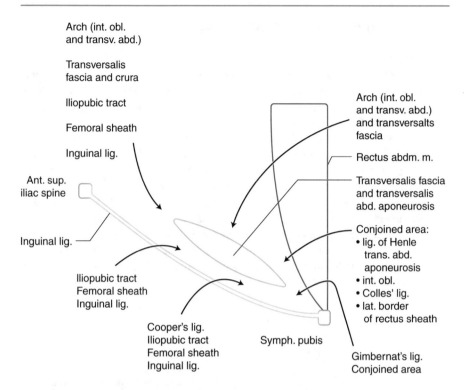

Arch (int. obl.
and transv. abd.)

Transversalis
fascia and crura

Iliopubic tract

Femoral sheath

Inguinal lig.

Ant. sup.
iliac spine

Inguinal lig.

Iliopubic tract
Femoral sheath
Inguinal lig.

Cooper's lig.
Iliopubic tract
Femoral sheath   Symph. pubis
Inguinal lig.

Arch (int. obl.
and transv. abd.)
and transversalts
fascia

Rectus abdm. m.

Transversalis fascia
and transversalis
abd. aponeurosis

Conjoined area:
• lig. of Henle
  trans. abd.
  aponeurosis
• int. obl.
• Colles' lig.
• lat. border
  of rectus sheath

Gimbernat's lig.
Conjoined area

Fig. 4.17 Highly diagrammatic presentation of the surgical ellipse

> **Remember**
> • The transversalis fascia and transversus abdominis aponeurosis together
>   are "good stuff" for open **repair** of inguinofemoral herniation.

Femoral Canal and Its Sheath

The femoral canal—within the groin area, below the inguinal ligament—is 1.25–2 cm long and occupies the most medial compartment of the femoral sheath. The femoral sheath is formed anteriorly and medially by the transversalis fascia and some transversus aponeurotic fibers, posteriorly by the pectineus and psoas fasciae and laterally by the iliacus fascia. The sheath forms three compartments, the most medial of which is the femoral canal, through which a femoral hernia may pass. The boundaries are:

- Lateral: a connective tissue septum and the femoral vein
- Posterior: the pectineal ligament (Cooper)
- Anterior: the iliopubic tract or the inguinal ligament or both
- Medial: the aponeurotic insertion of the transversus abdominis muscle and transversalis fascia or, rarely, the lacunar ligament

Blood Supply of the Anterior Abdominal Wall

Arterial Supply

Where there have been no previous incisions, the blood supply to the abdominal wall creates no problem. Where scars are present, the surgeon should be familiar with the blood supply to avoid necrosis from ischemia to specific areas. If possible, the surgeon should proceed through an existing scar.

The lower anterolateral abdominal wall is supplied by three branches of the femoral artery. They are, from lateral to medial, the superficial circumflex iliac artery (Fig. 4.18), the superficial epigastric artery, and the superficial external pudendal artery. Branches of these arteries travel toward the umbilicus in the subcutaneous connective tissues. The superficial epigastric artery anastomoses with the contralateral artery and all three arteries have anastomoses with the deep arteries.

The deep arteries lie between the transversus abdominis and the internal oblique muscles. They are the posterior intercostal arteries 10 and 11, the anterior branch of the subcostal artery, the anterior branches of the four lumbar arteries, and the deep circumflex iliac artery.

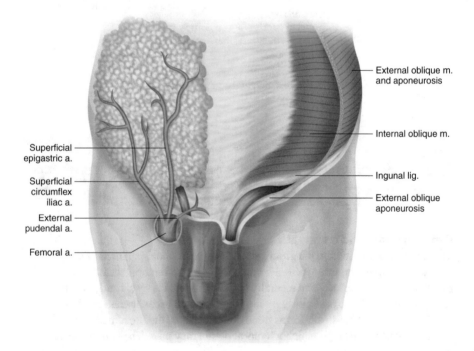

Fig. 4.18 The skin of the lower abdominal wall has been removed to show the superficial branches of the femoral artery

The rectus sheath is supplied by the superior epigastric artery, which arises from the internal thoracic artery, and the inferior epigastric artery, which arises from the external iliac artery just above the inguinal ligament.

The superior epigastric artery enters the upper end of the rectus sheath, deep to the rectus muscle. Musculocutaneous branches pierce the anterior rectus sheath to supply the overlying skin. The perforating arteries are closer to the lateral border of the rectus than to the linea alba. Creating an incision too far laterally will result in bleeding from the several perforating arteries; cutting the musculocutaneous nerves will cause muscle paralysis.

The inferior epigastric artery arises in the preperitoneal connective tissue. It enters the sheath at or below the level of the semicircular line of Douglas, passing between the rectus muscle and the posterior layer of the sheath.

Venous Drainage
The veins follow the arteries.

Nerve Supply of the Anterior Abdominal Wall

Both the anterolateral portion of the abdominal wall and the rectus abdominis muscle are supplied by anterior rami of the 7th to the 12th thoracic nerves and the 1st lumbar nerve (Fig. 4.19). A branch—the lateral cutaneous ramus—arises from each anterior ramus and pierces the outer two flat muscles, innervating the external oblique and forming the lateral cutaneous nerve. The anterior rami of the last six thoracic nerves enter the posterior layer of the rectus sheath, innervating the rectus muscle and sending perforating branches through the anterior layer of the sheath to form the anterior cutaneous nerves. The first lumbar nerve forms an anterior cutaneous nerve without passing through the sheath. These relationships are shown diagrammatically in Fig. 4.20. Rectus muscle paralysis, with weakening of the abdominal wall, will result from section of more than one of these nerves.

The nerves of the lower abdominal wall area are illustrated in Fig. 4.18.

Panorama of Laparoscopic Cadaveric Anatomy of the Inguinal Area (Figs. 4.21, 4.22, 4.23, 4.24, 4.25, 4.26, 4.27, 4.28, 4.29, 4.30, 4.31, 4.32, 4.33, and 4.34)

General Description of the Posterior (Lumbar) Body Wall

The lumbar area of the posterior body wall is bounded:

- Superiorly: by the 12th rib
- Inferiorly: by the crest of the ilium
- Posteriorly: by the erector spinae (sacrospinalis) muscles
- Anteriorly: by the posterior border of the external oblique muscle

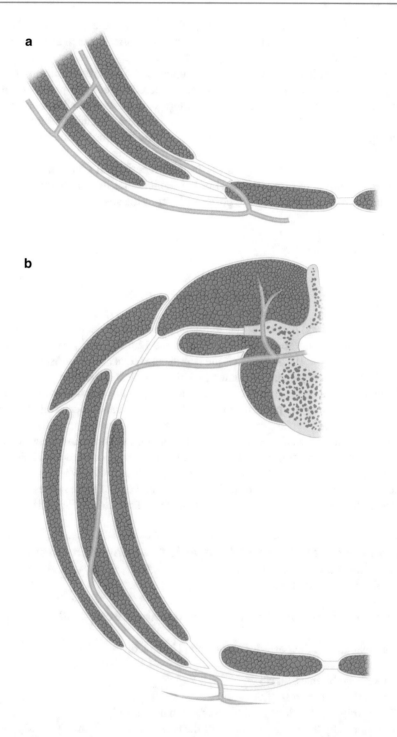

Fig. 4.19 The course of the anterior ramus of segmental nerves in the anterior body wall. (**a**) 7th to 12th thoracic nerves. (**b**) First lumbar nerve

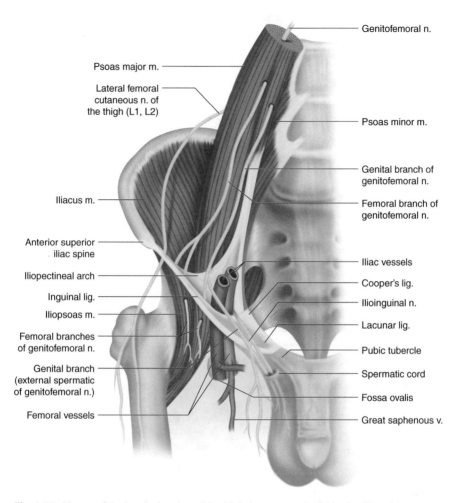

Fig. 4.20   Nerves of the inguinal region with which the surgeon should be familiar with

In this area, the body wall is composed of the following layers of muscle and fascia:

- Thick, tough skin.
- Superficial fascia: two layers of fibrous tissue with fat between them.
- A superficial muscle layer composed of the latissimus dorsi muscle posterolaterally and the external oblique muscle anterolaterally.
- Thoracolumbar fascia containing three layers: posterior, middle, and anterior. The posterior and middle layers envelop the sacrospinalis muscle, and the middle anterior layer envelops the quadratus lumborum. Another characteristic of the middle layer of the thoracolumbar fascia is its lateral continuation to the transversus abdominis aponeurosis by fusion of all three layers. Therefore, the transversus abdominis aponeurosis should be accepted on faith as part of the thoracolumbar fascia.

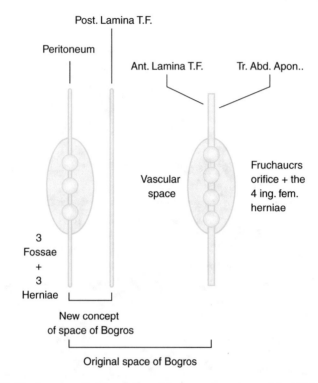

Fig. 4.21 Highly diagrammatic presentation of laparoscopic anatomy of the inguinal area demonstrating layers, fossae, and spaces

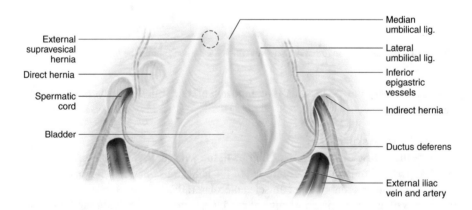

Fig. 4.22 Laparoscopic topographic anatomy of the inguinal region. In men, the spermatic vessels join the vas deferens to form the spermatic cord. The presence of a fascial defect lateral or medial to the inferior epigastric vessels defines an indirect or a direct hernia, respectively

- A middle muscular layer of the sacrospinalis, internal oblique, and serratus posterior inferior muscles.
- The deep muscular layer composed of the quadratus lumborum and psoas muscles.
- Transversalis fascia.
- Preperitoneal fat.
- Peritoneum.

Within this area, two triangles may be described: the inferior lumbar triangle (Petit) and the superior lumbar triangle (Grynfeltt).

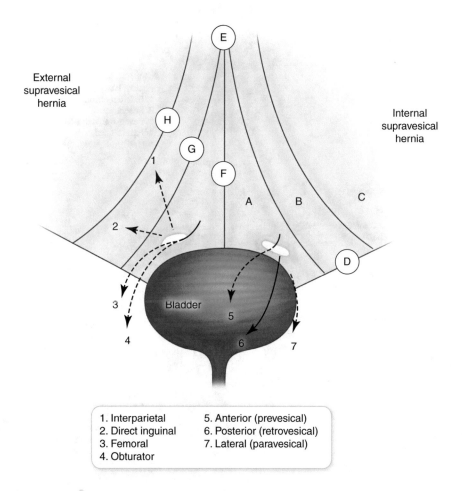

1. Interparietal
2. Direct inguinal
3. Femoral
4. Obturator
5. Anterior (prevesical)
6. Posterior (retrovesical)
7. Lateral (paravesical)

Fig. 4.23 The bladder and anterior abdominal wall viewed posteriorly. Possible pathways of external supravesical hernias are shown on the *left* and those of internal supravesical hernias are shown on the *right*. (**a**) Supravesical fossa with mouth of supravesical hernia. (**b**) Medial fossa. (**c**) Lateral fossa. (**d**) Inguinal ligament. (**e**) Umbilicus. (**f**) Middle umbilical ligament (obliterated urachus). (**g**) Lateral umbilical ligament (obliterated umbilical artery). (**h**) Inferior (deep) epigastric artery

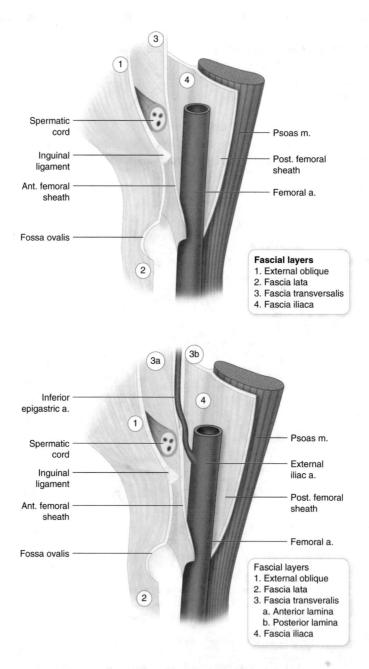

Fig. 4.24 (Top panel) Highly diagrammatic drawing of the transversalis fascia and femoral sheath (old concept). (Bottom panel) Highly diagrammatic drawing of the transversalis fascia and femoral sheath (new concept), emphasizing the bilaminar nature of the transversalis fascia in the inguinal area

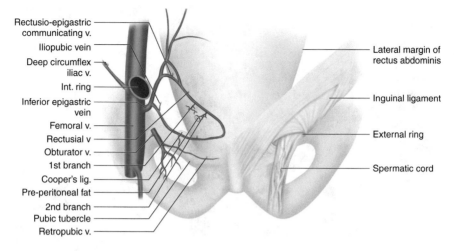

Fig. 4.25 The deep inguinal vasculature within the space of Bogros

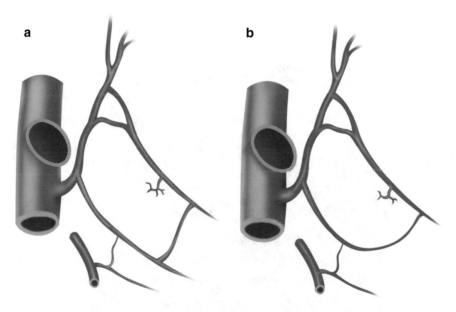

Fig. 4.26 (a–d) Variations in the vasculature of the deep inguinal venous system

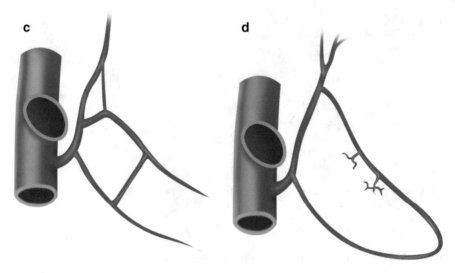

Fig. 4.26 (continued)

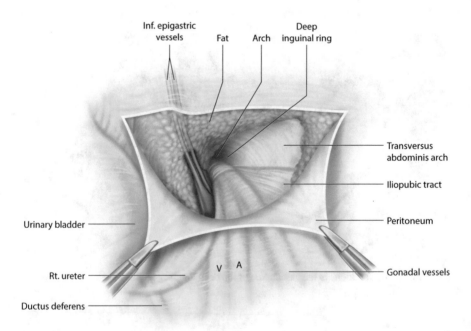

Fig. 4.27 After incising and retracting the peritoneum, the inferior epigastric vessels (the most superficial anatomical entities) will be seen. The arch and the iliopubic tract may or may not be seen

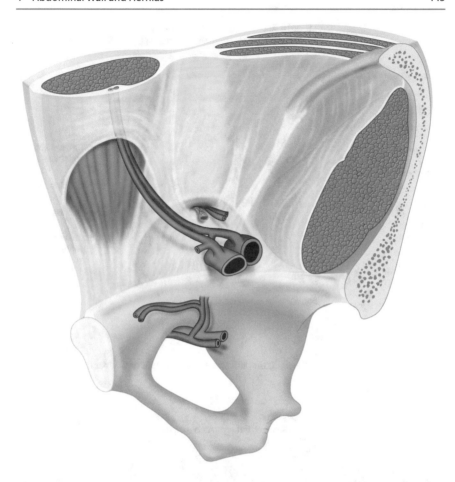

Fig. 4.28 Posterior view of myopectineal orifice of Fruchaud. The boundaries are as follows: superior, the arch; lateral, iliopsoas muscle; medial, lateral edge of rectus abdominis muscle; and inferior, pubic pecten

The base of the inferior lumbar triangle is the iliac crest. The anterior (abdominal) boundary is the posterior border of the external oblique muscle. The posterior (lumbar) boundary is the anterior border of the latissimus dorsi muscle. The floor of the triangle is formed by the internal oblique muscle with contributions from the transversus abdominis muscle and the posterior lamina of the thoracolumbar fascia. The triangle is covered by superficial fascia and skin.

The base of the superior lumbar triangle is the 12th rib and the serratus posterior inferior muscle. The anterior (abdominal) boundary is the posterior border of the internal oblique muscle; the posterior (lumbar) boundary is the anterior border of the sacrospinalis muscle. The floor of the triangle is formed by the aponeurosis of the transversus abdominis muscle arising by fusion of the layers of the thoracolumbar fascia. The roof of the triangle is formed by the external oblique and latissimus dorsi muscles.

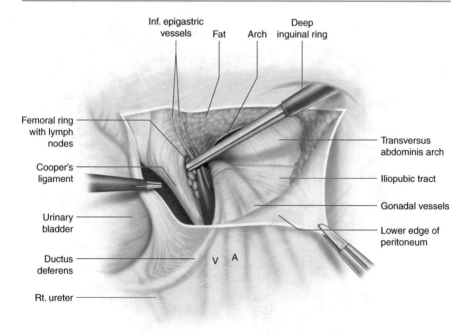

Fig. 4.29 With more cleaning the arch, iliopubic tract, and ligament of Cooper can be seen

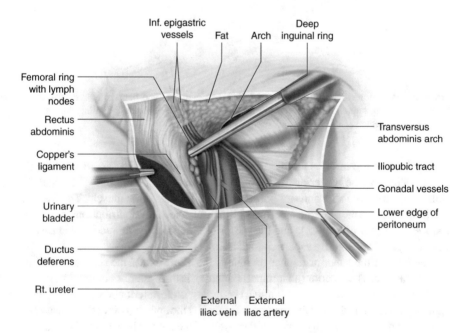

Fig. 4.30 With further cleaning, more entities will be seen: the spermatic cord and the iliac vessels

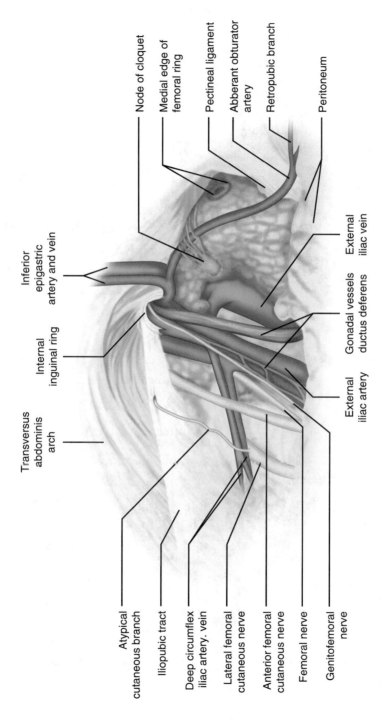

Fig. 4.31 Another panoramic laparoscopic view of the anatomy of the inguinal area

The triangle of doom

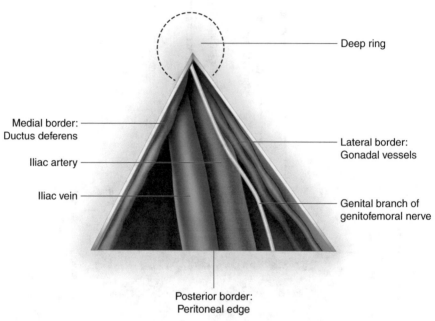

- Deep ring
- Medial border: Ductus deferens
- Iliac artery
- Iliac vein
- Lateral border: Gonadal vessels
- Genital branch of genitofemoral nerve
- Posterior border: Peritoneal edge

Fig. 4.32 The triangle of doom

Traingle of pain

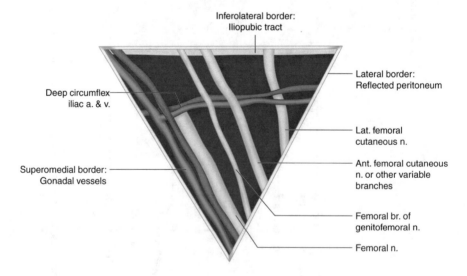

- Inferolateral border: Iliopubic tract
- Lateral border: Reflected peritoneum
- Deep circumflex iliac a. & v.
- Lat. femoral cutaneous n.
- Ant. femoral cutaneous n. or other variable branches
- Superomedial border: Gonadal vessels
- Femoral br. of genitofemoral n.
- Femoral n.

Fig. 4.33 The triangle of pain

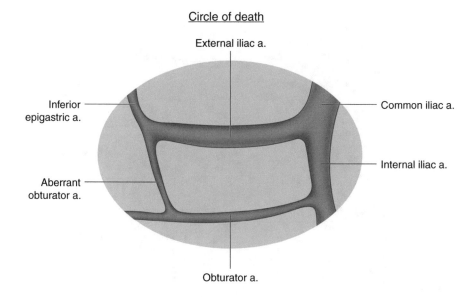

Fig. 4.34 The circle of death

The two triangles can be compared as follows:

Inferior triangle	*Superior triangle*
Upright triangle (apex up)	Inverted triangle (apex down)
Smaller	Larger
Less constant	More constant
Less common site of lumbar hernia	More common site of lumbar hernia
No nerves	12th thoracic nerve
No nerves	First lumbar nerve
Vascular	Avascular
Covered by superficial fascia and skin	Covered by latissimus dorsi muscle
Floor: thoracolumbar fascia, internal oblique muscle, and (partially) transversus abdominis muscle	Floor: union of the layers of the thoracolumbar fascia to form the aponeurosis of the transversus abdominis

In *hernias through the inferior lumbar triangle* (Fig. 4.35), the boundaries are as follows: if the hernia is small, the ring is formed by the thoracolumbar fascia and fibers of the internal oblique muscle; if it is larger, the ring may include the boundaries of the whole inferior triangle. Enlargement of the ring is by section of the fascia.

In *hernias through the superior lumbar triangle* (Fig. 4.35), the boundaries are as follows: if the hernia is small, the hernial ring is formed by the aponeurosis of the transversus abdominis only; if it is large, it may occupy the entire superior triangle. It may be necessary to enlarge the ring by a medial or lateral incision, or both, midway between the 12th rib and the crest of the ilium.

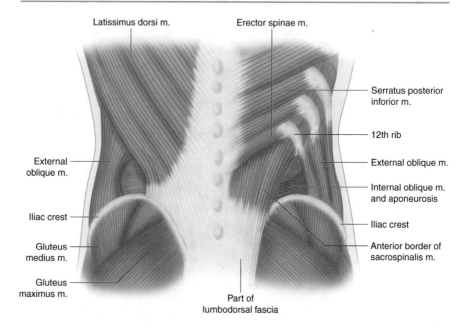

Fig. 4.35 *Left*: an inferior hernia through Petit triangle. The base of the triangle is formed by the iliac crest. *Right*: a superior hernia through Grynfeltt triangle. The base of the inverted triangle is formed by the 12th rib

Hernia anterolateral abdominal wall	Definition	Boundaries
Epigastric (ventral)	Defect of linea alba anywhere from xiphoid to umbilicus	Medial edge of right or left rectus sheath (anterior and posterior laminae as well as lateral edge of muscle between) may form lateral border
Umbilical	Incomplete closure of early natural umbilical defect; absence of umbilical fascia	Superior and inferior—linea alba Lateral—rectus abdominis muscle
Omphalocele	Herniation of intraperitoneal viscera into open umbilical ring	Umbilical cord; hernial sac covered by double layer of membranes (amniotic outside, peritoneum inside, Wharton jelly in between)
Gastroschisis	Defect of anterior abdominal wall to right or left of the midline	Layers of the abdominal wall

Spigelian	Herniation along the linea semilunaris of Spieghel (line of transition between the muscular fibers and the aponeurosis of the transversus abdominis muscle) anywhere above level of umbilicus lateral to the symphysis pubis	*If at intersection of linea semilunaris (Spieghel) and linea semicircularis (Douglas), or above the linea semicircularis but below and lateral to the umbilicus:* aponeurosis of internal oblique muscle and the aponeurosis of the transversus abdominis muscle *If above the level of the umbilicus:* ring is formed by tear in the transversus abdominis muscle and a defect of the aponeurosis of the internal oblique muscle
Groin—indirect	Herniation through the deep (internal) inguinal ring following the spermatic cord in male patients and the round ligament in female patients; may herniate through superficial (external) ring	*Boundaries of deep ring:* anterior and posterior—thickening of transversalis fascia "sling" inferior—iliopubic tract *Boundaries of superficial ring:* triangular opening of aponeurosis of external oblique composed of superior (medial) and inferior (lateral) crura; base of triangle is pubic crest
Groin—direct	Herniation through floor of inguinal canal—covered by transversalis fascia and aponeurosis of the transversus abdominis muscle	Located at medial fossa
Groin—external supravesical	Herniation between midline and lateral umbilical ligament	Partially or totally occupying the supravesical fossa
Femoral	Herniation through femoral canal (consisting of proximal ring and distal ring)	*Proximal ring:* anterior—iliopubic tract, inguinal ligament, or rarely, both Posterior—ligament of Cooper (pectineal ligament) Lateral—femoral vein Medial—insertion of iliopubic tract *Distal ring:* anterior—fascia lata Posterior—pectineal fascia Lateral—femoral sheath Medial—iliopubic tract or lacunar ligament

Posterolateral abdominal wall (Lumbar)		
	Herniation through superior and inferior lumbar triangles	*Superior triangle:* base—12th rib and serratus posterior inferior muscle Anterior—posterior border of the internal oblique muscle Posterior—anterior border of sacrospinalis muscle Floor—aponeurosis of transversus abdominis muscle
		Roof—external oblique and latissimus dorsi muscle *Inferior triangle:* base—iliac crest Anterior—posterior border of external oblique muscle Posterior—anterior border of latissimus dorsi muscle Floor—internal oblique with transversus abdominis muscle and posterior lamina of thoracolumbar fascia of internal oblique
Incisions	Varies according to the incision	Various
Pelvic walls and perineum		
Sciatic—suprapiriformic	Herniation through greater sciatic foramen above piriformis muscle	Anterior—sacroiliac ligament Inferior—upper border of piriformis muscle Lateral—ilium Medial—sacrotuberous ligament and upper part of sacrum
Sciatic—infrapiriformic	Herniation through greater sciatic foramen below piriformis muscle	Above—lower border of piriformis muscle Below—sacrospinous ligament Posterior—sacrotuberous ligament Anterior—ilium
Sciatic—subspinous	Herniation through lesser sciatic foramen	Anterior—ischial tuberosity Superior—sacrospinous ligament and ischial spine Posterior—sacrotuberous ligament
Obturator	Herniation through the obturator canal	Superior and lateral—obturator groove of the pubis Inferior—free edge of obturator membrane and the internal and external obturator muscles
Perineal—anterior	Herniation anterior to the superficial transverse perineal muscle	Medial—bulbospongiosus muscle Lateral—ischiocavernosus muscle Posterior—transverse perineal muscle
Perineal—posterior	Herniation posterior to the superficial transverse perineal muscle	Ring formed through levator ani, or between the levator ani and coccygeus muscles
Diaphragm		

Hiatal esophageal (sliding or paraesophageal)	Herniation through diaphragmatic crura	In 50%, right and left limbs or the right crus; in remainder, both right and left crura are involved
Diaphragmatic rings		
Congenital—Bochdalek (posterolateral)	Herniation through the lumbocostal trigone (above and lateral to left lateral lumbocostal arch)	Located at the posterior portion of the diaphragm close to 10th and 11th ribs; if large, the central tendon is involved
Congenital—Morgagni (retrosternal)	Herniation through the sternocostal triangles (foramina of Morgagni)	Anterior—costal cartilage and xiphoid process Lateral and posterior—diaphragm Medial—diaphragm Ring located at fusion of central tendon and pericardium
Pericardial ring	Herniation through the central tendon of the diaphragm and the pericardium	Various
Peritoneal cavity and anatomical entities within		
Transomental	Herniation through greater omentum	Bordered entirely by omental tissues
Transmesenteric	Herniation through mesentery of small bowel, transverse mesocolon, pelvic mesocolon, or the falciform ligament	Ring may be located in mesentery of small bowel, the transverse mesocolon, or the sigmoid mesocolon; at least one free edge of the ring is usually formed by a branch of the superior mesenteric or inferior mesenteric artery
Foramina or Fossae		
Epiploic foramen of Winslow	Herniation through the foramen	Superior—caudate process of liver and inferior layer of coronary ligament Anterior—hepatoduodenal ligament Posterior—inferior vena cava Inferior—first part of duodenum and transverse part of hepatic artery
Right paraduodenal	Herniation through right paraduodenal fossa	Superior—duodenum Anterior—superior mesenteric artery or ileocolic artery Posterior—lumbar vertebrae
Left paraduodenal	Herniation through left paraduodenal fossa	Superior—duodenojejunal flexure or the beginning of the jejunum, pancreas, and renal vessels Anterior—inferior mesenteric vein and left colic artery Right—aorta Left—left kidney

Superior ileocecal	Sac under right mesocolon or descending colon	Ileocolic (ileocecal) fold: formed by an anteriorly located semilunar elevation of the ileocolic mesentery by the anterior branch of the ileocecal artery
Inferior ileocecal	Sac under cecum	Anterior ileoappendicular fold
Paracolic	Sac under proximal ascending colon	Paracolic fold located in the right gutter
Internal supravesical		
Anterior supravesical	Herniation of the supravesical fossa in front of the bladder	Superior—the upward continuation of the vesical fascia and its fusion with the transversalis fascia and the peritoneum Inferior—fold of vesical fascia and peritoneum Lateral—lateral umbilical ligament and peritoneum Medial—medial umbilical ligament and peritoneum
Retrovesical (posterior supravesical)	Herniation of the supravesical fossa behind the bladder	Superior and anterior—vesical fascia and peritoneum of posterior bladder wall Inferior and posterior—transverse vesical fold
Postsurgery		
After retrocolic gastrojejunostomy	Two potential spaces are created; upper: above the mesocolon; lower: posterior to the gastric remnant	Anterior—gastrojejunostomy and efferent or afferent jejunal loop Posterior—posterior parietal peritoneum Superior—transverse mesocolon and posterior wall of the gastric remnant Inferior—ligament of Treitz and duodenojejunal peritoneal fold
Postsurgery		
After antecolic gastrojejunostomy (when afferent loop is attached to the lesser curvature of the stomach)	Rare, but more common than herniation of loop to greater curvature	Anterior—afferent jejunal loop with its mesentery Posterior—omentum, transverse colon, and mesoduodenojejunal peritoneal fold Inferior—jejunum with its mesentery
After antecolic gastrojejunostomy (when afferent loop is attached to the greater curvature of the stomach)	Information is scant because the herniation is so rare	Anterior—gastrojejunostomy and afferent jejunal loop Posterior—omentum and mesocolon Superior—transverse colon and mesocolon Inferior—ligament of Treitz and duodenojejunal peritoneal fold

Technique

Incisions of the Anterior Abdominal Wall

Principles

There are three requirements for a proper abdominal incision:

- Accessibility
- Extensibility
- Viability

A surgeon must plan the incision, taking personal preferences into account. The following rules should be observed where they apply:

- The incision should be long enough for a good exposure and for room to work but short enough to avoid unnecessary complications.
- Where possible, skin incisions should follow Langer's lines.
- Excise existing scars and proceed, rather than making incisions parallel to the scars.
- Split muscles in the direction of their fibers, rather than transecting them. The rectus muscle is an exception, because it has a segmental nerve supply and therefore no risk of denervation.
- Do not superimpose the openings formed through different layers of the abdominal wall.
- Wherever possible, avoid cutting nerves.
- Retract muscles and abdominal organs toward, not away from, their neurovascular supply.
- Insert drainage tubes in separate small incisions. Insertion in the main incision may weaken the wound.
- Pay close attention to cosmetic considerations, but not at the expense of the requirements of accessibility, extensibility, and viability, as noted previously.
- Be sure closure follows anatomical topography.
- Viability dictates using care in patients with multiple abdominal incisions. New incisions must be placed such that skin necrosis is avoided.

Surgical Anatomy of Specific Incisions

Abdominal incisions are legion. Some have descriptive names; others are eponymous. For practical purposes, we will describe only the major types of incisions without discussing their many variations (Fig. 4.36).

Vertical Incisions

Upper Midline Incision

Incisions of the linea alba and the transversalis fascia may reveal abundant and well-vascularized fat in the upper midline (Fig. 4.37a). We suggest that the incisions of

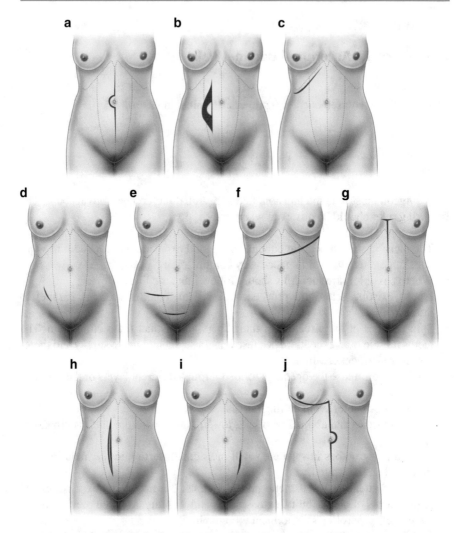

Fig. 4.36 Varieties of abdominal incisions. (**a**) Midline (linea alba) incision. (**b**) Paramedian (rectus) incision with muscle retraction. (**c**) Subcostal incision. (**d**) McBurney incision. (**e**) Transverse abdominal incision. (**f**) and (**g**) Two types of thoracoabdominal incisions. (**h**) Paramedian (rectus) incision with muscle splitting. (**i**) Pararectus incision. (**j**) "Hockey stick" (thoracoabdominal) incision

the peritoneum be made slightly to the left of the midline to avoid the ligamentum teres in the edge of the falciform ligament. If it is encountered, it may be ligated and divided. Close the linea alba from above downward. Alternatively, closing from caudal to cranial may be easier and cause less evisceration as you approach the costal margin.

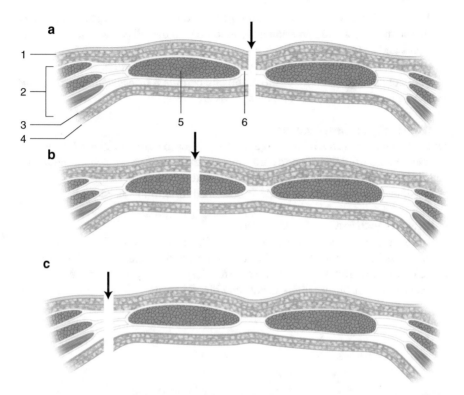

Fig. 4.37 Vertical incisions. (**a**) Incision through the linea alba. (**b**) Incision through the rectus muscle (paramedian) splitting the muscle. (**c**) Incision lateral to the rectus sheath (pararectus). Segmental nerves to the rectus muscle (*broken line*) will be cut. (**1**) Skin, (**2**) three flat muscles and their aponeuroses, (**3**) transversalis fascia, (**4**) peritoneum, (**5**) rectus abdominis muscle, (**6**) linea alba

A *thoracic extension* of a midline abdominal incision may be made through the eighth intercostal space as far as the scapula. In this procedure, the midline incision is exploratory, and the need for the thoracic extension depends on the pathology revealed by the exploration.

Sternal splitting may be used to continue the midline incision superiorly.

A lateral extension to one or even both sides may be L- or T-shaped.

A downward continuation of an upper midline incision is always an available option.

Lower Midline Incision

There are some anatomical differences in the midline above and below the umbilicus. The linea alba is narrow and more difficult to identify below. Remember that the bladder must always be decompressed.

An *upward extension* of a lower midline incision is always available to the surgeon. The incision should go around the umbilicus to the left to avoid the ligamentum teres and an unclean umbilicus.

Lateral extensions are the same as those of upper midline extensions.

Occasionally the anatomy of the umbilicus permits a *transumbilical extension*. The surgeon must be sure the umbilical folds are clean.

Rectus (Paramedian) Incision

This incision is preferred by the surgeon who wishes to close the abdominal wall in layers (Fig. 4.37b). It does not destroy muscle tissue or nerves. Retract the rectus muscle laterally to prevent tension on vessels and nerves (Fig. 4.38).

Feasible extensions may be made as described for midline incisions.

Pararectus Incision

The incision is made along the lateral border of the rectus sheath. This is an *undesirable incision* because it cuts across the nerve supply to the rectus muscle (Fig. 4.37c). The blood supply from the inferior epigastric artery also may be compromised.

Extensions will further injure nerves and blood vessels.

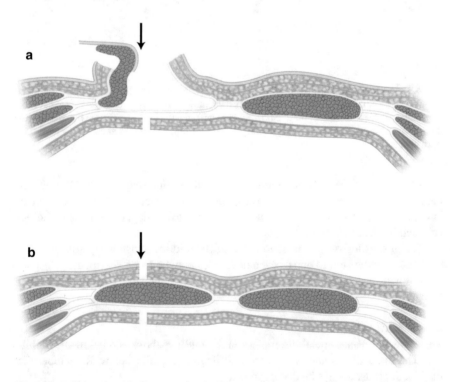

Fig. 4.38 Incision through the rectus sheath without muscle splitting. (**a**) Lateral retraction of the rectus muscle following incision of the anterior layer of the sheath. (**b**) Release of traction allows intact muscle to bridge the incision through the sheath (compare with Fig. 4.37b)

Transverse Incisions

In this type of incision, both rectus sheath and muscle are cut. All the transverse incisions may be extended in the midline.

Upper Abdomen

The rectus muscle and the flat muscles may be cut in the line of the skin incision.

Lower Abdomen (Pfannenstiel Incision)

This incision is made horizontally just above the pubis. The anterior rectus sheaths and the linea alba are transected and reflected upward 8–10 cm. The rectus muscles are retracted laterally, and the transversalis fascia and the peritoneum may be cut in the midline. The iliohypogastric nerve must be identified and protected (Fig. 4.39).

The lower abdominal incision may be extended laterally by dividing the tendinous attachment of the rectus muscle to the pubis. Lateral extension also may be attained by leaving the rectus muscle attached but retracting it medially and splitting the muscles of the anterolateral wall. This usually requires ligation of the inferior

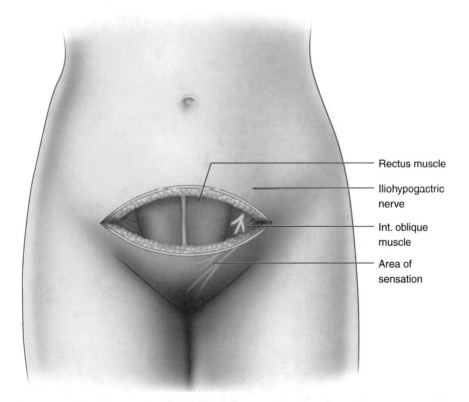

Rectus muscle

Iliohypogastric nerve

Int. oblique muscle

Area of sensation

Fig. 4.39 Pfannenstiel transverse abdominal incision showing the iliohypogastric nerve between the internal oblique muscle and the external oblique aponeurosis just lateral to the border of the rectus muscle

epigastric vessels. Extension too far laterally may jeopardize the iliohypogastric and ilioinguinal nerves (Fig. 4.40).

Oblique Incisions

An oblique **incision** can be extended laterally to the contralateral side of the body or to the same side by following the costal arch and avoiding the nerves. It may be extended upward or downward on the linea alba. It may be extended obliquely upward through the costal arch if it is necessary to convert it to a thoracoabdominal incision.

Subcostal Incision

The rectus sheath is incised transversely. The rectus muscle is cut, and the external oblique muscle is split and retracted. The incision should extend laterally no further than necessary in order to avoid cutting intercostal nerves. The operator usually sees the small eighth and the larger ninth nerves. The latter should be retracted and preserved.

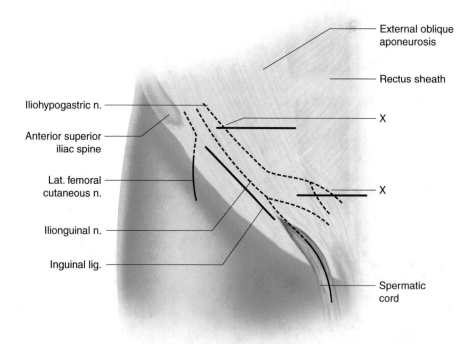

Fig. 4.40 The courses of the iliohypogastric and ilioinguinal nerves. Transverse incisions carried too far laterally may cut the iliohypogastric nerve. Inguinal incisions may injure the ilioinguinal nerve directly or it may be inadvertently included in a suture during closure of the incision

The external oblique, internal oblique, and transversus abdominis muscles usually can be split. Occasionally, the external oblique fibers must be cut laterally and downward.

A subcostal incision two fingerbreadths below and parallel to the right costal margin is the incision most frequently used.

McBurney Incision

The skin is incised for about 8 cm starting 4 cm medial to the right anterior superior iliac spine and extending downward on a line from the spine to the umbilicus. The aponeurosis of the external oblique and the internal oblique and transversus abdominis muscles are split in the direction of their fibers. The iliohypogastric nerve, deep to the internal oblique muscle, must be identified and preserved.

A McBurney incision may be extended upward and laterally for several centimeters without cutting muscles. Medial extension requires transecting the rectus sheath and muscle. In some instances, it is easier to close the incision and make a new one.

Thoracoabdominal Incisions

Various incisions have been reported for exposure of lesions in the upper abdomen and lower thorax. Thoracic incisions have been made through intercostal spaces 5–9 or by resection of ribs 7–9. The abdominal portion of the incision has been either a midline or a transverse continuation of the thoracic incisions. It may or may not extend into the rectus abdominis.

Use this incision only if it is absolutely necessary.

Dehiscence of the Incision

Obesity, prolonged ileus or bowel obstruction, and wound infection are important factors of dehiscence. Dehiscence is caused by poor quality of the tissue or suturing with bites that are too small, placed too far apart, or tied too tightly. Because wounds in patients with hypoproteinemia heal slowly, hyperalimentation is recommended for those whose protein intake is at all questionable.

In contaminated cases, secondary closure of the skin 4–5 days later is a mature surgical decision. The sutures at the initial closure may be placed, but not tied until later. Good hemostasis, debridement, irrigation, good approximation of skin, absence of tension, and avoidance of dead spaces all contribute to good healing without wound dehiscence, postoperative incisional hernia, or a disfiguring scar.

Incisional Hernias

Location

Incisional hernias may be located in any part of the abdominal wall, since they are the result of incisions made for some type of surgery. The usual sites are as follows:

- Upper midline
- Umbilical
- Lower midline

- Lateral upper quadrant
- Lateral lower quadrant
- Suprapubic, transverse
- Lumbar

Overall Etiology and Pathogenesis
- Surgery: dehiscence, infection, and poor anatomical knowledge or technique
- Obesity
- Pregnancy
- Straining or severe cough
- Abdominal distention
- Collagen synthesis disorder
- Diabetes
- Malnutrition
- Ascites
- Concomitant steroid therapy

Preoperative Evaluation and Care
- BMI 40
- HgA1C < 7% for 2 months
- Cessation of smoking 1 month prior to surgery
- Albumin >3.0 g/dL
- Consider CT scan, gastrointestinal and small bowel series, and barium enema
- Bowel prep, if indicated
- Cleansing of the abdominal wall with Hibiclens or pHisoHex 12 and 1 h prior to surgery
- Shaving the abdominal wall in the operating room
- Intravenous antibiotics in the operating room prior to making the incision and for the first 24 h postoperatively

Operating Room Strategies
I always try to repair these hernias with a nonabsorbable mesh. Most of these repairs are approached robotically which is essentially a laparoscopic repair. If the defect is of moderate size and essentially midline then I will opt for a retrorectus repair with mesh. If we are dealing with a significantly larger defect than this will require a repair utilizing a transversus abdominis release (TAR) with mesh, pioneered by Dr. Yuri Novitsky. If I feel that the patient has had the retro rectus space previously violated, then I will do an intraperitoneal onlay mesh (IPOM). There are some surgeons that eschew the use of any mesh intraperitoneally; however sometimes we do not have that luxury to be so dogmatic. In fact, there is no data yet to suggest that a TAR procedure is superior to an IPOM. If I am dealing with what I would term a hostile abdomen with no easy way to enter the peritoneal space, then I would consider a primary closure with an onlay mesh. This is not ideal, but in experienced hands such as those of Dr. Guy Voeller, it can be a good way out of a difficult situation.

Regarding the anterior component separation for repair of hernias, this is a procedure that I have used less and less over the years. The indications for using this technique are for large abdominal wall defects including multiple recurrent ventral hernias with a hostile abdomen which would make a laparoscopic approach very difficult. This procedure can be paired with an onlay mesh for a little more peace of mind.

With regard to infected mesh, the mesh usually needs to be removed, and, depending on the degree of infection, repair is done using an absorbable synthetic mesh such as phasix or synecor. These are both fairly new products and show promising results with regard to recurrence rates. In most cases I would opt for an IPOM. If, however, there is significant infection with the mesh engulfed in pus, then I would remove the mesh and perform a primary closure with the anticipation of the patient developing a recurrence and another trip to the operating room a year later.

Primary Closure
- **Step 1.** Remove scar by elliptical incision (Fig. 4.41).
- **Step 2.** Dissect skin flaps and subcutaneous tissue on both sides of defect down to the aponeurotic area, approximately 3–4 cm around the defect (Fig. 4.42).
- **Step 3.** If possible, avoid opening the sac. If this is not possible, remove sac and carefully palpate the defect or defects. Remove all scars and attenuated tissues.
- **Step 4.** Close the defect vertically or transversely with interrupted No. 0 Nurolon, with bites 2–2.5 cm from the ring.
- **Step 5.** Close in layers.

Open IPOM (Intraperitoneal Only Mesh)
For larger defects Ventralex ST or Ventrio ST patch repair is highly recommended: it consists of implanting a prosthesis deep to the muscles of the abdominal wall (Figs. 4.43, 4.44, 4.45, and 4.46). The Ventrio ST patch has the advantage of "pockets," which can be tacked easily to the overlying fascia by the use of either interrupted sutures or a laparoscopic tacking device (Fig. 4.47). The Ventralex has a strap that can be pulled up through the defect, thus pulling the patch tight against the anterior abdominal wall. The straps are then sutured to the overlying fascia or fascial ring. It is important to use a mesh size that allows for a 5 cm overlap between the fascial edge and the edge of the mesh. Close fascia over the mesh.

- **Step 1.** Remove scar.
- **Step 2.** Dissect down to sac and remove. If necessary, lyse adhesions, clearing anterior abdominal wall.
- **Step 3.** Choose an appropriate size piece of mesh. My first choice is a Bard Ventrio ST. This is placed into the defect, thus intraperitoneally. It is then secured circumferentially with the laparoscopic tacking device of your choice.
- **Step 4.** The overlying fascia is then reapproximated with an interrupted nonabsorbable suture such as 0 Nurolon or Proline.
- **Step 5.** Layered closure of the skin.

Note: Alternatively, any appropriately sized piece of coated mesh can be used for this repair with the mesh "parachuted" into the abdomen, secured with transfascial sutures.

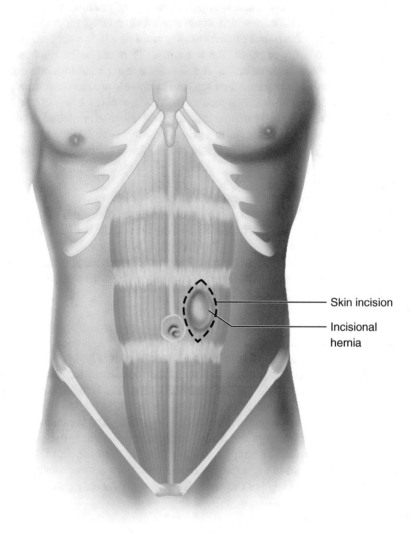

Fig. 4.41 Herniation at the site of a left rectus incision

Note
- When infected mesh is removed, it should be replaced with an absorbable product instead of nonabsorbable mesh. Expect to re-operate on these patients in a few years to repair their recurrent hernia.
- When placing nonabsorbable mesh, interrupted transfascial sutures are mandatory. Allow for at least a 5 cm overlap of mesh and fascia.
- When placing a Ventrio patch, use the laparoscopic tacking device, which should be inserted in the anterior pocket of the patch (Fig. 4.47). This placement will fix the patch circumferentially to the overlying fascia. Close fascia over mesh.

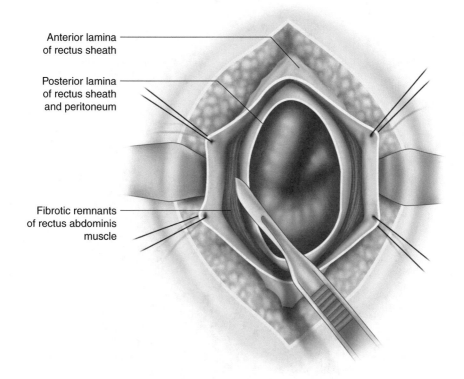

Anterior lamina
of rectus sheath

Posterior lamina
of rectus sheath
and peritoneum

Fibrotic remnants
of rectus abdominis
muscle

Fig. 4.42 Dissection around the ring

- Don't hesitate to view the repair with the laparoscope and to place more tacks as needed.
- For larger defects utilize transfascial fixation.
- The description of the anatomical fixation of a large prosthesis is *only approximately* as follows:
- Upper midline: costal arch, lateral flat muscles, or rectus sheath.
- Umbilical: lower costal arch; anterior superior iliac spine (if possible); lateral flat muscles; or rectus sheath.
- Lower midline: linea semicircularis, pectineal ligament, space of Retzius, rectus sheath, lateral flat muscles, pubic tubercles, and symphysis pubis.
- Lateral upper: costal arch, anterior superior iliac spine (if possible), rectus sheath, myoaponeurotic flat muscles, or lateral flat muscles.
- Spigelian: anatomical closure of defect. Remember that the sac is under the aponeurosis of the external oblique.
- Lateral lower: iliac crest, right and left ligaments of Cooper, rectus sheath, or lateral flat muscles.
- Lumbar: external oblique, latissimus dorsi, or iliac crest.
- On occasion, I have placed bone screws with attached sutures to fix the mesh to the pelvis.

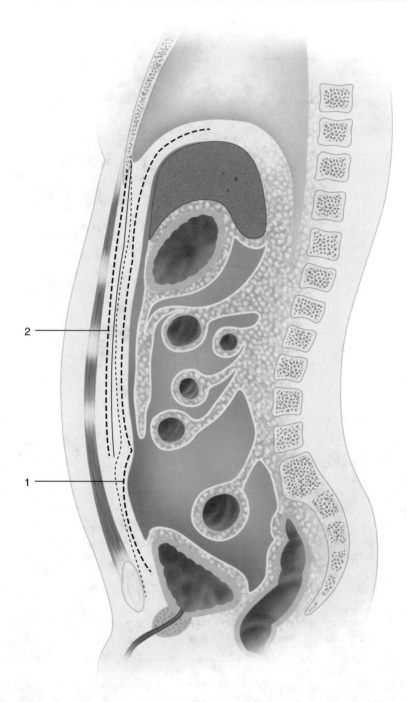

Fig. 4.43 Schematic representation of a paramedial sagittal cross section of the trunk, showing the two retroparietal cleavable spaces used for prosthetic repair of large hernias. *Broken line 1*, the retrofascial preperitoneal space used at the lower part of the wall. *Broken line 2*, the retrorectus space used at the supraumbilical part of the wall

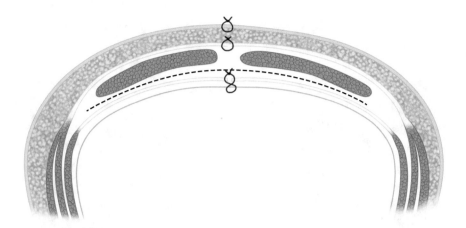

Fig. 4.44 Schematic representation of a horizontal cross section of the wall at its upper level, with a mesh prosthesis (*broken line*) in the retrorectus cleavable space

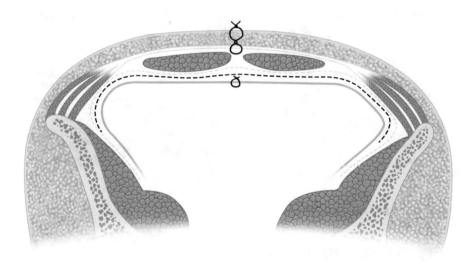

Fig. 4.45 Schematic representation of a horizontal cross section of the wall at its lower level, with a mesh prosthesis (*broken line*) in the retrofascial preperitoneal cleavable space

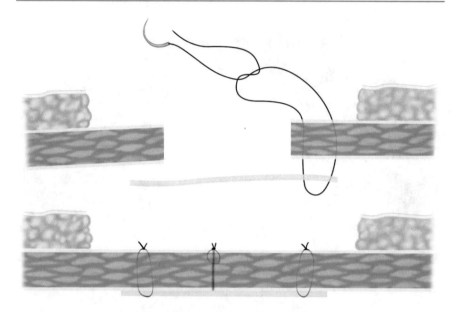

Fig. 4.46 *Above*: fixing the deep layer to the posterior surface of the transversalis fascia. *Below*: fixing a second layer to the anterior surface of the fascia

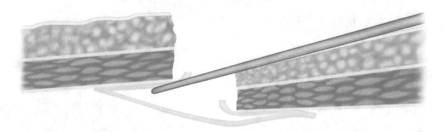

Fig. 4.47 Tacking the Ventrio ST patch

Component Separation (Fig. 4.48)

Anterior Component Separation

Component separation is required when the patient has a large incisional or ventral hernia or when infected mesh is being removed, resulting in a large defect. The goal is to place mesh deep to the muscles, secure it with transfascial sutures, and approximate the patient's fascia to the midline, over the mesh. This requires release of the abdominal wall components, the external oblique muscle, and rectus sheath bilaterally.

- **Step 1.** Excise the previous incision.
- **Step 2.** Debride scar tissue, peritoneum, and fatty fascia.

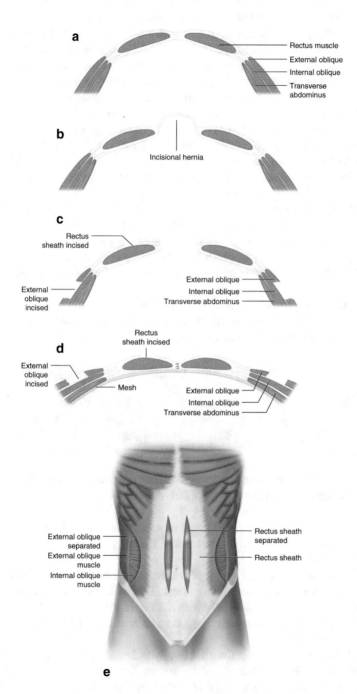

Fig. 4.48 (**a**) "Components" (external oblique muscle and rectus sheath) released. (**b–e**) Completed operation showing abdominal muscles approximated at the midline with mesh in place

- **Step 3.** Perform lysis of adhesions. Make sure that the peritoneum of the anterior abdominal wall is devoid of bowel or omental adhesions.
- **Step 4.** Elevate skin flaps on each side with a Bovie. It usually is necessary to go as far lateral as the anterior superior iliac spine, because this is where the external oblique muscle must be separated in order to advance the muscle flaps.
- **Step 5.** Using the Bovie, separate the external oblique muscle starting at the anterior superior iliac spine and ending at the costal margin. This should give 5–10 cm of advancement on each side. Again with the Bovie open the rectus sheath longitudinally 2 cm from the medial border (Fig. 4.48c).
- **Step 6.** Raise that medial portion of the anterior rectus sheath (Fig. 4.48d).
- **Step 7.** Choose an appropriately sized piece of mesh. The patient's fascia should be pulled to its midline position so that after the mesh is placed in the abdomen, the edge of the mesh will have a 5 cm overlay.
- **Step 8.** Secure the mesh circumferentially with transfascial sutures. Make sure that the fascia is pulled toward the midline when estimating where the sutures will be placed. In a successful mesh placement, the patient's fascia will approximate at the midline without causing any buckling of the mesh.
- **Step 9.** Close the anterior rectus sheath that has now been medialized at the midline.
- **Step 10.** Place a 10 mm Jackson–Pratt drain under each skin flap.
- **Step 11.** Close the wound in layers, using a 3 0 Vicryl for subcutaneous tissue and a 4 0 Vicryl for subcuticular tissue.

Note
- Depending on the circumstances it may be necessary to secure the mesh to the anterior superior iliac spine and the costal margin. This can be done with a 0 or #1 Prolene on a stout mayo needle, usually a #6.

Posterior Component Separation with Transversus Abdominis Muscle Release (Novitsky Repair)/ Retrorectus Repair

- **Step 1.** A midline incision is utilized. In most cases the midline scar is elliptically excised. A lysis of adhesions is done, freeing up bowel and omentum from the anterior abdominal wall.
- **Step 2.** Identify the medial border of the rectus muscle. The rectus sheath is then incised exposing the rectus muscle fibers. This incision on the rectus sheath is continued proximally and distally with the Bovie. At this point blunt finger dissection can continue to sweep away the rectus muscle fibers from the rectus sheath (Fig. 4.49).
- **Step 3.** The dissection is continued cranially and caudally. As one approaches the pelvis, the medial attachments of the arcuate line are divided thus facilitating entry into the preperitoneal space of the pelvis. The lateral dissection is continued until the perforators of the rectus muscle are encountered (Fig. 4.50).

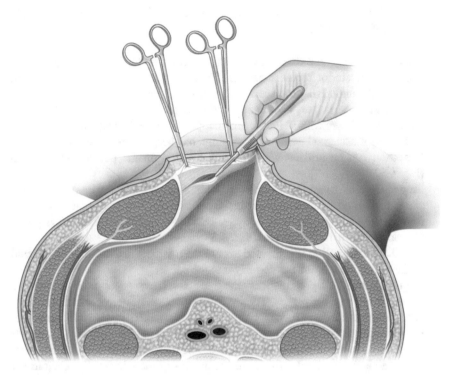

Fig. 4.49 Posterior sheath is incised lateral to the line alba

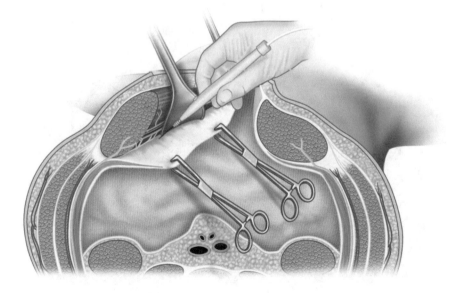

Fig. 4.50 Retrorectus dissection

Note: if one is doing a retrorectus repair, this is the point that this dissection is concluded. Proceed to step 9.

- **Step 4.** This is where division of the transversus abdominis muscle is undertaken. The posterior rectus sheath is divided just medial to these perforators, exposing the underlying transversus abdominis fibers (Fig. 4.51).
- **Step 5.** The transversus abdominis muscle is then divided with the Bovie by elevating the fibers with a right-angle clamp. The space between the transversus abdominis muscle and transversalis fashion has been entered. Once again finger dissection can be utilized while placing traction on the poster rectus sheath (Fig. 4.52).
- **Step 6.** Careful dissection is continued laterally employing finger or right-angle clamp dissection. If tears do occur in the peritoneum, they can be closed primarily with the 40 Vicryl figure of a suture. This dissection is as far lateral as possible usually to the psoas muscle (Figs. 4.53 and 4.54).
- **Step 7.** The dissection is continued toward the myopectineal orifice of Fruchaud as the dissection continues inferiorly into the pelvis.
- **Step 8.** Below the xiphoid process the linea alba prevents continuity of the two dissected retro rectus planes. The insertions of each posterior sheath cranially and laterally to the linea alba on both sides are incised. The posterior insertion of the posterior rectus sheath into the xiphoid process is also incised. This allows the connection the two retro rectus spaces. The most superior fibers of the transversus abdominis muscle which are just lateral to the edge of the xiphoid are divided.

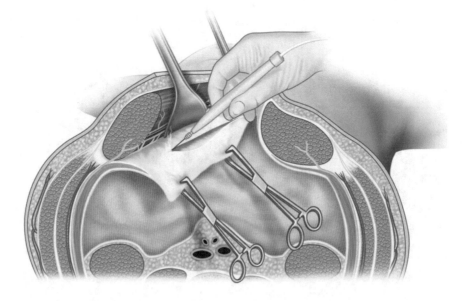

Fig. 4.51 Incising the lateral border of the rectus sheath

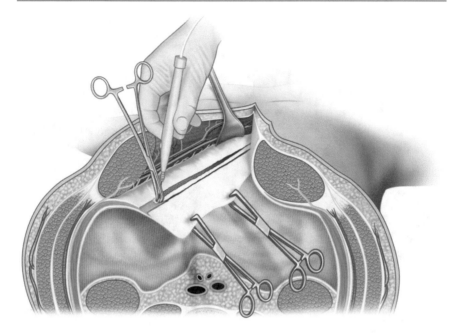

Fig. 4.52 Incising the transversus abdominis muscle

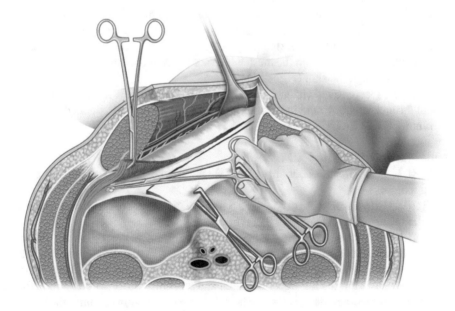

Fig. 4.53 Posterior component separation by dissecting deep or posterior to the divided transversus abdominis muscle

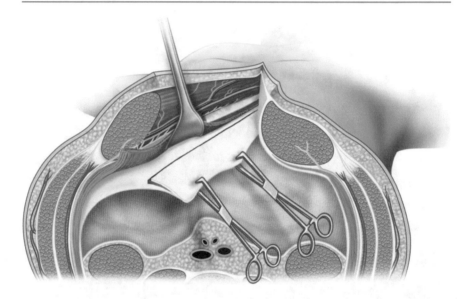

Fig. 4.54 With the transversus abdominis muscles disassociated from the posterior layers, they are medialized

- **Step 9.** The posterior rectus sheaths are then approximated with a running 0 V lock or STRATAFIX suture (Fig. 4.55).
- **Step 10.** An appropriately sized piece of mesh is then placed in this retro muscular space. It is fixed cooper's ligament inferiorly and superiorly to the costal margin laterally and to the xiphoid process as well as several additional trans abdominal sutures through the mesh which are brought out through separate stab wounds through the skin (Fig. 4.56).
- **Step 11.** A large round channel drain is than left on top of the mesh and brought out through a stab wound in the midline fascia is then re-approximated with the running #1 STRATAFIX suture (Fig. 4.57).

Laparoscopic/Robotic IPOM
- **Step 1.** Insufflate the abdomen using Veress needle inserted at the left costal margin.
- **Step 2.** Using an optical port, insert a 5 mm laparoscope. This is placed where I anticipate placing the da Vinci 8 mm trocar.
- **Step 3.** Survey the abdomen for adhesions. At this point da Vinci ports are placed in the left abdomen. The camera port is placed as far lateral as possible approximately halfway between the ASIS and the costal margin. Da Vinci ports are then placed in the left upper quadrant and left lower quadrant being mindful that placing these ports too close to the ASIS or costal margin can limit the range of motion of the instruments. This is my routine when dealing with midline defects. Before docking the robot, it may be necessary to take down adhesions,

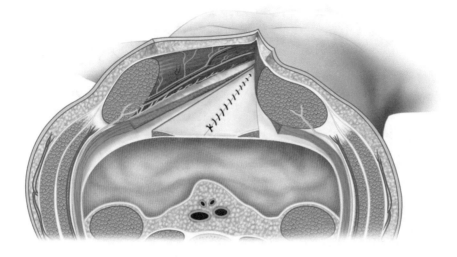

Fig. 4.55 Posterior layers are reapproximated at the midline with restoration of the visceral sac

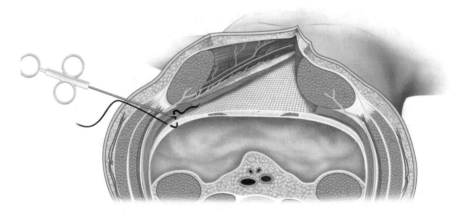

Fig. 4.56 Mesh is placed and fixed laterally with a suture passer

allowing working space for the robotic instruments. If that is not the case, proceed to docking the robot.

- **Step 4.** Lyse all adhesions to the anterior abdominal wall and hernia sac. Debridement of hernia sac, as necessary.
- **Step 5.** Primary closure of the defect is accomplished using a #1 STRATAFIX suture. This can be facilitated by decreasing the intraperitoneal pressure. If the defect is around 10 cm or less, this can usually be accomplished. If larger, then a retrorectus or tar procedure maybe necessary.

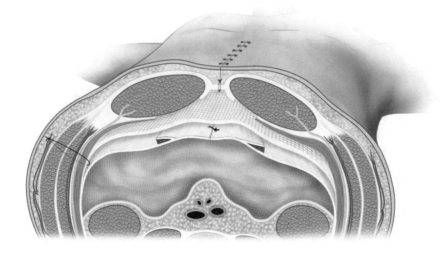

Fig. 4.57 Completed reconstruction of the abdominal wall with the linea alba medialized in the mesh posterior to it

- **Step 6.** Choose an appropriately sized piece of mesh such that at least 3 cm and preferably 5 cm overlap is achieved. My go to mesh is the Bard echo. This allows the mesh to be brought up against the anterior abdominal wall allowing for easier fixation.
- **Step 7.** The mesh is then secured circumferentially with the running 2–0 STRATAFIX suture. Alternatively, it can be tacked in circumferentially with two rows of the tacking device of your choice.
- **Step 8.** For transfascial sutures are placed in the 12, 3, 6, and 9 o'clock positions using the Carter Thompson suture passer.
- **Step 9.** The surgical site and abdomen are surveyed for bleeding. Trocars are removed, and if necessary fascial sutures placed and skin is closed.

Laparoscopic/Robotic TAPP
- **Steps 1–4:** As above
- **Step 5.** The peritoneum is incised at least 5 cm from the defect. This is continued proximally and distally. The preperitoneal plane is then developed, reducing the hernia sac using sharp and blunt dissection.
- **Step 6.** The defect is then closed with a running #1 STRATAFIX suture.
- **Step 7.** An appropriately sized piece of mesh is then placed and either sutured or tacked in place.
- **Step 8.** The peritoneal flap is then closed with a running 2–0 STRATAFIX suture.
- **Step 9.** All trocars removed, fascia closed as necessary, skin closed

Onlay Technique
- **Step 1.** Elliptical midline incision is made excising the old scar.
- **Step 2.** Skin flaps are raised on each side.
- **Step 3.** Assess approximation of fascial elements to the midline. If the fascia cannot be approximated to the midline, then the posterior rectus fascia on one side (you pick) is incised. If still not enough, then the contralateral posterior rectus fascia is similarly incised.
- **Step 4.** If there is still difficulty approximating the fascial elements to the midline, then external releases are done, first on one side and, then if necessary, on the other side. The factual elements are then approximated to the midline with a running # 1 Proline.
- **Step 5.** A lightweight mesh is used as the onlay. It should cover all the releases. Fiber and glue is then used to secure the mesh.
- **Step 6.** If external oblique muscle releases have been done, the mesh should be secured to the lateral edge of that release.
- **Step 7.** Drains are placed under the skin flaps and brought out for stab wounds and secured.
- **Step 8.** The skin is closed in layers.

Parastomal Hernia Repair
Repair of the parastomal hernia without mesh has a significantly higher recurrence rate compared to mesh repairs. The two procedures that I prefer are the Sugarbaker and keyhole procedures.

- **Step 1.** The abdomen is entered threat midline and all adhesions released from the anterior abdominal wall.
- **Step 2.** Herniated contents are reduced.
- **Step 3.** Mesh, usually some variety of PTFE, is placed over the defect and bowel lateralized as per Sugarbaker. Alternatively, the mesh can be keyholed around the bowel. If keyholed the slit mesh is then closed with a running 0 Proline.
- **Step 4.** The mesh is then secured with tacks and four transfascial sutures.
- **Step 5.** The midline is the enclosed per your routine.

Epigastric Through the Linea Alba
An epigastric hernia (or hernia through the linea alba) is a protrusion of preperitoneal fat or a peritoneal sac with or without an incarcerated viscus. It occurs in the midline between the xiphoid process and the umbilicus. The sac is covered only with skin and fat.

- **Step 1.** Make a vertical or transverse incision over the mass.
- **Step 2.** Dissect the fat down to the linea alba superiorly and inferiorly and to the anterior lamina of the rectus sheath laterally (Fig. 4.58).

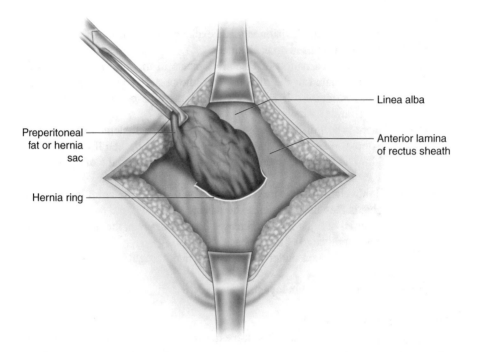

Preperitoneal fat or hernia sac

Hernia ring

Linea alba

Anterior lamina of rectus sheath

Fig. 4.58 Fat is dissected

- **Step 3.** Close the small defect in the linea alba transversely with interrupted 0 Nurolon suture (Fig. 4.59).
- **Step 4.** Close subcutaneous tissue and skin.

Note
- Alternatively, this repair can be performed using Ventrio or Ventralex patches, as previously described.

Umbilical Hernia

Small Umbilical Hernia (Fig. 4.60)

Step 1. Make an infraumbilical incision from the 3 o'clock position to the 9 o'clock position.

Step 2. Dissect the sac circumferentially to free it from the surrounding subcutaneous tissue (Fig. 4.60a, b).

Step 3. Divide the sac and excise the excess sac down to the ring (Fig. 4.60c).

Step 4. Use an interrupted 0 Surgilon to close the ring (Fig. 4.60d, e).

Step 5. Close the skin (Fig. 4.60f, g).

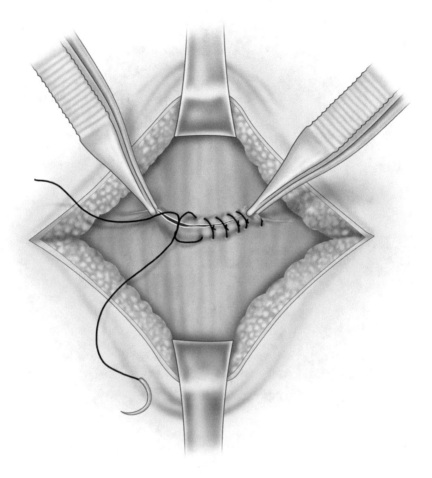

Fig. 4.59 Closure of the small defect

Note
- We use this technique when the defect is too small to accept a Ventralex patch.

Large Umbilical Hernia, Using Mesh (Fig. 4.61)
Umbilical hernias in adults may be the result of large, untreated infantile hernias that failed to close spontaneously. Umbilical hernias in the adult do not close spontaneously.

- **Step 1.** Make an infraumbilical incision from the 3 o'clock position to the 9 o'clock position.

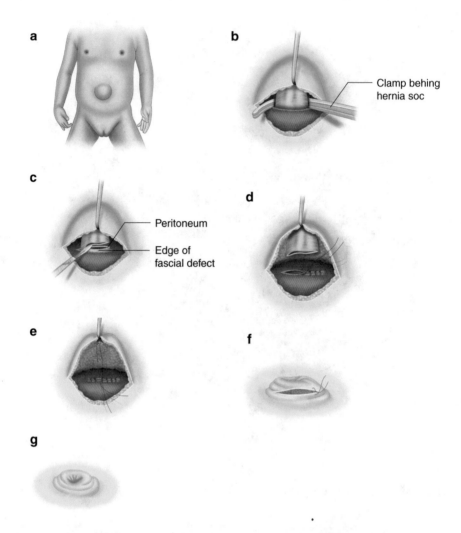

Fig. 4.60 Umbilical herniorrhaphy. (**a**) After umbilicus is grasped and elevated, incision is made in an infraumbilical skin crease. (**b**) Blunt dissection. Hernial sac encircled with clamp. (**c**) Sac opened and divided. Interrupted sutures placed and tied. (**d**) Absorbable sutures placed and tied to help obliterate dead space. (**e** and **f**) Skin is closed with subcuticular absorbable sutures. (**g**) Redundant skin is left alone

- **Step 2.** Using a Kelly clamp, dissect on each side of the umbilical sac, which usually is adherent to the overlying skin. Pass the Kelly clamp behind the hernia sac.
- **Step 3.** Dissect the hernia sac away from the overlying skin. Continue the dissection of the sac circumferentially down to and below the umbilical ring. Sometimes this is difficult or impossible; in that case, transect the sac.

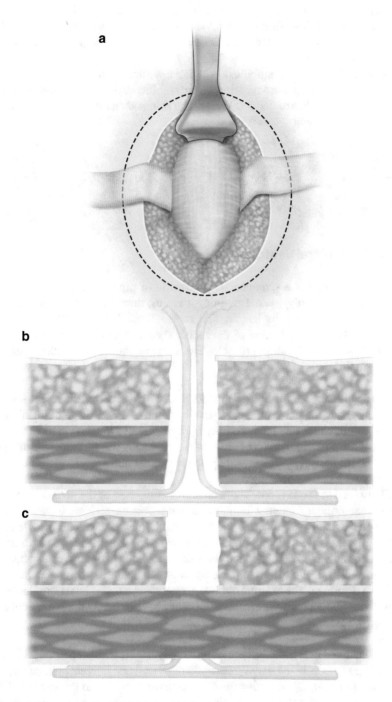

Fig. 4.61 (**a**) Insertion of patch. (**b**) Straps. (**c**) Suturing

- **Step 4.** An appropriately sized Ventralex patch can be inserted into and below the umbilical ring. The straps of the Ventralex patch are sutured to the overlying fascia with an interrupted 2-0 PDS suture. Usually, it is possible to close the fascia over the mesh.
- **Step 5.** The overlying umbilical skin flap is sutured down to the umbilical ring, thus reestablishing a normal-appearing umbilicus. The subcutaneous tissue is closed with an interrupted 3-0 Vicryl. The skin is then closed with a running 4-0 Vicryl subcuticular.

Note
- In almost all cases, larger umbilical hernias in adults are repaired using a mesh. This can be done in an open fashion as described above, employing a laparoscopic TAPP repair or a robotic retrorectus approach with mesh.

Spigelian (Lateral Ventral) Hernia

A spigelian hernia is a spontaneous protrusion of preperitoneal fat, a peritoneal sac, or, less commonly, a sac containing a viscus, through the spigelian zone (fascia) at any point along its length. The zone is bounded medially by the lateral margin of the anterior lamina of the rectus sheath and laterally by the muscular fibers of the internal oblique muscle. The surgeon should be familiar with three entities in this area:

- The semilunar line (of Spiegel) marks the lateral border of the rectus sheath. It extends from the pubic tubercle to the tip of the costal cartilage of the ninth rib.
- The semicircular line (arcuate line, fold, or line of Douglas) marks the caudal end of the posterior lamina of the aponeurotic rectus sheath, below the umbilicus and above the pubis. Unfortunately, the semilunar and semicircular lines are not easily seen in the operating room.
- The spigelian fascia (zone, aponeurosis) is composed of the aponeuroses of the external oblique, internal oblique, and transversus abdominis muscles. The region between these muscles and the lateral border of the rectus muscle defines the spigelian fascia. For all practical purposes, the spigelian fascia is formed by the approximation and fusion of the internal oblique and transversus abdominis aponeuroses. If the fusion of these aponeuroses is loose, a "zone" rather than a fascia is formed. The external oblique aponeurosis remains intact over the hernia. Anterior abdominal wall hernias can occur above or below the semicircular line (Fig. 4.62).

As illustrated in Fig. 4.63a, herniation usually begins with preperitoneal fat passing through defects in the transversus abdominis (A_1) and internal oblique (A_2) aponeuroses. In Fig. 4.63b, note that the transversus abdominis and the internal oblique are broken. However, the aponeurosis of the external oblique muscle remains intact and, with the skin, forms the covering of the hernia.

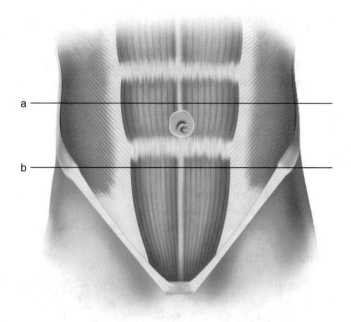

Fig. 4.62 Anterior abdominal wall hernias. (**a**) Hernia above the semicircular line. (**b**) Hernia below the semicircular line

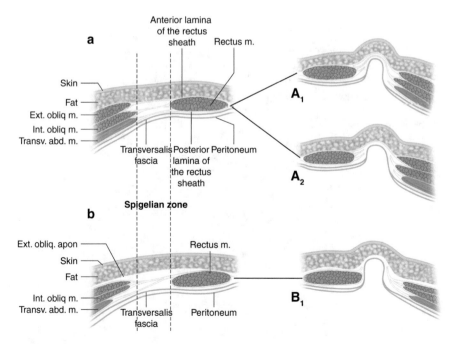

Fig. 4.63 (**a₁**) Transversus abdominis broken; (**a₂**) Transversus abdominis and internal oblique broken; (**b₁**) Transversus abdominis and internal oblique broken

Repair of Spigelian Hernia

- **Step 1.** Make a transverse or vertical incision through the aponeurosis of the external oblique muscle over the palpable mass. If the mass is not palpable at examination, make a midline or vertical rectus incision. If the hernia is incarcerated, the ring should be incised medially toward the rectus abdominis muscle.
- **Step 2.** Retract the aponeurosis of the external oblique muscle, revealing the internal oblique muscle and the hernial sac.
- **Step 3.** Open the sac; inspect its contents, ligate, and push the sac into the abdomen.
- **Step 4.** Free the ring of spigelian fascia from preperitoneal fat and peritoneal adhesions (Fig. 4.64).
- **Step 5.** Close the defect in the transversus abdominis and the internal oblique muscle with 0 Surgilon interrupted sutures.
- **Step 6.** Close the defect in the aponeurosis of the external oblique muscle with 2-0 Vicryl.
- **Step 7.** Close the skin with interrupted sutures or clips.

Note
- Alternatively, repair of this hernia can be done using a Ventrio patch as described in the section on incisional/ventral hernias or with a TAPP or Lap IPOM.

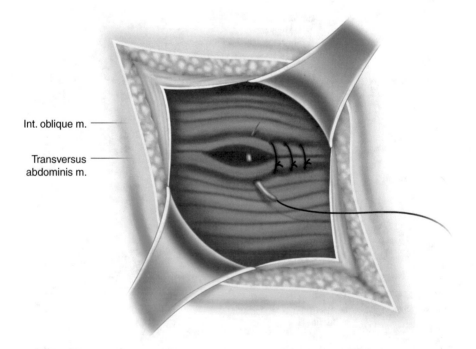

Int. oblique m.

Transversus abdominis m.

Fig. 4.64 Closure of defect

Groin Hernias

These hernias are best thought of as a failure of the anatomical structures of the myopectineal orifice of Fruchaud. Three types of hernia—indirect inguinal, direct inguinal, and external supravesical—may emerge through the abdominal wall above the inguinal ligament. A fourth type, femoral hernia, emerges beneath the inguinal ligament by way of the femoral canal. These four hernias make up 90% of all hernias. My go to for repair of these hernias is a TAP. This allows me to fully assess the entire myopectineal orifice as well as the contralateral side. However, there are other good open procedures yielding good results with low recurrence rates. I used to avoid previously operated on sites. So, if the patient had some type of posterior repair, then I would perform an open anterior repair. As I have become more adept with laparoscopy and the robot that is no longer the case. Most these repairs can be done laparoscopically/robotically either with a TEP or TAPP approach. There are special circumstances, however. Consider the patient with a strangulated hernia. You can always assume that this is an infected field and placing mesh is not the best idea. In those cases, I will use a McVay repair after having evaluated and dealt with compromised bowel. That is a durable repair with recurrence rates in the 5% range. The same applies to infected mesh. If the mesh is in an anterior position, it is removed, and then a good anterior approach without mesh, such as the aforementioned McVay repair, is used. If the infected mesh is in a pre-peritoneal position, then this is approached laparoscopically or robotically with mesh removal. In this instance I would repair with an absorbable synthetic mesh. For small indirect hernias in the younger patients, I think a Marcy repair is perfectly acceptable. This is essentially the same repair done in pediatric age patients which involves a high ligation of the sac with two or three sutures plicating the internal ring.

Direct Inguinal Hernia

A direct inguinal hernia passes through the floor of the inguinal canal in the Hesselbach triangle, which is covered by the transversalis fascia and the aponeurosis of the transversus abdominis muscle, if present.

External Supravesical Hernia

An external supravesical hernia leaves the peritoneal cavity through the supravesical fossa, which lies medial to the site of the direct inguinal fossae. Its subsequent course is that of a direct inguinal hernia (see above).

The repair procedure is the same as for direct inguinal hernia. The surgeon should be careful to protect the iliohypogastric nerve, which is located medial to the superior edge of the surgical ellipse.

Indirect Inguinal Hernia

An indirect inguinal hernia leaves the abdomen through the internal inguinal ring and passes down the inguinal canal a variable distance along with the spermatic cord or round ligament.

Several repairs are employed for indirect hernias when not using mesh. For younger patients with a small indirect hernia, a Marcy repair can work well. For larger indirect hernias in which the floor is involved, use a TEP or TAPP approach. If a laparoscopic approach cannot be done, then a McVay or Bassini repair can be used. A sliding indirect inguinal hernia contains the herniated viscus which makes up all or some of the posterior wall of the sac. The bladder, colon, ovaries, and uterine tube may be involved. Communicating and non-communicating sliding hernias are shown in Fig. 4.65. The internal ring is wider than usual due to the thick spermatic cord. Coincidental direct hernia or weakness of the posterior wall is a strong possibility. The hernial sac is located anterior and medial to the cord, as in an indirect hernia. The descending viscus forms the posterior wall of the empty processus vaginalis.

Femoral Hernia

A femoral hernia is a protrusion of preperitoneal fat or intraperitoneal viscus through a weak transversalis fascia into the femoral ring and the femoral canal. Figure 4.66 shows typical and atypical pathways taken by the femoral hernial sac, and Fig. 4.67

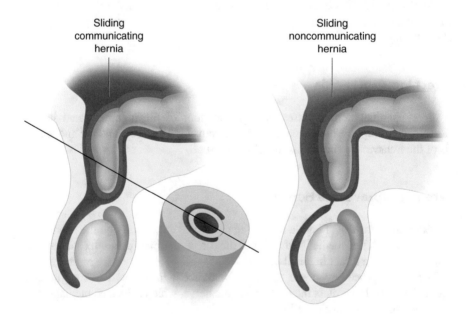

Fig. 4.65 Two types of sliding indirect inguinal hernia

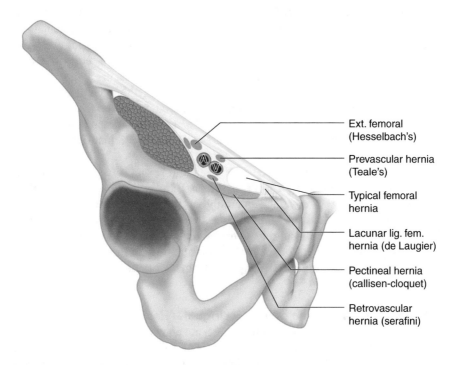

Fig. 4.66 Femoral hernia. Typical and atypical pathways taken by the femoral hernial sac. Note the possible relations to the femoral artery (A) and femoral vein (V)

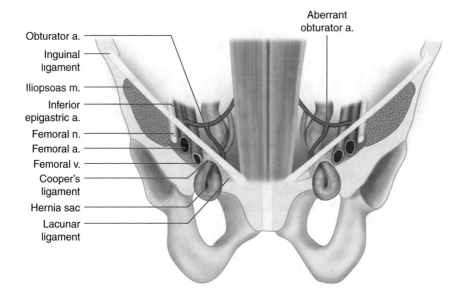

Fig. 4.67 Femoral hernia. The *left half* of the drawing shows an aberrant obturator artery (40%) passing medial to the hernial sac, making it dangerous to incise the lacunar ligament. The *right half* of the drawing shows an aberrant obturator artery passing lateral to the hernial sac, making it safe to incise the lacunar ligament

illustrates possible locations of aberrant obturator arteries. A femoral hernia can be approached in one of the several ways. Open: (1) repair through infrainguinal incision, (2) Cooper ligament repair, and (3) preperitoneal approach using the Nyhus method with mesh or the Kugel repair. Laparoscopic: TAPP. If a femoral hernia is to be repaired via a Cooper ligament repair, it is important that the floor of the canal be opened and the preperitoneal space be evaluated. Anything that is incarcerated in the femoral canal must be reduced. It is important that the transition suture between the inguinal ligament and Cooper ligament and the conjoined area be placed securely. It is that suture that prevents the femoral hernia from recurring.

The authors' preference for repair of a femoral hernia is to place mesh in the preperitoneal position using a TAPP approach. By placing a mesh in the preperitoneal space, there is coverage not only of the femoral canal but also the Hesselbach triangle and the internal ring. In short, the myopectineal orifice of Fruchaud is covered in its entirety. Quite often the femoral hernia is incarcerated and strangulated and therefore extremely difficult—if not impossible—to reduce without incising the inguinal (Poupart) ligament or the lacunar (Gimbernat) ligament.

Cooper Ligament Repair of Indirect Inguinal Hernia
- **Step 1.** Incise the skin approximately 2–3 cm above and parallel to the inguinal ligament (a transverse, gently curved incision following the lines of Langer is another option). With bilateral herniorrhaphy, both male and female patients will appreciate a symmetrical incision. Incise the subcutaneous fascia (Camper) and the fascia of Scarpa by sharp dissection. Open the aponeurosis of the external oblique muscle in the direction of its fibers. The external ring can be found with ease.

> **Remember**
> - Ligate the large veins (superficial epigastric, superficial circumflex, and external pudendal). Small vessels can be treated by electrocoagulation.
> - Protect the ilioinguinal nerve.
> - If the hernia is recurrent, it will be necessary to excise the preexisting scar, both for cosmetic reasons and for good healing.

- **Step 2.** Elevate the spermatic cord carefully and retract with a Penrose drain. Observe the floor of the inguinal canal (Fig. 4.68).
- **Step 3.** Identify the sac located anteromedial to the spermatic cord. Dissect it at the internal ring and lateral to the deep epigastric vessels.
- **Step 4.** Ligate and amputate the sac. Occasionally, if there is too much relaxation at the internal ring, the ligated sac should be fixed under the transversus abdominis muscle, which is the upper boundary of the internal ring. Leave the distal part of the sac in situ and open (Wantz procedure) to avoid anatomical complications.

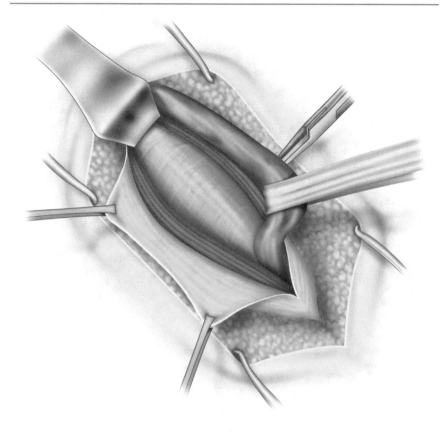

Fig. 4.68 Floor of inguinal canal

- **Step 5.** We agree with Nyhus that a single technique is not appropriate for all patients. The following steps illustrate our technique:
  - (a)   With 0 Surgilon, suture the conjoined area to the ligament of Gimbernat (Fig. 4.69).
  - (b)   Suture the conjoined area to the ligament of Cooper. This may require three sutures (Fig. 4.70).
  - (c)   The Cooper ligament dives deep, so a transition suture is required (Fig. 4.71). This will transition the repair from the Cooper ligament to the Poupart ligament. Without this transition suture, a femoral defect will be left, thus allowing for the possibility of a recurrence through the femoral canal. The transversus abdominis arch is sutured to the Poupart ligament, the iliopubic tract, and the Cooper ligament (Fig. 4.72).
  - (d)   The remainder of the sutures incorporates the arch and transversalis fascia, the iliopubic tract, and the inguinal ligament. The distal phalanx of the fifth finger should be inserted with ease into the deep ring, thereby ensuring that the closure is not too snug.

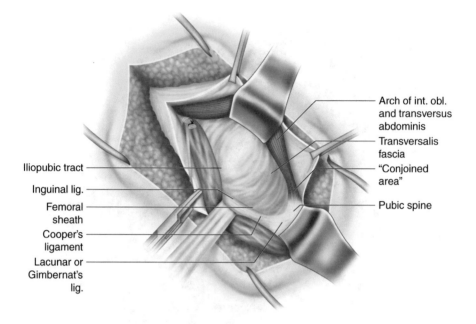

Fig. 4.69 Bulging of direct hernia (cord pulled laterally)

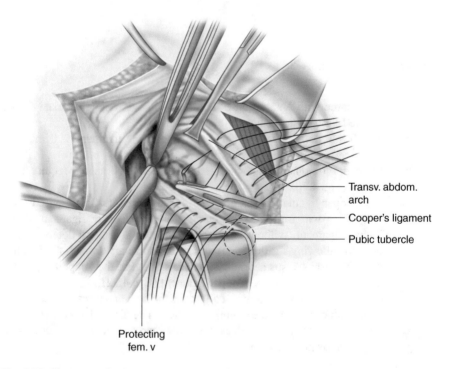

Fig. 4.70 Placement of sutures

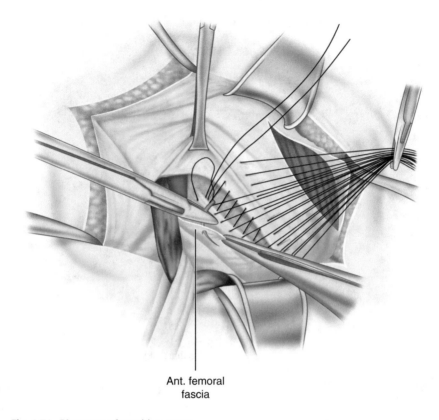

Ant. femoral
fascia

Fig. 4.71   Placement of transition suture

- **Step 6.** Tie all sutures.
- **Step 7.** Perform a relaxing incision. This is placed at the reflection of the external oblique aponeurosis medially. The lamellae are scored with the Bovie such that they separate, exposing the underlying rectus muscle.
- **Step 8.** Close the aponeurosis of the external oblique muscle with a running 2-0 PDS.
- **Step 9.** Close Scarpa fascia with interrupted 3-0 Vicryl. Close the skin.

Note: For a sliding hernia
- **Step 1.** Mobilize the sac and open it high and anteriorly. Do not dissect the viscus from the posterior wall of the sac (Fig. 4.73).
- **Step 2.** If there is excess anterior wall of the sac, trim it carefully (Fig. 4.74).
- **Step 3.** Close the remnants of the sac. Finish the repair as in McVay repair.

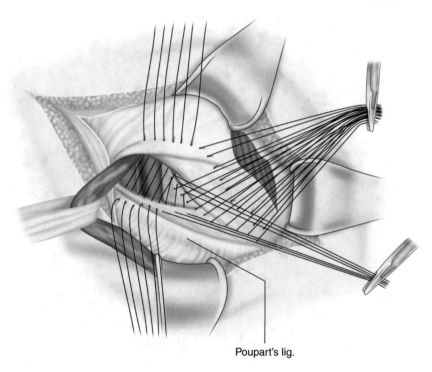

Poupart's lig.

Fig. 4.72 Closure of femoral canal

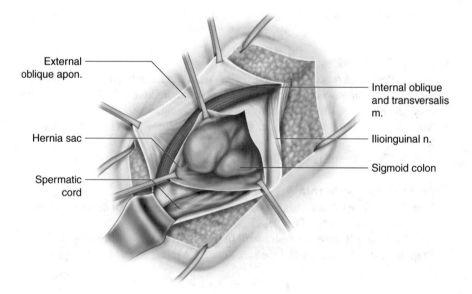

External oblique apon.

Hernia sac

Spermatic cord

Internal oblique and transversalis m.

Ilioinguinal n.

Sigmoid colon

Fig. 4.73 Location of hernia sac

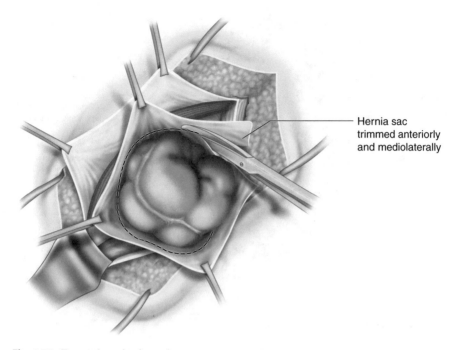

Hernia sac
trimmed anteriorly
and mediolaterally

Fig. 4.74 Excess tissue is trimmed

Shouldice Technique (Figs. 4.75, 4.76, 4.77, and 4.78)

Follow steps 1–4 for Cooper Ligament Repair of Indirect Inguinal Hernia, which is described previously in this chapter.

- **Step 5.** Incise the posterior wall of the inguinal canal from the internal ring, avoiding the deep epigastric vessels, and travel downward medially, ending at the pubic tubercle.
- **Step 6.** Elevate the narrower medial flap as much as possible, but do not elevate the lower lateral flap.
- **Step 7.** Start the first suture line at the pubic bone. Use stainless steel wire and approximate the deep part (white line) of the elevated medial flap to the free edge of the lateral flap. Tie the wire at the internal ring, but do not cut.
- **Step 8.** Using the same uncut wire suture, approximate the free edge of the medial flap in a continuous way to the shelving edge of the inguinal ligament, traveling downward from the internal ring to the pubic bone. Tie and cut the wire at the pubic bone.
- **Step 9.** Using steel wire, start the third suture line at the internal ring, approximating the internal oblique, transversus arch, and the conjoined area to the inguinal ligament. Tie the suture at the area of the pubic tubercle, but do not cut.

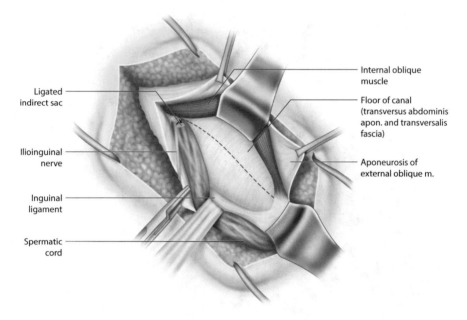

Ligated
indirect sac

Ilioinguinal
nerve

Inguinal
ligament

Spermatic
cord

Internal oblique
muscle

Floor of canal
(transversus abdominis
apon. and transversalis
fascia)

Aponeurosis of
external oblique m.

Fig. 4.75 Incision of posterior wall (floor)

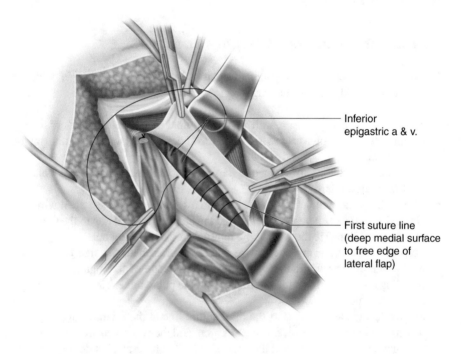

Inferior
epigastric a & v.

First suture line
(deep medial surface
to free edge of
lateral flap)

Fig. 4.76 Approximation of deep part

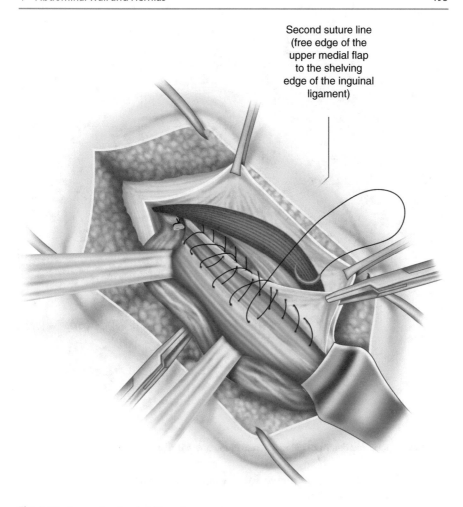

Second suture line
(free edge of the
upper medial flap
to the shelving
edge of the inguinal
ligament)

Fig. 4.77 Approximation (continued)

- **Step 10.** Using the same suture, reapproximate the same anatomical entities as in step 11 from the pubic tubercle to the internal ring.
- **Step 11.** Close the external oblique aponeurosis above the spermatic cord. Occasionally, if there is too much tension, the aponeurosis is closed under the spermatic cord.
- **Step 12.** Close the superficial fascia and skin as described previously.

Marcy Repair
Step 1. Make an oblique incision just medial to the inguinal ligament.
Step 2. Using the Bovie proceed through the subcutaneous tissue to the aponeurosis of the external oblique.

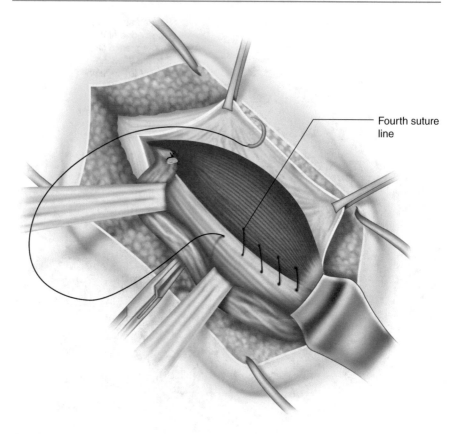

Fourth suture line

Fig. 4.78 Approximation from pubic tubercle to the internal ring

Step 3. Open the external oblique from a point just above the internal ring and through the external ring.

Step 4. Bluntly mobilize the spermatic cord and place a Penrose drain around it for traction.

Step 5. Open up the cremasteric fibers medially thus exposing the indirect sack.

Step 6. Place a hemostat on the sac and dissect it off of the chord down to the level of the inferior epigastric vessels.

Step 7. Perform a high ligation of the sac with a 0 Nurolon suture.

Step 8. Tighten up the internal ring with two or three sutures of 0 Nurolon.

Step 9. Close the external oblique aponeurosis with a running 2-0 Vicryl.

Step 10. Close the wound in layers.

Relaxing Incision (Fig. 4.79)

A great deal of tension can result from a newly created inguinal floor in a Cooper ligament repair. This tension can be relaxed using the relaxing incision.

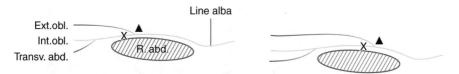

Fig. 4.79 Diagrammatic drawing of the relaxing incision. X, point of relaxing incision at the anterior lamina of the rectus sheath. (*black triangle*), "touchdown" of the external oblique aponeurosis, always between the linea alba and semilunar line

The surgeon should be familiar with the formation of the anterior lamina of the rectus sheath. Below the semicircular line (Douglas or arcuate), there is no posterior aponeurotic layer of the rectus sheath. The anterior layer is formed by the bilaminar aponeuroses of the internal oblique and transversus abdominis muscles and reinforced by the aponeurosis of the external oblique muscle. The aponeurosis of the external oblique muscle may "touch down," or attach, at the lateral or medial half of the anterior lamina. It almost never does so at the linea semilunaris (lateral border of the rectus abdominis) or at the linea alba.

The relaxing incision is made just lateral to the line of attachment ("touchdown") of the external oblique aponeurosis to the anterior lamina of the sheath. This is at the point where the fused internal oblique and transversus abdominis aponeuroses form the rectus sheath. The incision starts at the pubic crest and extends upward 5–8 cm. The length of the incision depends on the local anatomy and pathology.

A good anatomical relaxing incision will protect the external oblique aponeurosis and will not permit the rectus muscle to form a myocele. Avoid the iliohypogastric nerve. Also avoid a linea alba incision or an incision at the linea semilunaris by carefully elevating the medial flap of the aponeurosis of the external oblique muscle (Fig. 4.79).

When the direct or large indirect hernia repair is complete, the relaxing incision allows the transversus abdominis to slide inferiorly and laterally. As the incision opens, the rectus muscle is exposed but the overlying intact superficial lamina (external oblique aponeurosis) of the rectus sheath prevents the development of a hernia.

Femoral Hernia Repair Above the Inguinal Ligament
- **Step 1.** Make an incision above the inguinal ligament as in direct hernia. Incise the internal oblique muscle, the transversus abdominis muscle, and the transversalis fascia without entering the peritoneum. Blunt dissection in the preperitoneal space will direct the surgeon to the neck of the hernial sac, which should not be opened at this time.
- **Step 2.** Isolate the sac under the inguinal ligament at the fossa ovalis; with the index and middle finger of the other hand, gently push the unopened sac upward through the femoral canal into the inguinal canal (Figs. 4.80 and 4.81). If the hernia is not strangulated, this pressure is very useful. If the hernia is incarcerated or strangulated, the contents of the sac should be examined and not permitted to return to the abdominal cavity.

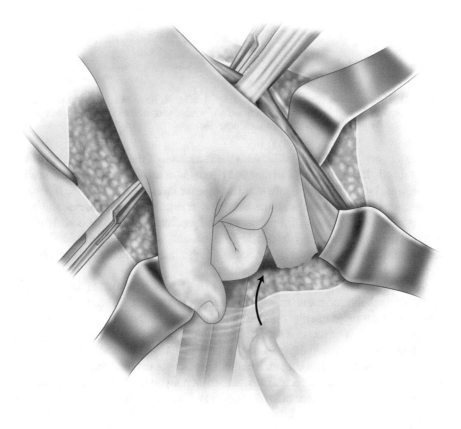

Fig. 4.80 Sac is manipulated through femoral canal into inguinal canal

• **Step 3.** Open the floor of the canal and proceed with a Cooper ligament repair.

Note
• An alternative method of reduction requires sectioning of the lacunar ligament. Before the ligament is incised, the surgeon must be certain that an aberrant obturator artery is not present. Gently manipulate the sac into the posterior wall without losing the contents. An assistant should hold the mass firmly with the thumb and index finger. Open the sac and inspect the contents. If the viscus is vital, trim and ligate the sac. Proceed with the repair as in direct inguinal hernia. If the viscus is not vital, follow resection and anastomosis with the usual repair.

Femoral Hernia Repair Below the Inguinal Ligament
• **Step 1.** Make a vertical or transverse incision just above the femoral swelling (Fig. 4.82).

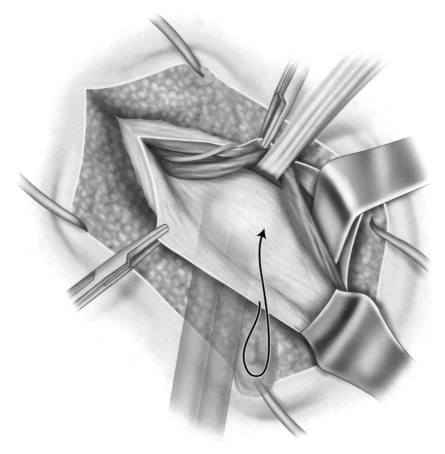

Fig. 4.81 Femoral hernia is now reduced, and sac seen in the inguinal canal

- **Step 2.** Isolate the swelling by careful sharp dissection and digital maneuver until the sac is exposed.
- **Step 3.** Carefully open the sac. Fluid (which is always present) is sent to the lab for culture and sensitivity testing (Fig. 4.83).
- **Step 4.** Inspect the contents of the sac. If viable, push the contents gently into the abdominal cavity. If constriction of the neck does not permit the return of the viscus into the peritoneal cavity, the hernial ring should be cut. It is our opinion that the best anatomical entity to sacrifice in this situation is the inguinal liga-ment, not the lacunar ligament.
- **Step 5.** Ligate the sac with 2-0 Vicryl and excise it. Gently push the sac into the peritoneal cavity so that the canal is as clean as possible.
- **Step 6.** Using 0 Nurolon, suture the inguinal ligament to the pectineal fascia or to Cooper ligament; we prefer Cooper ligament (Figs. 4.84 and 4.85).
- **Step 7.** Close the subcutaneous fat and the skin. If the contents of the sac (bowel) are not viable, the assistant should keep the loop in situ, holding it firmly. Make

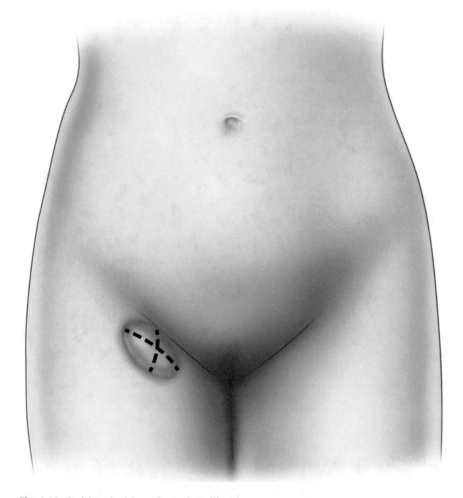

Fig. 4.82 Incision site (above femoral swelling)

a lower midline incision immediately; resection and anastomosis of the bowel must be done from above. Use of drains or closure of the wound depends on whether there was any contamination of the fossa ovalis or the peritoneal cavity.

Mesh Groin Hernia Repairs: Posterior Approach

Nyhus Procedure (Preperitoneal Approach)

Lloyd Nyhus popularized the open preperitoneal approach realizing that addressing the myopectineal orifice of Fruchaud would take care of direct, indirect, and femoral hernias. Dr. Kugel felt the same; however he wanted a less invasive method to

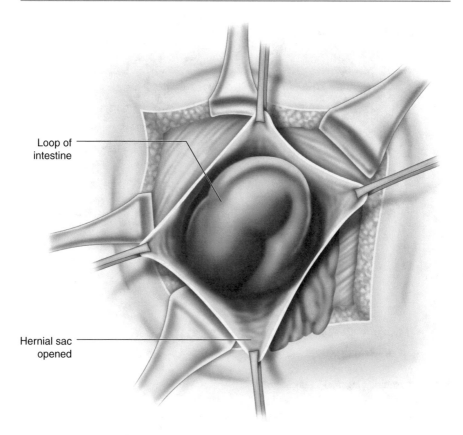

Loop of intestine

Hernial sac opened

Fig. 4.83 Sac opened and contents inspected

deliver a patch into the preperitoneal space. He designed an oval patch with memory so that it could be introduced into the preperitoneal space gently folded, and it would then spring open. With a little bit of manipulation by feel, the entire myopectineal orifice would be covered.

Figure 4.86 shows important anatomical structures of the posterior inguinal wall as seen from the preperitoneal approach. Figure 4.87 is the same view, demonstrating sites of groin hernias. Figure 4.88 shows the operative approach to the preperitoneal space. It is rarely necessary to ligate and sever the inferior epigastric artery and vein.

Nyhus Procedure for Direct, Indirect, and Femoral Inguinal Hernias

- **Step 1.** Two fingerbreadths above the symphysis pubis make a transverse skin incision 4–8 cm long.
- **Step 2.** After the skin and subcutaneous tissues have been incised and the rectus sheath exposed, estimate the level of the internal ring by inserting the left index finger into the external ring. This simple maneuver allows visualization of the location of the internal ring in the surgeon's mind's eye. The incision in the anterior rectus fascia should be placed so that it will pass just cephalad to the internal ring.

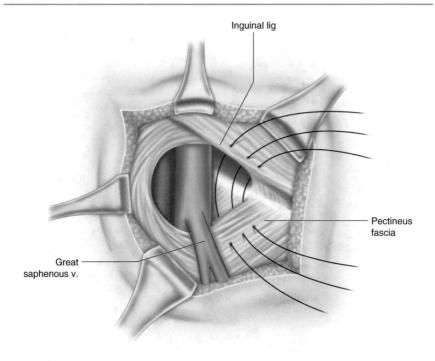

Fig. 4.84 Suturing inguinal ligament

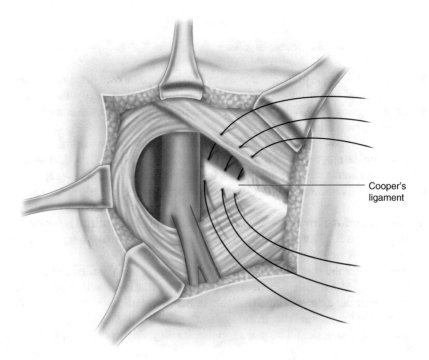

Fig. 4.85 Suturing inguinal ligament (Continued)

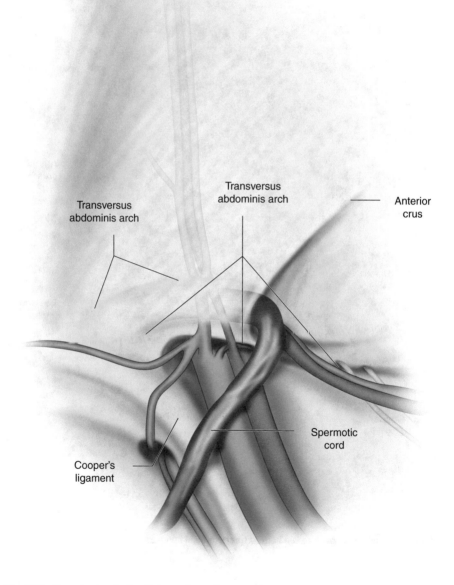

Fig. 4.86 Posterior inguinal wall (preperitoneal approach)

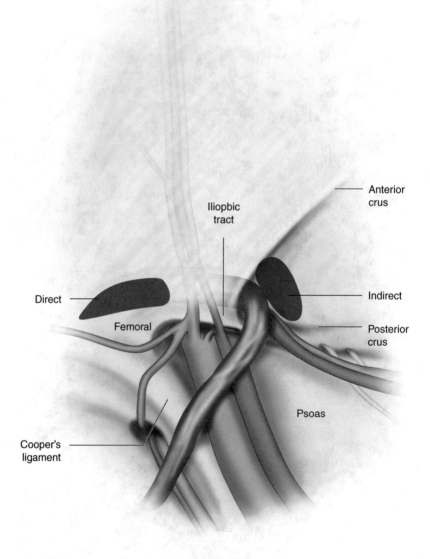

Fig. 4.87 Sites of common groin hernias (preperitoneal approach)

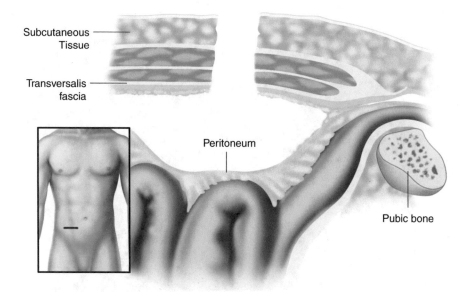

Subcutaneous Tissue

Transversalis fascia

Peritoneum

Pubic bone

Fig. 4.88 Operative approach to preperitoneal space. *Inset*: incision site

- **Step 3.** Make a transverse fascial incision beginning over the midrectus of the affected side (Fig. 4.89).
- **Step 4.** Enlarge the incision by separating and cutting the fascia and muscle fibers of the external oblique, internal oblique, and transversus abdominis muscles. The transversalis fascia is seen in the depth of the wound. When the transversalis fascia is cut, the preperitoneal space of Bogros is entered, and the proper plane of dissection is achieved.
- **Step 5.** Upon entering the space of Bogros, initiate blunt dissection using the finger and sponge on stick. Mobilize the spermatic cord with a Penrose drain. Dissect out the cord and reduce the sac or ligate and transect the sac. Leave the distal end open. If there is a direct sac, it will reduce with gentle traction using a sponge on stick.
- **Step 6.** Tailor a piece of Marlex mesh and place it such that the Hesselbach triangle, femoral canal, internal ring, and surgical incision will be covered by it. Suture the mesh inferiorly to the pubic bone and Cooper ligament. Make a 2–3 cm incision laterally in the mesh to allow the spermatic cord to pass through it. Close the opening such that there is just enough room for the cord to pass through. Bring the superior edge of the mesh underneath the superior edge of the wound. Close the wound with interrupted 0 Surgilon, incorporating the mesh into the closure.

Note
- This repair can be used for recurrent femoral and inguinal hernias because the mesh covers the entire myopectineal orifice of Fruchaud.

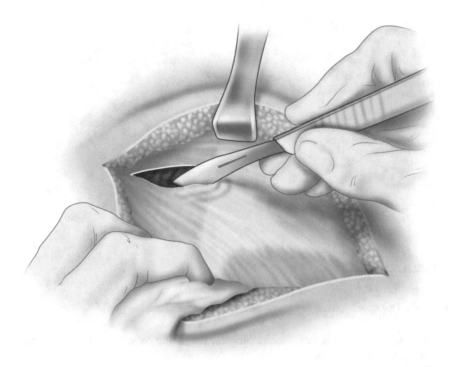

Fig. 4.89 Transverse fascial incision begins over midrectus muscle of the affected side

Kugel Hernia Repair (Preperitoneal Patch) (Figs. 4.90, 4.91, 4.92 and 4.93)

- **Step 1.** The preperitoneal space is entered through a muscle-splitting incision made at a point approximately halfway between the anterior superior iliac spine and the pubic tubercle (or a little higher).
- **Step 2.** Open the transversalis fascia vertically about 3 cm, and enter the preperitoneal space at a point just cephalad to the internal ring.
- **Step 3.** Use blunt dissection with finger or sponge on stick to free the peritoneum from the overlying transversalis fascia. Carefully separate the cord structures from the adjacent peritoneum and hernial sac ("posteriorization of the cord").
- **Step 4.** Dissect a preperitoneal pocket extending over to the symphysis medially, down over the iliac vessels posteriorly, about 3 cm lateral and superior to the transversalis incision, and roughly paralleling the inguinal ligament.

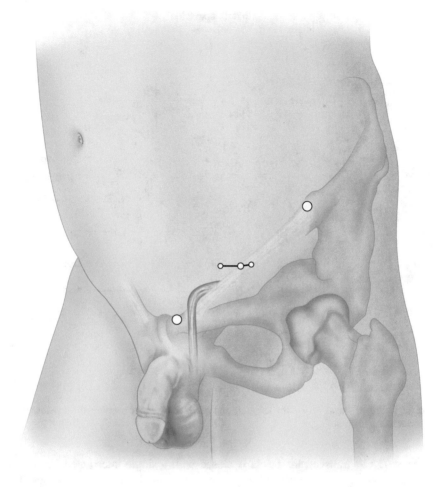

Fig. 4.90 External view showing anatomical landmarks used to locate point of incision

- **Step 5.** Insert the Kugel patch by passing the right index finger through the slit in the anterior layer of the patch, aiming toward the pubic bone (sliding the patch in over a narrow malleable retractor simplifies placement).
- **Step 6.** The patch should lie about three-fifths above the level of the inguinal ligament and two-fifths below it. When the mesh is properly placed in the space of Bogros, the peritoneum is deep to it; the cord structures are anterior and lateral to it. The mesh covers the Hesselbach triangle, internal ring, femoral canal, and the muscle-splitting incision that was made through the internal oblique and transversus abdominis muscles.

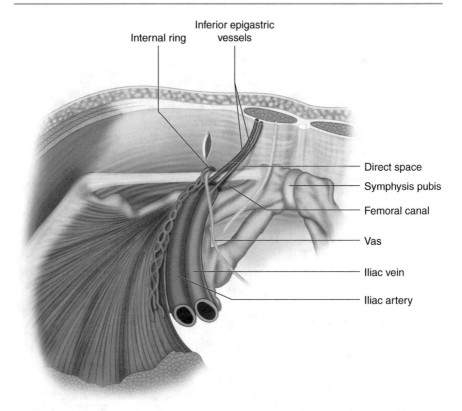

Fig. 4.91 Preperitoneal view of the left groin and pelvis showing the transversalis incision (*i*) just superior to the internal ring

- **Step 7.** The transversalis fascia is closed with a single interrupted absorbable suture "catching" the anterior layer of the patch near its superomedial edge. The patch should be anchored only in *a single* location. Close the remainder of the wound with absorbable suture. For very large direct hernias, we sometimes secure the patch to the pubic tubercle.

Laparoscopic/Robotic Inguinal Hernia Repair

The laparoscopic approach to repairing groin hernias allows "minimally invasive" access to the preperitoneal space for subsequent mesh herniorrhaphy. The rationale for this approach relies on two basic concepts. First, viewing the posterior inguinal wall through the preperitoneal space reveals the origin of all groin hernias and their close proximity within the myopectineal orifice (Fig. 4.94). A piece of mesh placed over the myopectineal orifice will repair all types of groin hernia simultaneously and without additional incisions or dissection (Fig. 4.95). Second, when repairing a defect with mesh, there are obvious mechanical advantages to placing the mesh behind the defect and against the pressures that are creating

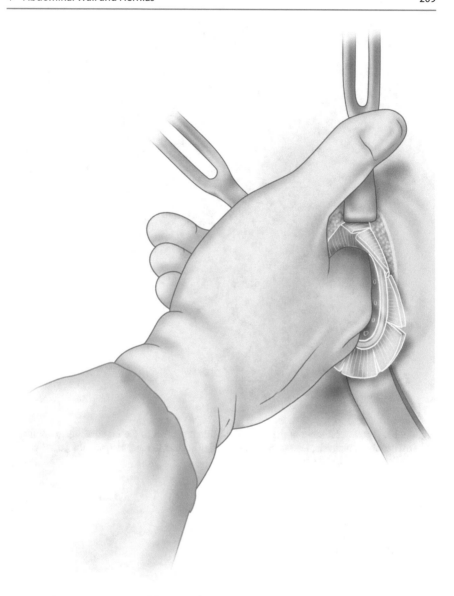

Fig. 4.92 Insertion of the patch through the open wound

herniation, rather than on top of the defect where it can easily be pushed away (Fig. 4.96). Laparoscopic access to the preperitoneal space allows placement of a large piece of mesh over the myopectineal orifice, for a truly "tension-free" repair, without the need for the larger incision used during the traditional preperitoneal repair of Nyhus. This "minimally invasive" technique allows patients to return to full activities immediately with a more comfortable recovery, when compared to other techniques of groin hernia repair. It is especially suited to recurrent or bilateral hernias.

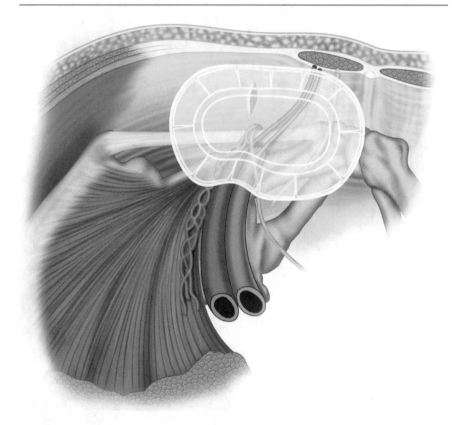

Fig. 4.93 Preperitoneal view of the patch in position: parallel to the inguinal ligament, medial edge over to the symphysis, lateral and superior edge beyond the incision, and the posterior edge lying back onto the iliac vessels

TEP

Position: Supine with both arms tucked
  Anesthesia: General
  Other: Biodrape

- **Step 1.** Through a 10 mm infraumbilical incision, expose the anterior surface of the anterior rectus sheath slightly to the left or right of the linea alba. Incise the anterior rectus sheath longitudinally and retract the rectus muscle fibers laterally, thereby exposing the anterior surface of the posterior rectus sheath.
- **Step 2.** Using the anterior surface of the posterior rectus sheath as a guide, insert a preperitoneal dissection balloon, Spacemaker by Covidien, into the preperitoneal space (Fig. 4.97), and advance it to position the end of the balloon just behind the symphysis pubis. Inflate the balloon to dissect the preperitoneal space (Fig. 4.98).

MYO - Pectineal orifice

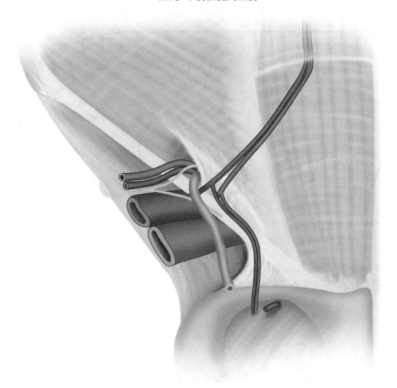

Fig. 4.94 Myopectineal orifice of Fruchaud

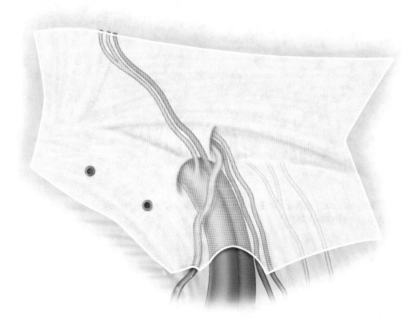

Fig. 4.95 Large mesh prosthesis covering the entire Myopectineal orifice of Fruchaud

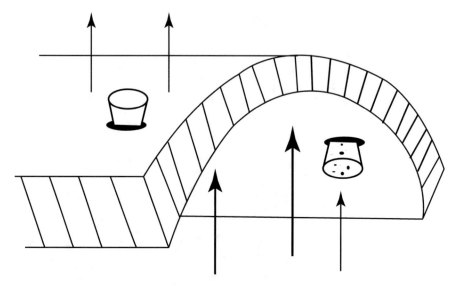

Fig. 4.96 Mechanical benefits of placing mesh behind defect (preperitoneal) to resist intra-abdominal forces promoting herniation

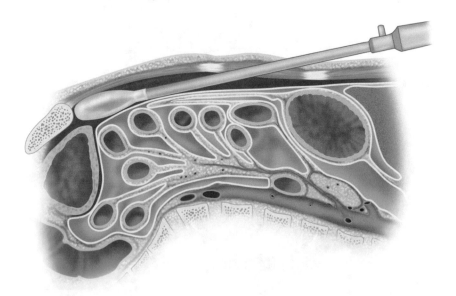

Fig. 4.97 Preperitoneal dissecting balloon inserted into the preperitoneal space and positioned just dorsal to symphysis pubis

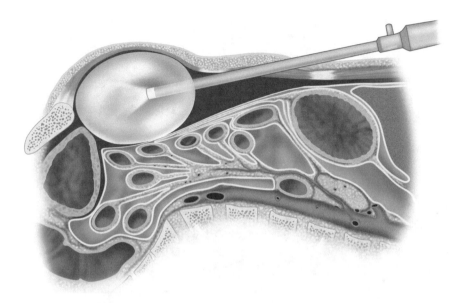

Fig. 4.98 Preperitoneal dissecting balloon inflated to dissect the preperitoneal space

- **Step 3.** Remove the balloon portion of the device leaving the trocar in place. Insufflate the preperitoneal space to a pressure of 10 mmHg. Place two 5 mm cannulas in the midline, one immediately suprapubic and the second midway between the umbilicus and symphysis pubis (Fig. 4.99).
- **Step 4.** Using a camera through the infraumbilical cannula and laparoscopic dissecting instruments through the two 5 mm cannulas, begin dissection of the preperitoneal space (Fig. 4.100).
- **Step 5.** Dissect and expose Cooper ligament from the symphysis pubis to just medial to the iliac vessels. This will expose Hesselbach triangle posteriorly, and during this dissection, any direct or femoral hernia can be identified and reduced. Be careful not to injure an aberrant obturator artery, which frequently crosses Cooper ligament near the femoral canal and adjacent to Gimbernat ligament.
- **Step 6.** While holding the epigastric vessels anteriorly and against the ventral abdominal wall with one hand, further dissect the preperitoneal space laterally and dorsally by pushing the peritoneum away from the abdominal wall. The peritoneum is loosely adherent to the ventrolateral abdominal wall up to the level of the arcuate line. Leave dissection of the cord structures for last.
- **Step 7.** Dissect the internal ring and look for the hernial sac of an indirect hernia. Reduce an indirect hernia by pulling the sac out of the internal ring. If this is difficult, the neck of the sac can be isolated and divided at the internal ring. Peel the peritoneum off the cord structures to complete the dissection of the myopectineal orifice.
- **Step 8.** The gonadal vessels and vas deferens should be protected throughout the dissection.

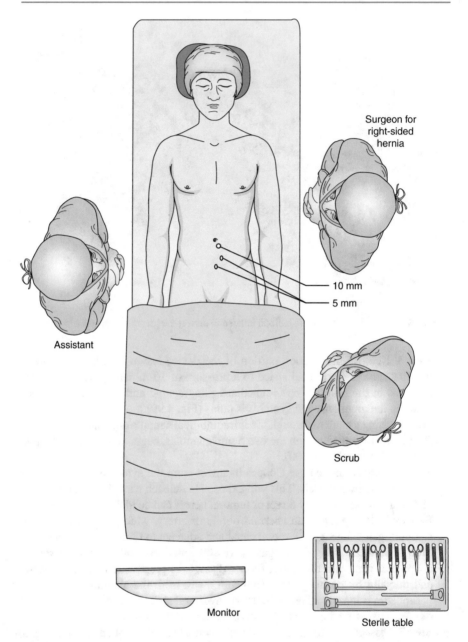

Fig. 4.99 Operating room setup and cannula sites for extraperitoneal laparoscopic inguinal herniorrhaphy

- **Step 9.** A piece of nonabsorbable mesh measuring 10 × 15 cm is rolled and placed within the peritoneal space through the 10 mm camera cannula. The mesh is unrolled and positioned over the myopectineal orifice. Alternatively, an anatomically shaped mesh can be used.

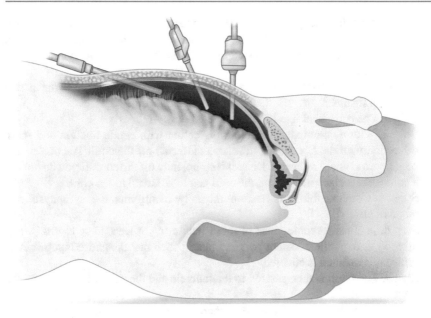

Fig. 4.100 Operating within the preperitoneal space laparoscopically

- **Step 10.** Affix the mesh using a laparoscopic tacking device. Place tacks along Cooper ligament from the symphysis pubis to just medial to the iliac vessels and along the ventral and lateral abdominal wall. Avoid the epigastric vessels. Do not place any tacks dorsal (or lateral and inferior to the cord structures) to the iliopubic tract laterally, where the femoral branch of the genitofemoral nerve, lateral femoral cutaneous nerve of the thigh, and genital branch of the genitofemoral nerve lie.
- **Step 11.** Desufflate the preperitoneal space while holding the dorsolateral corner of the mesh against the abdominal wall. The peritoneum will hold this corner of the mesh in place.
- **Step 12.** Remove the cannulas and close the fascia of the anterior rectus sheath with absorbable 0 suture. Close the skin on all cannula sites with a subcuticular 4-0 absorbable subcuticular suture.

> **Note**
> - If the patient has a large sac that extends into the scrotum and is difficult to remove, do not waste time trying to retrieve it. Transect it at the internal ring and close the resulting defect in the peritoneum using an Endoloop.

TAP

- **Step 1.** Position the patient as above.
- **Step 2.** Insufflate the abdomen with the Veress needle in the LUQ.

- **Step 3.** Next da Vinci ports are placed in the right and left upper quadrants, and a 12 mm camera port placed just off the midline above the umbilicus to the left. A fourth assistance port was placed in the RUQ. The robot is then docked, and the procedure started.
- **Step 4.** The peritoneum is incised with the hot shears from the ASIS to the medial umbilical ligament.
- **Step 5.** The peritoneal flap is then dissected down inferiorly.
- **Step 6.** With a combination of blunt dissection with gentle traction and sharp dissection with the hot shears, the sac is dissected off the cord. Traction on the cord lipoma should reduce it. Dissect it completely off the cord. If you do not see a cord lipoma place traction on the cord and look lateral to the cord.
- **Step 7.** Continue blunt dissection medially identifying the symphysis and pubic ramus.
- **Step 8.** A nonabsorbable piece of mesh measuring at least 15 × 10 cm is then inserted through the assistant port and placed such that the entire myopectineal orifice of Fruchaud is covered.
- **Step 9.** The mesh is then sutured to the tubercle and the ring if the defect with a 0 Vicryl.
- **Step 10.** The incised peritoneum is then closed with a running STRATAFIX suture. The surgical field is checked for bleeding.
- **Step 11.** The CO2 is then released under direct vision, and then all trocars removed. Trocar sites are then assessed for fascial closure. All skin wounds are closed with the 4-0 Vicryl subcuticular.

Note: Alternatively, a laparoscopic tacking device can be used to secure the mesh.

Mesh Groin Hernia Repairs: Anterior Approach

Lichtenstein Tension-Free Herniorrhaphy

Dissect out the spermatic cord as per indirect hernia repair. For the modified Lichtenstein repair, tailor your own mesh. Make sure the mesh extends 2 cm medially beyond the pubic tubercle, 3–4 cm above Hesselbach's triangle and 5–6 cm lateral to the internal ring. Suture the mesh to the pubic tubercle. Next, position the mesh on the floor of the canal and bring the cord through the "tails" of the mesh; cross the mesh tails and suture them to the internal oblique muscle above the internal ring. Suture the mesh to Poupart ligament, the conjoined area, and the arch (Fig. 4.101).

Bard Plug and Patch Repair
Over the years I have removed many of these Bard plugs that were causing pain or extruded into the inguinal canal or having migrated elsewhere resulting in erosion into surrounding structures such as a bowel or bladder. I have come to realize that a piece of mesh, whether it is nicely rolled or wadded, is not an elegant approach. I believe this is an approach that should be avoided.

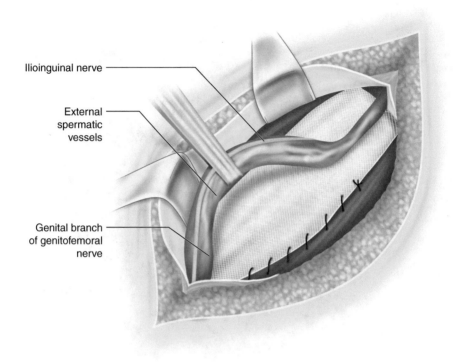

Ilioinguinal nerve

External
spermatic
vessels

Genital branch
of genitofemoral
nerve

Fig. 4.101   Lichtenstein repair

Other Repairs

Hydrocele

A hydrocele is a collection of abnormal fluid within the sac of the tunica vaginalis; it may be associated with a hernia. There are several varieties of hydrocele. We describe repair of adult non-communicating hydrocele. A communicating hydrocele—one that changes in size, as determined by patient observation—requires a high ligation of the sac in addition to partial excision of the hydrocele. Repair of pediatric hydrocele should be done by a pediatric surgeon.

Repair of Adult Non-communicating Hydrocele
- **Step 1.** For exploration, make a transverse incision. Because the terminal vascular branches in the scrotum lie transversely, this minimizes bleeding.
- **Step 2.** Carefully divide the three uppermost layers of the testis. Deliver the testis with its covering outside the scrotum.
- **Step 3.** Withdraw the fluid from the sac (Fig. 4.102) and observe the spermatic cord.

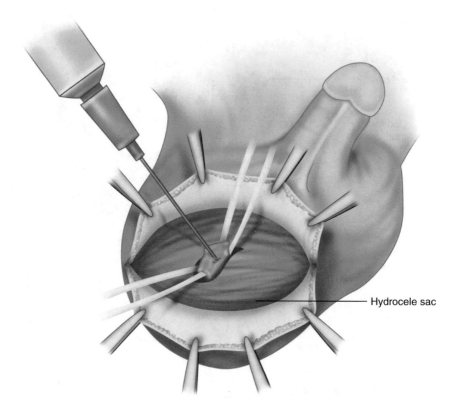

Fig. 4.102 Draining the hydrocele sac

- **Step 4.** Observe the covering of the spermatic cord.
- **Step 5.** Open the tunica vaginalis and perform a subtotal or total removal of the sac.
- **Step 6.** Approximate the dartos muscle and close the skin. Use only a few catgut sutures for the approximation, thereby avoiding skin inversion due to dartos retraction.

Lumbar Hernia Repair (Dowd-Ponka)

- **Step 1.** Make an incision—oblique or vertical—over the hernia site. Remember that in the upper hernia, the sac lies beneath skin, superficial fascia, and latissimus dorsi muscle (Fig. 4.103).
- **Step 2.** Dissect out the sac and reduce.
- **Step 3.** Place a Marlex or Prolene patch over the defect, and suture to the external oblique and latissimus dorsi muscles and lumbar periosteum using 3-0 inter-

Incisions:

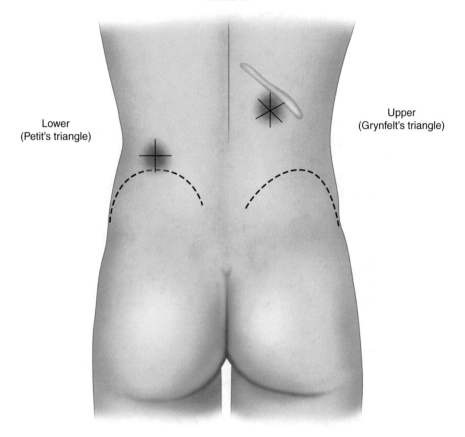

Lower
(Petit's triangle)

Upper
(Grynfelt's triangle)

Fig. 4.103 Lumbar hernia sites

rupted Surgilon (Fig. 4.104). Alternatively, place an appropriately sized Kugel patch subfascially and suture in an interrupted fashion.

- **Step 4.** Approximate the external oblique and latissimus dorsi muscles over the patch as far as possible without tension. Cut a flap of gluteal fascia, as shown by the dotted line in Fig. 4.105.
- **Step 5.** Use the flap of gluteal fascia turned up to cover the defect remaining and secure it to the present muscles with 0 Surgilon interrupted sutures (Fig. 4.106).
- **Step 6.** Close the subcutaneous fat and skin. Jackson–Pratt drains may be necessary.

Note
- Alternatively, repair of these hernias can be done using a Bard Ventrio mesh. Dissect out the sac and attenuated fascia from the surrounding tissue down to the hernial ring. Gently establish a space below the ring such that the mesh can reside with 3 cm of the overlap. Secure mesh.

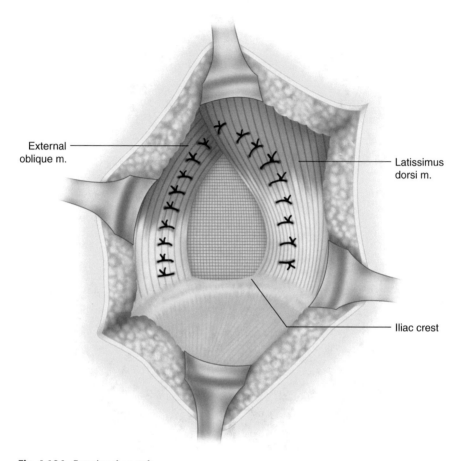

External
oblique m.

Latissimus
dorsi m.

Iliac crest

Fig. 4.104 Suturing the patch

Anatomical Complications of the Abdominal Wall and Hernia

Complications of Groin Hernia Repair

- Injury to vessels—the vessels usually involved are the inferior epigastric, external iliac vessels, or vessels of the spermatic cord. Less frequently involved vessels are the superficial epigastric artery and vein, the deep and superficial circumflex vessels, and obturator artery. In addition, injury to an aberrant obturator artery may occur when incising Gimbernat's ligament to relieve a strangulated femoral hernia.
- Injury to nerves injury to the iliohypogastric, ilioinguinal, or genitofemoral nerves may result. Postoperative neuralgia occurs in approximately 10% of patients. Chronic pain occurs much less. Injuries may be a result of suture placement, tack fixation, and scarring where the nerve becomes encumbered by scar

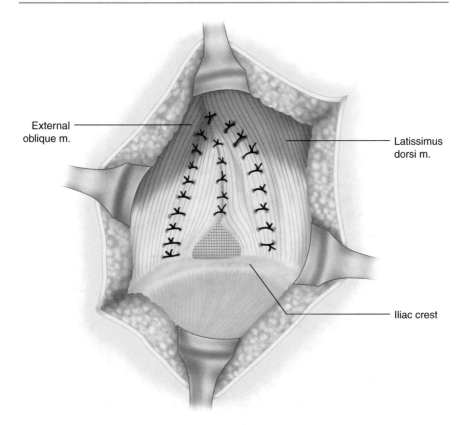

Fig. 4.105 Approximating the muscles

tissue or the nerve becoming enmeshed with the mesh. Any of these injuries can result in neuroma formation.
- Injury to the vast deferens.
- Injury to adjacent organs: small bowel, colon, and bladder. This would include not recognizing ischemia of the bowel from a strangulated hernia.
- Testicular atrophy from injury to the vessels of the spermatic cord.

Complications of Ventral Hernia Repair
Many complications of ventral hernia repairs can be linked to morbid obesity, diabetes with hemoglobin A-1 C greater than 7.5, and smoking. However, there are also complications of technique.

- Wound complications, necrosis of the skin edges, surgical site infection.
- Seroma formation.
- Hematoma formation usually from the epigastric vessels.
- Wound dehiscence.

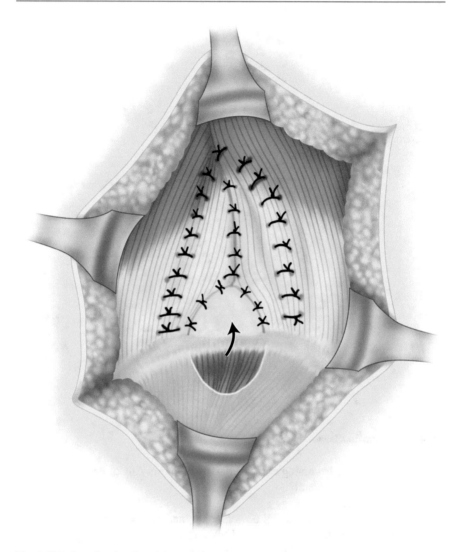

Fig. 4.106 Securing the gluteal fascia flap

- Bowel injury leading to fistula formation. This can be a result of mesh eroding into a bowel or an unrecognized injury.
- Mesh complications: mesh infection, mesh erosion into an adjacent hollow viscous, central mesh failure usually associated with the lightweight macroporous meshes.
- Iatrogenic hernia formation. This can occur when performing an anterior component separation procedure. When incising the external oblique laterally if that incision is taken too deep, a hernia may result. An intra-parietal hernia may result if the peritoneal sac is not properly closed. This can result in bowel protruding through the peritoneum but staying below the muscles.

Diaphragm

5

C. Daniel Smith

Anatomy

The diaphragm is a musculomembranous entity separating the thorax from the abdomen. The muscular part originates anteriorly from the xiphoid process, laterally from the inner surface of the six lower cartilages, and posteriorly from the medial and lateral lumbosacral arches, the median arcuate ligament, and the bodies of the three upper lumbar vertebrae. The muscular part inserts on the central tendon.

Crura

The crura arise from the anterior surface of the first to fourth lumbar vertebrae on the right, the first two or three lumbar vertebrae on the left, and from the intervertebral disks and the anterior longitudinal ligament. The crural fibers pass superiorly and anteriorly, forming the muscular arms that surround the openings for the aorta and the esophagus. They then insert on the central tendon. At their origins from the vertebrae, the crura are tendinous, becoming increasingly muscular as they ascend into the diaphragm proper (Fig. 5.1). Studies have found that in 90% of cadavers, posteriorly and medially, from their vertebral origins to the level of the tenth thoracic vertebra, the crura are tendinous. Sutures to approximate the crura should always be placed through the tendinous portions.

The pattern of the crural arms at the esophageal hiatus is variable. In one-half or more, both right and left arms arise from the right crus (Fig. 5.2a). In another one-third or more, the left arm arises from the right crus and the right arm arises from both crura (Fig. 5.2b). The remaining individuals present a variety of uncommon patterns. Hiatal hernia is not associated with any specific hiatal pattern.

C. D. Smith (✉)
Esophageal Institute of Atlanta, Atlanta, GA, USA
e-mail: cdsmith@esophageal.institute

© Springer Nature Switzerland AG 2021
L. J. Skandalakis (ed.), *Surgical Anatomy and Technique*,
https://doi.org/10.1007/978-3-030-51313-9_5

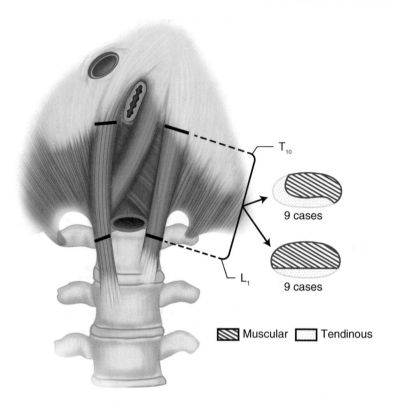

Fig. 5.1 The crura consist of both tendinous and muscular tissue; only the tendinous portion holds sutures. In nine out of ten persons, the medial edge of the crura is tendinous

Openings of the Diaphragm

Hiatus of the Inferior Vena Cava
The hiatus of the inferior vena cava lies in the right dome of the central tendon about 2.5 cm to the right of the midline and at the level of the eighth thoracic vertebra. The margins of the hiatus are fixed to the vena cava, which is accompanied by branches of the right phrenic nerve (Fig. 5.3).

Esophageal Hiatus
The elliptical esophageal hiatus is in the muscular portion of the diaphragm 2.5 cm or less to the left of the midline at the level of the tenth thoracic vertebra (Figs. 5.4 and 5.5). The anterior and lateral margins of the hiatus are formed by the muscular arms of the diaphragmatic crura. The posterior margin is formed by the median arcuate ligament (Fig. 5.6). The anterior and posterior vagal trunks and the esophageal arteries and veins from the left gastric vessels pass through the hiatus with the esophagus.

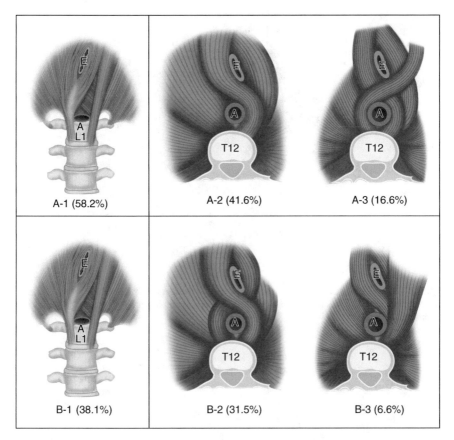

Fig. 5.2 The most common patterns of the diaphragmatic crura. (**a-1**) and (**b-1**) seen from below. (**a-2**, **a-3**) and (**b-2**, **b-3**) seen from above. *E* esophagus, *A* aorta

Regardless of its components, the normal hiatus should admit one or two of the surgeon's fingers if there is no folding of the peritoneum into the mediastinum.

The following means of narrowing the hiatus have been preferred:

- Vertical posterior approximation of the crura (Fig. 5.7a). This is a commonly used method.
- Vertical anterior approximation of the crura (Fig. 5.7b). Some surgeons recommend this type of repair. It has the following advantages: (1) it can be easier than posterior approximation, but care must be taken to avoid the nearby pericardium; (2) the crura are more tendinous anteriorly; and (3) the procedure accentuates the gastroesophageal angle.
- Horizontal narrowing of the hiatus (Fig. 5.7c). In some patients, a transverse defect is apparent; hence a horizontal approximation is appropriate.

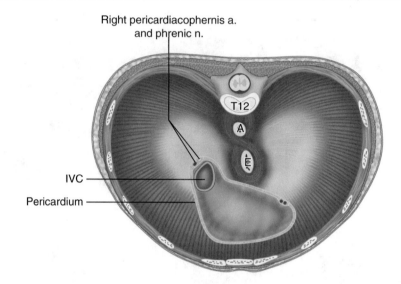

Fig. 5.3 The diaphragm viewed from above. The area in contact with the pericardium is indicated. The pericardial fibrous tissue is continuous with that of the diaphragm. *IVC* inferior vena cava, *E* esophagus, *A* aorta

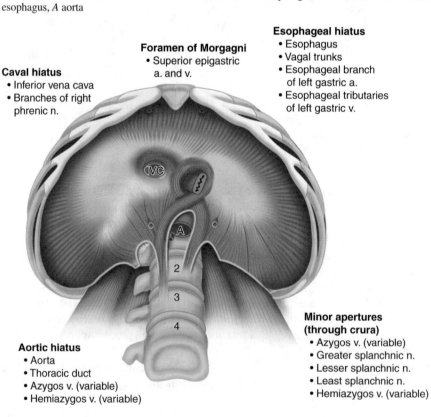

Fig. 5.4 The apertures of the diaphragm seen from below and the structures traversing them. *IVC* inferior vena cava, *A* aorta

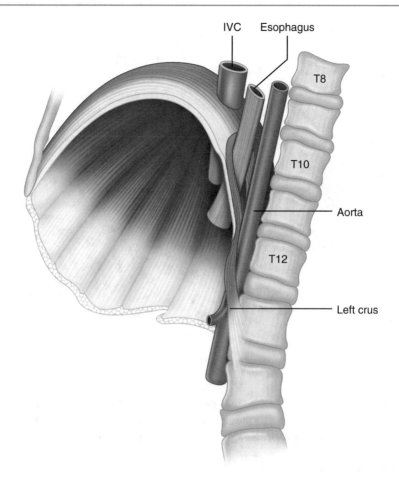

Fig. 5.5 The diaphragmatic openings for the inferior vena cava (IVC), the esophagus, and the aorta as seen from the left

Aortic Opening

The oblique course of the aorta takes it behind the diaphragm rather than through it (Fig. 5.5). The thoracic duct and (usually) the azygos vein accompany the aorta through the "opening." At the level of the twelfth thoracic vertebra, the anterior border of the opening is bridged by the median arcuate ligament. Laterally the diaphragmatic crura form the margins of the opening.

Other Openings in the Diaphragm

Anteriorly, the superior epigastric vessels pass through the parasternal spaces (foramina of Morgagni). In the dome of the diaphragm, the phrenic nerves pierce the upper surface to become distributed over the lower surface between the muscle and peritoneum.

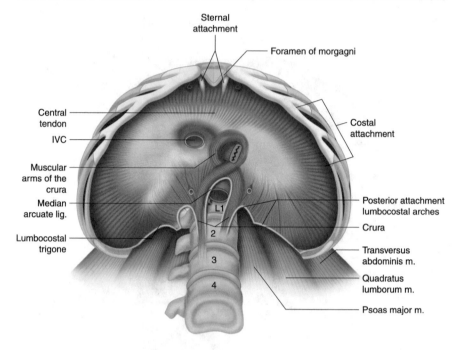

Fig. 5.6 The attachments of the muscles of the diaphragm seen from below. *IVC* inferior vena cava

The azygos vein may pass behind the diaphragm with the aorta (to the right of the right crus), or it may pierce the right crus. Also passing through the crura are the greater, lesser, and least thoracic splanchnic nerves (Fig. 5.4).

Median Arcuate Ligament

The esophageal hiatus is separated from the aortic hiatus by fusion of the arms of the left and right crura. If the tendinous portions of the crura are fused, the median arcuate ligament is present as a fibrous arch passing over the aorta, connecting the right and left crura. If the fusion is muscular only, the ligament is ill defined or absent.

The median arcuate ligament passes in front of the aorta at the level of the first lumbar vertebra, just above the origin of the celiac trunk (Fig. 5.6). In 16%, a low median arcuate ligament covers the celiac artery and may compress it.

In about 50% of cadavers with hiatal hernia studied, the ligament was sufficiently well developed to use in surgical repair of the esophageal hiatus. In the remainder, there was enough preaortic fascia lateral to the celiac trunk to perform a posterior fixation of the gastroesophageal junction (GEJ). At operation surgeons must avoid the celiac ganglion, which is just below the arcuate ligament.

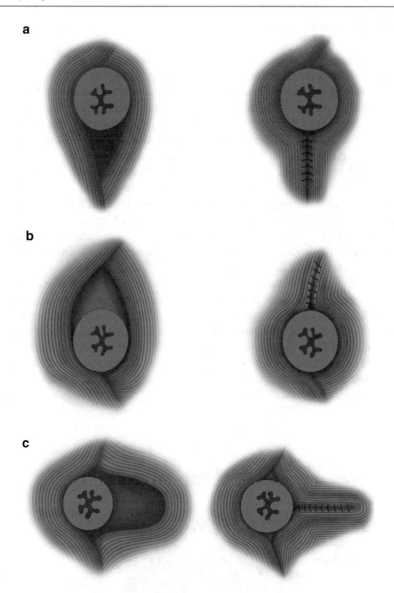

Fig. 5.7 Three methods of narrowing the esophageal hiatus. (**a**) Vertical with posterior approximation of the crura. (**b**) Vertical with anterior approximation of the crura. (**c**) Horizontal with shortening of one crus

Diaphragmatic-Mediastinal Relations

The fibrous tissue of the central tendon is continuous with the fibrous pericardium over much of the anterosuperior surface of the diaphragm (Fig. 5.3).

In addition to the pericardium, the mediastinum on the right contains the inferior vena cava; right phrenic nerve and pericardiophrenic vessels; right pulmonary ligament; esophagus with the right vagal trunk; thoracic duct; azygos vein and azygos arch; vertebral bodies; greater and lesser right thoracic splanchnic nerves; right sympathetic trunk; and right posterior intercostal arteries (Fig. 5.8).

In the left mediastinum are the pericardium; left phrenic nerve and pericardiophrenic vessels; esophagus; left vagal trunk; descending aorta; vertebral bodies; hemiazygos vein, accessory hemiazygos vein, highest intercostal vein; greater and lesser left thoracic splanchnic nerves; and left sympathetic trunk.

The triangle (of Truesdale) formed by the pericardium, aorta, and diaphragm contains the left pulmonary ligament and the distal esophagus. In sliding hiatus hernia, the stomach is in this triangle (Fig. 5.9).

The remainder of the superior surface of the diaphragm is covered with parietal pleura. The approximation of the right and left pleurae between the esophagus and the aorta forms the so-called mesoesophagus. The right pleura is in contact with the lower third of the esophagus almost as far down as the esophageal hiatus (Fig. 5.10). This proximity creates the risk of accidental entrance into the pleural cavity during abdominal operations on the esophageal hiatus. Even so, because surgeons work on the right side of the operating table, they are more likely to produce a pneumothorax or hemopneumothorax on the left.

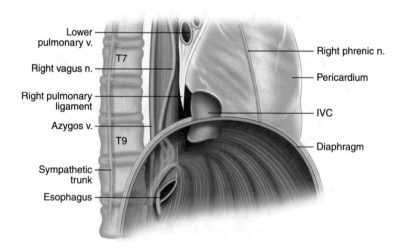

Fig. 5.8 Structures in the inferior portion of the right mediastinum. *IVC* inferior vena cava

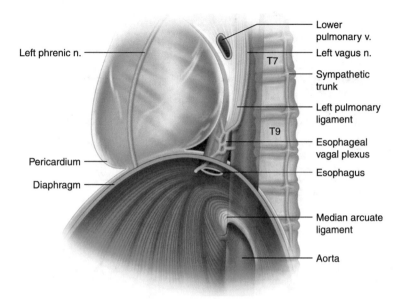

Fig. 5.9 Structures in the inferior portion of the left mediastinum

Vascular System of the Diaphragm

Arterial Supply
The arterial supply to the superior surface of the diaphragm consists of two branches from the internal thoracic arteries—the pericardiophrenic and musculophrenic arteries—and two branches from the thoracic aorta, the superior phrenic arteries. All these branches are small.

The major blood supply to the diaphragm is to the inferior surface. It comes from the inferior phrenic arteries, which arise from the aorta or the celiac axis just below the median arcuate ligament of the diaphragm. In a small percentage of individuals, the right inferior phrenic artery arises from the right renal artery. The inferior phrenic arteries also supply branches to the suprarenal glands (Fig. 5.11).

Venous Drainage
On the superior and inferior surfaces, the veins run with the arteries (Fig. 5.12).

Lymphatic Drainage
All the diaphragmatic lymph nodes lie on the superior surface of the diaphragm. These nodes can be divided into anterior, middle, and posterior groups (Fig. 5.13).

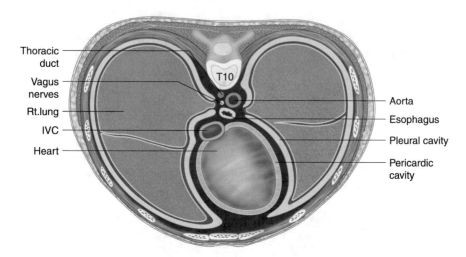

Fig. 5.10 Cross section through the thorax at the level of T$_{10}$ showing the relation of the pleura to the distal esophagus. *IVC* inferior vena cava

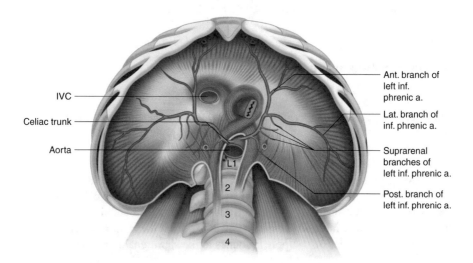

Fig. 5.11 Arterial supply of the diaphragm from below. The inferior phrenic arteries may arise from the celiac trunk or directly from the aorta. *IVC* inferior vena cava

They receive drainage from the upper surface of the liver, the gastroesophageal junction, and the abdominal surface of the diaphragm.

Efferent lymph vessels from these nodes drain upward to parasternal and mediastinal nodes anteriorly and to posterior mediastinal and brachiocephalic nodes posteriorly.

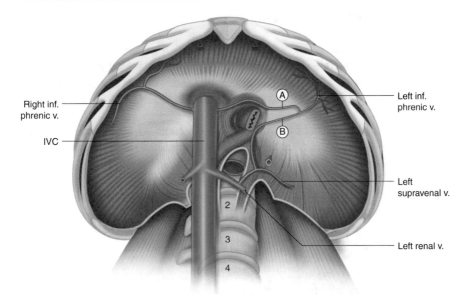

Fig. 5.12 Venous drainage of the diaphragm from below. The left inferior phrenic vein may enter the inferior vena cava (*A*), the left suprarenal vein (*B*), or both. *IVC* inferior vena cava

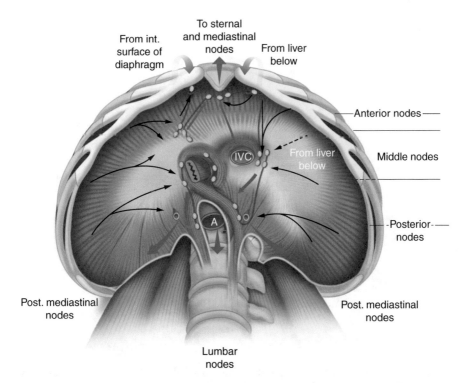

Fig. 5.13 Lymphatic drainage of the diaphragm seen from above. The diaphragm receives lymph from the liver below and sends it to ascending sternal, anterior, and posterior mediastinal nodes. *IVC* inferior vena cava, *A* aorta

Nerve Supply of the Diaphragm

The right phrenic nerve enters the diaphragm through the central tendon just lateral to the opening for the inferior vena cava. Occasionally it passes through that opening with the vena cava. The left phrenic nerve pierces the superior surface of the muscular portion of the diaphragm just lateral to the left border of the heart (Fig. 5.14).

The peripheral portions of the pleura and peritoneum have an independent sensory innervation that arises from the seventh to the twelfth intercostal nerves.

Structures at or Near the Esophageal Hiatus (Fig. 5.15)

Several structures lie close to the esophageal hiatus of the diaphragm and hence may be injured in surgical procedures on the hiatus. They are:

- Left inferior phrenic artery and left gastric artery
- Left inferior phrenic vein
- Left gastric (coronary) vein
- Aberrant left hepatic artery, if present
- Other vessels (celiac trunk, aorta, inferior vena cava)
- Vagal trunks (Fig. 5.16)
- Celiac ganglia
- Thoracic duct
- Subphrenic spaces
- Lower esophagus

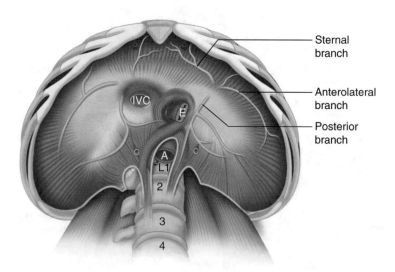

Fig. 5.14 The major branches of the phrenic nerves from below. Each phrenic nerve divides just before entering the diaphragm from above. *IVC* inferior vena cava, *E* esophagus, *A* aorta

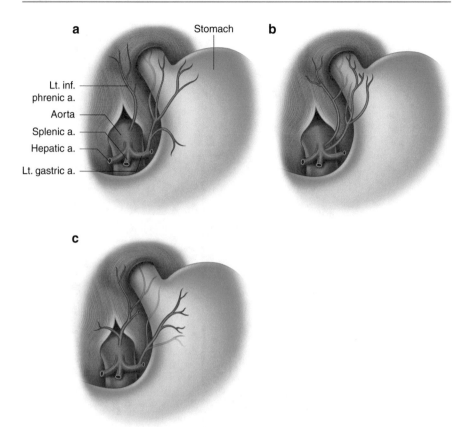

Fig. 5.15 Variations in the blood supply to the distal esophagus and the esophageal hiatus. (**a**) The inferior phrenic artery supplies the margin of the hiatus. An esophageal branch of the left gastric artery supplies the esophagus and anastomoses with the thoracic esophageal arteries. This is the most frequent pattern. (**b**) The esophagus is supplied by esophageal branches of the left gastric and the inferior phrenic arteries without cranial anastomoses. (**c**) The esophagus is supplied entirely by a branch of the inferior phrenic artery, which anastomoses with the thoracic esophageal arteries. This pattern is rare

Extensive mobilization or skeletonization of the lower esophagus may result in perforation during a surgical procedure, or afterward, from subsequent local ischemia.

Technique

Diaphragmatic Hernia

Normal anatomy of the esophageal hiatus is shown in sagittal section in Fig. 5.17a. *Hiatus hernia* is a protrusion of a portion of the stomach into the thoracic mediastinum through the esophageal hiatus of the diaphragm. It includes a hernial sac (Table 5.1).

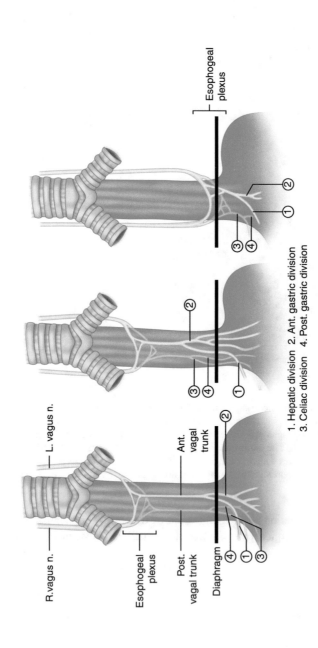

Fig. 5.16 Where four or more vagal structures emerge through the hiatus, they may be (**left**) divisions that have separated just above the diaphragm, (**center**) divisions and their branches that arise above the diaphragm, or (**right**) elements of the esophageal plexus that extend below the diaphragm. The vagal trunks are entirely within the abdomen

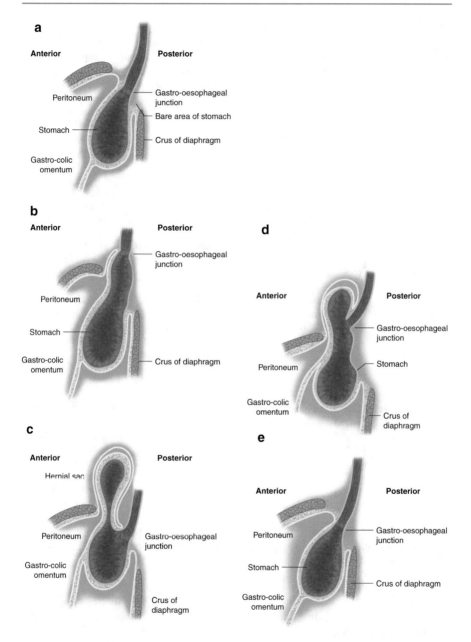

Fig. 5.17 Esophageal hiatus in sagittal section with (**a**) normal anatomy and (**b–e**) the various abnormalities described in the text: (**b**) sliding hiatus hernia, (**c**) paraesophageal hiatus hernia, (**d**) combined sliding and paraesophageal hiatus hernia, (**e**) congenital short esophagus

Table 5.1 Hernia through the esophageal hiatus

Hernia	Anatomy	Sac and contents	Remarks
Sliding hiatus hernia Fixed hiatus hernia	Congenital potential hernia. G–E junction and cardia are displaced upward to enter the mediastinum above the diaphragm. The phrenoesophageal membrane is attenuated. The herniated stomach may move freely or become fixed in the thorax	Sac lies anterior and to the left of herniated stomach. Contents: cardia, stomach	A large hiatus (admitting three fingers) may be a predisposing factor. Actual herniation usually occurs in middle life but has been seen in newborn
"Pure" paraesophageal hernia	Congenital potential hernia. The G–E junction and cardia are in normal position. The fundus has herniated through the hiatus into the thorax beside the esophagus	Sac lies anterior to esophagus and posterior to pericardium. Contents: cardia and fundus of stomach	An enlarged hiatus may be a predisposing factor. Actual herniation occurs in adult life
Combined sliding and paraesophageal hernia	Congenital potential hernia. The G–E junction, cardia, and much of the greater curvature of stomach have herniated into the thorax	Sac lies anterior to esophagus and posterior to pericardium in right posteroinferior mediastinum. Sac may contain fundus and body of stomach, omentum, transverse colon, and spleen	A hiatus already enlarged by a hiatus hernia. Progresses to complete thoracic stomach with volvulus
Congenital short esophagus	Congenital hernia. The G–E junction and cardia are displaced upwards and fixed in the thorax	No sac present	This lesion is rare. It appears to result from failure of the embryonic esophagus to elongate enough to bring the G-E junction into the abdomen

From SW Gray, LJ Skandalakis, and JE Skandalakis. Classification of hernias through the esophageal hiatus. In: Jamieson, GG (ed.) *Surgery of the Esophagus*. Edinburgh: Churchill Livingstone, 1988, pp. 143–148. (Reprinted with permission)

Several types of hiatus hernia are recognized today: sliding hiatus, paraesophageal hiatus, combined sliding and paraesophageal, congenital short esophagus, and traumatic diaphragmatic.

In sliding hiatus hernia, the esophagus moves freely through the hiatus, with the gastroesophageal junction in the thorax or in the normal position at different times. Sliding hernias make up 90% of all hiatus hernias (Fig. 5.17b). A sac is present. An uncommon type of sliding hernia is one that becomes secondarily fixed in the thorax by adhesions. The esophagus in such patients appears to be too short to reach the diaphragm because of contraction of the longitudinal muscle coat.

In paraesophageal hiatus hernia, the gastroesophageal junction remains in its normal location. The gastric fundus cardia and greater curvature bulge through the hiatus beside the esophagus; a sac is present. Volvulus of the herniated stomach is a major complication (Fig. 5.17c).

A combined sliding and paraesophageal hernia occurs when the gastroesophageal junction is displaced upward, as in a sliding hernia, and the fundus and greater curvature are herniated, as in a paraesophageal hernia (Fig. 5.17d).

Much debate centers around the classification of the congenital short esophagus. Three conditions must be considered. (1) In the *grossly normal esophagus*, the lower portion of the esophagus is lined by gastric mucosa (Barrett esophagus). This may be described also as heterotopic gastric mucosa. (2) In the *irreducible partially supradiaphragmatic true stomach*, the stomach has herniated into the thorax through an enlarged diaphragmatic esophageal hiatus and become fixed. This is true fixed hiatus hernia. (3) *Partially supradiaphragmatic true stomach* exists from birth and is not reducible. This is true "congenital short esophagus" (Fig. 5.17e) and is very rare.

Remember: When performing surgery for esophageal hernia, to
- Avoid injury to the vagus nerves.
- Avoid injury to the mediastinal pleura.
- Avoid injury to the left hepatic vein.
- Avoid perforation of the esophagus.
- Watch for an aberrant blood supply to the left triangular ligament.
- Watch for accessory bile ducts.
- Consider inserting a bougie.
- Consider gastropexy or gastrostomy.
- Consider an antireflux procedure.

Repair of Sliding Hiatus Hernia
- **Step 1.** A transverse, oblique, or vertical midline incision may be used. Incise the triangular ligament and retract the left lobe of the liver.
- **Step 2.** Develop a window starting on the right at the base of the crura and encircle all hiatal content including both left and right vagus nerves with a Penrose drain to allow safe manipulation of the herniated proximal stomach and distal esophagus.
- **Step 3.** While retracting on the Penrose drain, follow the crura circumferentially to mobilize the herniated content and hernia sac out of the mediastinum being careful to peal the sac off the pleura and pericardium thereby avoiding creating a pneumothorax or lung injury.
- **Step 4.** Dissect the greater curvature of the stomach, beginning at the cardia and continuing toward the gastrosplenic ligament and the vasa brevia. One or two vasa brevia may be divided, but damage to the spleen must be avoided (Fig. 5.18).

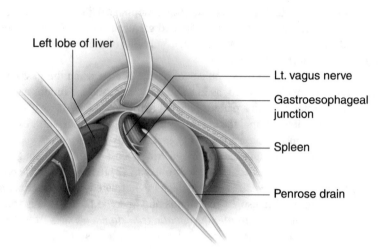

Fig. 5.18 Placement of Penrose drain

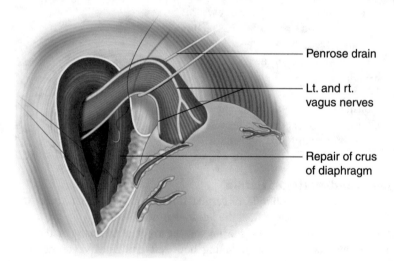

Fig. 5.19 Repair of hiatus

- **Step 5.** Dissect the diaphragm and the tissue beneath the esophagus. A widened hiatus can be repaired with 0 nonabsorbable sutures, carefully avoiding the underlying aorta, celiac axis, and pleura. Do not constrict the esophagus (Fig. 5.19).
- **Step 6.** Nissen Fundoplication. The anesthesiologist passes sequentially larger dilators into the esophagus until a No. 56 French dilator is positioned across the

gastroesophageal junction to prevent constriction by an excessively tight fundic wrap.

Remember
- Avoid the gas-bloat syndrome by protecting the vagus nerve and maintaining an adequate lumen in the distal esophagus through a loose fundoplication.
- If the vagus nerve is transected, perform a pyloroplasty.
- If the pylorus is stenotic, pyloroplasty is again recommended.
- If chronic peptic ulcer disease (duodenal ulcer) is present, vagotomy and pyloroplasty should be performed.
- It is nearly impossible to make a Nissen fundoplication too loose and very easy to make it too tight, so err on the side of the former.

Step 7. Wrap the fundus of the stomach 360° around the lower esophagus, and insert 2-0 silk sutures from the stomach to the esophagus to the stomach (Fig. 5.20).

Step 8. Place at least 2–4 sutures to complete the wrap such that it measures 2 cm in length (Fig. 5.21).

Step 9. In select patients in whom delayed gastric emptying is likely, perform a Stamm gastrostomy and close the abdominal wall.

Note
- When the wrap is completed, the surgeon should be able to place one finger between the wrap and the anterior esophageal area (see Fig. 5.27).

Repair of Paraesophageal Hernia

Procedure
- **Step 1.** Open the abdomen as for sliding hiatus hernia. Incise the left triangular ligament of the liver.
- **Step 2.** Reduce the stomach and esophagus into the abdomen (Fig. 5.22).
- **Step 3.** Open the hernia sac and expose the esophagus. Protect the anterior vagal trunk, and excise the sac (Fig. 5.23).
- **Step 4.** Perform anterior approximation of the crura with interrupted 0 nonabsorbable sutures (Fig. 5.24). Alternatively, perform posterior approximation of the crura. Occasionally the lesser curvature of the stomach is sutured to the left crus posteriorly with interrupted 2-0 silk sutures. The diaphragm should admit one finger between it and the esophagus (Figs. 5.25, 5.26, and 5.27).
- **Step 5.** The fundus of the stomach may be sutured to the undersurface of the diaphragm with 3-0 silk to add stability to the anatomical repair (Fig. 5.26).

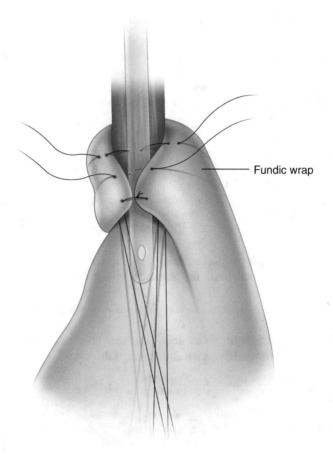

Fig. 5.20 Fundic wrap

- **Step 6.** A fundic wrap (see Nissen Fundoplication, step 4 of "Repair of Sliding Hiatus Hernia," earlier in this chapter) may be added to the repair in those unusual instances where a mixed paraesophageal hernia with reflux is present (Fig. 5.27).

Repair of Traumatic Diaphragmatic Hernia
- **Step 1.** Explore the abdomen through an upper midline incision.
- **Step 2.** Identify the defect and determine its extent. Inspect the intestines and other organs in the abdominal cavity for injury.
- **Step 3.** Approximate the edges of the diaphragm with interrupted 0 nonabsorbable sutures.
- **Step 4.** Insert a chest tube.

Laparoscopic Nissen Fundoplication
Various types of fundoplication have been used in the treatment of hiatal hernia and/or gastroesophageal reflux disease (GERD). Of these, the Nissen fundoplication

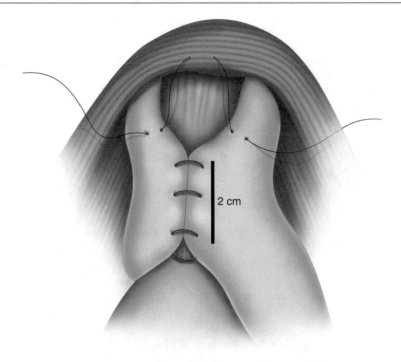

Fig. 5.21   Suturing the wrap

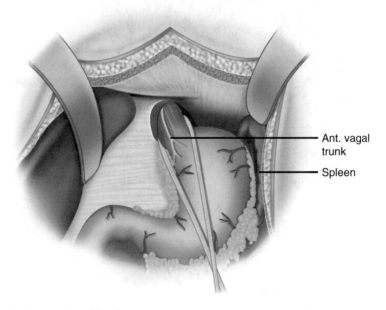

Fig. 5.22   Paraesophageal hernia

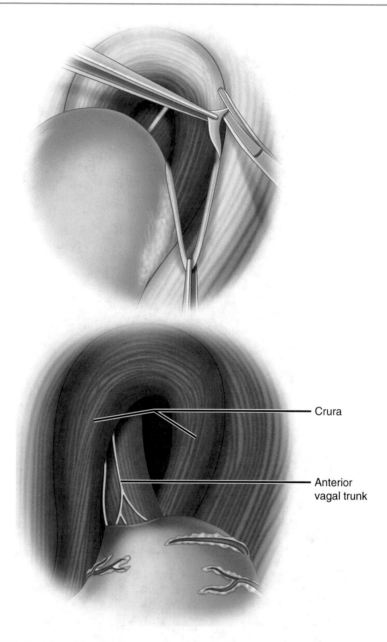

Fig. 5.23 Excision of the sac

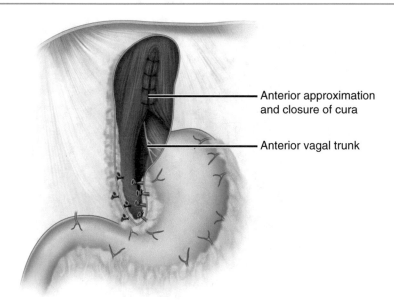

Fig. 5.24   Anterior approximation

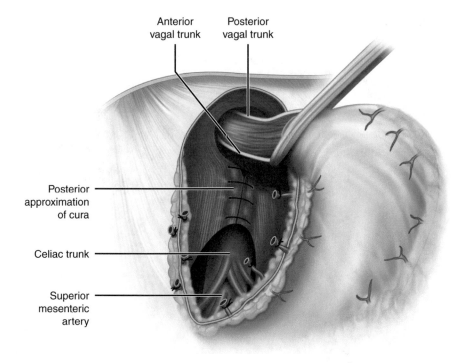

Fig. 5.25   Posterior approximation

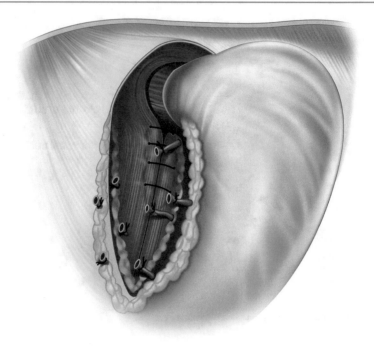

Fig. 5.26 Suturing of fundus

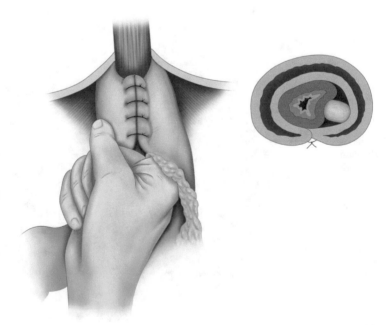

Fig. 5.27 Fundic wrap. Inset: cross section of repair

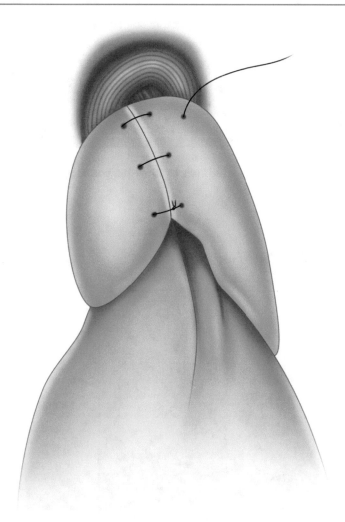

Fig. 5.28 The Nissen fundoplication with 360° fundic wrap. The completed wrap should be no greater than 2 cm in length

(360° wrap) (Fig. 5.28) has been the most widely performed and studied. It has been proven durable and effective in the control of GERD and in maintaining an intra-abdominal location of the gastroesophageal junction (GEJ) after hiatal hernia repair.

Since 1992, the laparoscopic technique of Nissen fundoplication has replaced the traditional open operation. It provides patients with a significantly enhanced postoperative recovery and excellent long-term outcomes. Rather than a hospital stay of 5–7 days and a 6-week postoperative convalescence—which is necessary with open fundoplication—patients who have had laparoscopic Nissen fundoplication remain hospitalized only 24 h and return to their usual activities within 1–2 weeks.

Preoperative: Mild laxative evening before surgery (e.g., one bottle of magnesium citrate orally)

Note
- Esophagoscopy and barium swallow should confirm diagnosis.
- 24-h esophageal pH monitoring or esophageal motility studies may be necessary.

Position: Supine with legs in stirrups to allow surgeon to operate from between the patient's legs (Fig. 5.29)

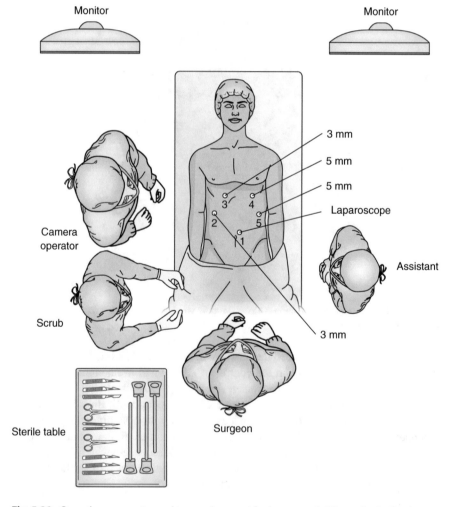

Fig. 5.29 Operating room setup and trocar placement for laparoscopic Nissen fundoplication

Anesthesia: General

Others: Foley catheter if operative expected to be more than 2 h and pneumatic compression hose

- **Step 1.** Prep and drape the patient so that either laparoscopy or open surgery can be performed.
- **Step 2.** Establish carbon dioxide pneumoperitoneum to 15 mmHg with a Veress needle inserted through a stab incision just below the umbilicus.
- **Step 3.** Insert five cannulas as detailed in Fig. 5.29.
- **Step 4.** Position liver retractor inserted through cannula No. 2 so that the left lobe of the liver is retracted ventrally, thereby exposing the anterior surface of the proximal stomach near the GEJ.
- **Step 5.** First assistant—using instrument inserted through cannula No. 5—grasps the anterior stomach just distal to the GEJ retracting caudally.
- **Step 6.** Operating through cannulas Nos. 3 and 4, use an energy hemostasis device (e.g., Harmonic Scalpel) to open the hepatogastric omentum over the caudate lobe of the liver and just above the hepatic branch of the vagus nerve (Fig. 5.30). This exposes the right crus of the diaphragm (**Note:** Either an accessory or replaced left hepatic artery may course within the hepatogastric omentum and should be sought and protected).
- **Step 7.** Be aware that the anterior vagus nerve can be injured during the following dissection; however, it is usually tight against the anterior wall of the esophagus and easily avoided. Continuing with a hemostatic energy device, carry this incision to the patient's left through the phrenoesophageal ligament anteriorly and over to the anterior surface of the left crus.
- **Step 8.** Dissect the right crus from its base through the crural arch. Similarly dissect the left crus from base through arch.
- **Step 9.** Dissect gently between the crura at their bases and thereby open the retroesophageal window. Look for and protect the posterior vagus nerve (Fig. 5.31). Pass a one-inch Penrose drain around the distal esophagus (Fig. 5.32), and use this Penrose as a handle for further dissection. Dissect the distal esophagus out of the chest until at least 2–3 cm of distal esophagus can be pulled below the diaphragm without tension.

> **Note**
> - By dissecting the right and left crura of the diaphragm and thoroughly dissecting the esophageal hiatus, the distal esophagus is safely isolated.
> - Compared to the anterior vagus nerve, the posterior vagus is often more distant from the esophagus and can be injured more easily during this dissection.
> - Once it is identified, the posterior vagus should be left within the Penrose to protect it from injury during esophageal mobilization.

- **Step 10.** Mobilize the gastric fundus. Enter the lesser sac one-third of the way down the greater curve of the stomach from the angle of His and isolate and

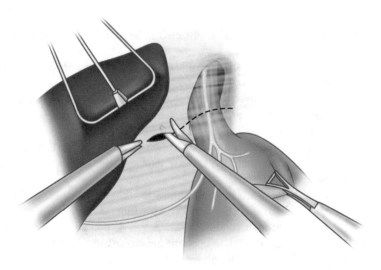

Fig. 5.30 Dissection begins by opening the hepatogastric omentum over the caudate lobe of the liver and cephalad to the hepatic branch of the vagus nerve. The incision is carried across the phrenoesophageal ligament (*broken line*)

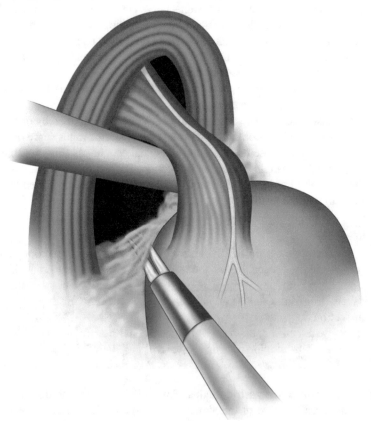

Fig. 5.31 By dissecting at the base of the crura, the retroesophageal window can be widely opened and the posterior vagus nerve identified and protected

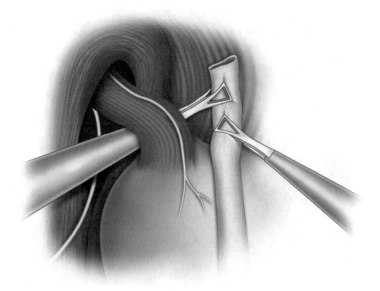

Fig. 5.32 A Penrose drain is used to encircle and retract the esophagus

divide short gastric vessels working back toward the GEJ (Fig. 5.33). This is best done with a hemostatic energy device (e.g., Liagasure). Divide any filmy attachments between the posterior wall of the proximal stomach and anterior surface of the pancreas.

> **Note**
> - Great care must be taken to avoid injury to the short gastrics or the spleen. Bleeding during mobilization of the gastric fundus may require laparotomy for control.
> - One or two "posterior" short gastric vessels or the left inferior phrenic artery are often encountered near the base of the left crus and should be expected. The Harmonic Scalpel should be used for the short gastric vessels.

Step 11. Bring the mobilized gastric fundus through the retroesophageal window and around the distal esophagus anteriorly to ensure adequate mobilization (Fig. 5.34).

> **Note**
> - When the hold on the gastric fundus is released, it should remain behind the esophagus and through the retroesophageal window. If the fundus exits the retroesophageal window and returns to its premobilized position, further mobilization is necessary (look for retrogastric connections or divide more short gastric vessels).

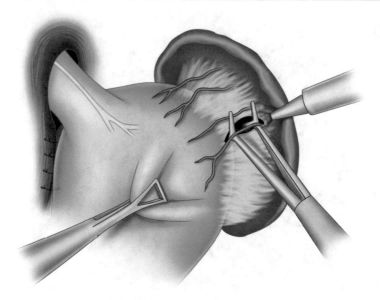

Fig. 5.33 The short gastrics are taken down beginning one-third of the way down the greater curvature of the stomach working cephalad

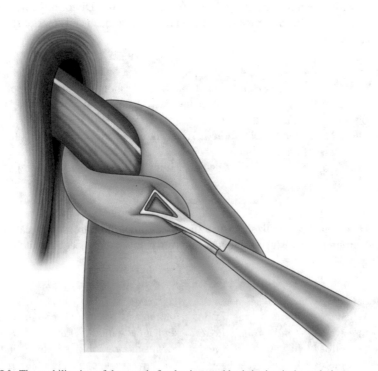

Fig. 5.34 The mobilization of the gastric fundus is tested by bringing it through the retroesophageal window anteriorly over the distal esophagus

- **Step 12.** Before completing fundoplication, reconstruct the esophageal hiatus by approximating the right and left crura behind the esophagus using interrupted 0 nonabsorbable suture. Use as many stitches as necessary to efface the crura with the distal esophagus (Fig. 5.35).
- **Step 13.** Complete the fundoplication around a 50–60 French esophageal dilator inserted by the anesthesiologist. Two to three 2-0 nonabsorbable sutures are placed with bites taking full-thickness gastric fundus and partial thickness anterior esophageal wall. When completed, the wrap should be no greater than 2 cm in length (see Fig. 5.28).

> **Note**
> - Avoid the anterior vagus nerve.
> - Sutures from the wrap to the diaphragm are optional.

Step 14. Remove cannulas and allow carbon dioxide insufflation to entirely escape the abdominal cavity.

Step 15. Close the fascia of the 10 mm incisions with an absorbable 0 suture and the skin with a subcuticular 4-0 absorbable suture.

Step 16. Patients are maintained on a soft diet and are limited to lifting no more than 10 pounds for 4 weeks postoperatively.

Linx Implantation

In 2013 the Food and Drug Administration approved magnetic sphincter augmentation with the Linx device (Fig. 5.36). This device is a bracelet of magnetic beads

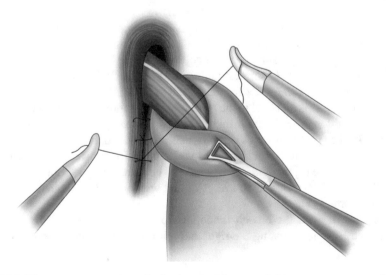

Fig. 5.35 The crura are approximated using interrupted sutures tied intra- or extracorporeally

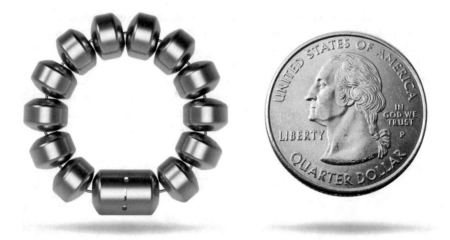

Fig. 5.36 Linx device

used in place of the Nissen fundoplication to augment the lower esophageal sphincter and thereby correct gastroesophageal reflux and help anchor the gastroesophageal junction below the diaphragm when used with hiatal hernia repair (Fig. 5.37).

The device offers outcomes comparable to a Nissen fundoplication and the following advantages over a Nissen fundoplication:

- Less invasive due to sparing use of the gastric fundus and the dissection and manipulation needed to mobilize the gastric fundus and wrap it 360 degrees around the gastroesophageal junction
- More reproducible performance in augmenting the sphincter
- Easier operation and more reproducible procedure and outcomes across a range of surgeon experience and skill (Nissen fundoplication typically requires a specialist to attain consistently good outcomes)
- More physiologic function allowing patients rto more readily belch and vomit and thereby avoiding the Nissen side-effect of gas bloat
- Easily reversible by a simple laparoscopic procedure for removal
- An overall lower rate to surgical failure and need for revisional surgery

The approach to using Linx for management of GERD and in association with hiatal hernia repair is identical to the Nissen fundoplication described above, except for Steps 10 through 13. In performing a Linx placement, Steps 10–14 are:

- **Step 10.** The posterior vagus nerve is identified and mobilized from the esophagus just proximal to its first branches which typically occur at or just below the gastroesophageal junction. This "window" between the posterior vagus nerve and the esophagus should be avascular and with only filmy tissue between the two structures (Fig. 5.38).
- **Step 11.** As with the Nissen fundoplication, the esophageal hiatus is reconstructed by approximating the right and left crura behind the esophagus using

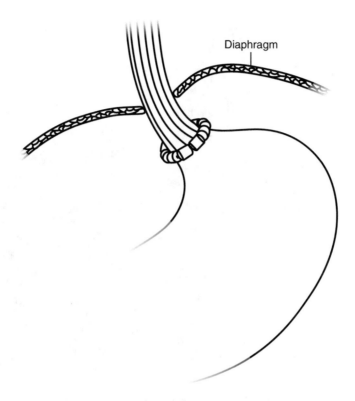

Fig. 5.37 Linx device in place around distal esophagus

interrupted 0 nonabsorbable suture, using as many stitches as necessary to achieve effacement of the crura to the non-retracted distal esophagus.
- **Step 12.** A sizing device is used to determine the appropriate size Linx device to place. Sizes vary based on the number beads that make up the bracelet. Sizing should result in a device that provides effacement with the esophagus without compression.

Note
- When considering size, err to the device being loose around the esophagus rather than compressing the esophagus.

- **Step 13.** An appropriate size device is then placed around the esophagus using the window that was created between the posterior vagus nerve and the esophagus. In this way the posterior vagus nerve is excluded from the device (Fig. 5.39).
- **Steps 14 and 15** remain the same as for the Nissen fundoplication.

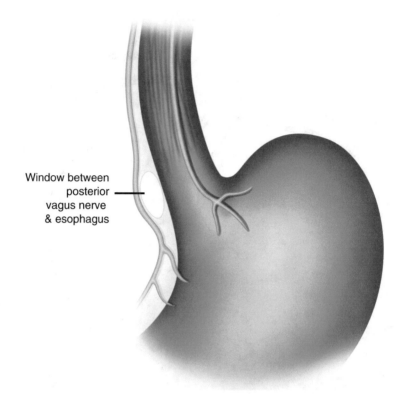

Window between
posterior
vagus nerve
& esophagus

Fig. 5.38 Dissection window between posterior vagus nerve and esophagus for Linx positioning

- **Step 16.** Patients are expected to eat some food of normal consistency every 3 h while awake starting immediately at hospital discharge. This is important to provide frequent opening and closing of the Linx device, while scar and healing are encapsulating the device. In this way the scar becomes flexible and allows the device to open and close easily with swallowing. This along with limiting lifting to no more than 10 pounds is necessary for the first 4 weeks after surgery. After this time patients can resume normal lift and physical activity and typically no longer need to eat every something every 3 h.

Note
- Eating something every 3 h is commonly referred to as "breaking-in" the device.
- This break-in period is usually complete after 4 weeks.
- Some patients need to continue the frequent small meals for more than 4 weeks when the scar takes longer to remodel and soften.

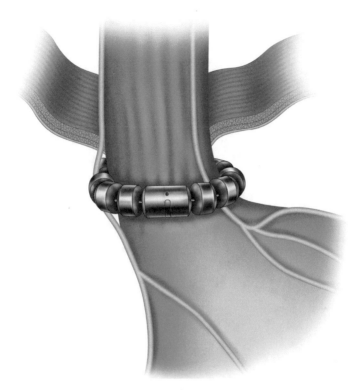

Fig. 5.39 Linx in place and relationship to posterior vagus nerve

Complications

Worldwide, the failure rate of Linx requiring removal is 3%. The most common reason for removal is dysphagia, followed by failure to control GERD, and rarely, esophageal erosion. All complications or failures of Linx are treated with device removal resulting in complete correction of the complication without need for further surgery. In the case of failure to control reflux, a Nissen fundoplication can be performed during the Linx removal procedure.

Erosion has been the most feared complication due to the perception that this leads to esophageal perforation. This condition occurs when the device erodes through the esophageal wall with device beads present in the esophageal lumen visualized during an upper endoscopy. Because this is a late complication, the device is entirely encapsulated with scar tissue when this occurs thereby preventing perforation into the abdominal cavity. Instead, an ulcer forms between the device and the esophageal lumen.

Erosion has occurred in 0.2% of patients, and all cases have been managed with an elective procedure to remove the device, either laparoscopically or endoscopically through the erosion tract, without any need for esophageal resection or major corrective surgery, and without any long-term or ongoing consequence.

Esophagus

6

C. Daniel Smith

Anatomy

General Description of the Esophagus

Length of the Esophagus

The esophagus is about 25 cm in length. The most useful reference point is the upper incisors, which are about 15 cm above the pharyngoesophageal junction; if the external nares are included, 7–9 cm must be added. In defining the esophagus, it is adequate to divide it into cervical, thoracic, and abdominal segments.

Constrictions of the Esophagus

Major Constrictions

There are three major constrictions:

- The cricopharyngeal or pharyngoesophageal constriction (diameters 1.7 × 2.3 cm).
- The bronchoaortic constriction. Anatomically there are two separate constrictions: the aortic at the level of T4 with diameters of 1.9 × 2.3 cm and the bronchial at the level of T5 with diameters of 1.7 × 2.3 cm.
- The diaphragmatic constriction at the level of T9 or T10 with a diameter of 2.3 cm.

These constrictions define two regions of dilatation: superior (between the cricopharyngeal and bronchoaortic constrictions) and inferior (between the bronchoaortic and diaphragmatic constrictions).

C. D. Smith (✉)
Esophageal Institute of Atlanta, Atlanta, GA, USA
e-mail: cdsmith@esophageal.institute

© Springer Nature Switzerland AG 2021
L. J. Skandalakis (ed.), *Surgical Anatomy and Technique*,
https://doi.org/10.1007/978-3-030-51313-9_6

Minor Constrictions (Seen Occasionally)

- A retrosternal constriction may lie between the pharyngoesophageal and the aortic constrictions.
- A cardiac constriction may lie behind the pericardium and is produced if right atrial enlargement is present, as in mitral stenosis.
- A supradiaphragmatic constriction may be produced by a tortuous, arteriosclerotic aorta.

Curves of the Esophagus

The esophagus has three gentle curves: in the neck, behind the left primary bronchus; below the bifurcation of the trachea; and behind the pericardium. In terms of vertebral levels, the esophagus is to the left of the midline at T1, to the right at T6, and to the left again at T10.

Remember the three Cs: three constrictions and three curves. Most esophageal pathology (e.g., lodgment of foreign bodies, burns from caustic chemicals, and cancer) is located at or close to these constrictions. The bronchoaortic constriction is the most frequently involved.

Topography and Relations of the Esophagus

The tubercle of the cricoid cartilage is the single constant landmark of the upper esophageal opening.

Pharyngoesophageal Junction

The muscular pharyngeal wall is formed by three overlapping muscles: the superior, middle, and inferior pharyngeal constrictors. The inferior constrictor muscle (Fig. 6.1) blends inferiorly with the sphincter-like transverse cricopharyngeal muscle, which blends with the circular, muscular esophageal wall. Between the two parts of the cricopharyngeal muscle is the weak area (triangle) of Killian. There is another weak area between the lower transverse and the muscular coat of the esophagus (Fig. 6.1). These weak areas may become the site of acquired pulsion diverticula (Zenker's, above; Laimer's, below). They also are the sites of possible perforation by an esophagoscope.

Two anatomical entities at this point contribute to narrowing of the esophageal lumen: internally the hypopharyngeal fold and externally the cricopharyngeal muscle. At this location perforation by instruments, lodging of foreign bodies, spasm, and neoplasms tends to occur.

The cricopharyngeal muscle and the lower border of the cricoid cartilage demarcate the end of the pharynx and the start of the esophagus. The so-called inferior constrictor of the pharynx, the cricopharyngeal muscle, originates from

Fig. 6.1 The lateral aspect of the pharyngoesophageal junction showing (**a**) the upper weak area; (**b**) the lower weak area; (1) the oblique fibers of the inferior constrictor muscle; (2) the cricopharyngeal muscle; (3) the muscularis of the esophagus

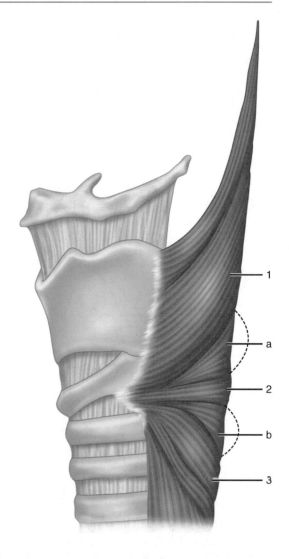

the thyroid and cricoid cartilages. It is composed of two parts, the upper oblique and the lower transverse; the lower transverse is probably the cricopharyngeal sphincter.

Logically, a diverticulum above the transverse portion of the cricopharyngeal muscle should be recognized as pharyngeal and one originating below as esophageal. However, in the literature this distinction is not always made (Fig. 6.2). For example, a diverticulum originating above the junction, which should be called Zenker's, may instead be referred to as pharyngoesophageal or esophageal, causing confusion.

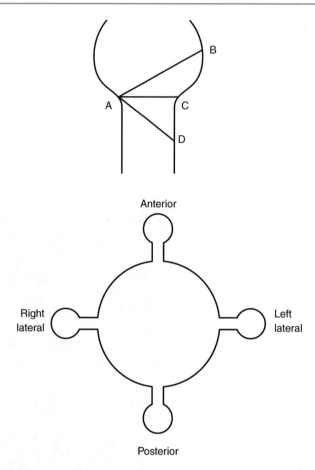

Fig. 6.2 *Top*: highly diagrammatic presentation of the musculature of the pharyngoesophageal junction. AB = oblique muscle; AC = transverse muscle; AD = muscular coat. Sites of potential diverticula are as follows: ABC = Killian's triangle (1908) = pharyngeal diverticulum; ABD = Zenker's diverticulum (1878) = pharyngoesophageal diverticulum; ACD = esophageal weakness = esophageal diverticulum. A congenital diverticulum has a wide neck and includes all layers. An acquired diverticulum has a narrow neck and no muscular coat. *Bottom*: highly diagrammatic presentation of diverticula. *Note*: The anterior diverticulum is a rare congenital condition

Cervical Esophagus

The cervical esophagus is approximately 5–6 cm long and extends from C6 to T1 or from the cricoid cartilage and cricopharyngeal muscle to the thoracic inlet at the level of the sternoclavicular joints. The carotid tubercle (of Chassaignac), which is the palpable anterior tuberosity of the transverse process of C6, is a good anatomical landmark. It projects somewhat to the left of the trachea, and incisions are commonly made on this side to approach the esophagus.

Anteriorly, the cervical esophagus is covered by the larynx and trachea.

Anterolaterally, there are four anatomical entities related to the esophageal wall on each side (see Fig. 2.15). From the periphery inward, they are the carotid sheath, the inferior thyroid artery, the lobe of the thyroid gland, and the recurrent laryngeal nerve. Also related to the distal cervical esophagus on the left side is the thoracic duct.

Posteriorly, the cervical esophagus is related to the alar fascia, the prevertebral fascia, the longissimus cervicis muscle, and the vertebrae.

Between the alar fascia and the prevertebral fascia is the retrovisceral space, the so-called danger space that extends down the mediastinum and ends approximately at the level of T4.

Pretracheal Space

The space in front of the trachea is not related directly to the esophagus. It is related clinically, however, since perforations of the anterior esophageal wall may open into the pretracheal space and therefore the mediastinum, producing a serious or even fatal mediastinitis.

Thoracic Esophagus

The thoracic portion of the esophagus extends from the level of T1 to T10 or T11. Successful esophageal surgery requires knowledge of the anatomy of the mediastinum; we remind the reader that the thoracic esophagus is located in the superior and posterior mediastinum. The key structure of the superior mediastinum is the aortic arch. The posterior mediastinum displays venous structures on the right and arterial structures on the left.

The anterior relations of the thoracic esophagus from above downward consist of the following structures: trachea and aortic arch, right pulmonary artery, left main bronchus, esophageal plexus below the tracheal bifurcation, pericardium and left atrium, anterior vagal trunk, esophageal plexus, and esophageal hiatus.

The posterior relations of the thoracic esophagus are vertebral column, longus colli muscle, right posterior intercostal arteries, left thoracic duct obliquely from T7 to T4, right pleural sac, azygos vein, hemiazygos vein, accessory hemiazygos vein, anterior wall of the aorta, esophageal plexus of the vagus nerve below the tracheal bifurcation, and sometimes the posterior vagal trunk.

The lateral relations on the right are mediastinal pleura, azygos vein, right main bronchus, root of right lung, right vagus nerve, and esophageal plexus (Fig. 6.3).

The lateral relations on the left are aortic arch, left subclavian artery, left recurrent laryngeal nerve, left vagus nerve, thoracic duct from T4 to C7, pleura, and descending thoracic aorta (Fig. 6.4).

The following structures are between the esophagus and the left mediastinal pleura: left common carotid artery, left subclavian artery, aortic arch, and descending aorta. The entire length of the thoracic esophagus is directly related to the right mediastinal pleura except where the arch of the azygos vein crosses above the right main bronchus.

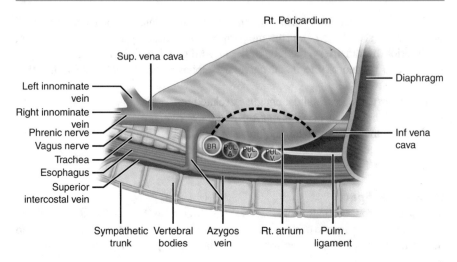

Fig. 6.3 Right mediastinum showing the disposition of its contents. *BR* bronchus, *PUL* pulmonary

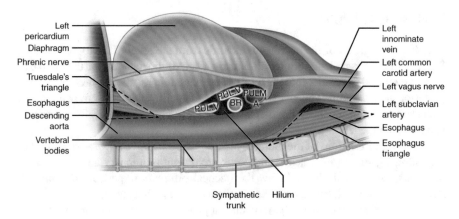

Fig. 6.4 Left mediastinum showing the disposition of its contents. *BR* bronchus, *PUL* pulmonary

Surgical Considerations
- From a surgical standpoint, lesions of the upper half of the thoracic esophagus should be explored through the right chest to avoid technical problems with the aortic arch. Lesions of the lower half of the thoracic esophagus can be explored through the left or right chest.
- With the right-sided approach, the azygos vein should be ligated and divided where it crosses the right wall of the esophagus to empty into the posterior wall of the superior vena cava. The azygos vein may be ligated with impunity. However, ligation of the superior vena cava between the atrium and the azygos vein cannot be tolerated if the azygos vein has been ligated.
- The esophageal triangle in the left side of the mediastinum is formed by the descending arch of the aorta, the subclavian artery, and the vertebral column. The

floor of the triangle is formed by the left mediastinal pleura beneath which the esophagus is located (Fig. 6.4).

- The lower end of the thoracic esophagus, which is covered by pleura, may be found in the triangle of Truesdale. The triangle of Truesdale is formed by the diaphragm below, the pericardium above and anteriorly, and the descending aorta posteriorly (Fig. 6.4). The posterior approximation of the right and left pleurae between the esophagus and the aorta forms the so-called meso-esophagus. The right pleura are in contact with the lower one-third of the esophagus, almost to the diaphragmatic hiatus. This proximity of the right pleura to the hiatus introduces the risk of pneumothorax during abdominal operations on the hiatus. The anterior approximation of the two pleurae is at the sternal angle (see Fig. 5.10).

Anatomic Weak Points

Two anatomically weak areas of the esophageal wall – one above and one below the cricoid muscle – have been mentioned. They can become the sites of pulsion diverticula. Another weak area, the left lateral posterior wall of the esophagus near the diaphragm, is occasionally the site of spontaneous idiopathic rupture of the healthy esophagus.

Abdominal Esophagus and Gastroesophageal Junction (Fig. 6.5)

External Junction

The gastroesophageal junction lies in the abdomen just below the diaphragm.

Fig. 6.5 Views of the "gastroesophageal junction" by four specialties. Each is correct

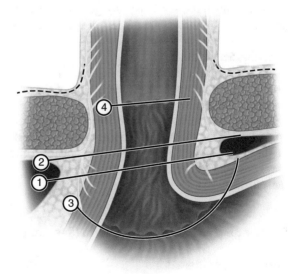

1. Anatomist   2. Surgeon
3. Radiologist   4. Endoscopist

The abdominal esophagus is said to be from 0.5 to 2.5 cm in length and occasionally as long as 7 cm. The surgeon has access to an appreciable length of esophagus below the diaphragm.

The abdominal esophagus lies at the level of the 11th or 12th thoracic vertebra and is partially covered by peritoneum in front and on its left lateral wall. Relations with surrounding structures are as follows:

Anterior: The posterior surface of the left lobe of the liver, the left vagal trunk, and the esophageal plexus

Posterior: One or both crura of the diaphragm, the left inferior phrenic artery, and the aorta

To the right: The caudate lobe of the liver

To the left: The fundus of the stomach

Internal Junction

The histological junction between the esophagus and stomach is marked by an irregular boundary between stratified squamous epithelium and simple columnar epithelium. Above the boundary, islands of columnar gastric epithelium may be present at all levels of the esophagus. The lower esophagus may occasionally be lined by gastric mucosa. A biopsy specimen to identify histologic changes in the mucosa should be taken more than 2 cm above the epithelial junction to avoid most of these patches.

Part of the problem of defining the gastroesophageal junction is the fact that this mucosal boundary does not coincide with the external junction described above. In the living patient, the situation is even less simple. The submucosal connective tissue is so loose that the mucosa moves freely over the underlying muscularis. Even at rest, the junctional level may change. Figure 6.5 shows the internal gastroesophageal junction from the point of view of four specialties.

"Cardiac Sphincter"

There is a sphincter at the cardiac orifice of the stomach that normally permits swallowing but not reflux. A slight thickening of the circular musculature of the distal esophagus has been described.

Several other structures have been held responsible for closing the cardia: the angle (of His) at which the esophagus enters the stomach, the pinchcock action of the diaphragm, a plug of loose esophageal mucosa (mucosal rosette), the phrenoesophageal membrane, and the sling of oblique fibers of the gastric musculature.

Esophageal Hiatus and the Crura (See Chap. 5)

Surgical Considerations

Placing permanent sutures deep in the crura, including the attached pleura, is absolutely necessary for narrowing the hiatus. The surgeon must be certain the sutures are in the tendinous portions of the crura and not in the muscular part only. Care must be taken to avoid placing sutures too deep at the most posterior portion of the hiatus as the aorta is immediately dorsal and can be injured or entrapped in a deep suture.

Phrenoesophageal Ligament

Where the esophagus passes from the thorax into the abdomen through the diaphragmatic hiatus, a strong, flexible, airtight seal is present – the phrenoesophageal ligament. The seal must be strong enough to resist abdominal pressure, which tends to push the stomach into the thorax, and flexible enough to give with the pressure changes incidental to breathing and the movement incidental to swallowing. A seal known as the phrenoesophageal ligament or membrane consists, in principle, of the following elements: pleura, subpleural (endothoracic) fascia, phrenoesophageal fascia (of Laimer), transversalis (endoabdominal subdiaphragmatic) fascia, and peritoneum (Fig. 6.6).

The first and last of these elements provide the requirement for airtightness; the middle three provide flexibility and strength. The ligament exists in infants, is attenuated in adults, and does not exist in adult patients with hiatal hernia.

The development of the phrenoesophageal ligament can be summarized as follows:

- In newborn infants, the phrenoesophageal ligament is present.
- In adults, the ligament is attenuated, and subperitoneal fat accumulates at the hiatus.
- In adults with hiatal hernias, the ligament for all practical purposes does not exist.

Surgical Considerations: Dividing the phrenoesophageal ligament will mobilize the cardia, but the surgeon undertaking a Hill procedure must be prepared to find the ligament ill-defined or absent.

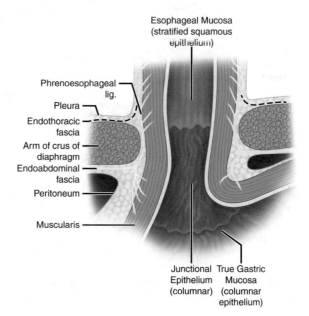

Fig. 6.6 Diagram of a coronal section through the gastroesophageal junction and the esophageal hiatus of the diaphragm

Esophageal Mucosa
(stratified squamous
epithelium)

Phrenoesophageal lig.

Pleura

Endothoracic fascia

Arm of crus of diaphragm

Endoabdominal fascia

Peritoneum

Muscularis

Junctional Epithelium (columnar)

True Gastric Mucosa (columnar epithelium)

Peritoneal Reflections

Hepatogastric (Gastrohepatic) Ligament: The abdominal esophagus is contained between the two layers of the hepatogastric ligament. The ligament contains the following structures: left gastric artery and vein; hepatic division of left vagus trunk; lymph nodes; occasionally, both vagal trunks; occasionally, branches of the right gastric artery and vein; and the left hepatic artery when it arises from the left gastric artery (in 23% of cases).

Gastrosplenic (Gastrolienal) Ligament: The hepatogastric ligament encloses the abdominal esophagus on the right; its leaves rejoin on the left of the esophagus to form the gastrosplenic ligament. The lesser sac lies behind these ligaments (for more information, see Chap. 15).

Gastrophrenic Ligament (See Chap. 7, Stomach)

The Structure of the Esophageal Wall (Fig. 6.7)

Mucosa

The esophagus is lined with a thick layer of non-keratinizing, stratified squamous epithelium continuous with the lining of the oropharynx.

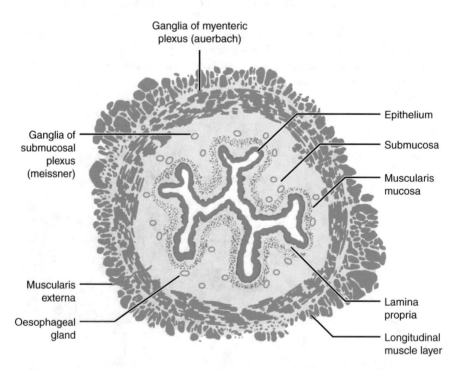

Fig. 6.7 Cross section of the esophagus showing the layers of the wall. The longitudinal and circular layers of the muscularis externa contain striated muscle fibers decreasing distally

Submucosa

A layer of loose connective tissue lies external to the mucosa. *The thick submucosa is the strongest part of the esophageal wall.* It is this layer with the lamina propria that the surgeon must count on for a sound esophageal anastomosis.

Muscularis Externa

The chief muscles of the esophagus are an internal circular layer and an external longitudinal layer. Both layers in the upper quarter of the esophagus are large striated (voluntary) muscle fibers. In the second quarter, striated and smooth (involuntary) fibers are mingled; the lower half contains only smooth fibers (Fig. 6.8).

Adventitia

The connective tissue of the mediastinum around the esophagus is not a true layer of that organ, and it does not provide the surgeon with a firm anchorage for sutures. It is the lack of a serosa that contributes to the complication of anastomotic disruption following esophageal resection and anastomosis.

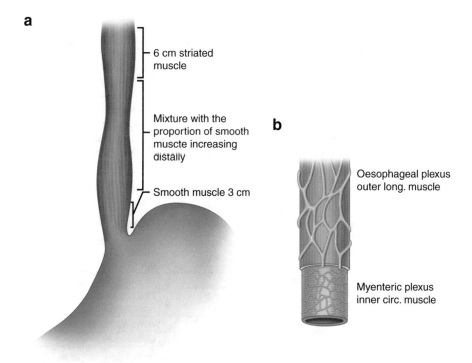

Fig. 6.8 (**a**) Relative distribution of smooth and striated muscle in the esophagus. (**b**) The extrinsic and intrinsic nerves of the esophagus

Nerve Supply to the Esophagus

Intrinsic Nerve Supply

Within the esophageal wall, there are two plexuses of nerves: Meissner's plexus in the submucosa and Auerbach's plexus in the connective tissue between the circular and longitudinal muscularis externa.

Extrinsic Nerve Supply

The esophagus receives nerves from three sources: cerebrospinal, sympathetic, and parasympathetic (vagal).

Blood Supply of the Esophagus

The blood supply, segmental or not, is adequate for intramural anastomoses. Poor technique, not poor blood supply, is responsible for leakage (Tables 6.1 and 6.2).

Table 6.1 Arterial supply of the esophagus

Esophageal segment	Primary	Secondary or occasional
Cervical	Br. of inferior thyroid aa.	Br. of pharyngeal aa.
	Anterior: Trachea and esophagus	Br. of subclavian a.
	Posterior: Esophagus and longitudinal trachea and transverse anastomoses	Br. of bronchial a. Superior thyroid a.
Upper thoracic	Br. of subclavian a. or lower branches of inferior thyroid a.	Ant. Esophagotracheal a. from aortic arch
Mid-thoracic	L. Bronchial a. ascending br. to esophagus and trachea; descending br. to esophagus	R. Internal thoracic R. Costocervical trunk R. Subclavian a.
	R. bronchial a. branches as L. but smaller	
	Ascending and descending branches may arise directly from aortic arch	
Lower thoracic	Superior and inferior esophageal aa. from aorta	Branches from R. intercostal aa.
Abdominal	Branches of L. gastric a.	Variable: R. inferior phrenic a.
	L. inferior phrenic a.	Branches from splenic a.
		Branches from superior suprarenal a.
		Accessory L. hepatic a.
		Celiac trunk

From JE Skandalakis, SW Gray, and LJ Skandalakis. Surgical Anatomy of the Esophagus. In: GG Jamieson. *Surgery of the Esophagus*. Edinburgh: Churchill Livingstone, 1988, pp. 19–35. Reprinted with permission

Table 6.2 Venous drainage of the esophagus

Esophageal segment	Venous drainage	Termination
Cervical and superior thoracic (upper 1/3)	Inferior thyroid vein Bronchial vein	Innominate vein Superior vena cava Highest intercostal vein
Thoracic (middle 1/3)	Azygos and hemiazygos veins	Superior vena cava
Inferior thoracic and abdominal (lower 1/3)	Left gastric vein Left inferior phrenic vein	Portal vein

From Skandalakis JE, Gray SW, Skandalakis LJ. Surgical anatomy of the oesophagus. In: Jamieson GG, ed. *Surgery of the Oesophagus*. Edinburgh: Churchill Livingstone, 1988. Reprinted with permission

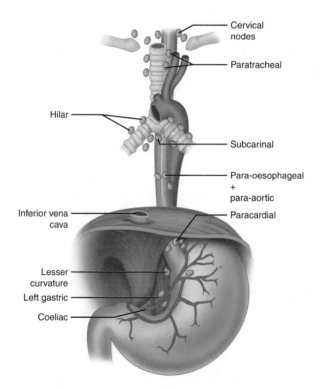

Fig. 6.9 Diagram of the groups of lymph nodes draining the esophagus. There is no standard terminology

Lymphatics of the Esophagus

The esophageal lymphatics form plexuses in the mucosa (lamina propria), submucosa, muscularis, and adventitia.

Lymph nodes are generously distributed along the esophagus, and groups of nodes have been named by their relations to adjacent organs (Fig. 6.9). "Skip areas" of up to 8 cm between lymph nodes involved in cancer may be encountered.

A few generalities about "unpredictable" drainage may be stated. Nodes of the cervical esophagus drain to internal jugular, supraclavicular, and upper paratracheal nodes. Nodes of the posterior thoracic region drain to posterior mediastinal, intercostal, and paraesophageal nodes. Nodes of the anterior thoracic region drain to tracheal, hilar, subcarinal, paracardial, and celiac nodes. Cancer involves paratracheal nodes on the right more often than those on the left. Posterior hilar nodes are more often involved than are other nodes at the carina.

Among patients with carcinoma of the cervical and upper thoracic esophagus, celiac nodes are involved in 10%. In cases of carcinoma of the middle one-third, the celiac nodes are involved in 44%. In view of the anatomical distribution of lymphatics, less than subtotal esophagectomy is not a sound procedure. For better results, esophageal resection from 6 to 10 cm above and below the tumor is mandatory.

Lymphatic Drainage of the Gastroesophageal Junction

It has been stated that cancer at the cardia spreads by lymphatics and usually appears first below the diaphragm among the gastrohepatic, gastrophrenic, gastrosplenic, and gastrocolic lymph nodes. Early metastasis to the liver may follow invasion of the gastric veins. Extension to the peripancreatic nodes is unusual. Isolated involvement of the diaphragm can occur. One study found that splenic hilar nodes were involved in 11% of spleens of patients with cancer of the gastroesophageal junction.

Metastatic spread above the diaphragm is less common, though not rare. Tumors of the esophagus just above the diaphragm may metastasize to the gastrohepatic nodes and liver.

Thus, the lymphatic channels at the cardia follow the arteries: the left gastric with its esophageal branches and the splenic with its left gastroepiploic and vasa brevia. Unorthodox dissemination, however, must not be overlooked.

Technique

Pharyngoesophageal Diverticulum

- **Step 1.** Incise as in thyroidectomy but with extension to the right or the left according to the location and presentation of the diverticulum and less extension to the opposite side. Divide the subcutaneous fascia (fat and platysma) and use special retractors for traction (Fig. 6.10).
- **Step 2.** Retract the sternocleidomastoid (SCM) muscle laterally and isolate the carotid sheath. The ansa hypoglossi, which is located in front of or within the sheath, should be saved if possible and sacrificed only if absolutely necessary. We like to divide the omohyoid muscle and ligate the middle thyroid vein. As in thyroidectomy, the thyroid lobe is retracted medially, and the recurrent nerve is found and protected. Ligate and divide the inferior thyroid vein if necessary (Fig. 6.11).
- **Step 3.** The upper part of the diverticulum may be seen medial to the SCM and lateral to the thyroid lobe and to the recurrent nerve but between the inferior pharyngeal constrictor above and the esophagus below (Fig. 6.12).

Fig. 6.10 Division of subcutaneous fascia

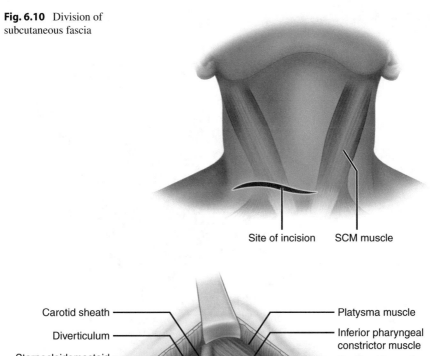

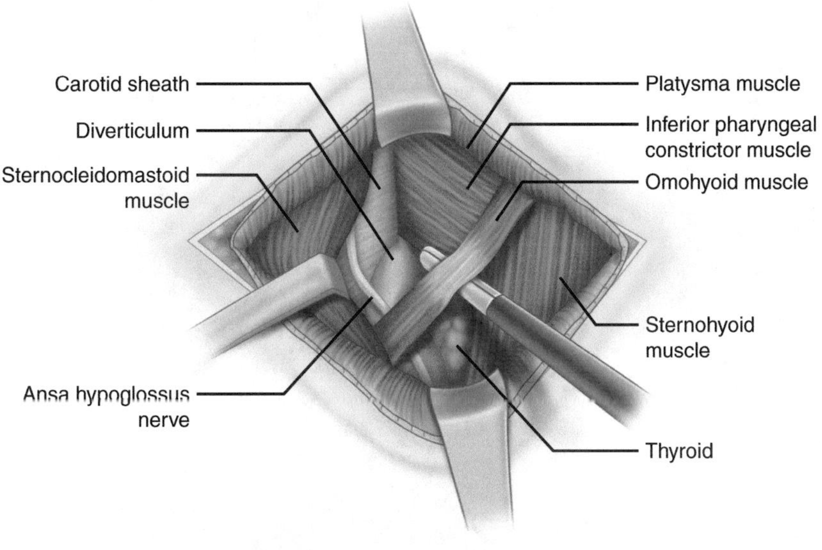

Site of incision   SCM muscle

Carotid sheath

Diverticulum

Sternocleidomastoid muscle

Ansa hypoglossus nerve

Platysma muscle

Inferior pharyngeal constrictor muscle

Omohyoid muscle

Sternohyoid muscle

Thyroid

Fig. 6.11 Division of omohyoid muscle

- **Step 4.** By blunt dissection, separate the diverticulum from all surrounding structures. Elevate it, carefully clean its neck, clamp it with two clamps, and remove it (Figs. 6.12 and 6.13).
- **Step 5.** Close the diverticulum base with 4–0 synthetic absorbable interrupted suture material. Close the cricopharyngeal muscle with mattress interrupted 3–0 synthetic nonabsorbable sutures (Fig. 6.14).
- **Step 6.** Close the wound as in thyroidectomy. Drainage is up to the surgeon.
  Another method of amputation of the diverticulum is the use of TA-30 or TA-55 staples longitudinally or transversely. Be sure to proceed as follows:

Fig. 6.12 Elevation of
diverticulum

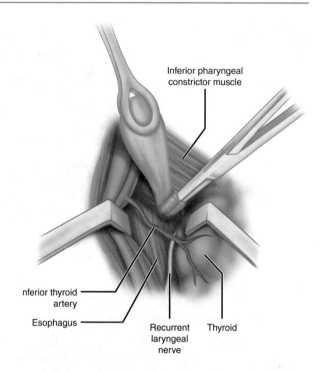

Inferior pharyngeal
constrictor muscle

nferior thyroid
artery

Esophagus

Recurrent
laryngeal
nerve

Thyroid

Fig. 6.13 Clamping of
diverticulum

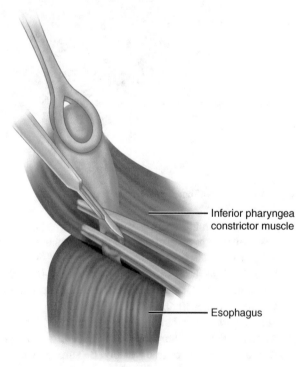

Inferior pharyngea
constrictor muscle

Esophagus

Fig. 6.14 Closure of
diverticulum base and
cricopharyngeal muscle

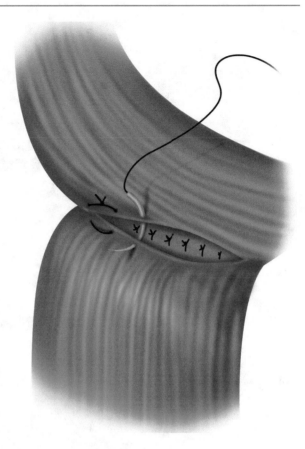

- **Step 1.** Establish good myotomy (Fig. 6.15).
- **Step 2.** Isolate the neck of the diverticulum if present.
- **Step 3.** Insert 40F Maloney dilator into the esophagus if it has not been inserted
  previously.

Achalasia or Cardiospasm

Laparoscopic Heller's Myotomy

- **Step 1.** Patient positioning, laparoscopic access, and dissection exposure of the
  gastroesophageal junction are identical to Steps 1–10 of laparoscopic Nissen
  fundoplication (see Chap. 5).
- **Step 2.** Using the Penrose drain, pull down to expose the anterior surface of the
  gastroesophageal junction anteriorly. Using an energy-assisted device (e.g., laparoscopic electrocautery), make a longitudinal incision through the longitudinal
  and circular muscle layers until the mucosal surface is exposed (dotted line in
  Fig. 6.16 indicates incision).
- **Step 3.** Extend the incision for 6 cm proximal to the gastroesophageal junction and at least 1 cm distal to this point. Care should be taken to avoid

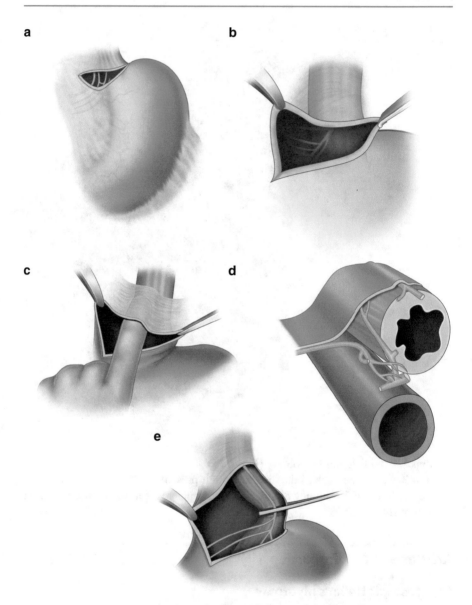

Fig. 6.15 Exposure of periesophageal space. (**a**) Incision. (**b**) Division of adventitial and adipose tissue. (**c**) Finger is used to identify abdominal esophagus. (**d**) The "stout" or dorsal meso-esophagus is disrupted by digital pressure and final perforation. If the meso-esophagus is "very stout," divide between clamps with direct vision, avoiding the posterior right esophageal wall. (**e**) The esophagus is retracted. At least 5 cm of the distal esophagus should be mobilized

injuring the anterior vagus nerve that often may cross the muscle incision (Fig. 6.17).
- **Step 4.** For a partial fundoplication, suture the gastric fundus to the left and right margin of the myotomy (Fig. 6.18).
- **Step 7.** Close the abdominal walls.

Fig. 6.16 Exposure of
mucosal surface

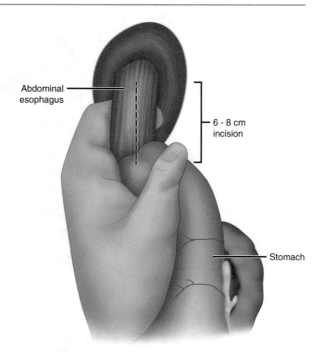

Fig. 6.17 Completed
esophagogastric myotomy

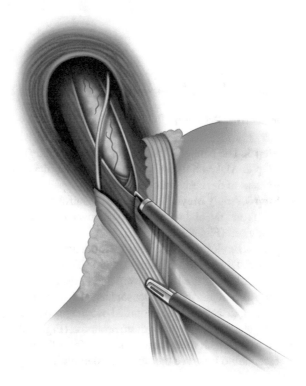

Fig. 6.18 Dimensions of
myotomy and completed
partial posterior
fundoplication

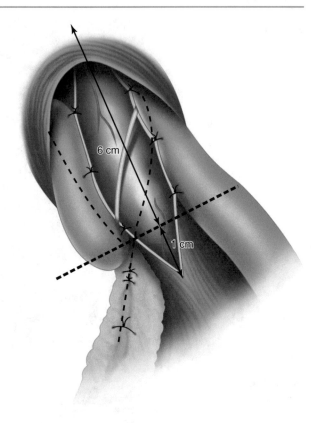

Transhiatal Esophagectomy

Abdominal Portion

- **Step 1.** The patient is placed in supine position. The head is turned to the right.
- **Step 2.** Make an upper midline abdominal incision from the left of the xiphoid process to the umbilicus (Fig. 6.19).
- **Step 3.** Apply Mayo Third Arm and Balfour retractors for better exposure of the hiatus and the abdominal cavity. A reverse Trendelenburg position of the patient is advised (Fig. 6.20).
- **Step 4.** Explore the abdomen to rule out metastatic disease and assess resectability.
- **Step 5.** Divide the left triangular and left coronary ligaments with cautery; retract the left lobe of the liver upward and to the right.
- **Step 6.** Divide the phrenoesophageal ligament. Identify the gastroesophageal junction. Encircle the abdominal esophagus by blunt palpation and sharp dissection, and place a Penrose drain around it (Fig. 6.21).
- **Step 7.** Detach the greater omentum from the stomach to the pyloric area; it is essential to preserve the right gastroepiploic and gastroduodenal vessels.

Fig. 6.19 Midline upper abdominal and oblique left cervical incisions

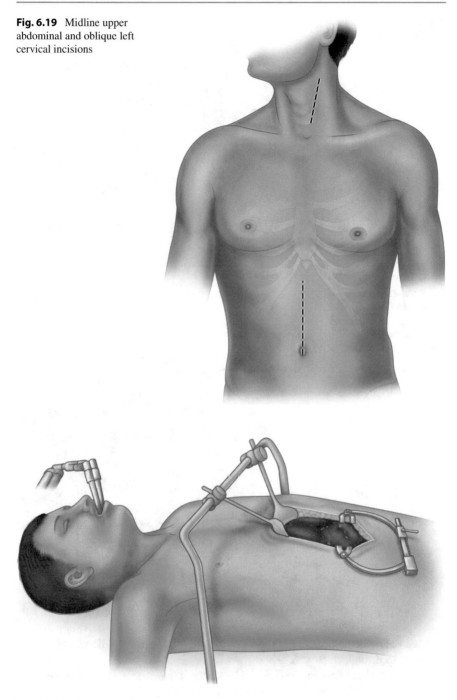

Fig. 6.20 Retractors in situ

Fig. 6.21 Penrose drain
around the esophagus

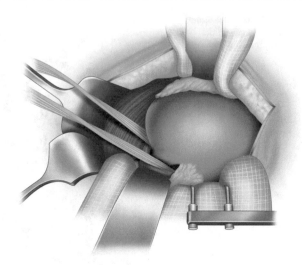

Fig. 6.22 Division of
short gastric and left
gastroepiploic vessels and
mobilization of
gastrosplenic ligament

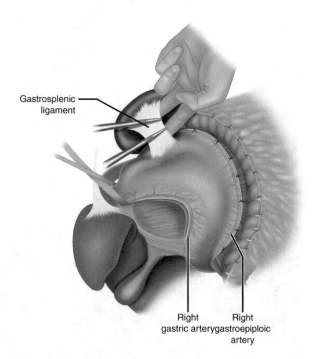

Gastrosplenic
ligament

Right
gastric artery

Right
gastroepiploic
artery

- **Step 8.** Divide and ligate the short gastric and left gastroepiploic vessels. Avoid injury to the spleen (Fig. 6.22).
- **Step 9.** Via the lesser sac, divide and ligate the left gastric vessels separately and sweep the nodal tissue toward the lesser curvature.
- **Step 10.** Perform kocherization of the duodenum and a drainage procedure (pyloromyotomy, pyloroplasty, or pyloric injection of 200 units of Botox).

Fig. 6.23 Mobilization of the stomach for esophageal replacement. The greater curvature has been mobilized, preserving the right gastroepiploic and right gastric arteries. The short gastric and left gastric arteries are divided, and a pyloromyotomy is performed

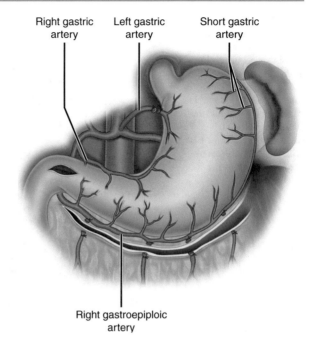

Right gastric artery   Left gastric artery   Short gastric artery

Right gastroepiploic artery

Preserve the right gastric and right gastroepiploic vessels. The stomach is now totally mobilized from the hiatus to the pylorus, and its vitality is secured by the right gastroepiploic and right gastric vessels.

- **Step 11.** Mobilize the abdominal esophagus distally by retracting on the Penrose drain (Figs. 6.23 and 6.24).
- **Step 12.** Enlarge the hiatus by partial division of the right crus. Continue mobilizing the esophagus up to the level of the carina. Avoid injury to the azygos vein and membranous trachea. If necessary, control minor bleeding with packing. Perforating vessels from the aorta can be divided under direct visualization.

Cervical Portion

- **Step 1.** Make an oblique left cervical incision along the medial border of the SCM muscle from the level of the sternal notch to just below the mandible.
- **Step 2.** Retract the SCM laterally, divide the omohyoid and sternothyroid muscles, and retract laterally the carotid sheath. Divide and ligate the inferior thyroid artery.
- **Step 3.** Carefully mobilize the esophagus. Identify the left recurrent laryngeal nerve and retract the trachea and thyroid gland medially. Enter the retroesophageal space medial to the carotid and jugular vessels. By blunt dissection, develop the posterior plane. Insert a Penrose drain around the esophagus. Avoid injury of the great auricular accessory recurrent laryngeal nerve (Fig. 6.25).

Fig. 6.24 Mobilization of the lower portion of the esophagus during transhiatal esophagectomy. A Penrose drain, encircling the esophagogastric junction, is used to provide countertraction, while the posterior midline dissection is performed with the volar aspects of the fingers against the esophagus

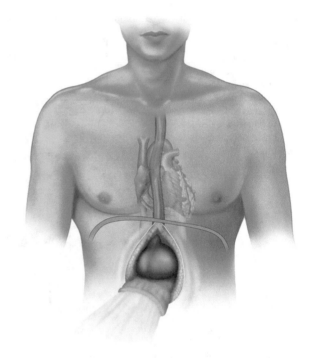

Fig. 6.25 An oblique cervical incision used for transhiatal esophagectomy. The platysma and omohyoid muscles are divided; the sternocleidomastoid muscle is retracted posteriorly, and a Penrose drain is placed around the cervical esophagus

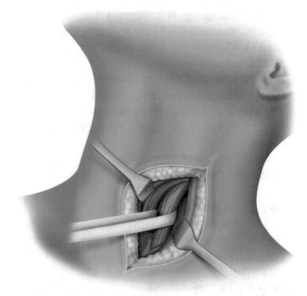

- **Step 4.** Slowly and carefully perform total anterior and posterior esophageal mobilization via cervical and hiatal approach using the right and left index fingers; they will meet each other close to or just above the carina (Fig. 6.26).
- **Step 5.** With an endoscopic gastrointestinal anastomosis (GIA) stapler, divide the cervical esophagus approximately 5 cm distal to the cricopharyngeal muscle (Fig. 6.27).

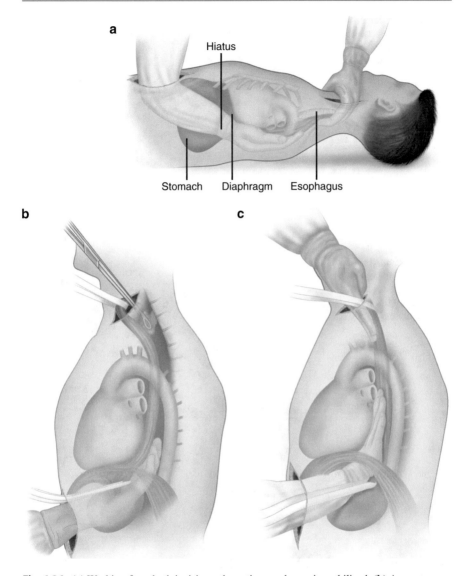

Fig. 6.26 (**a**) Working from both incisions, the entire esophagus is mobilized. (**b**) A sponge on a stick, inserted through the cervical incision into the posterior mediastinum, facilitates mobilization of the esophagus away from the prevertebral fascia. (**c**) Mobilization of the anterior aspect of the esophagus during transhiatal esophagectomy. The palmar aspects of the fingers are placed against the esophagus, and pressure is exerted posteriorly to minimize cardiac displacement and resultant hypotension

- **Step 6.** Suture a Penrose drain at the distal end of the divided cervical esophagus. If not using a stapler, apply stay sutures at the proximal end to keep the esophageal mucosa in situ.
- **Step 7.** Pull the Penrose drain down via the posterior mediastinum and deliver the esophagus into the abdominal wound via the diaphragmatic hiatus.

Fig 6.27 Division of the cervical esophagus with a gastrointestinal anastomosis (GIA) stapler

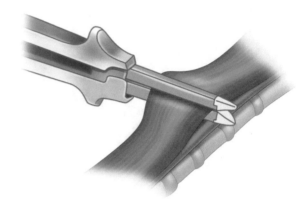

Fig. 6.28 After resection of the esophagus, the stomach is divided with sequential applications of the GIA stapler at least 4–6 cm away from palpable tumor

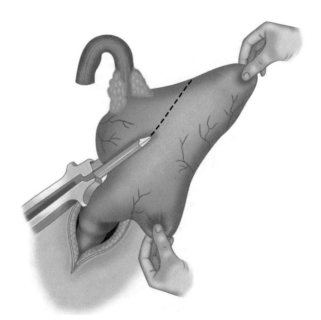

Preparation of the Gastric Conduit (Neoesophagus) and Anastomosis

- **Step 1.** Using a linear GIA 75 stapler, divide the stomach distal to the gastro-esophageal junction to remove a portion of the greater curvature and the adjacent lymph nodes (Fig. 6.28). Over sewing the staple line with 3–0 interrupted silk Lembert sutures is optional. The resection specimen will contain approximately 90% of the esophagus and proximal one-third of the stomach. Obtain frozen section analysis of esophageal and stomach margins prior to anastomosis.
- **Step 2.** Position the gastric conduit (neoesophagus) gently from below into the posterior mediastinum and push it up to the cervical incision, making sure that no rotation of the stomach (stapled portion of stomach to the patient's right) has occurred (Fig. 6.29).

Fig. 6.29 The final position of the intrathoracic stomach after transhiatal esophagectomy. The gastric fundus is suspended from the prevertebral fascia several centimeters above the cervical anastomosis, and the pyloromyotomy is located 2–3 cm below the diaphragmatic hiatus

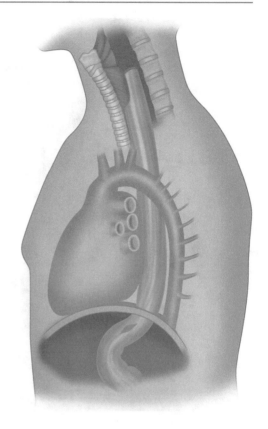

- **Step 3.** In an end-to-side technique with single-layer interrupted 4–0 PDS, double-layered 3–0 silk, or a combined endoscopic GIA stapler and sutures, anastomose the stomach to the oblique opening of the cervical esophagus (Fig. 6.30). It is paramount for the anastomosis to have good blood supply, no tension, and no evidence that residual cancer or Barrett's esophagus is present at the anastomosis.
- **Step 4.** Place a flat, closed-system suction drain in the retroesophageal space, and bring it out through a separate stab incision laterally. Carefully inspect the abdominal cavity and posterior mediastinum for bleeding.
- **Step 5.** Close incisions. If the pleural cavity is violated, place chest tubes bilaterally.

Postoperative Care

Notwithstanding which surgical approach is chosen, the nasogastric tube is kept on low suction. It is usually removed on the fifth postoperative day. Chest tubes are removed in the absence of an air leak when pleural drainage is less than 200 cc/day.

A water-soluble radiographic contrast swallow study is performed on the fifth postoperative day. If no leakage or obstruction is noted over the subsequent 3 days, the patient's diet is advanced to a postgastrectomy diet.

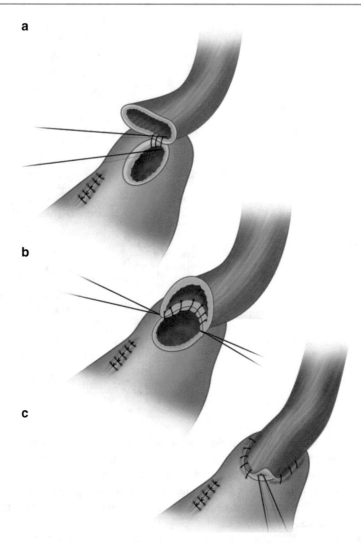

Fig. 6.30 (**a**) and (**b**). Construction of an end-to-side cervical esophagogastric anastomosis. The posterior portion is completed with knots tied on the inside. (**c**) The last anterior sutures are placed with a 46-French bougie (not shown) in place and tied with the knots on the outside

Ivor Lewis Approach

Approximately 17,500 new cases of carcinoma of the esophagus occur each year in the United States. Surgical resection continues to play an important role in the treatment of this disease and can be performed in a variety of ways. In 1946, Ivor Lewis described an operative approach for neoplasms of the distal esophagus including an abdominal procedure to surgically stage the tumor and mobilize the stomach, followed by a right thoracotomy to resect the involved esophagus and stomach and reestablish gastrointestinal continuity with an esophagogastric anastomosis in the chest. Currently, the Ivor Lewis approach is widely applied for any carcinoma occurring in the middle and lower esophagus or gastroesophageal junction.

All patients with upper- and mid-esophageal tumors should undergo either rigid or fiberoptic bronchoscopy prior to resection to rule out tumor invasion into the membranous trachea. Tracheal invasion is an absolute contraindication to resection.

Abdominal Portion

- **Step 1.** Intubate the patient with a double-lumen endotracheal tube and place patient in a supine position for the abdominal portion of the procedure. An upper midline incision is made extending from the xiphoid process to just above the umbilicus (Fig. 6.31a).

a   b

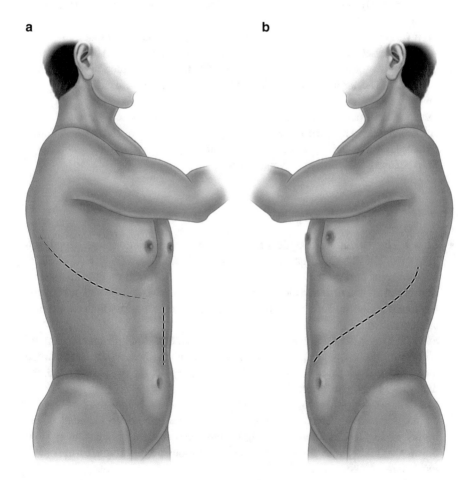

Fig. 6.31 (**a**) Abdominal and right posterolateral thoracotomy. (**b**) Thoracoabdominal incision

- **Step 2.** Explore the abdomen thoroughly to rule out metastases of the liver, peritoneum, and omentum; these would preclude resection. Abdominal retractors such as the Buchwalter or Omni-Tract can be used to facilitate exposure of the stomach.
- **Step 3.** Divide the left triangular and left coronary ligaments of the liver with electrocautery. The left lobe of the liver can then be retracted to the right with the abdominal retractor. Divide the phrenoesophageal ligament and encircle the esophagus, at the hiatus, with a large Penrose drain. The right crus of the diaphragm can be divided to ensure that four fingers can easily fit through the hiatus, thus avoiding any compression on the gastric conduit.
- **Step 4.** Detach the greater omentum from the stomach, taking care not to injure the right gastroepiploic artery.
- **Step 5.** Divide the short gastric vessels. This can be done by first ligating the vessels or by using a coagulating/cutting device such at the LigaSure (Valleylab, Boulder, CO) or the Harmonic Scalpel (Ethicon Endo-Surgery, Inc., Cincinnati, OH).
- **Step 6.** The stomach is then retracted cephalad, and the left gastric artery and vein are dissected close to the aorta and inferior vena cava. All nodal tissue should be swept toward the stomach to ensure that it is included in the resected specimen. The artery and vein are individually ligated with silk sutures and divided.
- **Step 7.** Perform a Kocher maneuver to mobilize the duodenum. Since the stomach is denervated by the esophagectomy, a pyloromyotomy or Heineke–Mikulicz pyloroplasty is usually performed at this point.
- **Step 8.** Insert a feeding jejunostomy tube.

Thoracic Portion

- **Step 9.** The patient is placed in a left lateral decubitus position, re-prepped, and re-draped, and the right lung is deflated to facilitate the esophageal dissection. Make a right posterolateral thoracotomy through the fourth or fifth interspace. The serratus anterior muscle is usually not divided but reflected anteriorly. Explore the chest to rule out pulmonary or pleural metastases which would preclude resection (Fig. 6.32).
- **Step 10.** Going from distal to proximal, open the mediastinal pleura anterior and posterior to the esophagus. Avoid injury to the thoracic duct, which lies between the aorta, vertebrae, and azygos vein. When thoracic duct injury is suspected, the duct should be ligated at the hiatus.
- **Step 11.** Encircle the esophagus with a Penrose drain below the level of the carina. All periesophageal tissue and lymph nodes should be included in the resection. Ligate and divide the azygos vein. Dissect the esophagus away from the airway, taking care not to injure the membranous portion of the carina or left main stem bronchus (Fig. 6.33).

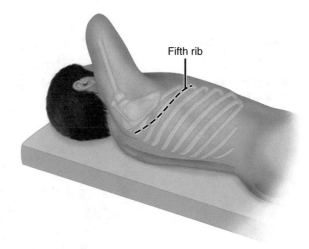

Fig. 6.32 Right thoracotomy

Fifth rib

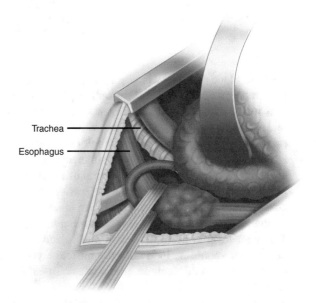

Fig. 6.33 Mobilization of mid-esophageal tumor through a right thoracotomy. A Penrose drain is placed around the esophagus, which is dissected away from the posterior membranous trachea. Division of the azygos vein facilitates the dissection

Trachea

Esophagus

- **Step 12.** Mobilize the stomach into the chest taking care to keep the lesser curvature positioned laterally. For distal tumors, transect the esophagus above the level of the azygos vein; for more proximal tumors, transect higher up. Oncologic principles dictate a margin that is a minimum of 9 cm from the tumor.
- **Step 13.** Use a linear stapler (GIA) to divide the stomach beginning at the angle of His and extending toward the lesser curvature. Ligate and divide the left gastroepiploic artery after its second or third branch; the gastric transection is continued through this area on the lesser curve of the stomach. The gastric staple line may be over sewn with a running 3–0 absorbable suture.

Fig. 6.34 An intrathoracic esophagogastric anastomosis is placed at the apex of the right chest after the gastric fundus is suspended from the prevertebral fascia

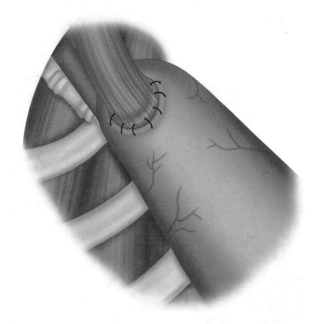

- **Step 14.** Place a Satinsky clamp several centimeters above the point of esophageal transection and divide the esophagus with a scalpel. The specimen is then sent for proximal and distal frozen section margins. With an electrocautery, make a linear gastrotomy the same width as that of the esophagus. Perform the esophagogastric anastomosis in single- or double-layer fashion. Single-layer anastomoses are constructed using interrupted 3–0 silk suture. For a two-layer anastomosis, sew the posterior portion of the outer layer first, followed by the inner layer, and finally the anterior portion of the outer layer. Double-layer anastomoses can be constructed with an inner layer of 3–0 absorbable suture in a running fashion or with 3–0 nonabsorbable suture in an interrupted fashion. The outer layer is performed with interrupted 3–0 nonabsorbable suture. The outer layer should include only the muscle layer of the esophagus, while the inner layer should include the mucosa in addition to the muscle layers (Fig. 6.34).
- **Step 15.** Prior to completing the anastomosis, a nasogastric tube should be advanced through the anastomosis into the stomach. Place two pleural tubes: one near the anastomosis and one near the diaphragm. Close the chest.

Minimally Invasive Esophagectomy (MIE)

Adhering to the principles outlined in the above techniques for esophagectomy, today nearly all of the surgical maneuvers described can be affected using minimally invasive techniques (thoracoscopy and laparoscopy). Except in advanced cases where a minimally invasive technique would likely compromise a curative resection (e.g., advanced malignancy) or safe dissection of critical structures would be dangerous (e.g., prior chest surgery or infection), most centers who specialize in esophageal surgery offer some type of minimally invasive esophagectomy (MIE).

Abdominal Portion

- **Step 1.** Intubate the patient with a double-lumen endotracheal tube and place patient in a supine position for the abdominal portion of the procedure. Laparoscopic access is obtained as described for performance of laparoscopic Nissen fundoplication (see Fig. 5.29).
- **Step 2.** Explore the abdomen thoroughly to rule out metastases of the liver, peritoneum, and omentum; these would preclude resection.
- **Step 3.** The left lobe of the liver is retracted ventrally using the same technique as for laparoscopic Nissen fundoplication. Divide the phrenoesophageal ligament and encircle the esophagus, at the hiatus, with a large Penrose drain (see Fig. 5.32). The right crus of the diaphragm can be divided to enlarge the hiatus, thus avoiding any compression on the gastric conduit.
- **Step 4.** Divide the gastrocolic ligament outside of the gastroepiploic arcade starting at the right gastroepiploic artery and continue up to the short gastric vessels (Fig. 6.35). It is critical to preserve the gastroepiploic arcade since the blood supply to the neoesophagus will from the right gastric artery and the gastroepiploic arcade (Fig. 6.36).

Fig. 6.35 Dividing the gastroepiploic ligament preserving the gastroepiploic artery

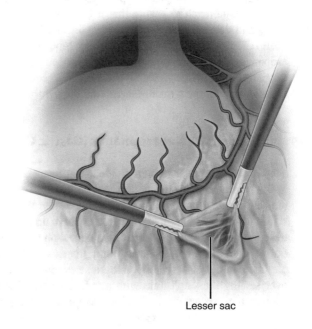

Lesser sac

Fig. 6.36 The blood
supply to the neoesophagus
based on the right gastric
artery and
gastroepiploic arcade

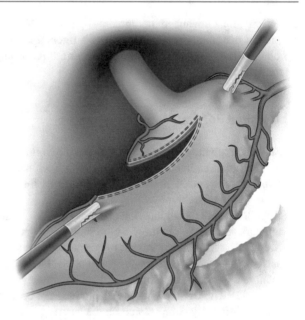

- **Step 5.** Divide the short gastric vessels using a coagulating/cutting device such at the LigaSure (Valleylab, Boulder, CO) or the Harmonic Scalpel (Ethicon Endo-Surgery, Inc., Cincinnati, OH).
- **Step 6.** The lesser sac is opened completely, and the stomach mobilized to expose the left gastric artery and vein from both posteriorly through the lesser sac and anteriorly through the gastrohepatic ligament. All nodal tissue should be swept toward the stomach to ensure that it is included in the resected specimen. The artery and vein are then divided with a linear GIA stapler with a vascular load.
- **Step 7.** The duodenum is then mobilized. Since the stomach is denervated by the esophagectomy, some type of drainage procedure is performed, typically either a laparoscopic pyloroplasty or endoscopic injection of 200 Units of Botox, 50 Units in each of the 4 quadrants around the pylorus.

Preparation of the Neoesophagus (Gastric Conduit)

- **Step 8.** Using a linear stapler, divide the stomach transversely starting just distal to the gastroesophageal junction and on the lesser curve side at approximately the fourth lesser curve arterial branch and then through a series of subsequent staplings progress parallel to the greater curve up to the angle of HIS. In this way the stomach is tubularized creating a neoesophagus with its blood supply based off the right gastroepiploic artery and greater curve arcade (Fig. 6.37). This staple line can be reinforced by using a sleeve guard over the staple cartridges or over sewing the staple line with a V-Loc suture. The resection specimen will contain approximately 90% of the esophagus and proximal one-third of the stomach. Obtain frozen section analysis of esophageal and stomach margins prior to anastomosis.

Fig. 6.37 Creation of neoesophagus (gastric conduit) by dividing the stomach from the lesser curve side transversely and parallel to the greater curve ending at the angle of HIS

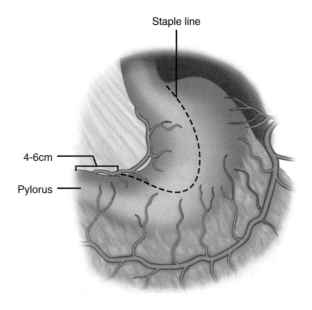

Staple line

4-6cm

Pylorus

Fig. 6.38 Proximal end of gastric conduit sutured to the distal end of the surgical specimen

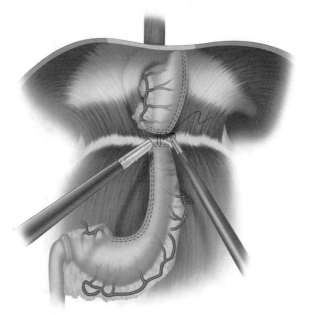

- **Step 9.** Suture the proximal end of the gastric conduit to the distal end of the surgical specimen such that when the esophagus and proximal stomach are retracted into the chest, the gastric conduit will be drawn into the chest. Position the gastric conduit (neoesophagus) gently from below through the enlarged esophageal hiatus and into the posterior mediastinum making sure that no rotation of the stomach (stapled portion of stomach to the patient's right) has occurred (Fig. 6.38).

- **Step 10.** A feeding jejunostomy tube is often used, especially in patients who are nutritionally compromised or in whom a delay in oral intake is anticipated.
- **Step 11.** Trocars are removed, and the fascia of any trocar site larger than 5 mm is closed and skin on all incisions closed.

Thoracic Portion

- **Step 12.** The patient is placed in a left lateral decubitus position, re-prepped, and re-draped, and the right lung is deflated to facilitate the esophageal dissection. Four trocars are placed as depicted in Fig. 6.39.
- **Step 13.** Going from distal to proximal, open the mediastinal pleura anterior and posterior to the esophagus. Avoid injury to the thoracic duct, which lies between the aorta, vertebrae, and azygos vein. When thoracic duct injury is suspected, the duct should be ligated at the hiatus.
- **Step 14.** Encircle the esophagus with a Penrose drain below the level of the carina. All periesophageal tissue and lymph nodes should be included in the resection. Ligate and divide the azygos vein. Dissect the esophagus away from the airway, taking care not to injure the membranous portion of the carina or left main stem bronchus (Fig. 6.40).

Fig. 6.39 Trocar placement for thoracoscopic esophageal resection and anastomosis

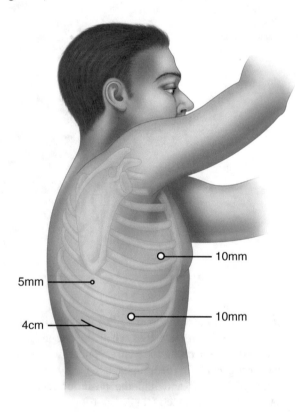

5mm

4cm

10mm

10mm

- **Step 15.** With the thoracic portion of the esophagus completely mobilized, the distal esophagus and proximal stomach with the attached gastric conduit are retracted into the chest. The entire gastric conduit is pulled into the chest ensuring adequate length to reach the proximal esophagus for subsequent anastomosis.
- **Step 16.** A linear stapler is used to divide the esophagus proximally at or slightly above the azygous vein. The sutures connected to the gastric conduit are cut and the specimen placed in a specimen removal bag and removed through an enlarged trocar site incision. Before progressing with fashioning an anastomosis, the proximal and distal margin of the specimen is assessed through immediate frozen section analysis by pathology to ensure the proximal margin is free of any abnormal malignant cells.
- **Step 17.** An esophagogastrostomy can be created using a hand-sewn technique similar to what is described above for the Ivor Lewis esophagectomy. More commonly an anastomosis is created using a circular stapler. The anvil is passed orally and the spike on the anvil placed through the end of the remaining esophagus (Fig. 6.41) and the handle passed through a gastrotomy in the gastric conduit (Fig. 6.42). The handle and anvil are then connected, and the stapler closed (Fig. 6.43) and fired creating a circular stapled anastomosis. The gastrotomy in the gastric conduit is closed with a linear stapler.
- **Step 18.** After completing the anastomosis, a nasogastric tube should be advanced through the anastomosis into the gastric conduit positioning the tip just past the pylorus. Also, an EGD is performed to assess the anastomosis and the pyloroplasty if performed. Place two pleural tubes: one near the anastomosis and one near the diaphragm, reinflate the right lung and close the trocar site incisions.

Fig. 6.40 Mobilization of mid-esophageal tumor through right thoracoscopy. A Penrose drain is placed around the esophagus, which is dissected away from the posterior membranous trachea and the azygous vein is ligated

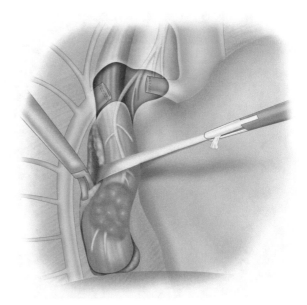

Fig. 6.41 Positioning the anvil of a circular stapler in the reaming esophagus with the spike perforating the esophagus for subsequent connection to the stapler handle

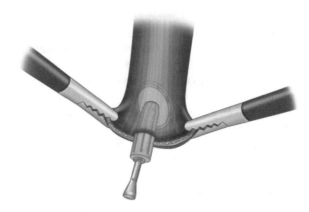

Fig. 6.42 Position the handle of the circular stapler through a gastrotomy in the gastric conduit

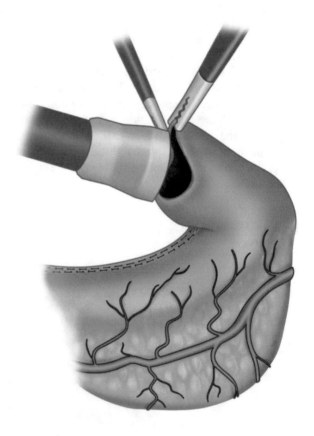

Fig. 6.43 Connecting the handle and anvil of the circular stapler for subsequent closure, firing and creation of anastomosis

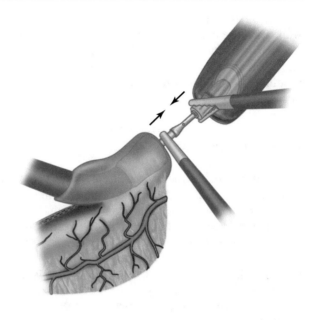

Other Approaches (Summarized)

Ivor Lewis–McKeown (Three-Stage) Esophagectomy

This procedure utilizes the incisions of the Ivor Lewis esophagectomy with an added left cervical incision for the anastomosis. The procedure is used for proximal tumors where an intrathoracic anastomosis would not allow for an acceptable margin. This approach also allows for a cervical lymph node dissection. The abdominal and thoracic portions are performed in the same manner as in the Ivor Lewis esophagectomy except that the right chest portion is performed first followed by the abdominal portion and ending with the cervical portion. The cervical portion follows the same technique described in the transhiatal esophagectomy.

Left Thoracoabdominal Esophagectomy

This approach was the original approach to esophagectomy and is still employed for distal tumors. This procedure does not allow for a very proximal anastomosis because of the presence of the aortic arch, and therefore it is not useful for more proximal tumors.

The patient is placed in a right lateral decubitus position, and a left posterolateral thoracotomy is performed through the seventh interspace (Fig. 6.31b). The incision may be extended across the costal margin, and the rectus muscle is divided. The diaphragm is opened in a radial fashion leaving a 2-cm rim of diaphragm on the chest wall. This avoids injury to the phrenic nerve branches while leaving enough diaphragm on the chest wall to facilitate closure. The rest of the esophagectomy is performed in a manner similar to the Ivor Lewis esophagectomy. The benefits of this approach are that it avoids the need for a separate abdominal incision and for repositioning of the patient, as required in an Ivor Lewis esophagectomy.

Colon Interposition

The colon may be used as an esophageal substitute in situations where the stomach is not usable. The left, right, or, less commonly, transverse colon may be used. The blood supply to the left and right colonic conduits is based on the ascending branch of the left colic artery and the middle colic arteries, respectively. If the ileocolon is to be used, the right colic artery, in addition to the middle colic artery, must be spared.

- **Step 1.** Mobilize the colon by dividing the lateral peritoneal reflection of the right or left colon extending to the hepatic or splenic flexure.
- **Step 2.** Detach the greater omentum from the transverse colon, taking care not to injure the middle colic vessels.
- **Step 3.** Assess the colon's arterial vascular supply by holding up the transverse colon and transilluminating the mesocolon. Place atraumatic vascular clamps across all arteries that are to be divided. For example, if the left colon will be used, clamps should be placed on the middle colic artery and across the vascular arcades at the proximal and distal points of colonic transection. This acts as a good test of the remaining blood vessel (ascending branch of left colic artery, for a left colon conduit) (Fig. 6.44). The clamps should be left on for 10–15 min and the colon serially inspected for color, pulse, and peristalsis. If the colon does not look viable, a different conduit should be used.
- **Step 4.** Divide the colon with a GIA stapler. When using the left colon, divide it proximal to the middle colic vessels and distal to the ascending branch of the left colic artery. The middle colic artery should be divided close to the superior mesenteric artery to avoid injuring the marginal artery and its arcades. When using the right colon, divide it distal to the middle colic artery and proximal to either the terminal ileum or the cecum. If the ileum is to be used, both the right and middle colic arteries must be retained. If the distal ileum is not used, divide the right colic artery as it branches off the superior mesenteric artery and retain the middle colic artery.
- **Step 5.** Perform an end-to-end colocolonic anastomosis (Fig. 6.45) to reestablish colonic continuity. Bring the colonic conduit through the chest and anastomose it to the remaining esophagus. The colonic conduit can be placed in a substernal position or, preferably, in the posterior mediastinum.

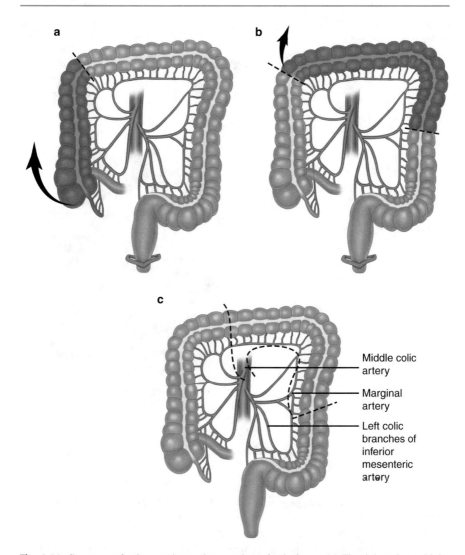

Fig. 6.44 Segments of colon can be used as esophageal substitutes. (**a**) The right colon, with its vascular supply, which is based on the right branch of the middle colic artery, is rotated as an isoperistaltic segment. (**b**) The left colon, with its vascular supply, which is based on the ascending branch of the left colic artery, is brought up in an isoperistaltic fashion. (**c**) The vascular anatomy of the transverse and descending colon. Division of the transverse colon at the right of the middle colic vessels [(**a**) and (**b**)]

Fig. 6.45 Colocolonic
end-to-end anastomosis.
Note the vascular pedicle
of the colonic segment

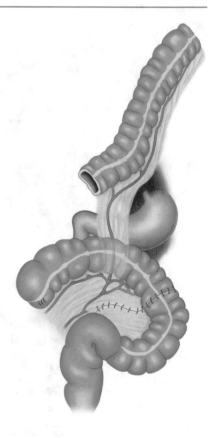

Anatomical Complications

- Injury of the recurrent laryngeal nerve may cause paralysis of a vocal cord. This nerve is especially vulnerable just below the point where it passes under the inferior constrictor muscles to become intralaryngeal.
- Injury or transection of the vagus nerve will cause gastric atony and lack of pyloric relaxation. Damage to the vagus nerve in an antireflux surgery will cause dumping, decreased gastric emptying, failure of relaxation of the pyloric outlet, and diarrhea. The interior vagus nerve is at risk when performing laparoscopic antireflux surgery as it is poorly visualized under the phrenoesophageal membrane.
- Injury of the intercostal nerve may result in chronic chest pain.
- Injury of the thoracic duct will result in chylothorax.
- The azygos vein can be injured especially during a transhiatal approach.

Stomach

7

Mohammad Raheel Jajja and Snehal Patel

Anatomy

Two Gastric Units

From the viewpoint of a surgeon, the stomach is part of two almost-separate organ systems, each with its special pathology and surgical approach. The first can be called the "proximal gastric surgical unit." It contains the proximal stomach, distal esophagus, and esophageal hiatus of the diaphragm (Fig. 7.1). The second is the "distal gastric surgical unit," which includes the gastric antrum and pylorus, together with the first part of the duodenum (Fig. 7.2).

Proximal Gastric Surgical Unit
The length of the abdominal esophagus ranges from 0.5 to 2.5 cm. Its relations with surrounding structures are:

Anterior: Posterior surface of left lobe of liver

Posterior: Right crus of diaphragm and aorta

Right: Segment 1 (caudate or spigelian lobe) of liver

Left: Fundus of stomach

The cardiac orifice is the gastroesophageal junction. The fundus, for all practical purposes, is the upper part of the body which, in the supine position, augments upward. The body is the part of the stomach between the antrum and the fundus.

M. R. Jajja
Department of Surgery, Winship Cancer Institute, Emory University, Atlanta, GA, USA

S. Patel (✉)
Department of Surgery, Emory University, Atlanta, GA, USA
e-mail: snehal.patel@emory.edu

© Springer Nature Switzerland AG 2021
L. J. Skandalakis (ed.), *Surgical Anatomy and Technique*,
https://doi.org/10.1007/978-3-030-51313-9_7

Fig. 7.1 The proximal gastric surgical unit. The two ends of the stomach acquire different lesions, and operations require different methods

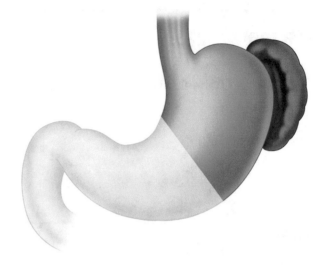

Fig. 7.2 The distal gastric surgical unit. Most gastric surgery takes place in this area

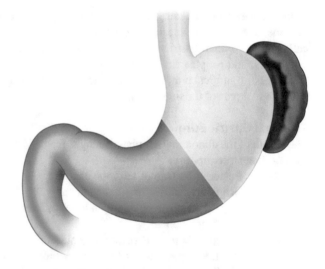

Distal Gastric Surgical Unit

The gastric antrum, pylorus, and first portion of the duodenum form a unit from an embryologic, physiologic, and, certainly, surgical viewpoint.

Gastric Antrum

In the opened stomach, the antrum is easily distinguished from the body of the stomach by its mucosa, which is flatter and without rugae. It is histologically distinct, being without chief or parietal (acid-producing) cells. The margin of the antrum is irregular, but definite. Externally the antrum is difficult to demarcate. The boundary on the lesser curvature usually lies at the incisura angularis; it is usually found in textbook drawings, but in the operating room it is inconstant and often absent.

Surgeons not planning a gastrotomy to locate the antral margin can use the "crow's foot" of the anterior descending vagal trunk as a landmark. The antrum can be expected to begin 3–4 cm cranial to the crow's foot, about 8–10 cm proximal to the pylorus. On the greater curvature, there is no good landmark. In most cases the boundary extends from a point on the lesser curvature 2/5 of the way from the pylorus to the esophagus to a point on the greater curvature 1/8 of the distance from the pylorus to the esophagus.

Pylorus

The pylorus is a muscular region of the stomach; proximally, it merges into the gastric antrum without a definite external boundary; distally, it ends abruptly at the thin-walled duodenum.

At the pyloroduodenal junction, the continuity of the circular musculature is interrupted by an annular septum that arises from the connective tissue of the submucosa. Proximal to this ring, the circular muscle layer is thickened to form the pyloric sphincter. Distal to the ring, the circular muscle coat at the duodenum is thinner.

First Part of the Duodenum

The distal gastric surgical unit includes only the first 2.5 cm of the duodenum (for more information, see Chap. 8.)

Relations of the Distal Gastric Surgical Unit

Posteriorly the unit is related to the:

- Floor of lesser sac
- Transverse mesocolon
- Head and neck of pancreas
- Aorta and celiac trunk and its branches
- Celiac ganglion and plexus
- Hepatic triad
- Gastroduodenal artery

Anteriorly the unit is related to the:

- Anterior abdominal wall
- Medial sector (segment 4) of left lobe and anterior sector (segments 5 and 8) of right lobe of the liver
- Transverse mesocolon
- Neck of gallbladder (if stomach is empty)

Gastric Wall

The gastric wall consists of the serosa, the muscular layer, submucosal layer, and mucosal layer.

The distal esophagus is lined by stratified squamous epithelium; the abdominal esophagus is lined with mucous cells. Simple columnar cells compose the mucosal layer of the cardia. The mucosal layer of the fundus and body consists of two types of cells: parietal (oxyntic) acid-secreting cells and chief pepsin-secreting cells.

Ligaments

Hepatogastric Ligament (Lesser Omentum)

The hepatogastric ligament (also known as pars flaccida) is the proximal part of the lesser omentum. It extends from the porta hepatis to the lesser curvature of the stomach and upward as the ventral mesentery of the abdominal esophagus. The ligament contains:

Regularly: Left gastric artery and vein; hepatic division of the anterior vagal trunk; anterior and posterior gastric divisions of the vagal trunks (nerves of Latarjet); lymph nodes and vessels.

Occasionally: An aberrant left hepatic artery (23% of individuals) in proximal part of hepatogastric ligament; distally and to the right, branches of the right gastric artery and vein. In this region also are the common hepatic artery and portal vein; here they rise ventrally to gain their positions in the hepatoduodenal segment of the lesser omentum.

Hepatoduodenal Ligament
The hepatoduodenal ligament is the distal part of the lesser omentum, extending from the liver to the first 2.5 cm of the duodenum. The free edge envelops the hepatic triad (the proper hepatic artery, portal vein, and extrahepatic biliary ducts) as well as the hepatic plexus and lymph nodes.

Gastrocolic Ligament
The gastrocolic ligament is a portion of the greater omentum passing from the greater curvature of the stomach and the first part of the duodenum to the transverse colon.

Gastrosplenic Ligament
See Chap. 15.

Gastrophrenic Ligament
The gastrophrenic ligament is continuous with the hepatogastric ligament to the left of or, perhaps, opposite the esophagus. It has an avascular area through which the surgeon's finger can safely pass and through which a Penrose drain can be inserted around the cardia to pull down the esophagus. This is a useful maneuver in vagotomy. The upper part of the ligament is avascular, and the lower part contains short gastric arteries and veins and lymph nodes.

Vascular System of the Stomach (Fig. 7.3)

Arterial Supply

Following is a summation of all the arteries that supply the stomach. Each of the principal arteries of supply originates from the celiac trunk.

- Left gastric
  - Ascending branch (gives rise to esophageal)
  - Descending branch (gives rise to gastric)
- Hepatic
  - Right gastric
  - Gastroduodenal
- Anterior superior pancreaticoduodenal
- Retroduodenal
- Posterior superior pancreaticoduodenal
- Supraduodenal
- Right gastroepiploic (major branches)
- Splenic
  - Posterior gastric
  - Short gastrics
  - Left gastroepiploic (major branches)

The stomach can survive after ligation of all but one of its primary arteries, and extragastric ligation will not control bleeding from a gastric ulcer.

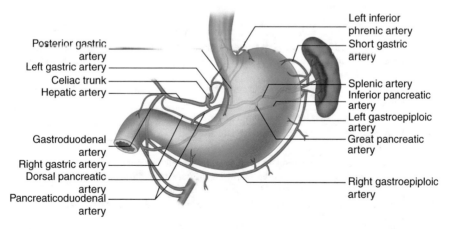

Fig. 7.3 The arterial supply to the stomach: L. Inf Ph left inferior phrenic artery, SG short gastric artery, L. GE left gastroepiploic artery, R. GE right gastroepiploic artery, S splenic artery, GP great pancreatic artery, Inf P inferior pancreatic artery, PD pancreaticoduodenal artery, DP dorsal pancreatic artery, GD gastroduodenal artery, R. G right gastric artery, H hepatic artery, CT celiac trunk, L. G left gastric artery, Post G posterior gastric artery

Venous Drainage

The veins, for all practical purposes, follow the arteries.

Lymphatic Drainage

The lymphatic drainage of the stomach consists of 20 stations, and these are classified into four groups (Fig. 7.4):

D1: Perigastric nodes directly attached along the lesser curvature and greater curvatures of the stomach (stations 1–6, N1 level)

D2: Nodes along the left gastric artery (station 7), common hepatic artery (station 8), celiac trunk (station 9), splenic hilus, and splenic artery (station 10 and 11)

D3: Lymph nodes at stations 12 through 14, along the hepatoduodenal ligament and the root of the mesentery (N3 level)

D4: Stations 15 and 16 in the para-aortic and the paracolic region (N4 level)

Station	Definition
1	Right paracardial LNs, including those along the first branch of the ascending limb of the left gastric artery
2	Left paracardial LNs including those along the esophagocardiac branch of the left subphrenic artery
3a	Lesser curvature LNs along the branches of the left gastric artery
3b	Lesser curvature LNs along the second branch and distal part of the right gastric artery
4sa	Left greater curvature LNs along the short gastric arteries (perigastric area)
4sb	Left greater curvature LNs along the left gastroepiploic artery (perigastric area)
4d	Rt. greater curvature LNs along the second branch and distal part of the right gastroepiploic artery
5	Suprapyloric LNs along the first branch and proximal part of the right gastric artery
6	Infrapyloric LNs along the first branch and proximal part of the right gastroepiploic artery down to the confluence of the right gastroepiploic vein and the anterior superior pancreatoduodenal vein
7	LNs along the trunk of left gastric artery between its root and the origin of its ascending branch
8a	Anterosuperior LNs along the common hepatic artery
8p	Posterior LNs along the common hepatic artery
9	Coeliac artery
10	Splenic hilar LNs including those adjacent to the splenic artery distal to the pancreatic tail and those on the roots of the short gastric arteries and those along the left gastroepiploic artery proximal to its first gastric branch
11p	Proximal splenic artery LNs from its origin to halfway between its origin and the pancreatic tail end
11d	Distal splenic artery LNs from halfway between its origin and the pancreatic tail end to the end of the pancreatic tail
12a	Hepatoduodenal ligament LNs along the proper hepatic artery, in the caudal half between the confluence of the right and left hepatic ducts and the upper border of the pancreas

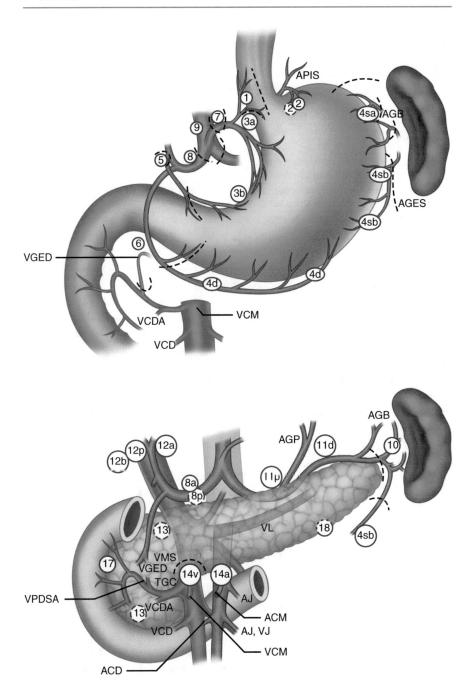

Fig. 7.4 Diagram of the lymphatic drainage of the stomach

Station	Definition
12b	Hepatoduodenal ligament LNs along the bile duct, in the caudal half between the confluence of the right and left hepatic ducts and the upper border of the pancreas
12p	Hepatoduodenal ligament LNs along the portal vein in the caudal half between the confluence of the right and left hepatic ducts and the upper border of the pancreas
13	LNs on the posterior surface of the pancreatic head cranial to the duodenal papilla
14v	LNs along the superior mesenteric vein
15	LNs along the middle colic vessels
16a1	Paraaortic LNs in the diaphragmatic aortic hiatus
16a2	Paraaortic LNs between the upper margin of the origin of the celiac artery and the lower border of the left renal vein
16b1	Paraaortic LNs between the lower border of the left renal vein and the upper border of the origin of the inferior mesenteric artery
16b2	Paraaortic LNs between the upper border of the origin of the inferior mesenteric artery and the aortic bifurcation

Parasympathetic Nerves (Vagus Nerves)

The left and right vagus nerves descend parallel with the esophagus and contribute to a rich external esophageal nerve plexus between the level of the tracheal bifurcation and the level of the diaphragm. From this plexus, two vagal trunks—anterior and posterior—form and pass through the esophageal hiatus of the diaphragm. Each trunk subsequently separates into two divisions (Fig. 7.5).

From the anterior vagal trunk, the hepatic division passes to the right in the lesser omentum, branching before it enters the liver. One branch turns downward to reach the pylorus and, sometimes, the first part of the duodenum. The second division, the anterior gastric, descends along the lesser curvature of the stomach, giving branches to the anterior gastric wall.

From the posterior trunk arise the celiac division, which passes through the celiac plexus, and the posterior gastric division, which supplies branches to the posterior gastric wall.

Identification of Vagal Structures at the Hiatus

The basic configuration and variations of the vagus nerves at the esophageal hiatus are well known, but the thoracic pattern is not visible to the abdominal surgeon, who must proceed on the basis of the structures that can be seen. A study of components of the esophageal hiatus in 100 cadavers found two vagal structures only, 88% of the time (Fig. 7.5). The usual structures at the esophageal hiatus are the anterior and posterior vagal trunks, which have not yet split to form the four typical divisions discussed above. Both trunks are usually to the right of the midline of the esophagus. The posterior trunk lies closer to the aorta than to the esophagus (Fig. 7.6).

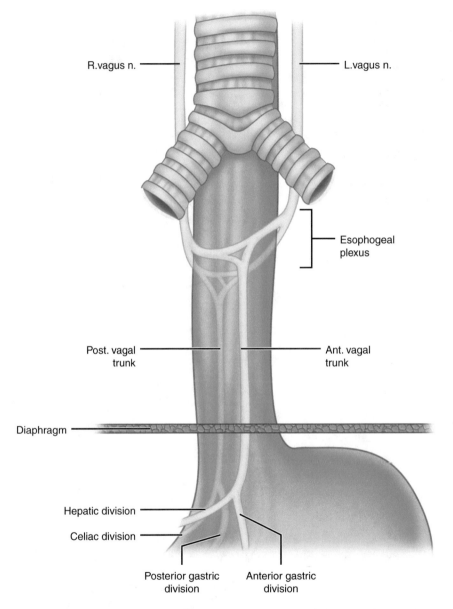

Fig. 7.5 The terminology of vagal structures of the thorax and abdomen. In this example, two vagal trunks pass through the hiatus to enter the abdomen

Rarely four vagal structures (7%) (Fig. 5.16a) or more than four structures (5%) (Fig. 5.16b) were identified at the hiatus. The four or more divisions of the vagal trunks (hepatic, celiac, anterior gastric, and posterior gastric) appear when division has occurred above the diaphragm.

Fig. 7.6 The relation of the anterior and posterior vagal trunks to the aorta and the esophagus, showing the number of specimens with vagal trunks lying to the right or left of the midline. In most but not all of the 88 specimens, the trunks are to the right of the midline. Note that the anterior trunks are closer to the esophagus than are the posterior trunks

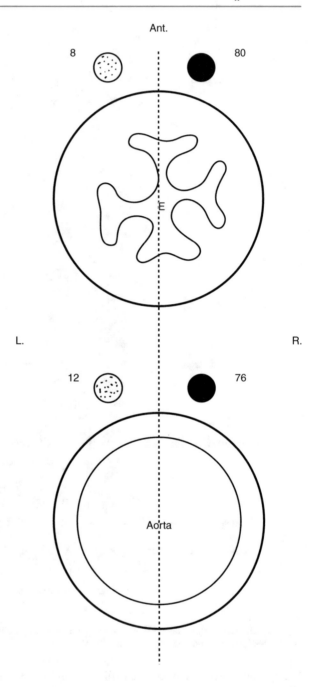

Distribution of the Vagus Nerves to the Stomach

Anterior Gastric Division

The separation of the anterior gastric and hepatic divisions occasionally occurred above the diaphragm, but the divisions usually lay on the abdominal esophagus or the cardia.

In almost all cases, a major branch of the anterior gastric division formed the principal anterior nerve of the lesser curvature (anterior nerve of Latarjet). It usually lay from 0.5 to 1.0 cm from the lesser curvature.

From 2 to 12 branches pass from the principal nerve to the stomach wall. The average in the subjects in the abovementioned study was six.

Constant landmarks on the stomach are difficult to obtain. The position of the incisura angularis often has to be estimated. Although we have often seen the nerve of Latarjet branch in the "crow's foot" formation, this pattern is far from constant, being equivocal in some cases and absent in many (Fig. 7.7).

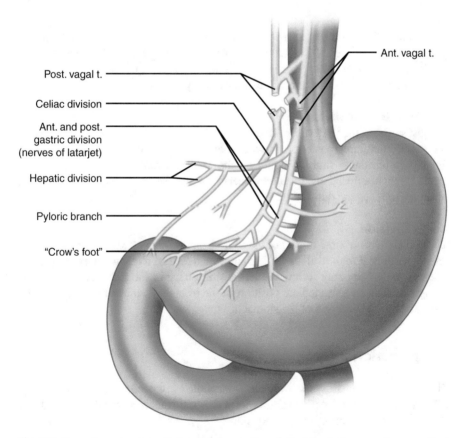

Fig. 7.7 Truncal vagotomy results in vagal denervation of all abdominal organs. A concomitant drainage procedure is required for gastric stasis

Fig. 7.8 "Typical"
distribution of anterior
gastric and hepatic
divisions of the vagus

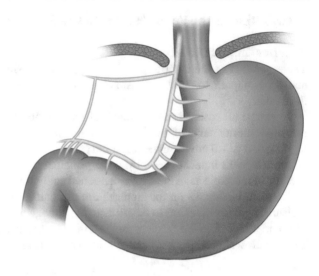

Hepatic Division

The hepatic division of the anterior vagal trunk usually separates from the anterior gastric division at the level of the abdominal esophagus (Fig. 7.8). It lies between the leaflets of the avascular portion of the hepatogastric ligament. It is frequently found in multiple branches that are usually closely parallel.

Posterior Gastric Division

In most subjects, the posterior gastric division forms the principal posterior nerve of the lesser curvature (posterior nerve of Latarjet). As a rule, the posterior nerve appears to terminate slightly higher on the lesser curvature and possesses fewer gastric branches than does the anterior nerve. In no case has a posterior nerve been observed to reach the duodenum.

Celiac Division

The celiac division is the largest of the four vagal divisions. It lies in the gastropancreatic peritoneal fold. In all cases, it is single and leads directly to the celiac plexus. The celiac division may follow the left gastric artery or the right crus of the diaphragm or take an intermediate position in the triangle bounded by the artery, the crus, and the right margin of the stomach.

Sympathetic Nerves

The sympathetic chains, the thoracic splanchnic nerves containing afferent and efferent fibers, and the celiac ganglia form the basic elements for the sympathetic innervation of the stomach and duodenum.

Technique

Gastrostomy

Percutaneous Endoscopic Gastrostomy (Pull-Technique)

1. The abdominal skin is prepped in usual sterile manner and draped to expose the upper abdomen (below the costal margin).
2. Esophagogastroduodenoscopy (EGD) is performed with a standard upper endoscope. The stomach is insufflated generously via the air channel on the endoscope.
3. The abdominal wall is transilluminated using the endoscope light. This is visible externally as a bright light on the abdominal wall.
4. Finger pressure is applied at the point of maximal transillumination, and the focal indentation is visualized endoscopically on the gastric lumen.
5. The selected area should be at least 2 cm below the costal margin and away from the xiphoid process.
6. A needle (with outer plastic catheter) attached to a syringe is passed from the abdominal wall into the stomach (confirmed by endoscopic visualization). The needle is removed with the catheter left in place.
7. Next, the blue wire is passed through the plastic catheter into the stomach. The snare wire is passed from the endoscope into the stomach as well.
8. The guidewire is then snared and brought out through the oral cavity. The snare is separated from the guidewire. The guidewire is attached to the gastrostomy tube and pulled into the stomach.
9. The endoscope is reintroduced into the stomach. A scalpel is used to make a horizontal incision (0.5–1.0 cm wide, 2–3 mm deep) on the needle entry site on the skin. The plastic catheter is removed, and the guidewire is gently pulled through with the attached tube under direct visual guidance.
10. Once the bumper is flush with gastric mucosa and easily rotatable, the gastrostomy tube is secured to the skin using the external bumper (1–2 cm from the skin).
11. The excess portion of the tube, including the terminal dilator, is then cut away with the scissors, leaving approximately 15–20 cm of the tube behind. Dressing is applied and tube can be used 4 h after placement.

Stamm Gastrostomy

A small upper-midline incision is favored, which may be extended, if necessary.

- **Step 1.** With Babcock clamps, elevate the anterior wall of the stomach approximately 6–10 cm from the gastroduodenal junction. Place and tie two purse-string sutures of 3–0 silk or Vi cryl 120° from each other (Fig. 7.9).
- **Step 2.** Make a very small stab incision (usually 0.5 cm in length) in the center of the designated area of the purse-string sutures and insert an 18–22 Foley balloon catheter (alternatively a Malecot catheter can be used) (Fig. 7.9).

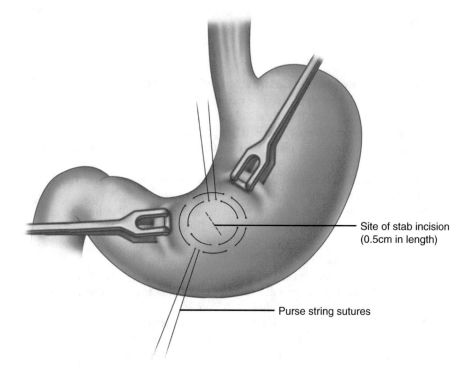

Site of stab incision
(0.5cm in length)

Purse string sutures

Fig. 7.9 Purse-string sutures at anterior wall of stomach

- **Step 3.** Insert the catheter and inflate the balloon. Tie the inner purse string very tightly, then tie the outer purse string; do not cut it or remove the needles (Fig. 7.10).
- **Step 4.** Pull the catheter until it reaches the gastric mucosa at the gastric stab wound. Use gentle movements to ensure that the balloon is well attached to the gastric mucosa. Stitch the purse-string sutures to the anterior abdominal wall at the three and nine o clock positions. To make certain that dead space does not exist, use 3–0 silk suture to fix the gastric wall to the anterior abdominal wall at the 6 and 12 o'clock positions. Close the skin and use a 2–0 silk suture to secure the gastrostomy tube to the skin of the abdominal wall.

Note
- There are other types of gastrostomies, including Witzel and Janeway. They are seldom used today.

Fig. 7.10 Placement of
catheter (Inset: detail of
catheter and balloon)

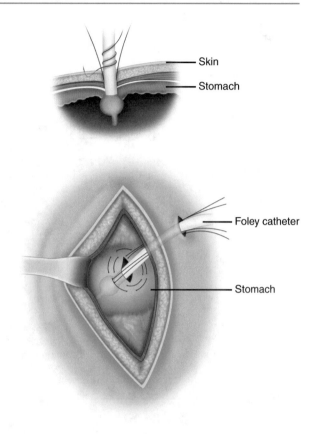

Skin

Stomach

Foley catheter

Stomach

Gastrojejunostomy

Retrocolic

- **Step 1.** Make an upper-midline incision or incision of the surgeon's choice.
- **Step 2.** The location of the stoma should be close to the pylorus at the most dependent area of the greater curvature. Place a Babcock clamp in an oblique fashion at the lesser curvature and at the greater curvature (Fig. 7.11).
- **Step 3.** Lift the transverse colon to evaluate its mesocolon. Protect the middle colic artery by noting its location. Identify an avascular area and incise it; in most cases, it will be to the left of the middle colic artery. The posterior wall of the stomach projects through the opening in such a way that the lesser curvature is located at the lowest corner of the mesenteric opening. Using interrupted 4–0 silk, suture the mesentery to the gastric wall at this point (Fig. 7.12).
- **Step 4.** Again using interrupted 4–0 silk sutures, attach to the gastric wall (proximal to the lesser curvature) a jejunal loop that is approximately 15 cm distal to the ligament of Treitz. Anastomose the loop to the posterior gastric wall in two

Fig. 7.11 Clamps placed
at lesser curvature

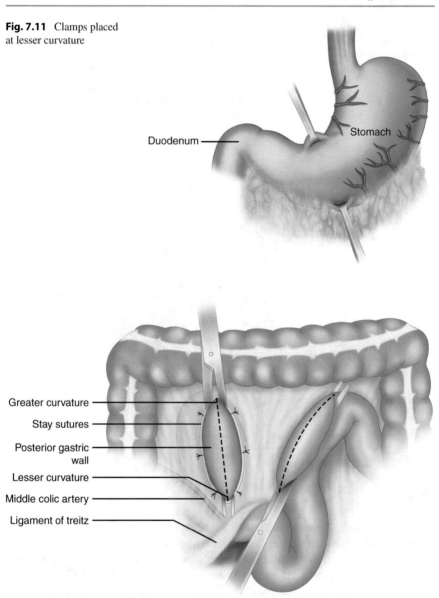

Fig. 7.12 Locating the avascular area prior to incision

layers using a running 3–0 PDS suture for the mucosal layer and a 3–0 silk interrupted suture for the seromuscular layer (Figs. 7.13, 7.14, and 7.15).

Note
- Alternatively, a stapled anastomosis is acceptable.

Step 5. Close the abdominal wall.

Fig. 7.13 Mesentery is sutured to gastric wall. Note location of ligament of Treitz

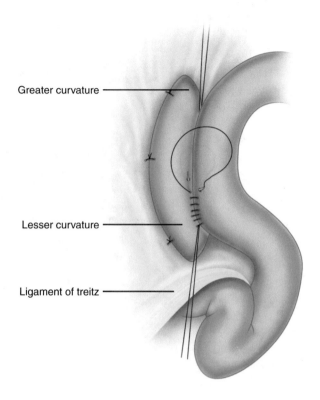

Greater curvature

Lesser curvature

Ligament of treitz

Fig. 7.14 Enterotomy and gastrotomy

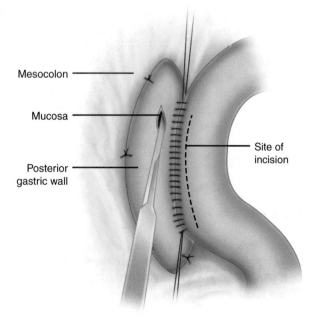

Mesocolon

Mucosa

Posterior gastric wall

Site of incision

Fig. 7.15 Anastomosing the jejunal loop to the posterior gastric wall

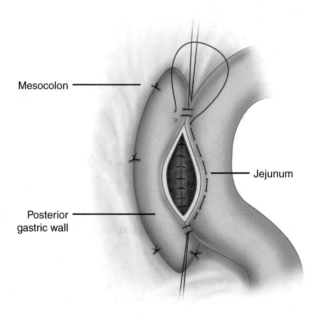

Mesocolon

Jejunum

Posterior gastric wall

Fig. 7.16 Antecolic gastrojejunostomy

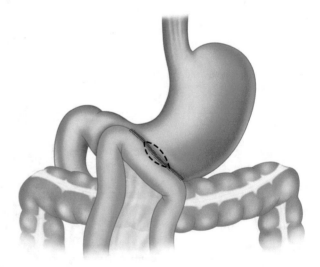

Antecolic (Fig. 7.16)

Follow steps as in the retrocolic gastrojejunostomy. The jejunal loop is anterior to the colon; therefore, attach it to the posterior wall of the stomach at the most dependent part of the greater curvature through an opening of the gastrocolic ligament (Table 7.1).

Table 7.1 Type of gastric ulcers

Type	Suggested operation
I	Distal gastrectomy with Billroth I
II, III	Distal gastrectomy (Billroth II) with truncal vagotomy
IV	Sub-total gastrectomy (Csendes or Pauchet resection)
V	Diffuse ulcers throughout gastric body, pharmacologic management recommended, total gastrectomy if refractory

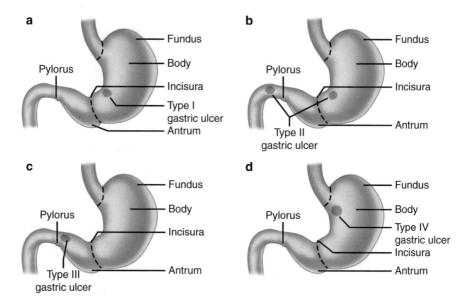

Fig. 7.17 Types of gastric ulcers

Perforated Ulcers (Fig. 7.17)

Perforated Peptic Ulcers

Graham Patch (Figs. 7.18 and 7.19)
- **Step 1.** Perform detailed and complete cleansing by irrigating the peritoneal cavities. Pay special attention to the suprahepatic and subhepatic areas: the right and left pericolic gutters should be cleaned and the pelvis should be irrigated vigorously. **Identify the perforation site and send a full thickness section of mucosa for pathological analysis of h-pylori.**
- **Step 2.** Using no more than two or three sutures, plug the perforated ulcer with vascularized piece of omentum. Then, using a 3–0 silk or synthetic absorbable, take a full-thickness bite of duodenum on each side of the perforation. Tie the sutures above the omental piece.

Fig. 7.18 Attaching
omental plug

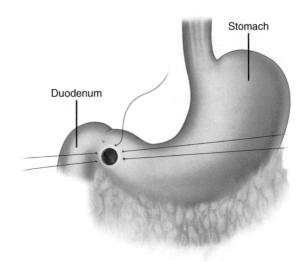

Fig. 7.19 Closure
in layers

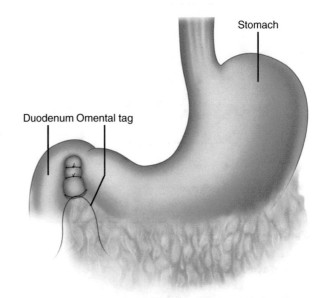

- **Step 3.** Irrigate, and then close in layers using repeated irrigation. Drainage is
  individualized to patient status (immunocompromised, elderly or large defect).
  Intravenous antibiotics, which were started prior to surgery, should be continued
  for at least 48 h (we recommend continuing anti-h-pylori regimen until pathology results are back).

Note

- Occasionally the perforated ulcer is associated with partial obstruction, bleeding, or both. Sometimes, especially 6 h after the onset of perforation, local edema exists and interferes with approximating or closing the perforation with sutures. In this case an antrectomy and Billroth II anastomosis may be necessary. The ulcer should be included in the specimen. If the duodenum is too inflamed or scarred to close, a Malecot catheter is placed in it and closed around it.
- If bleeding is present, it is probably arising from a posterior wall ulcer penetrating the gastroduodenal artery. Therefore, the patient has two problems: an anterior perforated ulcer and a posterior bleeding ulcer. Suture the artery superficially. Remember that the duct of Santorini is under the artery and in 10% of cases it is the only duct of the exocrine pancreas. If the suture incorporates the duct, pancreatitis can result. Occasionally in early perforation a truncal or superselective vagotomy with pyloroplasty could be indicated or perhaps a truncal vagotomy with Billroth II procedure.
- Be sure to administer intravenous antibiotics prior to incision and for 24–48 h postoperatively.

Perforated Gastric Ulcers

Since most gastric neoplasms are malignant, the surgeon should always remember that a perforated gastric ulcer could be of benign or malignant origin.

- **Step 1.** Clamp the perforated ulcer with a Babcock clamp. After the peritoneal cavity has been thoroughly cleansed, remove the ulcer and send it to the lab for frozen section. During this time, irrigation of the peritoneal cavity continues, and the surgeon devises the patient's treatment strategy.
- **Step 2.** If the ulcer is benign, close the gastric wall in two layers: the first with through-and-through PDS 3–0 suture and the second with Lembert seromuscular suture of 3–0 or 4–0 silk. A stapling device can also be used to close the gastric wall. (If the ulcer is malignant, the surgeon should consider performing a subtotal gastrectomy only for patients in good condition and with localized peritonitis, as well as without any sign of shock and comorbidity. In the absence of a staging work-up and new guidelines which suggest multimodal management of gastric cancer, it may be prudent to address the perforation and peritonitis only at this stage and leave cancer management after appropriate work-up has been done).

Note

- It is the authors' policy to excise the ulcer in toto and send it to the lab for frozen section.

An ulcer of the *high anterior gastric wall* may be excised by making a circumferential incision around it. The procedure is aided by deep seromuscular sutures proximal and distal to the ulcer. Close in two layers.

When working with an ulcer of the *high posterior gastric wall*, which is very high and close to the gastroesophageal junction, establish good proximal mobilization of the stomach and abdominal esophagus. Turn the stomach in such a way that the greater curvature lies posterior and the lesser curvature lies anterior. From this point, the procedure is the same as for an anterior gastric wall ulcer excision. Again, additional procedures depend upon the benignity or malignancy of the ulcer.

Pyloric Stenosis (Fig. 7.20)

Although this procedure is usually performed by a pediatric surgeon, we will present the technique because it is done occasionally by general surgeons.
- **Step 1.** Make a right upper quadrant muscle-splitting incision.
- **Step 2.** Deliver the pylorus and the pyloric tumor from the peritoneal cavity.
- **Step 3.** Hold the tumor firmly with the thumb and index finger in such a way that the proximal duodenum is pushed up to the distal pylorus, protecting the duodenal mucosa.
- **Step 4.** Carefully incise the serosa and pyloric muscle. Using the Benson spreader with extreme care, further separate the muscle. With the pyloric mucosa exposed, check for mucosal perforation and, if present, close with 4–0 silk.
- **Step 5.** Close the abdominal wall.

Pyloroplasty

Heineke–Mikulicz Pyloroplasty

- **Step 1.** Perform a Kocher maneuver. Place two sutures, one superior and one inferior to the middle of the proposed longitudinal pyloroduodenal incision (Fig. 7.21).
- **Step 2.** Close the transverse duodenotomy in a longitudinal fashion. Apply traction on the two previously placed sutures and close in two layers using 3–0 PDS and 3–0 silk.

Finney Pyloroplasty (Fig. 7.22)

- **Step 1.** Mobilize the first and second portions of the duodenum by performing a Kocher maneuver.
- **Step 2.** With interrupted Lembert suture of 3–0 silk, appose the pyloric area of the stomach and the first portion of the duodenum.

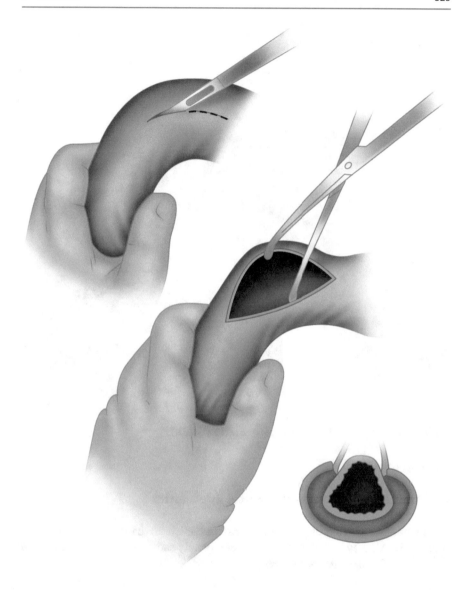

Fig. 7.20 Pyloric stenosis. Top: Muscle-splitting incision. Middle: Pylorus and pyloric tumor are delivered. Bottom: Exposed mucosa

- **Step 3.** Make a U-shaped, inverted incision to include the distal pyloric antrum and the proximal second portion of the duodenum. Locate the ulcer and excise it.
- **Step 4.** Close the gastroduodenal opening in layers, inner layer with a running PDS 3–0 stitch and outer with interrupted 3–0 silk Lemberts. Truncal vagotomy may be done if surgery is performed immediately after the perforation of the ulcer.

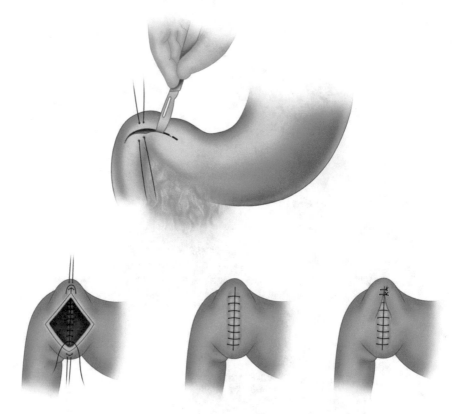

Fig. 7.21 Heineke–Mikulicz pyloroplasty (see text for details)

Gastrectomies

Determination of Some Anatomical Boundaries

Following are some arbitrary guidelines on which to base gastric resections (Fig. 7.23). All may be helpful; none are completely satisfactory. *All are described from the lesser curvature to the greater curvature.*

Guideline for 75% Gastric Resection
- A line extending from the first branch of the left gastric artery to a point approximately 2.5 cm below the spleen or to a point in the avascular area between the short gastric artery and the left gastroepiploic artery (Fig. 7.23).

Guidelines for 50% Gastric Resection
- A line extending from the third vein below the gastroesophageal junction on the lesser curvature (which is near the descending branch of the left gastric artery) to the midpoint of the left gastroepiploic artery where it comes closest to the gastric wall on the greater curvature.
- See Guidelines for Antrectomy (below) and Fig. 7.23.

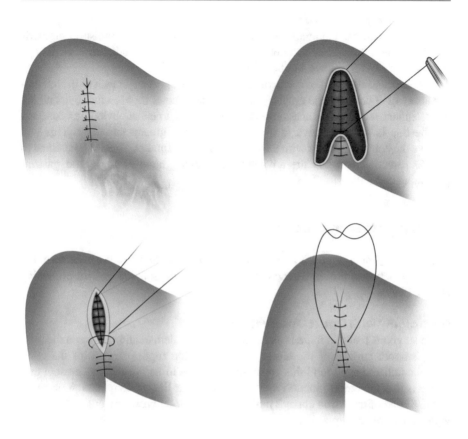

Fig. 7.22 Finney pyloroplasty (see text for details)

Fig. 7.23 Some arbitrary landmarks for partial gastric resection: (line 1) 75% resection; (line 2) 50% resection

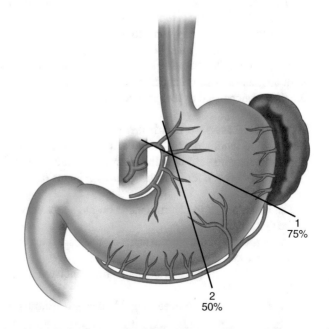

Guidelines for Antrectomy

The classic external landmarks for the antrum have been the incisura angularis proximally and the pyloric sphincter distally. The proximal landmark is vague and inconsistent. An alternative solution follows:

A line extending from the origin of the ascending esophageal branch of the left gastric artery (2–3 cm from the esophagus) to the anastomosis between the right and left gastroepiploic arteries. This anastomosis is, unfortunately, neither obvious nor constant.

The line is usually drawn at the midpoint of the greater curvature. This will remove the antrum together with a small cuff of distal fundus. This is about equal to a 50% resection and has the advantage of leaving none of the antral gastrin-producing cell area (Fig. 7.23).

Location of the Antral Boundary

Deciding how much stomach to resect would be easy if one knew the location of the boundary between the acid-producing gastric glands and the gastrin-producing pyloric glands.

Gastrotomy with Direct Observation

Some surgeons feel that there is an internally visible demarcation between the relatively smooth surface of the antral mucosa and the rugose surface of the body mucosa. Others have found this apparent difference to be misleading. Present evidence is that the antral junction may be an irregular line of demarcation or, more often, a zone of transition about 2 mm wide at the lesser curvature and about 3 mm wide at the greater curvature.

Estimation Based on Averages

On the lesser curvature the boundary between the antrum and the body is 2/5 of the distance from the pylorus to the cardia; on the greater curvature the boundary is 1/8 of the distance from the pylorus to the cardia.

Some other factors must be considered (Fig. 7.24). The position of the junction may shift with the pathologic state of the stomach. Also, the area of gastrin-producing antral mucosa appears to expand in the presence of a gastric ulcer, while remaining unchanged in the presence of a duodenal ulcer.

Estimation Based on Landmarks

There are no landmarks on the greater curvature, but on the lesser curvature three landmarks may be used to help determine the junction of the antrum and body: the pylorus, the "crow's foot" of the gastric divisions of the vagus nerve, and the incisura angularis.

- The boundary of the antrum starts on the lesser curvature 6–10 cm proximal to the pyloric valve.
- The boundary of the antrum starts on the lesser curvature 3–4 cm proximal to the "crow's foot" (Fig. 7.7).
- The boundary of the antrum starts at the incisura angularis (which may or may not be present).

As one can see, the preceding guidelines are arbitrary and unsatisfactory.

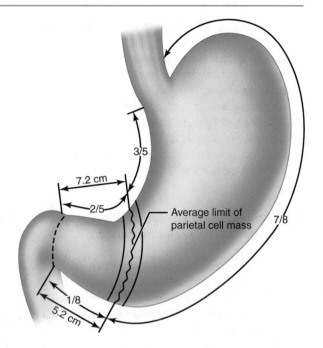

Fig. 7.24 The antrum–body junction in the "average stomach" is found at 2/5 of the distance from the pylorus to the cardia along the lesser curvature and 1/8 of the same distance along the greater curvature

Mobilization of the Stomach

Mobilization of the stomach may be obtained by (1) incising the gastrosplenic ligament and leaving the spleen in place, (2) mobilizing the spleen and preserving the short gastric arteries, or (3) removing the spleen.

Further mobilization of the stomach may be achieved by incision of the phrenoesophageal ligament to permit the distal esophagus to be brought into the abdomen. Inconstant avascular adhesions between the posterior surface of the stomach and the pancreas may require division.

Mobilization of the Duodenum

The first step is the method of Kocher. The peritoneum lateral to the duodenum is sectioned from the epiploic foramen downward, and the duodenum and head of the pancreas are raised from the underlying vena cava. A laparotomy pad may be placed behind the duodenum and pancreas. Further mobilization may be obtained by separating the first part of the duodenum from the pancreas.

In performing an esophagoduodenectomy after total gastrectomy, as much as 3.5 cm can be gained by sectioning the cystic duct and artery (with removal of the gallbladder), partially releasing the common bile duct, and allowing the duodenum to be rotated.

Complications of Ligation of the Left Gastric Arteries

Ischemia of the Gastric Remnant

Following a radical subtotal gastrectomy, the blood supply to the remaining gastric pouch comes from:

- Ascending branches of the left gastric artery
- Anterior short gastric arteries
- Left inferior phrenic artery
- Descending branches from thoracic esophageal branches
- Posterior gastric artery

Ischemia Resulting in Gastric Necrosis with Subsequent Anastomotic Leakage and Peritonitis

T-Closure of Stomach or Duodenum

T-closures of the stomach or duodenum are not recommended because the blood supply to the resulting corners may be inadequate. A long gastrotomy incision for the management of massive upper gastrointestinal bleeding should not extend past the pylorus, so that if a subsequent gastric resection seems desirable, a T-closure of the duodenal stump may be avoided. Similarly, if the surgeon believes a pyloroplasty may be required, a long exploratory incision might force her or him to make a T-closure of the pylorus. Figure 7.25 shows the recommended exploratory incisions for evaluating gastroduodenal hemorrhage.

It has been demonstrated that the entire stomach can be perfused through the right gastroepiploic artery alone.

Ischemia of the Duodenal Cuff

The duodenal branches of the pancreaticoduodenal arcades should be treated as end arteries and preserved if possible. This may be especially important in those patients having few, widely spaced (2–3 cm) duodenal branches (Fig. 7.26).

To be within the zone of safety, the minimum length required for anastomosis is 1–2 cm.

Control of Hemorrhage from the Gastroduodenal Artery

The rich submucosal vasculature of the stomach and duodenum becomes a disadvantage in the control of massive hemorrhage from ulcerative erosion of the gastroduodenal artery.

Careful suture ligation of the bleeding site from the inside is the only procedure recommended.

The retroduodenal portion of the gastroduodenal artery is about 2.5 cm from the pylorus and separated by about 0.8 cm (range 0.4–1.2 cm) of pancreatic tissue.

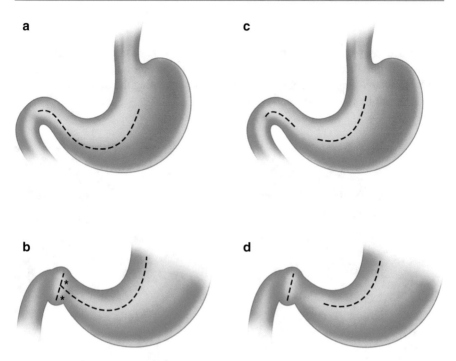

Fig. 7.25 Gastrostomy incisions: (**a**) Long incision extending into pylorus. (**b**) Closure of long incision resulting in corners (x) that may become ischemic. (**c**) Two separate incisions. (**d**) Closure avoids the corners of the preceding incision

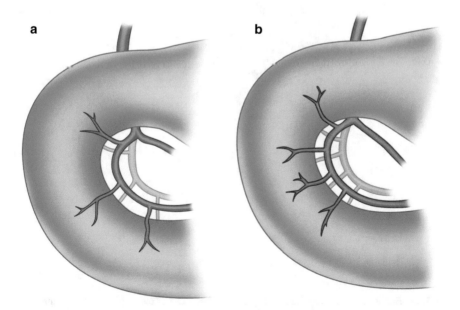

Fig. 7.26 Variations of arteries to the duodenum. (**a**) Widely spaced arterial branches. (**b**) Closely spaced arterial branches. These branches should be treated as end arteries and as many as possible should be preserved

Middle Colic Artery

A gastrectomy requires the surgeon to enter the lesser peritoneal cavity. Typically, entrance is obtained through the anterior leaf of the greater omentum (Fig. 7.27a). With reasonable care, the surgeon usually avoids perforating the transverse mesocolon, in which lies the middle colic artery.

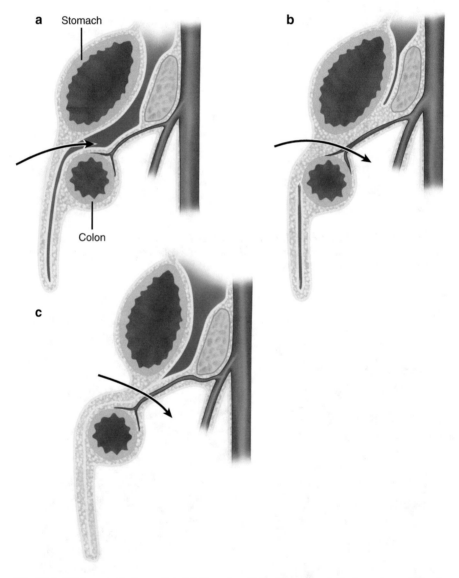

Fig. 7.27 Entrance to the lesser sac. (**a**) Normal anatomy. The arrow indicates entrance through the greater omentum. The middle colic artery in the transverse mesocolon is in no danger. (**b**) Pathological fixation of the omentum and posterior wall of the stomach with the transverse mesocolon. (**c**) Normal anatomy, but entrance so far inferior may injure the middle colic artery

In the presence of pathology, such as gastric ulcer or pancreatitis, the posterior leaf of the greater omentum and the posterior wall of the stomach may have become fixed to the transverse mesocolon and pancreas, thus eliminating the cavity of the lesser sac and giving the surgeon no warning that the mesocolon has been penetrated (Fig. 7.27b).

Even in the absence of abnormal fixation, should surgeons attempt to enter the lesser sac too far inferiorly, they will pass through the fused anterior leaf and transverse mesocolon (Fig. 7.27c). Under either circumstance, the middle colic vessels may be inadvertently ligated and divided along with the gastroepiploic branches.

Posterior Gastric Artery

A posterior gastric artery as much as 2 mm in diameter may arise from the proximal or middle third of the splenic artery. It supplies the posterior wall of the upper body, the fundus, and the cardia. Unrecognized, it may be a source of troublesome hemorrhage.

Because there are numerous types of gastrectomies and modifications (antecolic, retrocolic, large stoma [Polya's], small stoma [Hofmeister], Roux-en-Y, etc.), presentation of all of them is not possible within the scope of this book (Figs. 7.28 and 7.29). We have included subtotal distal gastrectomy (Billroth I and II), the difficult duodenal stump, total gastrectomy for cancer, vagotomy, and highly selective (or proximal gastric) vagotomy.

Subtotal Distal Gastrectomy

Billroth I (Figs. 7.30, 7.31, and 7.32)

Step 1. Mobilize the distal stomach by careful ligation of the arteries and veins of the lesser and greater curvature, distal to the point of the gastric transection. The surgeon now decides whether to perform a 75 or 50% gastrectomy or antrectomy and ligates the vessels accordingly.

   (a) Ligation of the gastrocolic ligament: Start in the vicinity of the origin of the left gastroepiploic vessels by carefully dividing the ligament between clamps. Ligate with 2–0 silk, proceeding from left to right to reach the gastroduodenal junction. The Harmonic Scalpel, also, can be used here.

   (b) Remember that the middle colic artery is within the leaflets of the transverse mesocolon. Carefully separate the transverse mesocolon from the posterior gastric wall to avoid injuring this vessel, which occasionally is not anastomosed with the marginal artery and, therefore, may cause problems for the transverse colon.

   (c) Use small, curved mosquito clamps to skeletonize the gastroduodenal area by ligating the vessel with 3–0 or 4–0 silk.

Step 2. Ligate the vessels of the lesser curvature and the right gastric artery (to avoid duodenal ischemia, ligate only the number of vessels necessary to perform the

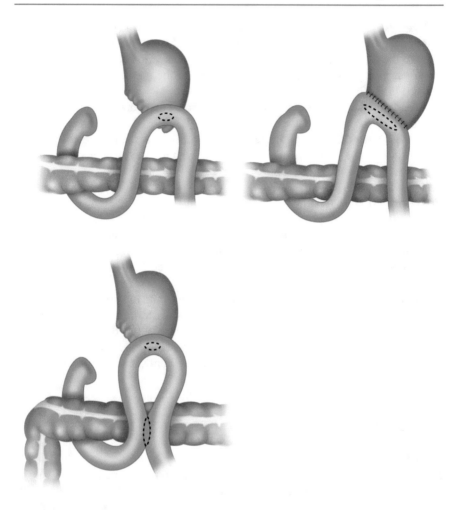

Fig. 7.28 Partial gastrectomies: gastric resections and variations

anastomosis). Continue dissecting and ligating toward the left gastric artery, which should be doubly ligated.

Step 3. Place two seromuscular sutures just below the duodenal transection line and a Kocher clamp just distal to the pylorus, but not in the duodenum. Divide the duodenum just distal to the Kocher clamp; this will ensure that no gastric mucosa is left at this level. We prefer not to use any clamps at the duodenum.

Step 4. At the designated line of gastric division, place clamps: noncrushing proximally and crushing (Kocher) distally, directed toward the lesser curvature. Divide the stomach and remove the specimen. Place a suture, as an indicator, at a point of the noncrushing clamp designating the two areas of the gastric remnant, one toward the lesser curvature (which will be closed), and one toward the greater curvature (which will be anastomosed to the duodenum). The first area should be

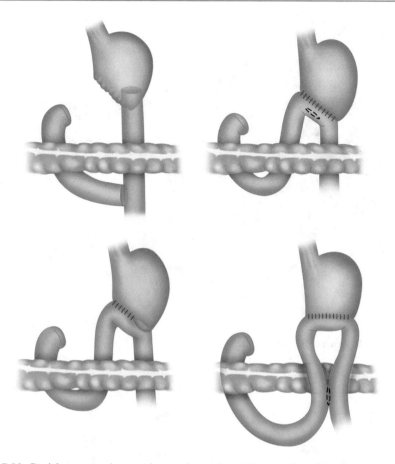

Fig. 7.29 Partial gastrectomies: gastric resections and variations (continued)

Fig. 7.30 Transection of distal stomach

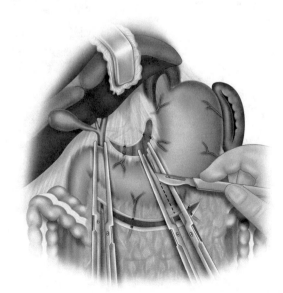

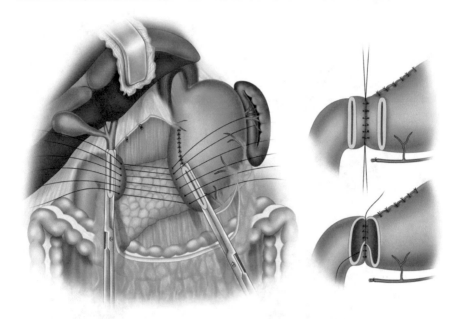

Fig. 7.31 Stomach is divided. Closure in two layers

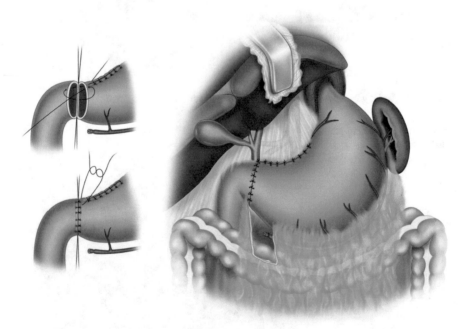

Fig. 7.32 Gastric and duodenal walls approximated. Gastric wall is anastomosed to duodenum

closed with two layers, using 3–0 PDS continuous oversewn, and after removal of the clamp, with 3–0 interrupted silk. Alternatively, a TA-90 stapler may be used for closing the lesser curvature. We like to cover the staple line with 3–0 silk Lembert sutures.

Step 5. Because of some peculiar mobility of the gastric mucosa, we apply Babcock clamps, bringing the mucosal and submucosal layers together so the gastric mucosa will not retract. Obtain hemostasis. Using interrupted 3–0 silk, approximate the gastric and duodenal wall posteriorly. Remove clamps and anastomose the gastric opening (including the gastric wall in toto) to the duodenum. Use a running 3–0 PDS for the mucosae and interrupted 3–0 silk seromuscular for the outside.

Remember the Angle of Sorrow
- This is where three suture lines come together at the lesser curvature area when the stomach and duodenum are anastomosed. It should be reinforced with 3–0 silk, taking seromuscular bites of both sides of the lesser curvature and the duodenum (Fig. 7.33).

Billroth II

- **Step 1.** Mobilize the stomach for 75 or 50% gastrectomy or antrectomy as described previously for Billroth I. Also, mobilize the first portion of the duodenum to allow enough room for a two-layer closure or for use of the TA-55 stapler across the duodenum. The staple line can be supported with interrupted 3–0 silk Lembert sutures. Also, we like to cover the suture line with viable omentum that may be present in the vicinity.

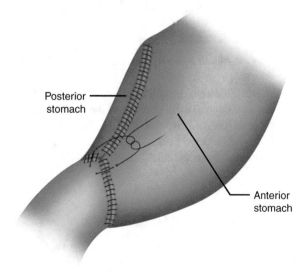

Fig. 7.33 Angle of sorrow. Reinforcing the juncture

Posterior stomach

Anterior stomach

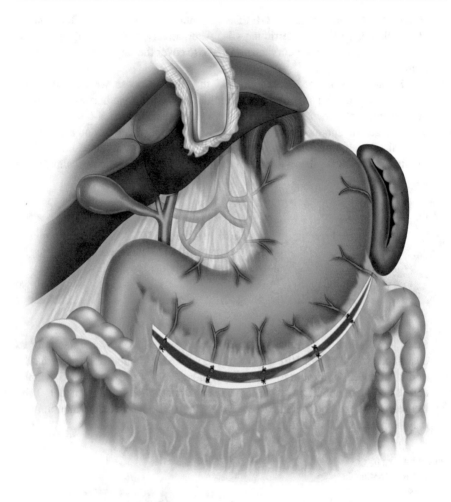

Fig. 7.34 Mobilization of the stomach and first part of the duodenum

- **Step 2.** There are many modifications of the Billroth II gastrectomy. The surgeon may decide to use the opening of the gastric remnant in toto or to use part of it as we described in Billroth I. In Figs. 7.34, 7.35, 7.36, 7.37, 7.38, 7.39, 7.40, 7.41, 7.42, and 7.43 we present the retrocolic method, but the antecolic method (not illustrated) is acceptable on rare occasions.

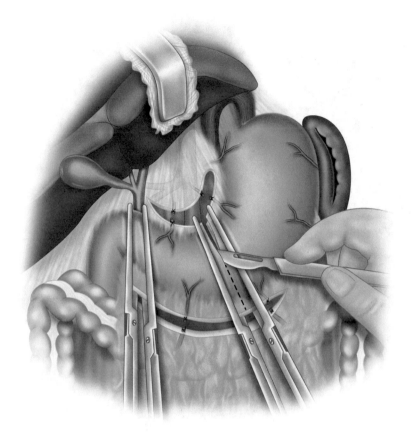

Fig. 7.35 Transect and remove the distal stomach and a small part of the first portion of the duodenum

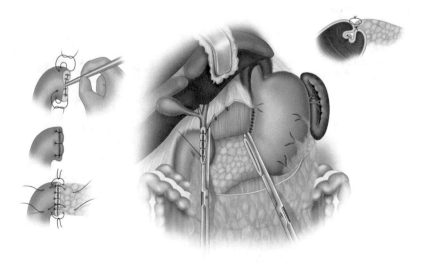

Fig. 7.36 The specimen is removed and the duodenal opening is closed in two layers

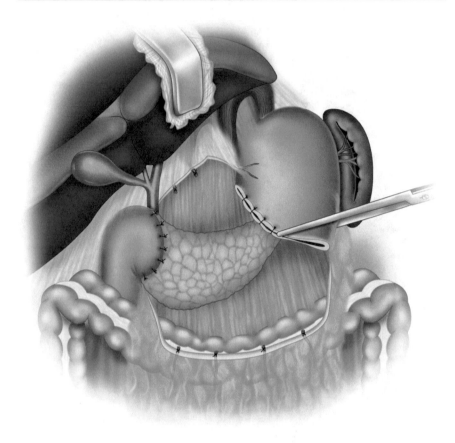

Fig. 7.37 Partial closure of the gastric opening at the lesser curvature side

Fig. 7.38 Elevate the transverse colon. If preparing a retrocolic anastomosis, insert a proximal jejunal loop through an avascular area of the mesocolon

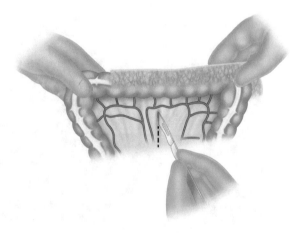

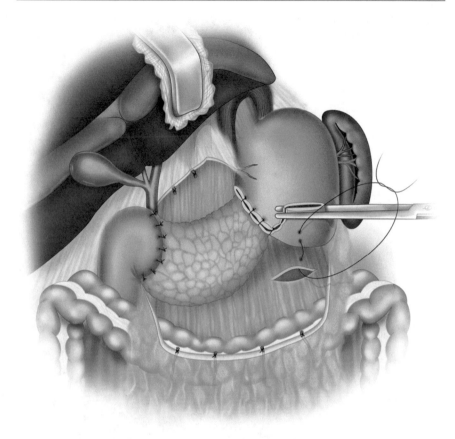

Fig. 7.39 Suturing of the mesocolon to the posterior gastric wall close to the opening

Fig. 7.40 The proximal loop is inserted through the opening of the mesocolon

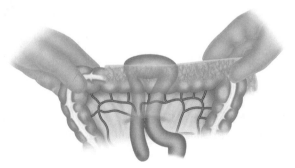

Fig. 7.41 The four-layer anastomosis (see also Fig. 7.42)

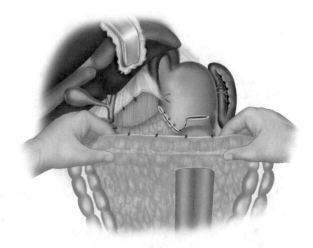

Fig. 7.42 Completion of the four-layer anastomosis

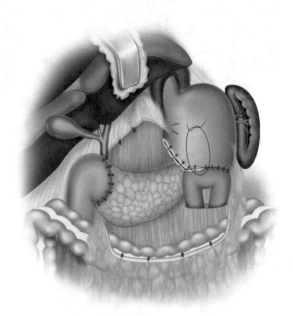

Difficult Duodenal Stump

- **Step 1.** Close the duodenal stump as perfectly as possible (Table 7.2).

Total Gastrectomy for Cancer

The specimen should include the following (Fig. 7.44):
- Gastroesophageal junction
- Lesser omentum (hepatogastric and partial hepatoduodenal ligaments)

Fig. 7.43 (**a**) and (**b**) An alternative method of anastomosis, bringing the stomach down the mesocolic opening and securing the gastric wall with interrupted sutures to the transverse mesocolon

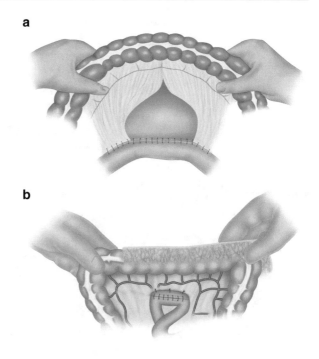

Table 7.2 Siewart classification of GEJ tumors

Siewert type	Epicenter of the lesion
I	Within 1 to 5 cm above the anatomic GEJ
II	Within 1 cm above and 2 cm below the GEJ (i.e. true carcinoma of the cardia)
III	Between 2 to 5 cm below the GEJ, infiltrating GEJ and esophagus from below (subcardial carcinoma)

Type I and II are treated as esophageal primary tumors. Type III is considered a gastric tumor and treated with total gastrectomy and D2 lymphadenectomy

- Distal pancreas, as required
- Greater omentum, including gastrocolic ligament, but protecting the transverse mesocolon, which contains the middle colic artery
- Spleen
- D1 and D2 lymph node stations, with nodes along hepatoduodenal ligament and the upper border of the pancreas also removed (referred to as D2+ lymphadenectomy)
- **Step 1.** Approach the gastroesophageal area and, with the index finger, penetrate the local avascular ligaments (Fig. 7.45). Insert a Penrose drain for traction of the abdominal esophagus.
- **Step 2.** Elevate the greater omentum and carefully separate it from the transverse colon (Figs. 7.46 and 7.47). Treat the duodenum and the lower pole of the spleen with care. If the surgeon decides to perform a splenectomy, the splenic veins and

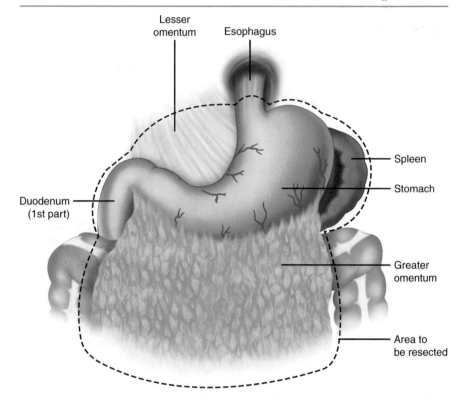

Fig. 7.44 Resection site for total gastrectomy

ligaments should be ligated and cut. Continue the upward dissection of the greater omentum, with ligation of the upper short gastric vessels.

- **Step 3.** Remove the lesser omentum. Ligate doubly the right and left gastric arteries. We prefer sharp and blunt dissection, pushing all the tissues from the porta hepatis toward the greater curvature (Fig. 7.48).
- **Step 4.** With complete gastric mobilization from the gastroesophageal junction to the proximal portion of the second part of the duodenum, divide the duodenum and the abdominal esophagus (Fig. 7.49). Place 3–0 silk stay sutures on each side of the esophagus (Fig. 7.50). Remove the specimen.
- **Step 5.** Perform duodenal closure as described previously. Gastrointestinal continuity is accomplished by a Roux-en-Y esophagojejunal anastomosis as follows. Divide the jejunum between the GIA stapler. Sacrifice one (preferably) or two arterial arcades. Pass the distal end of the divided bowel through a small hole of the transverse colon. Anastomose end to side with the esophagus using 4–0 interrupted silk (Fig. 7.51). Be careful that the esophageal mucosa retracts upward, and be sure to include all the esophageal layers in your bites. Before the

Fig. 7.45 Blunt
penetration

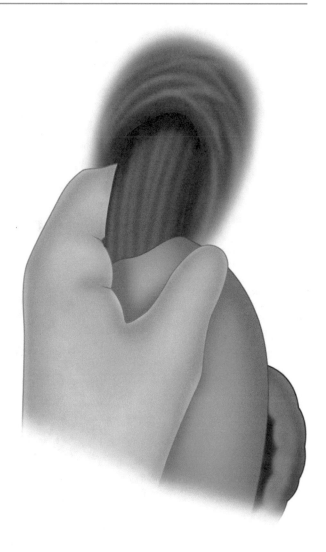

anterior layer is closed, pass the nasogastric tube into the jejunal loop. We protect
the anastomosis with two or three interrupted silk sutures, anchoring the jejunal
wall just below the suture line to the esophageal hiatus.
- **Step 6.** Anastomose the opening of the proximal jejunum to the jejunal loop in
  two layers. Fix the opening of the transverse mesocolon to the jejunum with a
  few 4–0 silk interrupted sutures (Fig. 7.52).
- **Step 7.** Close the abdomen.

Fig. 7.46 Greater omentum elevated

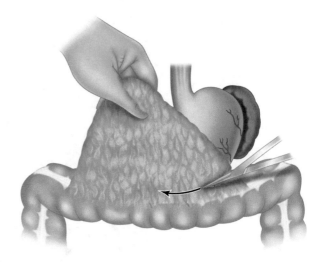

Fig. 7.47 Relationship of omentum to transverse colon. X = points of separation

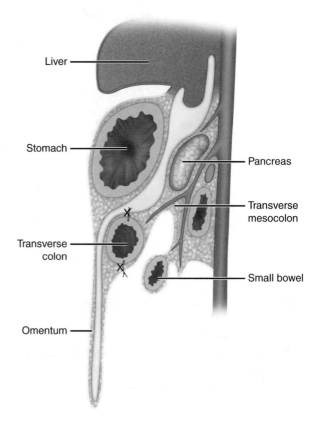

Fig. 7.48 Removal of lesser omentum

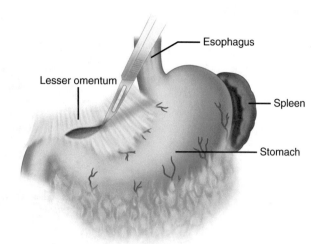

Fig. 7.49 Stomach divided from abdominal esophagus and the duodenum

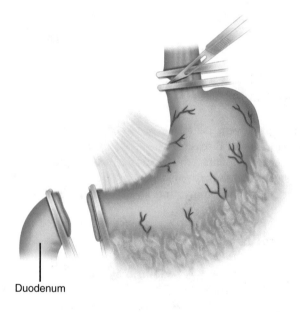

Fig. 7.50 Placement of
stay sutures

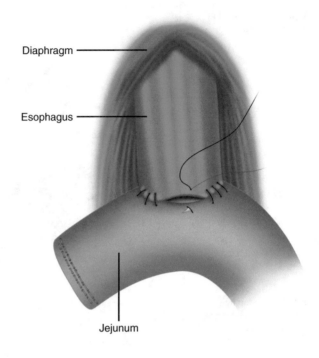

Diaphragm

Esophagus

Jejunum

Vagotomies

Since the advent and extensive use of proton pump inhibitors, the role of surgeons in gastric ulcer disease has declined significantly. However, we may still on occasion encounter intractable ulcers that need surgical management, and it is important to understand the anatomical and physiologic basis of these operations. There are four types of vagotomy: truncal, selective, parietal cell, and extended proximal.

Truncal Vagotomy

A truncal vagotomy is performed by sectioning the anterior and posterior trunks within the abdomen (Fig. 7.7). This procedure destroys the vagal innervation to the stomach and all other abdominal viscera. Identification is subordinate in this procedure; complete transection is the goal. Complete skeletonization of the abdominal esophagus is mandatory, and pyloric drainage is usually necessary.

Selective Vagotomy

In selective vagotomy, only the anterior and posterior descending nerves of the gastric divisions (nerves of Latarjet) are divided (Fig. 7.53). The hepatic branch of the

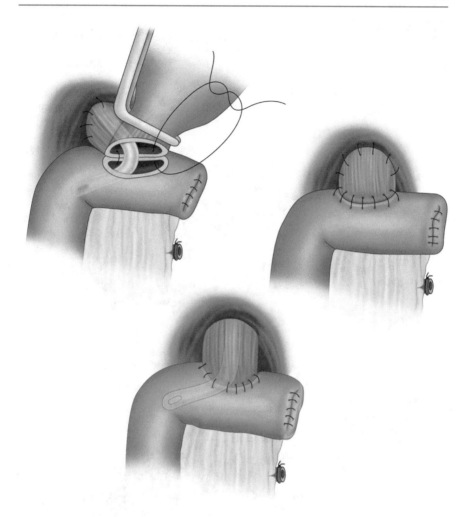

Fig. 7.51 Duodenal closure (see text)

anterior division, including the pyloric branch, and the celiac branch of the posterior division are preserved. Thus, the stomach is denervated, while the vagal fibers to the pylorus, the biliary tract, and the intestines remain intact.

Parietal Cell Vagotomy

A parietal cell vagotomy may also be called "highly selective vagotomy," "superselective vagotomy," "proximal gastric vagotomy," or "acidosecretive vagotomy." The goal is denervation of the proximal two-thirds of the stomach only, preserving the antral and pyloric innervation as well as the hepatic and celiac divisions (Fig. 7.54). Denervation is accomplished by sectioning of the proximal gastric branches of the

Fig. 7.52 Completed
end-to-side
esophagojejunal and
jejunojejunal anastomoses

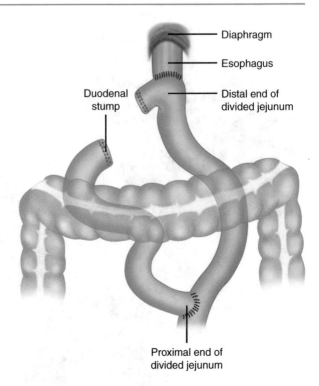

Fig. 7.53 Selective
vagotomy preserves the
celiac and hepatic divisions
but will not denervate the
pylorus, biliary tract, and
remaining intestinal tract

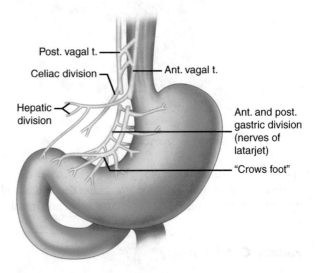

descending anterior and posterior nerves of Latarjet while preserving the distal
branches to the antrum and pylorus.

The distal extent of a highly selective vagotomy is to the left of the "crow's foot,"
about 7 cm from the pylorus. This may or may not coincide with the location of the
boundary between the antrum and the body of the stomach. Various authors state
that the distal limit of dissection should be between 5 and 10 cm from the pylorus.

Fig. 7.54 Parietal cell (superselective) vagotomy preserves antropyloric as well as celiac and hepatic innervation. There is some risk of perforation as a result of ischemia of the lesser curvature

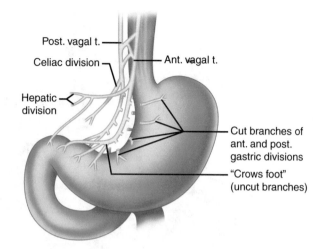

Post. vagal t.

Celiac division

Ant. vagal t.

Hepatic division

Cut branches of ant. and post. gastric divisions

"Crows foot" (uncut branches)

Extended Proximal Vagotomy

Extended proximal vagotomy for complete gastric denervation as shown in Fig. 7.55 consists of vagal denervation of the gastric fundus and greater curvature.

> **Remember**
> - Vagotomy may be said to be complete if no areas of parietal cell activity can be found with a pH probe; if activity is found, the vagotomy is incomplete. Clinically, vagotomy may be considered complete if there is no recurrence of an ulcer.
> - Gastric branches arising from vagal trunks proximal to the separation of the major division may be present and, if so, must be sectioned. The first and highest of such posterior branches is the "criminal nerve of Grassi."

Truncal Vagotomy

- **Step 1.** Mobilize the abdominal esophagus by peritoneal incision of the gastroesophageal junction. Palpate the abdominal esophagus. Locate the anterior vagus nerve and mobilize it with a nerve hook. Remove a segment of the nerve, clip the proximal and distal ends, and send the specimen to the lab for frozen section (Fig. 7.56).
- **Step 2.** Palpate the posterior area. The nerve may be located close to the aorta between the right and left diaphragmatic crura and slightly right of the midline. Again, remove a segment of the nerve, clip the proximal and distal ends, and send to the lab for frozen section (Fig. 7.57).
- **Step 3.** Because the vagus nerve exhibits many vagaries, it is important to skeletonize the esophagus.

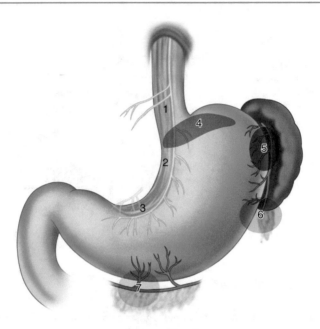

Fig. 7.55 The seven areas of vagotomy. Preganglionic efferent vagus nerves reach the parietal cell mass in seven areas. Area 1 is the periesophageal region; area 2 is the lesser curve of the stomach; area 3 is the crow's foot area; area 4 is represented by the broken line, as the gastropancreatic fold is not visible anteriorly; area 5 is the region of short gastric vessels; area 6 is the left gastroepiploic pedicle; and area 7 is the right gastroepiploic pedicle. Areas 3, 4, 6, and 7 are divided routinely during extended highly selective vagotomy. Area 5 is preserved because the nerves at this site cannot be divided without sacrificing essential blood supply to the proximal part of the stomach

Fig. 7.56 Sectioning of anterior vagus nerve

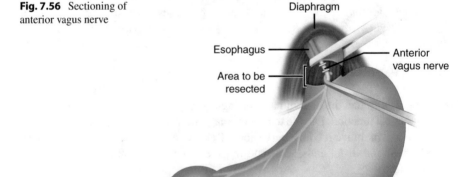

Fig. 7.57 Sectioning of posterior vagus nerve

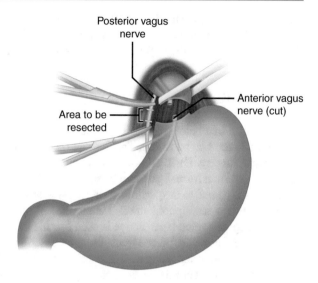

Posterior vagus nerve

Anterior vagus nerve (cut)

Area to be resected

Parietal Cell Vagotomy

- **Step 1.** Mobilize the abdominal esophagus at the periesophageal space. Localize the right and left vagus nerves, which should be protected. Localize the nerves of Latarjet. Protect the hepatic division and celiac divisions.
- **Step 2.** Mobilize the distal half of the greater curvature. Starting approximately 6 cm from the pylorus, begin an upward dissection of the neurovascular elements between the inner curve and the nerve of Latarjet, by dividing and ligating them with 4–0 silk. Continue dissection toward the cardiac angle.

Remember
- Protect the trunks
- Protect the nerves of Latarjet
- Protect the pyloric branch
- Protect the crow's foot

- **Step 3.** Re-peritonealize the lesser curve by approximating the anterior and posterior walls with interrupted 3–0 silk.

Minimally Invasive Approaches to Gastric Resection

With the extensive use of laparoscopy and now robotic techniques by general surgeons in the past decade, it is prudent to mention some basic minimally invasive approaches to the stomach. It is pertinent to mention that the fundamental operation does not change, but the method of conducting that operation may show slight variations. Sticking to good surgical principles as described above is paramount. MIS techniques in stomach are most commonly used for bariatric surgical procedures with extension now to cancer resections and lymph node dissections.

Sleeve Gastrectomy

We have described below the most common surgical procedure for morbid obesity performed in the United States. The authors recommend using the NIH guidelines for bariatric surgery. For BMI > 45, we do not recommend sleeve gastrectomy and prefer to perform a formal gastric bypass surgery.

1. Access is gained to the peritoneal cavity using the optical trocar entry technique 15 cm below the xiphoid and 2–3 cm to the left of midline.
2. A 45-degree angled laparoscope is used for this procedure.
3. Remaining ports are placed in positions as described in Fig. 7.58.
4. The liver is elevated using a Nathanson liver retractor inserted through a subxiphoid insertion (in this instance the right lateral most port doesn't need to be placed initially). Alternatively, the liver can be elevated using a closed grasper to prop-ip the left lateral sector of the liver.
5. The pylorus of the stomach is then identified, and the greater curve of the stomach elevated.

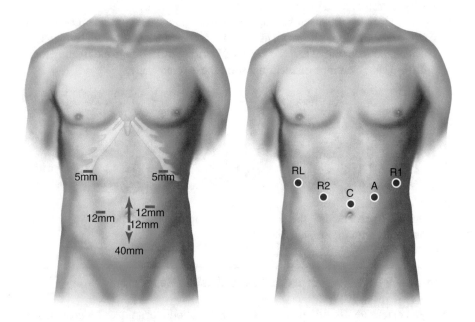

Fig. 7.58 Left panel – Port Placement for laparoscopic gastrectomy. Right panel – Port placement for robotic gastrectomy*. *Given the significant differences in robotic platforms from different generations this is a generalized overview of port placement

6. The greater sac is entered after dividing the greater omentum. The greater curvature of the stomach is then dissected free from the omentum and the short gastric blood vessels using the laparoscopic ultrasonic scalpel.
7. The dissection is started 5 cm from the pylorus and proceeds to the Angle of His.
8. A standard endoscope (10 mm gastroscope) is then passed under direct vision through the esophagus, stomach, and into the first portion of the duodenum.
9. The gastroscope is aligned along the lesser curvature of the stomach and used as a bougie to perform the vertical sleeve gastrectomy beginning 2 cm proximal to the pylorus and extending to the Angle of His.
10. An endoscopic linear cutting stapler (the authors prefer with seam guards) is used to serially staple and transect the stomach staying just to the left and lateral to the endoscope.
11. The gastrectomy is visualized with the endoscope during the procedure. The transected stomach, which includes the greater curvature, is completely freed and removed from the peritoneum through the left flank port incision.
12. The staple line along the remaining tubularized stomach is then tested for any leak through insufflations with the gastroscope, while the remnant stomach is submerged under irrigation fluid.
13. The staple line is concurrently evaluated for bleeding both intraperitoneally with the laparoscope as well as intraluminally with the gastroscope.
14. The authors do not routinely leave a drain in place after standard sleeve gastrectomy. Drain placement should be individualized based on patient and intraoperative factors. Ports are closed in standard fashion with all 12 mm ports having fascia closed.

Anatomical Complications

Stomach

- Complications related to vagotomy
- Hemorrhage related to vagotomy
- Ischemia of the distal esophagus from skeletonization which could lead to stenosis, dysphasia, or perforation
- Injury to the spleen usually from excessive traction on the gastrosplenic or front a splenic ligament
- Preparation of pleura leading to pneumothorax
- Bleeding from the left lobe of the liver after mobilization
- Inadequate vagotomy

Complications Related to Hiatal Hernia Repair

- Vascular injuries
- Injury to left hepatic vein

- Injury to accessory vessels or to bile ducts extending into the left triangular ligament
- Injury to the left inferior phrenic artery which crosses the left crus and passes behind the esophagus
- Injury to the left inferior phrenic vein
- Injury to left gastric artery
- Injury to left gastric (coronary) vein
- Injury to the aorta and celiac truck
- Injury to inferior vena cava
- Injury to an aberrant left hepatic artery

Organ Injuries

- Injury of the pleura which is in contact with the lower third of the esophagus resulting in a pneumothorax
- Injury to the liver during its mobilization and excessive retraction
- Injury to the hepatic division of the vagus nerve when dissecting the hepatogastric ligament
- Thoracic duct injury
- Pericardial sac injury
- Injury to the posterior branches of the phrenic nerve
- Esophageal perforation

Complications Related to Gastrectomy

- Vascular injuries
  - 25% of patients most or all of the hepatic arterial blood supply comes from the left gastric artery. Ligation of this artery may result in ischemia to all or a portion of the liver
  - Ischemia of the gastric remnant. The blood supply to the gastric remnant comes from ascending branches of the left gastric artery, anterior short gastric arteries, left inferior phrenic artery, descending branches from thoracic esophageal branches and the posterior gastric artery.
  - Ischemia of the distal esophagus can result from ligation of the left gastric artery.
  - Inadvertent celiac and hepatic vagotomy.
  - Ischemia resulting in gastric necrosis. See preceding section.
  - Ischemia of the duodenal cuff.
  - Injury to gastroduodenal artery, middle colic artery, and the posterior gastric artery.
- Adjacent organ injuries
  - Esophagus. Perforation can be a result of aggressive dissection looking for the vagus nerve.

- Liver. See above.
- Omentum. Ligation of the blood supply, right and left gastroepiploic arteries, can result in infarction. If not removed it can result in fever and infection with abscess formation.
- Spleen. Avulsion-type injuries can result in bleeding.
- Common bile duct. This can occur during mobilization of the duodenum.
- Accessory pancreatic duct of Santorini. In approximately 10% of patients the accessory duct is the sole drainage of part of the pancreas. Injury of this duct can occur when ligating the gastroduodenal artery.
- Pancreas. Inversion of the duodenal following a Billroth II procedure could obstruct the accessory pancreatic duct or the main pancreatic duct.
- Colon. Blood supply to the transverse colon can be interrupted if the middle colic artery is injured. This can occur when entering the lesser sac.

Duodenum

8

David R. Elwood

Anatomy

General Description of the Duodenum

The duodenum measures approximately 25–30 cm in length, giving rise to the name, "duodenum" or breadth of twelve fingers. "Duodenal sweep" refers to the first and second portions of the duodenum.

The first, or superior, portion (5 cm long) passes upward from the pylorus to the neck of the gallbladder. The proximal half of the first portion is intraperitoneal, movable, and enclosed by the same peritoneal layers that invest the stomach. It is attached to the undersurface of the right lobe of the liver via the hepatoduodenal ligament. This segment is more distensible, having only a few longitudinal mucosal folds rather than the circumferential folds that line the rest of the duodenum. It is commonly referred to as the duodenal "bulb" or "cap," and it can have a triangular appearance on radiologic imaging. The bulb is in intimate contact posteriorly with the common bile duct and gastroduodenal artery. The distal half of the first portion becomes retroperitoneal. It forms the inferior boundary of the epiploic foramen, or "Foramen of Winslow." The duodenum is separated from the inferior vena cava by a small amount of connective tissue.

The second, or descending, portion (7.5 cm long) lies posterior to the transverse mesocolon and anterior to the right kidney and inferior vena cava. The left border is attached to the head of the pancreas. The common bile and pancreatic ducts open into the left side of this portion of the duodenum.

The third and fourth portions of the duodenum lie inferior to the transverse mesocolon. Their cranial surfaces are in contact with the uncinate process of the

D. R. Elwood (✉)
Division of General and Gastrointestinal Surgery, Department of Surgery, Emory University, Atlanta, GA, USA
e-mail: david.elwood@emory.edu

© Springer Nature Switzerland AG 2021
L. J. Skandalakis (ed.), *Surgical Anatomy and Technique*,
https://doi.org/10.1007/978-3-030-51313-9_8

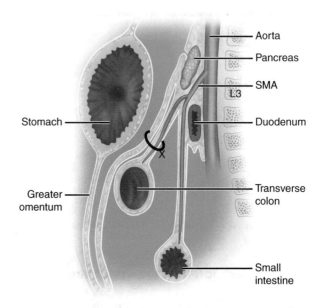

Fig. 8.1 Diagrammatic sagittal section showing the position of the duodenum in relation to the aorta and the superior mesenteric artery. The transverse mesocolon is marked by an X. *SMA* superior mesenteric artery

pancreas (Fig. 8.1). The parietal peritoneum covering the fourth portion of the duodenum contains folds beneath which are blind recesses or paraduodenal fossae.

The third, or horizontal, portion of the duodenum (10 cm long) passes to the left and slightly upward, crossing anterior to the inferior vena cava and posterior to the superior mesenteric artery and vein. The fourth, or ascending, portion (2.5 cm long) passes upward and slightly to the left, crossing the spine anterior to the aorta. It may cover the origin of the inferior mesenteric artery from the aorta. The duodenum ends at the duodenojejunal flexure, which usually lies immediately to the left of the aorta.

At the gastroduodenal junction, the continuity of the circular musculature is interrupted by a ring-shaped septum of connective tissue derived from the submucosa. Proximal to this ring, the circular muscle layer thickens to form the pyloric sphincter of the stomach; distal to the ring there is an abrupt decrease in the thickness of the circular muscle to form the relatively thin-walled duodenum. This decrease results in a pyloric "os pylorus" surrounded by a duodenal fornix. This arrangement must be kept in mind when performing pyloromyotomy.

The gastroduodenal junction is marked internally by the submucosal glands of Brunner. This may not correspond to the muscular junction. The submucosal glands may extend a few centimeters into the pylorus, and occasionally, antral gastric mucosa may prolapse through the pylorus to produce a radiological finding, but not a true clinical syndrome.

The duodenojejunal junction is marked externally by the attachment of the suspensory ligament of Treitz. This ligament is a fibromuscular band that arises from the right crus of the diaphragm, inserting on the upper surface of the duodenojejunal flexure. It passes posterior to the pancreas and the splenic vein and anterior to the left renal vein.

Usually the suspensory ligament inserts on the duodenal flexure and the third and fourth portions of the duodenum (Fig. 8.2b). Alternatively, it may insert on the flexure only (Fig. 8.2a) or on the third and fourth portions only (Fig. 8.2c), or there may be multiple attachments (Fig. 8.2d).

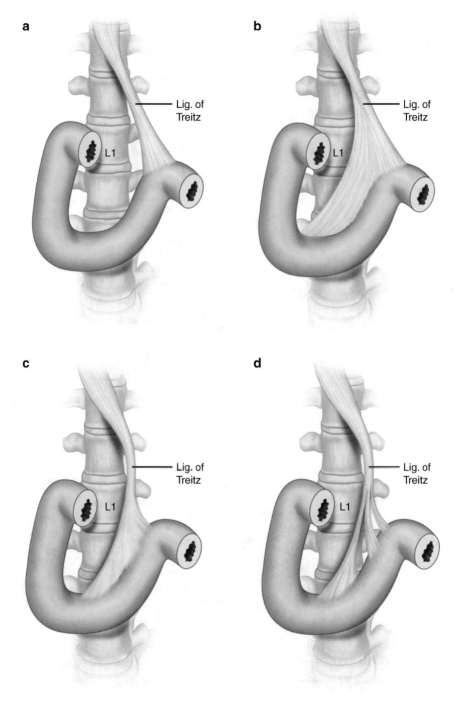

Fig. 8.2 Four configurations of the suspensory ligament of Treitz: (**a**) attachment to the duodeno-jejunal flexure. (**b**) Attachments to the flexure and the third and fourth portions of the duodenum. (**c**) Attachments to the third and fourth portions only. (**d**) Multiple separated attachments of the suspensory ligament

Vascular System of the Duodenum

Arteries

The blood supply of the duodenum is confusing due to the diverse possibilities of origin, distribution, and individual variations (Figs. 8.3, 8.4, and 8.5). This is especially true of the blood supply of the first portion of the duodenum.

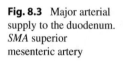

Fig. 8.3 Major arterial supply to the duodenum. *SMA* superior mesenteric artery

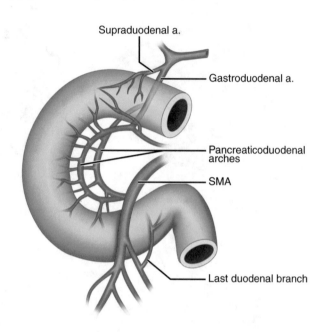

Supraduodenal a.

Gastroduodenal a.

Pancreaticoduodenal arches

SMA

Last duodenal branch

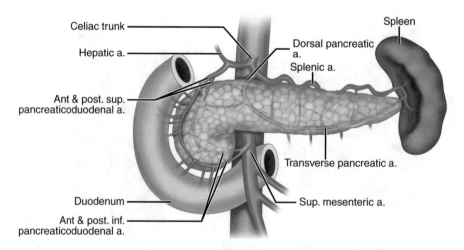

Celiac trunk

Hepatic a.

Ant & post. sup. pancreaticoduodenal a.

Dorsal pancreatic a.

Splenic a.

Spleen

Transverse pancreatic a.

Duodenum

Ant & post. inf. pancreaticoduodenal a.

Sup. mesenteric a.

Fig. 8.4 Anterior view of arterial supply of the duodenum and pancreas

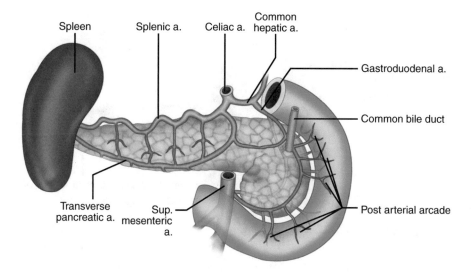

Fig. 8.5 Posterior view of arterial supply of the duodenum and pancreas

The first part of the duodenum is supplied by the supraduodenal artery and the posterior superior pancreaticoduodenal branch of the gastroduodenal artery (retroduodenal artery as described by Edwards, Michels, and Wilkie), which is a branch of the common hepatic artery.

The remaining three parts of the duodenum are supplied by an anterior and a posterior arcade. Pancreatic and duodenal branches spring from the arcades. Those supplying the duodenum are called arteriae rectae; they may be embedded in the substance of the pancreas.

Four arteries contribute to the pancreaticoduodenal vascular arcades:

- The anterior superior pancreaticoduodenal arteries (commonly two in number) arise from the gastroduodenal artery on the ventral surface of the pancreas.
- The posterior superior pancreaticoduodenal (retroduodenal) artery usually crosses in front of the common bile duct, then spirals to the right and posterior to the duct, descending deep to the head of the pancreas. Several of the retroduodenal artery branches anastomose inferiorly with rami from the posterior branch of the inferior pancreaticoduodenal artery.
- Third and fourth, the anterior inferior pancreaticoduodenal artery and the posterior inferior pancreaticoduodenal artery arise from the superior mesenteric artery or its first jejunal branch, either separately or from a common stem.

The surgeon should be sure to ligate only one of the two arcades—superior or inferior.

Veins

The venous arcades draining the duodenum follow the arterial arcades and tend to lie superficial to them (Figs. 8.6 and 8.7). The veins of the lower first part of the duodenum and the pylorus usually open into the right gastroepiploic veins.

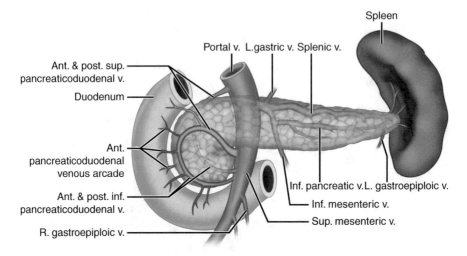

Fig. 8.6 The venous drainage of the duodenum and pancreas: anterior view

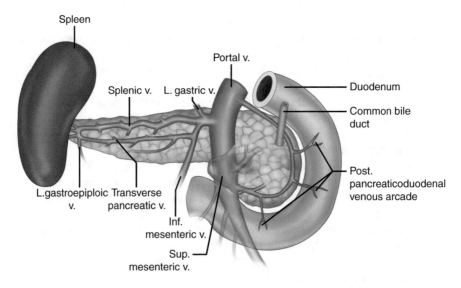

Fig. 8.7 The venous drainage of the duodenum and pancreas, and formation of the hepatic portal vein: posterior view

Lymphatic Drainage

The duodenum is richly supplied with lymphatics (Fig. 8.8). Collecting trunks pass over the anterior and posterior duodenal wall toward the lesser curvature to enter the anterior and posterior pancreaticoduodenal lymph nodes.

The lymphatics of the duodenum have received very little attention, even though some studies of the lymphatics of the pancreas have been conducted.

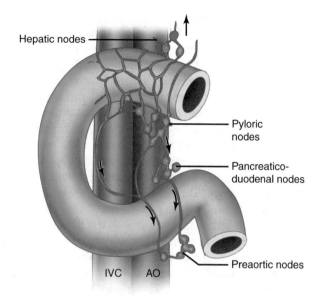

Fig. 8.8 Diagrammatic presentation of duodenal lymphatica. *Ao* aorta, *IVC* inferior vena cava

Hepatic nodes

Pyloric nodes

Pancreatico-duodenal nodes

Preaortic nodes

IVC   AO

Nerve Supply of the Duodenum

Within the duodenal wall are the two well-known neural plexuses of the gastrointestinal tract. Meissner's plexus is in the submucosa, and Auerbach's plexus is between the circular and longitudinal layers of the muscularis externa. In 6 of 100 specimens studied, nerves from the hepatic division of the anterior vagal trunk gave rise to one or more branches that innervated the first part of the duodenum. In most specimens, some branches could be traced upward toward the gastric incisura. The vagaries of the vagus nerve are well known.

Technique

Surgery of the duodenum includes duodenotomy, duodenostomy, duodenal resection, and partial anastomosis with stomach or jejunum. Most of these surgical techniques are described in other chapters in connection with other organs such as the stomach (see Chap. 7) and the pancreas (see Chap. 9). The author presents here maneuvers for duodenal exposure, surgical treatments for superior mesenteric artery syndrome, and proper ligation of the gastroduodenal artery within a bleeding duodenal ulcer.

Surgical Applications

Good results from surgical procedures in the first part of the duodenum can be anticipated if surgeons have sound anatomical knowledge and if they practice good technique and conservative skeletonization. The blood supply to this area is limited.

Excessive vascular skeletization beyond 2 cm can lead to ischemia and "blow out" of a duodenal stump or failure of a B1gastroduodenal anastomosis.

The second and proximal third portions of the duodenum are difficult to deal with because of their relationship to the head of the pancreas and the uncinate process. It is important to be aware of the superior mesenteric vessels, the transverse mesocolon with its marginal artery and the middle colic artery, and the inferior mesenteric artery, which the third portion of the duodenum covers in most cases. The surgeon should proceed slowly when dealing with the uncinate process, which is closely related to the superior mesenteric vessels. The inferior pancreaticoduodenal arcades yield many small vessels; small branches from the superior mesenteric artery are present.

The fourth portion of the duodenum is related to two important anatomical entities: the ligament of Treitz and the inferior mesenteric vein, located to the left of the paraduodenal fossae. This portion is a useful place to begin exploring the distal duodenum (third and fourth portions), and the surgeon should remember that mobilization of the right colon and transection of the ligament of Treitz are necessary for good exposure of the distal duodenum. The divisions of the intestinal branches of the superior mesenteric artery provide the blood supply, which is similar to that of the rest of the small bowel. The arteries have no collateral circulation, and the wall has the least efficient blood supply in the antimesenteric border. (The duodenum does not have a mesentery; the middle of the anterior wall, which is covered by peritoneum, should be considered "antimesenteric.")

Exposure and Mobilization of the Duodenum
(Figs. 8.9, 8.10, and 8.11)

It may be necessary to expose the duodenum to search for traumatic injury, to perform pancreatic procedures, to explore the distal common bile duct, to section the suspensory ligament for relief of duodenal compression, or to reduce a redundant proximal loop of a gastrojejunostomy above the transverse mesocolon. Exposure can be accomplished by the following maneuvers:
- Mobilization of the first, second, and proximal third portions of the duodenum is accomplished by incising the parietal peritoneum from the epiploic foramen downward along the descending duodenum (second portion) and retracting it medially; this is the Kocher maneuver. The posterior wall of the duodenum can be examined, and the retroduodenal and pancreatic portions of the common bile duct can be explored.
- An incision through the transverse mesocolon or the gastrocolic omentum exposes the third portion of the duodenum. Alternatively, the Cattell maneuver can be performed by reflecting the right side of the colon medially and incising the line of fusion between the small bowel mesentery and retroperitoneum to

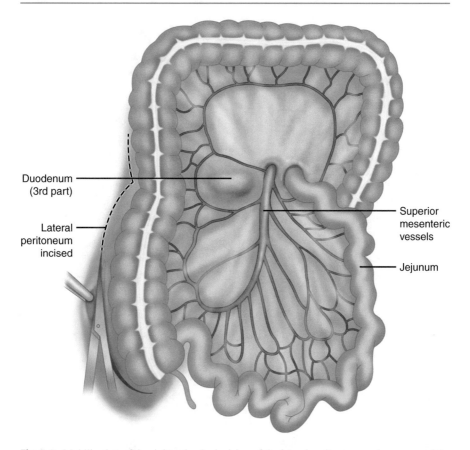

Duodenum
(3rd part)

Lateral
peritoneum
incised

Superior
mesenteric
vessels

Jejunum

Fig. 8.9 Mobilization of the right colon by incision of the lateral peritoneum and exposure of the third part of the duodenum by incision of the transverse mesocolon. Note that the superior mesenteric vein is not identified

reveal the third portion of the duodenum proximal to the superior mesenteric vessels (Figs. 8.9, 8.10, and 8.11).

- Incision through the gastrocolic omentum and further reflection of the right colon, combined with a Kocher maneuver extended to the parietal fold just inferior to the paraduodenal fossa, will expose the entire duodenum. This is the Cattell-Braasch maneuver (Fig. 8.12). When incising the peritoneum at the duodenojejunal flexure, attention must be paid to avoiding injury to the inferior mesenteric vein. The duodenum can be further mobilized by transection of the suspensory ligament.

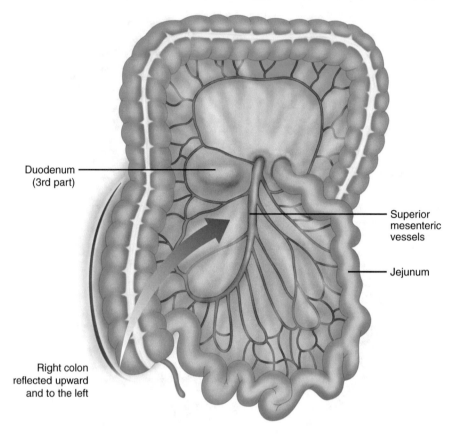

Duodenum
(3rd part)

Superior
mesenteric
vessels

Jejunum

Right colon
reflected upward
and to the left

Fig. 8.10 *Arrow* indicating medial retraction of the right colon. Note that the superior mesenteric vein is not identified

Repair of Vascular Compression of the Duodenum
(Figs. 8.13, 8.14, 8.15, 8.16, and 8.17)

The fourth portion of the duodenum lies within the crook formed by the aorta and the origin of the superior mesenteric artery. The normal angle between these two structures is between 38 and 65 degrees. When that angle is decreased to less than approximately 25 degrees, compression of the duodenum can lead to obstruction, termed superior mesenteric artery syndrome or Wilkie syndrome. Two strategies for treating the obstruction include ligament of Treitz release and bypass.

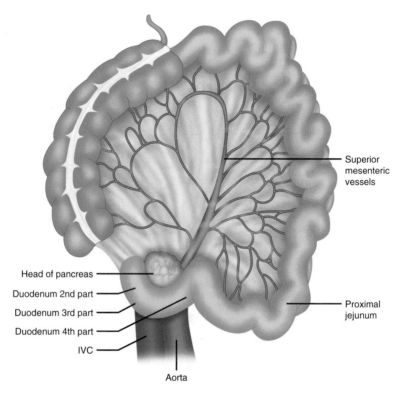

Superior
mesenteric
vessels

Head of pancreas

Duodenum 2nd part

Duodenum 3rd part

Duodenum 4th part

IVC

Proximal
jejunum

Aorta

Fig. 8.11 Cattell maneuver. *IVC* inferior vena cava

Fig. 8.12 Cattell-Braasch
maneuver

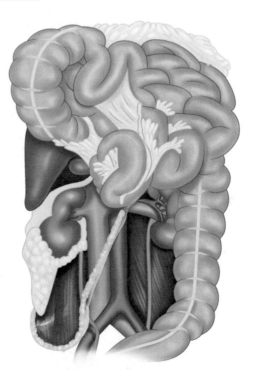

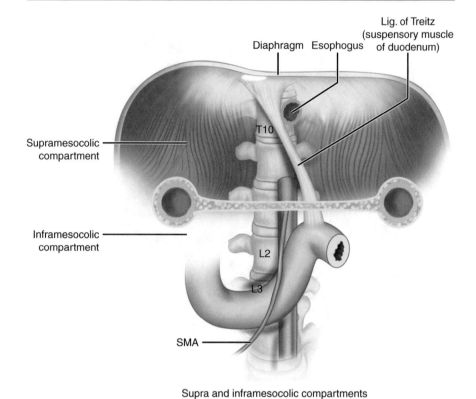

Supra and inframesocolic compartments

Fig. 8.13 Normally, the duodenum crosses the spine at the level of the third lumbar vertebra. It is suspended in this position by the ligament of Treitz. *SMA* superior mesenteric artery

In order to release the ligament of Treitz, this structure is isolated, ligated, and divided. This allows the duodenum to drop far enough for the surgeon to insert two fingers between the duodenum and the origin of the superior mesenteric artery. The duodenojejunal junction can be further mobilized to the right of the mesentery root; this is the Strong procedure.

Currently, bypass of the obstruction is the preferred surgical intervention for superior mesenteric artery syndrome. The third portion of the duodenum is exposed via the transverse mesocolon, and an antiperistaltic duodenojejunostomy is created. This is increasingly accomplished by laparoscopic or robotic approaches.

Ligation of the Gastroduodenal Artery Within a Posterior Duodenal Ulcer

A penetrating ulcer in the posterior first portion of the duodenum can lead to life-threatening upper gastrointestinal hemorrhage. The gastroduodenal artery typically courses immediately posterior to the duodenal bulb where it is susceptible to

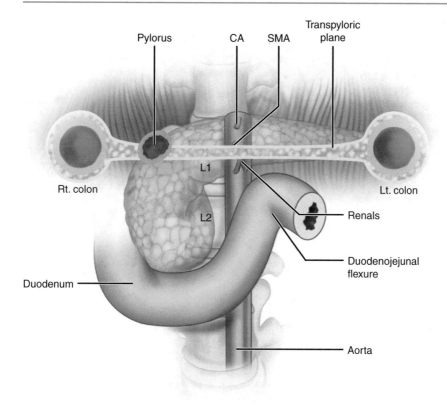

Fig. 8.14 The superior mesenteric artery arises at the level of the first lumbar vertebra, between the celiac axis and the renal arteries. *CA* colic artery, *SMA* superior mesenteric artery

Fig. 8.15 Diagrammatic sagittal section showing the duodenum between the superior mesenteric vessel and the aorta. *MCA* middle colic artery, *SMA* superior mesenteric artery

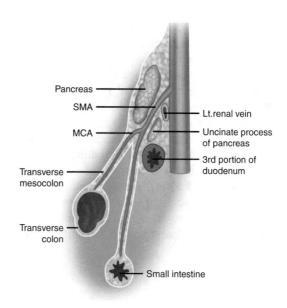

Fig. 8.16 Section of the ligament of Treitz will usually allow the duodenum to drop far enough to admit two fingers between the superior mesenteric artery and the aorta

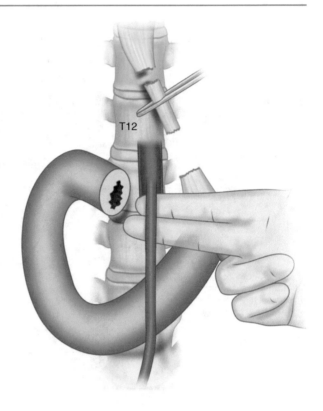

erosion and bleeding when exposed by an overlying ulcer. A thorough understanding of the regional anatomy is essential to achieve an expeditious and safe exposure and ligation of the bleeding vessel.

A Kocher maneuver is performed to mobilize the first and second portions of the duodenum. This optimizes exposure and provides tissue laxity for eventual closure of the duodenotomy.

A 2–3 cm longitudinal incision is made along the anterior aspect of the duodenal bulb, across the pylorus and then proximally 2–3 cm onto the gastric antrum. Retention sutures placed at the edges of the duodenotomy are useful for exposing the posterior wall.

Three-point ligation is performed with permanent suture (Fig. 8.18). The cephalad and caudal horizontal stitches must be deep enough to encircle the gastroduodenal artery proximal and distal to the erosion. It is critical that these are not placed too wide or too deep in order to prevent entrapment of the common bile duct. A third vertical stitch is placed medially to ligate the transverse pancreatic artery, which can cause postoperative retrograde bleeding if ignored. No stitch is placed laterally, as the common bile duct typically lies lateral and posterior to the gastroduodenal artery (Fig. 8.19).

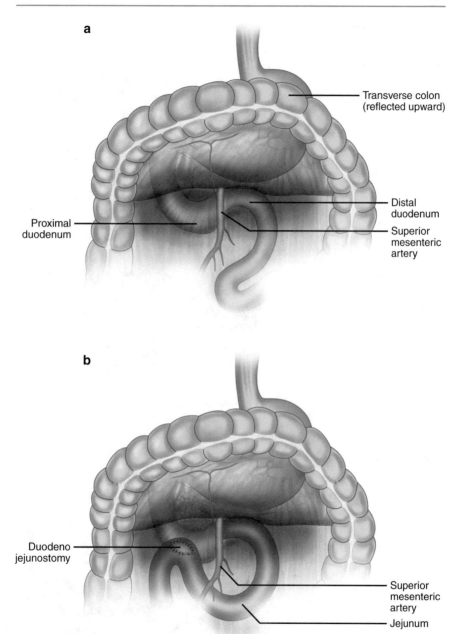

Fig. 8.17 (**a**) Note the dilated proximal duodenum. (**b**) Duodenojejunostomy bypassing the obstruction

Fig. 8.18 Three-point ligation of gastroduodenal artery

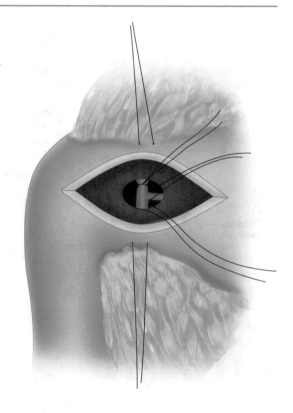

Fig. 8.19 Relationship between gastroduodenal artery and common bile duct

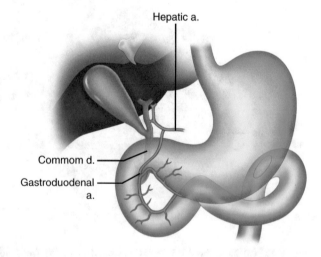

Closure of the duodenotomy can usually be completed in transverse fashion with a Heineke-Mikuliez pyloroplasty (Fig. 8.20). However, if there is significant fibrosis and narrowing of the duodenal bulb, this may result in gastric outlet obstruction. In this situation, a Finney pyloroplasty should be performed (Fig. 8.21).

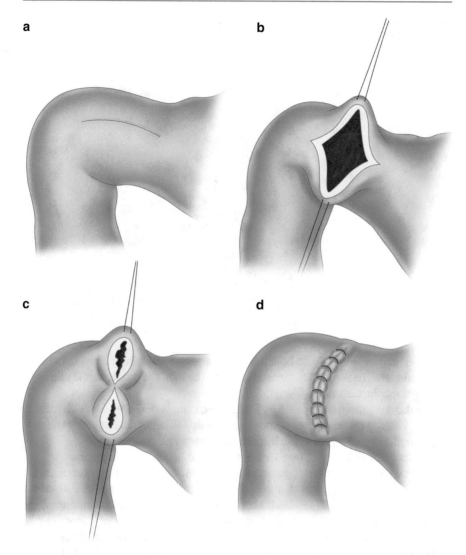

Fig. 8.20 Heineke-Mikuliez pyloroplasty. (**a**) 2–3 cm longitudinal incision along the anterior aspect of the duodenal bulb across the pylorus. (**b**) Retention sutures placed at the edges of the duodenotomy to aid with exposure of the posterior wall. (**c**) Duodenotomy edges approximated. (**d**) Transverse closure

Surgical Notes to Remember

- It is impossible to perform duodenectomy alone because the head of the pancreas is fixed to the duodenal loop; the only practical procedure is pancreaticoduodenectomy.
- No more than 2 cm of the first part of the duodenum should be skeletonized. If more is skeletonized, a duodenostomy may be necessary to avoid "blowout" of the stump secondary to poor blood supply.

Fig. 8.21 Finney
pyloroplasty

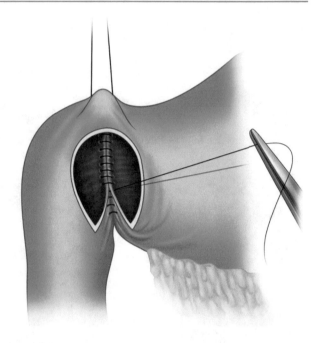

- It is important not to ligate both the superior and the inferior pancreaticoduode-nal arteries. The result may be necrosis of the head of the pancreas and of a large part of the duodenum.
- The duodenum can be exposed by the Kocher, Cattell, or Cattell-Braasch maneu-vers. When it is necessary to expose the fourth portion of the duodenum, care is required to avoid injury to the inferior mesentery vein.
- The suspensory ligament may be transected and ligated with impunity.
- When dealing with a large, penetrating posterior duodenal or pyloric ulcer, the surgeon should remember that the proximal duodenum shortens because of the inflammatory process (duodenal shortening); the anatomical topography of the distal common bile duct, as well as the opening of the duct of Santorini (the minor duodenal papilla) and the ampulla of Vater (the major duodenal papilla), is distorted; and leaving the ulcer in situ is a wise decision. Useful procedures include careful palpation or visualization of the location of the ampulla of Vater or common bile duct exploration with a catheter insertion into the common bile duct and the duodenum.
- The common bile duct, in most cases, is located to the right of the gastroduo-denal artery at the posterior wall of the first portion of the duodenum. Three-point ligation is required to secure the exposed gastroduodenal artery. These stitches must be diligently placed close to the edge of the ulcer. In many cases, the artery crosses the supraduodenal portion of the common bile duct anteri-orly or posteriorly, a phenomenon also observed with the posterior superior pancreaticoduodenal artery, which crosses the common bile duct ventrally and dorsally.

- The accessory pancreatic duct (of Santorini) passes under the gastroduodenal artery. To avoid injury to or ligation of the duct, ligate the artery away from the anterior medial duodenal wall where the papilla is located. "Water under the bridge" applies to the gastroduodenal artery and the accessory pancreatic duct as well as to the relation of the uterine artery and ureter. In 10% of cases, the duct of Santorini is the only duct draining the pancreas; therefore, it would be catastrophic if the duct were ligated accidentally along with the gastroduodenal artery.

Anatomical Complications

- Injury of the left gastric artery and vein during dissection of gastrohepatic ligament
- Injury to middle colic artery during dissection of gastrocolic ligament
- Bleeding from pancreaticoduodenal arcades from an aggressive Kocher maneuver
- Bleeding from portal vein during exploration of the neck of the pancreas as the surgeons fingers are passed behind the neck
- Injury to an aberrant common hepatic artery arising from superior mesenteric artery or one of its branches
- Injury to an aberrant right hepatic artery arising from the superior mesenteric artery
- Injury to an aberrant left hepatic artery. This artery presents a problem only when arising from the right side superior mesenteric artery or from the gastroduodenal artery.
- Injury to an aberrant middle colic artery passing through the head of the pancreas or between the head and the duodenum
- Injury to the cisterna chyli resulting in chylous ascites

Pancreas

9

Kimberly M. Ramonell and Snehal Patel

Anatomy

General Description of the Pancreas

The pancreas lies transversely in the retroperitoneal sac, between the duodenum on the right and the spleen on the left. It is related to the omental bursa above, the transverse mesocolon anteriorly, and the greater sac below. For all practical purposes, the pancreas is a fixed organ.

Anteriorly, the pancreas is related to other organs from right to left as follows (Fig. 9.1):

Above: Duodenum, pylorus, liver, stomach, and spleen

Below: Duodenum, jejunum, transverse colon, and spleen

Intermediate: Transverse colon, mesocolon, transverse mesocolon, and spleen

On the anterior surface of the head of the pancreas and across the duodenum, the transverse mesocolon is very short, so that the colon itself is attached to the underlying organ.

The second and third parts of the duodenum are overlapped by the head of the pancreas; therefore, there is a pancreatic "bare area" of the duodenum (Fig. 9.2) that is not covered by peritoneum. A second bare area exists on the anterior surface of the second portion of the duodenum, where the transverse colon is attached. With

K. M. Ramonell
Department of General Surgery, Emory University, Atlanta, GA, USA

S. Patel (✉)
Department of Surgery, Emory University, Atlanta, GA, USA
e-mail: snehal.patel@emory.edu

© Springer Nature Switzerland AG 2021
L. J. Skandalakis (ed.), *Surgical Anatomy and Technique*,
https://doi.org/10.1007/978-3-030-51313-9_9

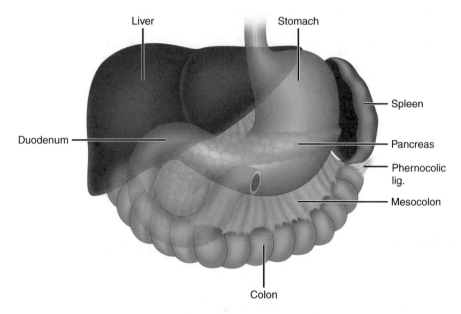

Fig. 9.1 Anterior relationships of the pancreas

Fig. 9.2 Bare areas of the duodenum. The entire concave surface is in intimate contact with the pancreas; the attachment of the transverse mesocolon crosses the anterior surface of the second portion

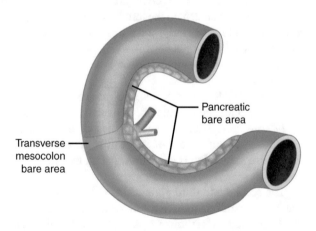

pancreatic cancer or pancreatitis, the pancreas and the mesocolon, together with its middle colic artery, become firmly fixed.

Posteriorly the pancreatic bed in the retroperitoneal space consists of an area between the hilum of the right kidney, the hilum of the spleen, the celiac artery, and the inferior mesenteric artery. From right to left, the area contains the hilum of the right kidney, the inferior vena cava, the portal vein, the superior mesenteric vein, the aorta, the left kidney, and the hilum of the spleen (Fig. 9.3).

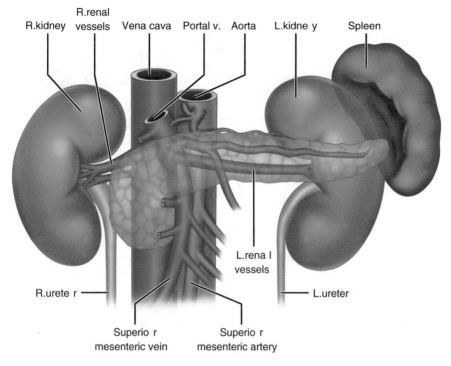

Fig. 9.3 Posterior relationships of the pancreas. Anterior view

Parts of the Pancreas

The pancreas may be arbitrarily divided into five parts: head, uncinate process, neck, body, and tail (Fig. 9.4).

Head

The head of the pancreas is that portion lying to the right of the superior mesenteric artery and vein. The head adheres to the medial aspect of the duodenal loop.

The anterior pancreaticoduodenal arcade can be seen along the ventral surface of the head of the pancreas, coursing roughly parallel with the duodenal curvature. The posterior pancreaticoduodenal vascular arcade is a major entity on the posterior surface of the head. This surface is close to the hilum and medial border of the right kidney, right renal vessels and the inferior vena cava, the right crus of the diaphragm, and the right gonadal vein. The head may be in close association to the third part of the common bile duct in a variety of ways.

Fig. 9.4 The five parts of the pancreas. The line between the body and the tail is arbitrary

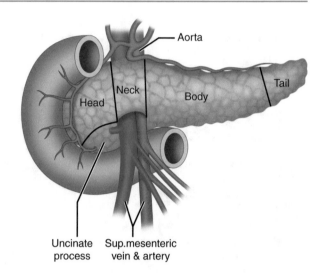

Uncinate Process

The uncinate ("hooklike") process is an extension of the head of the pancreas and is highly variable in size and shape. It passes downward and slightly to the left from the principal part of the head. It further continues behind the superior mesenteric vessels and in front of the aorta and inferior vena cava. In sagittal section, the uncinate process lies between the aorta and the superior mesenteric artery, with the left renal vein above and the duodenum below.

The uncinate process may be absent or may completely encircle the superior mesenteric vessels (Fig. 9.5). If the process is well developed, the neck of the pancreas must be dissected from the front to avoid injury to the vessels. Short vessels from the superior mesenteric artery and vein supply the uncinate process and must be carefully ligated.

Neck

The pancreatic neck, ranging from 1.5 to 2 cm in length, can be defined as the site of passage of the superior mesenteric vessels and the beginning of the portal vein cephalad to the pancreas.

The gastroduodenal artery passes to the right of the neck and provides origin for the anterior superior pancreaticoduodenal artery. Posterior to the neck, the portal vein is formed by the confluence of the superior mesenteric and splenic veins. Near the inferior margin of the pancreatic neck, one can often see the terminations of the inferior pancreaticoduodenal vein and right gastroepiploic vein where they drain into the superior mesenteric or splenic veins or into the portal vein proper.

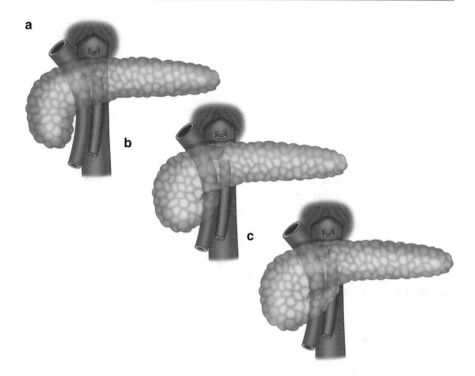

Fig. 9.5 Variations in the extent of the uncinate process of the pancreas. (**a**) Does not reach superior mesenteric vessels. (**b**) Reaches across superior mesenteric vein almost to superior mesenteric artery. (**c**) Reaches beyond superior mesenteric artery

The inferior mesenteric vein drains, with essentially equal frequency, into the splenic vein, the superior mesenteric vein, or the site of formation of the portal vein. Careful elevation of the neck and ligation of anterior tributaries, if present, are necessary. Bleeding can make it difficult to evaluate the structures lying beneath the neck.

The portal vein receives the posterior superior pancreaticoduodenal, right gastric, left gastric and pyloric veins. It is fairly common for an anomalous vein to enter the anterior surface.

Body

The anterior surface of the body of the pancreas is covered by the double layer of peritoneum of the omental bursa that separates the stomach from the pancreas. The body is related to the transverse mesocolon, which divides into two leaves: the superior leaf covers the anterior surface, and the inferior leaf passes inferior to the pancreas. The middle colic artery emerges from beneath the pancreas to travel between the leaves of the transverse mesocolon.

Posteriorly, the body of the pancreas is related to the aorta, the origin of the superior mesenteric artery, the left crus of the diaphragm, the left kidney and its vessels, the left adrenal gland, and the splenic vein (see Fig. 9.3). Small vessels from the pancreas enter the splenic vein and, during pancreatectomy, must be ligated in order to preserve the vein and the spleen.

Tail

The tail is relatively mobile. Its tip reaches the hilum of the spleen in 50% of cases. Together with the splenic artery and the origin of the splenic vein, the tail is contained between two layers of the splenorenal ligament.

The outer layer of this ligament is the posterior layer of the gastrosplenic ligament. Careless division of this ligament may injure the short gastric vessels. The ligament itself is almost avascular, but digital manipulation should stop at the pedicle. Commonly a caudate branch arises from the left gastroepiploic or an inferior splenic polar branch and passes to the tip of the tail of the pancreas. Anticipate this branch in the pancreaticosplenic ligament.

Pancreatic Ducts

The main pancreatic duct (of Wirsung) and the accessory duct lie anterior to the major pancreatic vessels. Pathological ducts are readily palpated and opened from the anterior surface of the pancreas.

Because of the developmental origin of the two pancreatic ducts, several variations are encountered; most can be considered normal. The usual configuration is seen in Fig. 9.6a.
- Both ducts open into the duodenum (Fig. 9.6a).
- The duct of Wirsung carries the entire secretory contents; the duct of Santorini ends blindly (Fig. 9.6b).
- The duct of Santorini carries the entire secretion; the duct of Wirsung is small or absent (Fig. 9.6c).

The greatest diameter of the main pancreatic duct is in the head of the pancreas, just before the duct enters the duodenal wall.

Less than 3 ml of contrast medium will fill the main pancreatic duct in the living patient, and 7–10 ml will fill the branches and the smaller ducts.

Duodenal Papilla

The duodenal papilla (of Vater) lies at the end of the intramural portion of the common bile duct. It is on the posteromedial wall of the second part of the duodenum, to the right of the second or third lumbar vertebra in most cases. On endoscopy, the papilla was found to the right of the spine at the level of the second lumbar vertebra

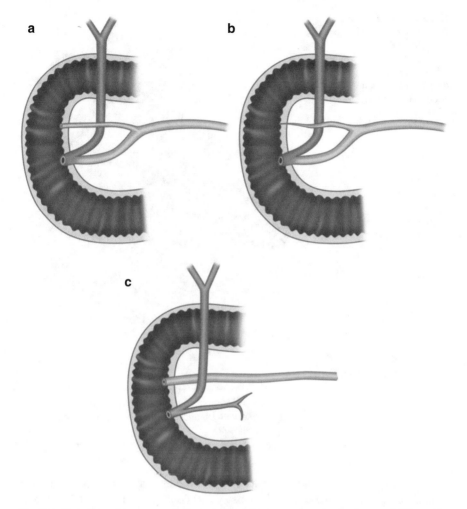

Fig. 9.6 Variations of the pancreatic ducts. (**a**) Both ducts open into the duodenum. (**b**) The accessory duct ends blindly in the duodenal wall. (**c**) The main duct is smaller than the accessory duct, and they are not connected

in most patients. The distance of the papilla from the pylorus is highly variable, ranging from 1.5 to 12 cm. Inflammation of the proximal duodenum may shorten the distance making the pylorus an unreliable landmark.

The present concept of musculature is that there is a complex of four sphincters composed of circular or spiral smooth muscle fibers surrounding the intramural portion of the common bile and pancreatic ducts. The complex may be broken into four separate sphincters, as shown in Fig. 9.7.

The sphincteric complex varies from 6 to 30 mm in length, depending on the obliquity of the ducts. In some individuals, the complex may extend into the pancreatic portion of the common bile duct. This is important to know, because complete

Fig. 9.7 Diagram of the four entities composing the sphincter of Boyden (measurements from White TT. Surgical anatomy of the pancreas. In: Carey LC, editor. The Pancreas. St Louis: CV Mosby Co; 1973)

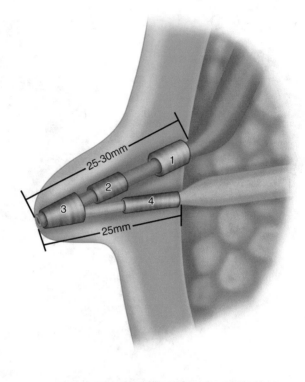

1. Superior sphincter   3. Sphincter ampullae
2. Inferior (submucosal 4. Pancreatic sphincter
   sphincter)

anatomical transection of all elements of the complex may not be necessary for satisfactory function. Incision by 5-mm steps while testing with a suitable dilator will help limit the incision to the shortest length necessary to obtain the desired results. On the mucosal surface of the duodenum, the duodenal papilla of Vater is found where a longitudinal mucosal fold meets a transverse fold to form a T (Fig. 9.8).

These are some practical considerations:

- Too much lateral or distal traction on the opened duodenum may erase the folds and distort the T.
- The papilla is often covered by a transverse fold. One must gently elevate the folds in the assumed location.
- If the T is not apparent and the papilla cannot be palpated, the common bile duct must be probed from above.
- A duodenal diverticulum lying close to the papilla may present difficulties for the surgeon or the endoscopist. The papilla has been found in a diverticulum; it separated from the duodenal wall and was immediately reimplanted.

Fig. 9.8 The T
arrangement of mucosal
folds of the duodenum
indicates the site of the
major duodenal papilla.
Mucosal fold may cover
orifice of papilla in some
cases. Major papilla is
rarely this obvious

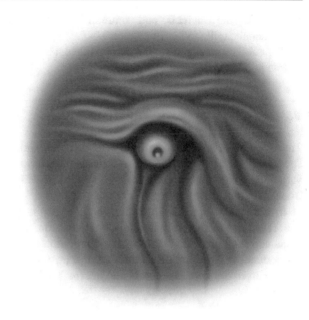

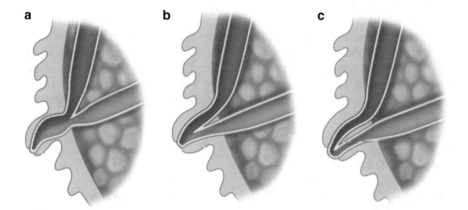

Fig. 9.9 Diagram of the relations of the pancreatic and common bile ducts. (**a**) Minimal embryonic absorption of the ducts into the duodenal wall; an ampulla is present. (**b**) Partial embryonic resorption of the ducts; no true ampulla is present. (**c**) Maximum embryonic resorption of the ducts; two separate orifices open on the papilla

The ampulla is the common pancreaticobiliary channel below the junction of the ducts within the papilla (Fig. 9.9a). If the septum between the ducts extends to the orifice of the papilla, there is no ampulla.

The most useful classification is as follows:
- **Type 1.** The pancreatic duct opens into the common bile duct at a variable distance from the orifice of the major duodenal papilla. The common channel may or may not be dilated (85%) (Fig. 9.9a, b).

- **Type 2.** The pancreatic and common bile ducts open separately on the major duodenal papilla (5%) (Fig. 9.9c).
- **Type 3.** The pancreatic and common bile ducts open into the duodenum at separate points (9%).

Vascular System of the Pancreas

The vascular system of the pancreas is complex and nontypical. Nevertheless, a "general plan" is shown in the previous chapter; most importantly, remember that variations are common. The pancreas is supplied with blood from both the celiac trunk and the superior mesenteric artery.

In general, it appears that the blood supply is greatest to the head of the pancreas, less to the body and tail, and least to the neck. The head of the pancreas and the concave surface of the duodenum are supplied by two pancreaticoduodenal arterial arcades (anterior and posterior). Ligation of both vessels will result in duodenal ischemia and necrosis. All major arteries lie posterior to the ducts.

Pancreatic Arcades

The gastroduodenal artery divides to form the anterior superior and posterior superior pancreaticoduodenal arteries. The anterior inferior pancreaticoduodenal artery arises from the superior mesenteric artery at or above the inferior margin of the pancreatic neck. It may form a common trunk with the posterior inferior artery. Ligation of the jejunal branch itself will endanger the blood supply to the fourth part of the duodenum.

Dorsal Pancreatic Arcade

The dorsal pancreatic arcade lies posterior to the neck of the pancreas and, often, posterior to the splenic vein.

Transverse Pancreatic Artery

The transverse (inferior) pancreatic artery is the left branch of the dorsal pancreatic artery, and it supplies the body and tail of the pancreas.

Branches of the Splenic Artery

The splenic artery is located on the posterior surface of the body and tail of the pancreas (see Fig. 8.5). From two to ten branches of the splenic artery anastomose with the transverse pancreatic artery. The largest of these, the great pancreatic artery (of von Haller), is the main blood supply to the tail of the pancreas. Ligation of the splenic artery does not require splenectomy, but ligation of the splenic vein does.

Caudal Pancreatic Artery

The caudal pancreatic artery arises from the left gastroepiploic artery or from a splenic branch at the hilum of the spleen.

Venous Drainage

In general, the veins of the pancreas parallel the arteries and lie superficial to them. Both lie posterior to the ducts in the body and tail of the pancreas. The drainage is to the portal vein, splenic vein, and superior and inferior mesenteric veins (see Figs. 8.6 and 8.7).

The hepatic portal vein is formed behind the neck of the pancreas by the union of the superior mesenteric and splenic veins (see Fig. 8.7).

The portal vein lies behind the pancreas and in front of the inferior vena cava, with the common bile duct on the right and the common hepatic artery on the left.

Lymphatic Drainage

Figure 9.10 shows the chief groups of lymph nodes receiving lymphatic vessels from the pancreas. Lymphatic drainage may prove to be as complex and nontypical as the arterial supply.

Nerve Supply of the Pancreas

Innervation of the pancreas occurs by the sympathetic division of the autonomic nervous system through the splanchnic nerves and by the parasympathetic division through the vagus nerve. In general, these nerves follow blood vessels to their destinations.

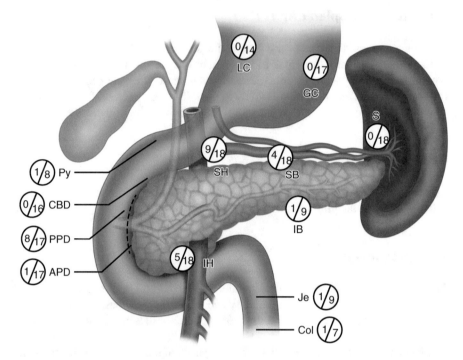

Fig. 9.10 Chief groups of lymph nodes receiving lymphatic vessels from the pancreas. *SH* superior head, *IH* inferior head, *PPD* posterior pancreaticoduodenal, *APD* anterior pancreaticoduodenal, *SB* superior body, *IB* inferior body, *S* splenic, *GC* greater curvature, *LC* lesser curvature, *Py* pylorus, *CBD* common bile duct, *Je* jejunum, *Col* colon. In the Whipple resection (indicated by the stippled vertical line), the SB, IB, and S groups usually are not removed

The celiac ganglion is the central station of both sympathetic and parasympathetic innervation. Extirpation—surgical or chemical—of the celiac ganglion should interrupt afferent fibers of both sympathetic and parasympathetic systems.

Ectopic and Accessory Pancreas

Pancreatic tissue in the stomach, duodenal wall, ileal wall, Meckel's diverticulum, or at the umbilicus is not unusual. Less common sites are the colon, appendix, gallbladder, omentum or mesentery, and in anomalous bronchoesophageal fistula. Most such pancreatic tissue is functional. Islet tissue is often present in gastric and duodenal heterotopia, but it is usually absent in accessory pancreatic tissue elsewhere in the body. Figure 9.11 shows the possible sites of heterotopic pancreatic tissue.

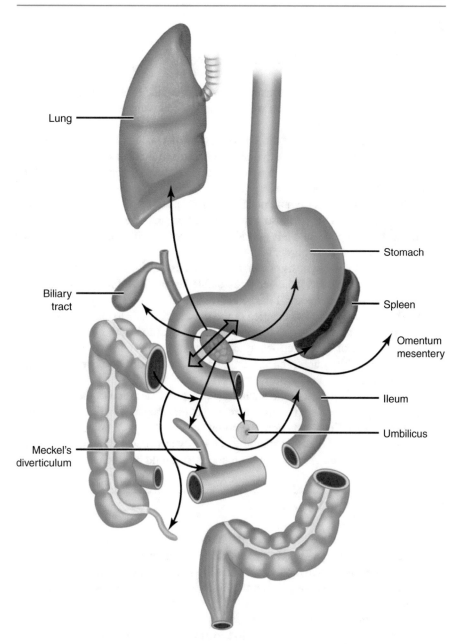

Fig. 9.11 Sites of pancreatic heterotopia. The relative frequency is indicated by the width of the arrows. The stomach and duodenum are by far the most common sites

Technique

Evaluation of Resectability of the Pancreas

The authors strongly advise intravenous contrast-enhanced axial imaging of the pancreas prior to surgery. Also, we suggest the following steps in the operating room:

1. Good general exploration of the abdomen with special attention to the pancreas.
2. Attention to specific areas of lymph node drainage that are accessible without further incision. These are the pyloric and pancreaticoduodenal nodes and the nodes at the root of the mesentery (Fig. 9.10).
3. Further investigation of lymph nodes, which requires some incision of the hepatogastric omenta. This will also require a Kocher maneuver. Inspect the pancreaticoduodenal, celiac, and left gastric nodes, together with nodes of the superior and inferior pancreatic borders.
4. Assuming that the diagnosis of cancer has been determined and that the exploration outlined above has indicated a resectable lesion, these final steps should be undertaken before the start of the actual resection:
   (a) Further exploration of the area of the muscle of Treitz to ensure mobility of the fourth part of the duodenum and the first portion of the jejunum.
   (b) Evaluation of the posterior surface of the head of the pancreas and the distal comm0on bile duct to ensure that there is no fixation to underlying structures, including the inferior vena cava.
   (c) Gentle examination of the uncinate process and elevation of the neck of the pancreas with one or two fingers to ensure that they are not fixed to the superior mesenteric vessels or to the portal vein.
   (d) Final review of the local anatomy to identify any previously undetected vascular anomalies. Any available angiograms should be studied.

Exploration of the Pancreas

There are several possible routes to exploration of the pancreas, which may be used individually or in combination, each with particular advantages and disadvantages:

- Through the gastrocolic ligament. This is the route used by most surgeons.
- Through the hepatogastric omentum. This is useful in patients with exceptionally ptotic stomachs.
- Detaching the greater omentum from the transverse colon. This is time-consuming, but it gives better visualization of the entire lesser sac.
- Through the mesocolon. This gives only limited exposure of the pancreas and risks injury to the middle colic blood vessels.
- Kocher maneuver. This provides good exposure of the posterior surface of the head of the pancreas.
- Mobilizing the splenic flexure, the spleen, and tail of the pancreas. This is appropriate when partial pancreatectomy and splenectomy or splenic preservation is seriously contemplated.

Puestow Procedure

PRIOR TO SURGERY: Endoscopic retrograde cholangiopancreatography; bowel preparation.

POSITION: Supine.

ANESTHESIA: General.

OTHER: Insert nasogastric tube and Foley catheter.

- **Step 1.** To enter the lesser sac, divide the gastrocolic ligament using clamps and ligate the vessels (Fig. 9.12).
- **Step 2.** Kocherize the duodenum. Perform detailed palpation of the pancreas. Visualize and palpate the dilated pancreatic duct that snakes obviously at the anterior surface of the pancreas.
- **Step 3.** Using an 18-gauge needle, aspirate the pancreatic duct with a syringe. Incise the pancreatic duct enough to insert a small, right-angle, curved mosquito clamp into the lumen of the duct. Incise along its length with electrocautery. The pancreatic incision should be 6–8 cm or more if there is ductal dilatation at the head of the pancreas with formation of pancreatic lakes (Fig. 9.13).
- **Step 4.** Locate the ligament of Treitz and transect a loop of jejunum approximately 30 cm from it. Ligate the mesenteric vessels. Divide the jejunum with a gastrointestinal anastomosis (GIA) stapler (Fig. 9.14).
- **Step 5.** Elevate the transverse colon and incise an avascular area of the transverse mesocolon to permit the previously closed distal jejunal limb (Roux-en-Y) to pass into the lesser sac (Fig. 9.15).

Fig. 9.12 Exposure of lesser sac. Dashed line represents line of incision along gastrocolic ligament

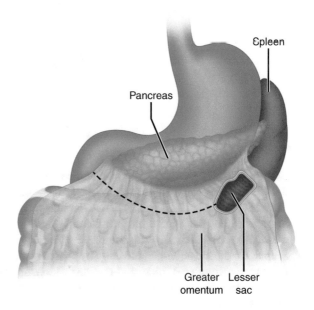

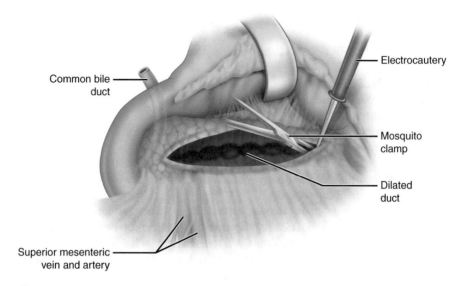

Fig. 9.13 Incision with electrocautery

Fig. 9.14 Division
of jejunum

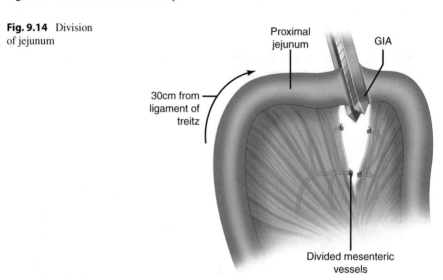

- **Step 6.** Perform a side-to-side pancreaticojejunostomy by placing interrupted 3–0 silk sutures between the seromuscular layer of jejunum and the pancreatic capsule (Figs. 9.15, 9.16, and 9.17). A running suture is acceptable.
- **Step 7.** Suture the jejunal loop to the edges of the opening of the transverse mesocolon with a few 4–0 silk sutures (Fig. 9.17).
- **Step 8.** Create the jejunojejunostomy by anastomosing the proximal jejunal segment to the Roux-en-Y in an end-to-side fashion, approximately 45 cm distal to the pancreaticojejunostomy. The anastomosis is done in standard two-layer fashion (Fig. 9.18).

Fig. 9.15 Incision of transverse mesocolon

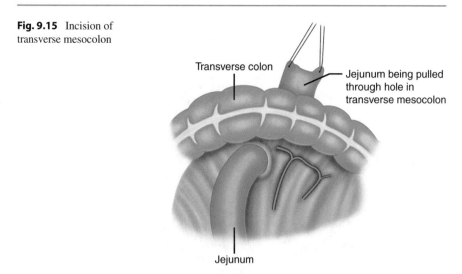

Transverse colon

Jejunum being pulled through hole in transverse mesocolon

Jejunum

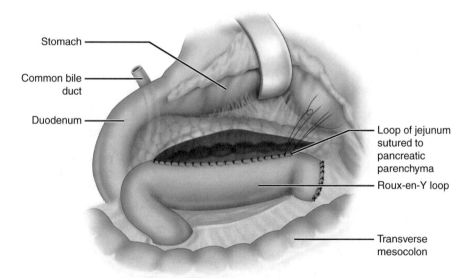

Stomach

Common bile duct

Duodenum

Loop of jejunum sutured to pancreatic parenchyma

Roux-en-Y loop

Transverse mesocolon

Fig. 9.16 Side-to-side pancreaticojejunostomy

- **Step 9.** Figure 9.19 shows the completed anastomoses. Perform cholecystectomy, insert Jackson–Pratt drain, and close in layers.

Note:
- The pancreaticojejunostomy is not a mucosa-to-mucosa anastomosis.

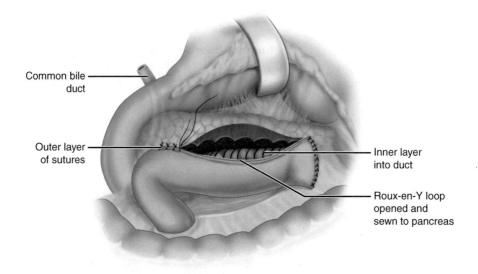

Fig. 9.17 Jejunal loop is sutured

Fig. 9.18
Jejunojejunostomy

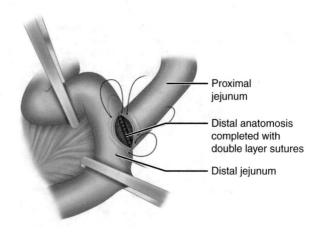

Fig. 9.19 Completion of
Puestow procedure

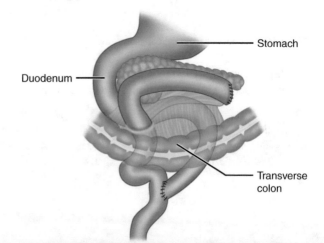

Pancreatectomies

Embryologically, anatomically, and surgically, the head of the pancreas, the common bile duct, and the duodenum form an inseparable unit. Their relations and blood supply make it impossible for the surgeon to remove completely the head of the pancreas without removing the duodenum and the distal part of the common bile duct. The only alternative procedure, the so-called 95% pancreatectomy, leaves a rim of pancreas along the medial border of the duodenum to preserve the duodenal blood supply.

Ninety-Five Percent Distal Pancreatectomy for Chronic Pancreatitis

In spite of the procedure's name, far more than 5% of the pancreas usually remains after performing 95% distal pancreatectomy (orientation: Fig. 9.20). The percentage depends on the size of the head and the presence or lack of the uncinate process.

Step 1. Explore and intubate the common bile duct and perform cholecystectomy.

Step 2. Mobilize the head, uncinate process, body, and tail of the pancreas. The uncinate process should be treated carefully if present. Care must also be taken with the following vessels: splenic artery, splenic vein, superior mesenteric vein, and tributaries. Using 4–0 silk, carefully ligate small veins without traction. Mobilize the neck by dissecting bluntly with the index fingers between the posterior surface of the pancreas and the underlying superior mesenteric vessels (Fig. 9.21).

Step 3. Using electrocautery, divide the head of the pancreas from the remaining gland very close to the duodenal loop (Fig. 9.22). For the duodenum and thin pancreatic rim to survive, it is very important to protect the superior and inferior pancreaticoduodenal arteries. One of these vessels can provide sufficient blood, so if the other is accidentally injured and ligated, no harm results; but *do not*

Fig. 9.20 Partial pancreatectomy: 95% pancreatectomy; 85% pancreatectomy; Whipple procedure; distal pancreatectomy. Distal pancreatectomy includes resection from any point between 4 and 5 to the tip of the tail

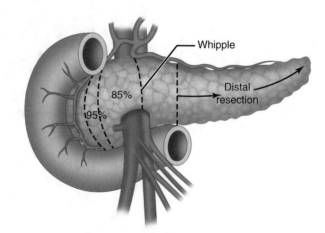

Fig. 9.21 Exploration of the pancreas. The surgeon's index fingers are passed behind the neck of the pancreas. The neck should separate easily from the underlying vessels

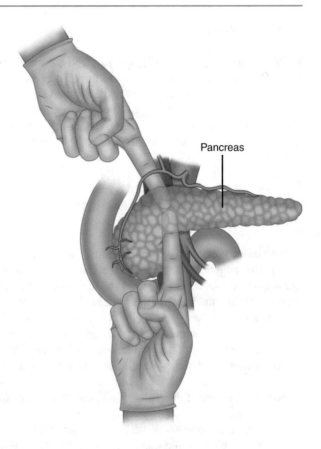

Fig. 9.22 Division of head of pancreas

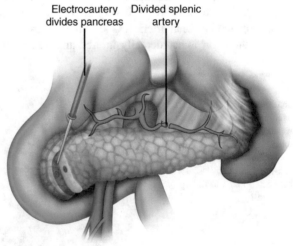

Fig. 9.23 Preparation for splenectomy

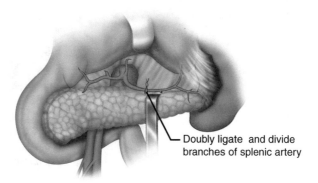

Doubly ligate and divide
branches of splenic artery

Fig. 9.24 Division of
splenic artery

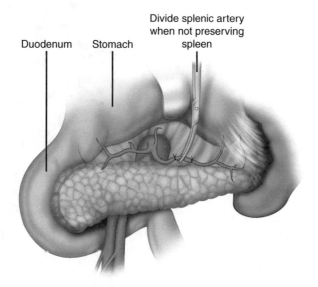

Divide splenic artery
when not preserving
spleen

Duodenum   Stomach

ligate both. Palpate and preserve the third and fourth portions of the common bile duct.

Step 4. Identify the divided pancreatic duct and close it with a mattress suture of 4–0 nonabsorbable material. Doubly ligate the splenic artery, the splenic vein, and t12heir tributaries, and perform splenectomy (Figs. 9.23, 9.24, 9.25, and 9.26). Remove specimen consisting of distal pancreas and spleen.

Step 5. Insert Jackson–Pratt drain, and close the abdominal wall in layers.

Distal Pancreatectomy (With or Without Splenectomy)

For orientation see Fig. 9.12. Keep in mind all the technical steps of the previously discussed pancreatic procedures when performing the following:

Fig. 9.25 Preparing
splenic vein tributaries

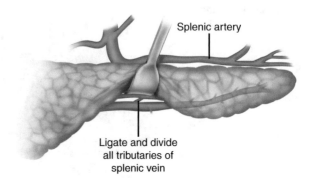

Splenic artery

Ligate and divide
all tributaries of
splenic vein

Fig. 9.26 The
ligated vessels

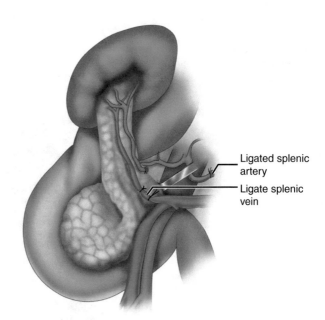

Ligated splenic
artery

Ligate splenic
vein

- **Step 1.** Transect the pancreas approximately where it crosses the portal vein
  (Fig. 9.27).
- **Step 2.** Create a Roux-en-Y loop by anastomosing the pancreatic head or part
  of the remaining body by invagination to a divided jejunal loop approximately
  45 cm from the ligament of Treitz (as described in step 11 of the procedure for
  pancreaticoduodenectomy, below) using an end-to-end pancreaticojejunostomy. Fashion an end-to-side jejunojejunostomy (Fig. 9.28), producing continuity of the gastrointestinal tract plus a defunctionalized limb of
  approximately 60 cm.

Note:
- An alternative method is to oversew the pancreas and drain the area.

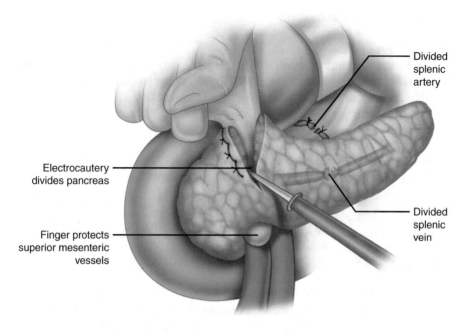

Fig. 9.27 Transection of pancreas

Fig. 9.28 End-to-end
pancreaticojejunostomy

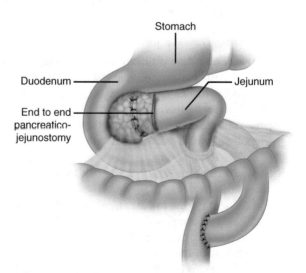

Total Pancreatectomy (With or Without Splenectomy)

- **Step 1.** The pancreas is not divided; therefore, there is no pancreaticojejunostomy. Remove both the spleen and the pancreaticoduodenal duo in continuity.
- **Step 2.** With 3–0 silk, carefully ligate all arterial or venous branches connecting the spleen, pancreas, and duodenum. These vascular collections are totally unpredictable, and the surgeon should be careful to avoid traction. Occasionally a splenopancreatic ligament is present and should be ligated close to the pancreas.

Pancreaticoduodenectomy

Whipple Procedure

There are many modifications of the Whipple procedure. To present all of them, step by step is beyond the scope of this book. We present our technique below.

The specimen of a typical Whipple operation includes:
- Distal stomach
- Duodenum
- Part of the proximal jejunum
- Head, neck, and uncinate process of the pancreas
- Distal biliary tree (distal common hepatic duct, gallbladder, common bile duct).

Note:
- The biliary duct resection depends on the extension of the tumor and the insertion of the cystic duct.

PREPARATION PRIOR TO SURGERY: (1) Celiac and superior mesenteric artery arteriography may be useful. Have the films in the operating room. (2) Antibiotics: both prior to and during surgery. (3) Bowel preparation.

INDICATIONS: (1) Pancreatic malignancy. (2) Duodenal malignancy. (3) Distal common bile duct malignancy.

POSITION: Supine.

ANESTHESIA: General.

- **Step 1.** Make a bilateral subcostal or long midline incision.
- **Step 2.** General exploration, the last evaluation being the pancreaticoduodenal area including hepatogastroduodenal ligament and celiac axis.
- **Step 3.** Duodenal mobilization by full kocherization and elevation of the duodenopancreatic duodenum from the retroperitoneal space and the great vessels. The gastrocolic ligament may be divided now or later, and the lesser sac should be explored.
- **Step 4.** Identify elements of the hepatic triad:
  - Common bile duct
  - Portal vein: medial to the common bile duct. (Dissection of the portal vein is facilitated by dividing the gastroduodenal artery.)
  - Hepatic artery: medial to the portal vein
  - Identify, also, the superior mesenteric vein by blunt and sharp dissection, since no venous branches are inserted into the anterior surface of the superior mesenteric vein. The dissection of the superior mesenteric vein can be started at the inferior border of the pancreas.
  - If both the portal vein and the superior mesenteric vein are fixed, this means tumor involvement, unresectability, and, perhaps, the possibility of a bypass procedure.
  - Continue with the following two procedures:

Fig. 9.29 Protecting the head of the pancreas

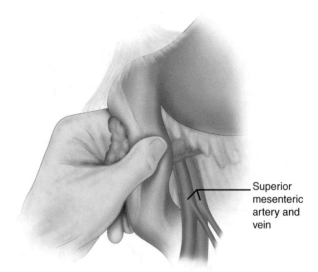

Superior mesenteric artery and vein

(a) Duodenal kocherization and insertion of the index finger under the head of the pancreas, the distal phalanx reaching the great vessels (Fig. 9.29).

(b) Dissection of the portal vein at the superior and inferior borders of the pancreas. The surgeon should be able to approximate both index fingers as indicated in Fig. 9.21.

- Good separation by both procedures of the duodenum and pancreas means resectability. If a transduodenal-pancreatic biopsy is being considered, this may be a good time to do it.

- **Step 5.** As in distal gastrectomy, divide lesser and greater omentum. Apply TA-90 stapler just proximal to antrum and divide stomach.

- **Step 6. Arterial steps**: If the anatomy is typical and orthodox and no replacing right hepatic artery is present, localize, isolate, ligate, and divide the gastroduodenal artery close to its origin from the hepatic artery. Do the same to the right gastroepiploic artery (see Fig. 7.3).

- **Step 7. Biliary steps**: Mobilize the gallbladder. Localize, isolate, divide, and clamp the common hepatic duct with a small noncrushing clamp proximally and a small mosquito clamp distally, just above the exodus of the cystic duct or in that vicinity. Divide the common hepatic duct, and ligate with 3–0 silk close to the cystic duct (Fig. 9.30).

- **Step 8. Pancreaticoduodenectomy steps**: After total exposure of the superior mesenteric vein, and with the left index finger under the neck of the pancreas, divide the pancreatic parenchyma using electrocautery (Fig. 9.31). Ligate the small veins and arteries. Shave the remaining distal pancreas, and send the specimen to the lab for frozen section.

- **Step 9.** Localize the ligament of Treitz in the paraduodenal fossae. Using the GIA stapler, divide the jejunum approximately 10–12.5 cm distal to the ligament of Treitz. Be careful not to injure the inferior mesenteric vein, which is located

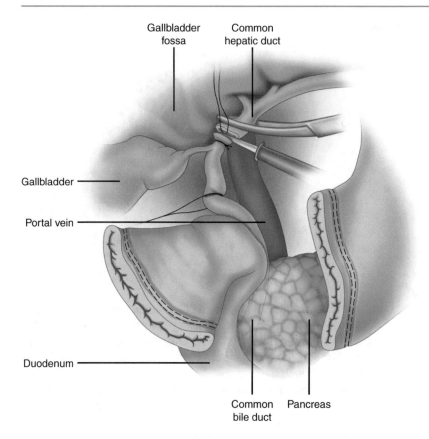

Fig. 9.30 Preparing the common hepatic duct

to the left of the paraduodenal fossae. Clamp, divide, and ligate the mesentery at the mesenteric border of the proximal jejunal limb. With careful digital elevation of the proximal jejunum and fourth and third portions of the duodenum, push the jejunal loop gently under the vessels and to the right (Fig. 9.32).

- **Step 10.** If the uncinate process is still attached and if the uncinate process ligament is present, it should be divided between clamps, and the distal part should be ligated (Fig. 9.33). Carefully dissect the uncinate process from the portal vein and the superior mesenteric vein. Send the specimen to the lab for more frozen sections.
- **Step 11.** The anastomoses to be formed: pancreaticojejunostomy, hepatojejunostomy (choledochojejunostomy), and gastrojejunostomy (Figs. 9.34, 9.35, and 9.36).
  - (a) End-to-end pancreaticojejunal anastomosis is accomplished by invagination of the pancreas into the intestinal lumen using two-layer closure of interrupted silk.

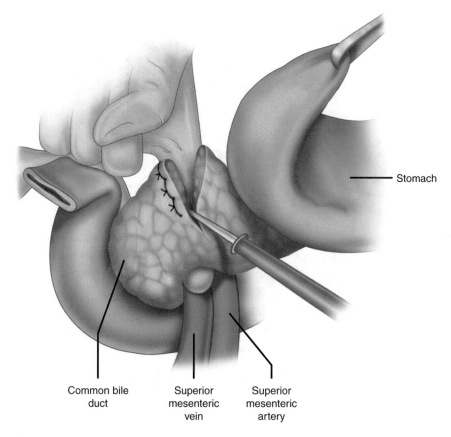

Stomach

Common bile
duct

Superior
mesenteric
vein

Superior
mesenteric
artery

Fig. 9.31 Division of parenchyma

(b) Perform a single-layer, end-to-side choledochojejunostomy using 4–0 interrupted synthetic absorbable material. Tack the jejunum to the abdominal surface of the liver with a few 4–0 silk sutures.

(c) Form an end-to-side gastrojejunostomy in the usual manner, in two layers, using 3–0 chromic and 3–0 silk.

- **Step 12.** Insert a Jackson–Pratt drain to drain Morison's pouch and the area of the pancreaticojejunostomy. Close the abdomen in layers.

  For more details, we advise the reader to use the following textbooks:

- Cameron JL. Atlas of surgery. Philadelphia: Decker; 1990.
- Chassin JL. Operative strategy in general surgery. 2nd ed. New York: Springer; 1994.
- Skandalakis JE, Gray SW, Rowe JS Jr. Anatomical complications in general surgery. New York: McGraw-Hill; 1983.

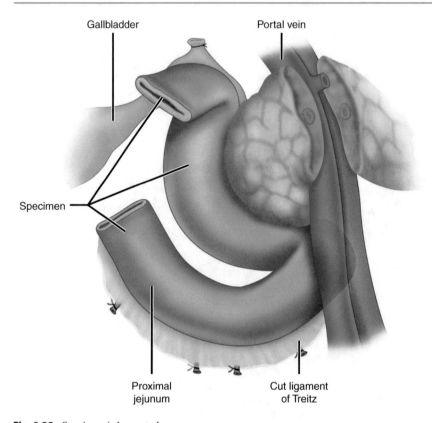

Fig. 9.32 Specimen is harvested

Fig. 9.33 Division of
uncinate process

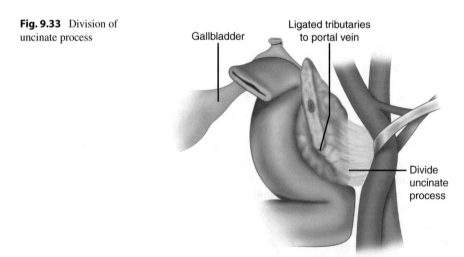

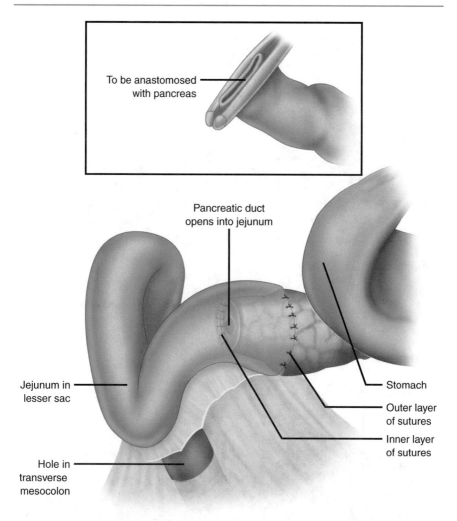

Fig. 9.34 Placement of sutures

Laparoscopic Distal Pancreatectomy

In comparison to the laparoscopic resection of other solid organs (spleen, kidney, adrenal, liver), laparoscopic pancreatic resection (LPR) has been relatively slow to progress. However, with advances in surgical technology (ultrasonic scalpel, electrothermal bipolar vessel-sealing (EBVS) devices and endovascular staplers), LPR has evolved to achieve excellent patient outcomes as well as shorter length of stay, earlier patient convalescence, and less postoperative pain (equivalent to other minimally invasive solid organ surgery). We present here the indications for LPR, patient positioning, operative set up, trocar site and hand port positioning, as well as the operative technique and steps of the operation.

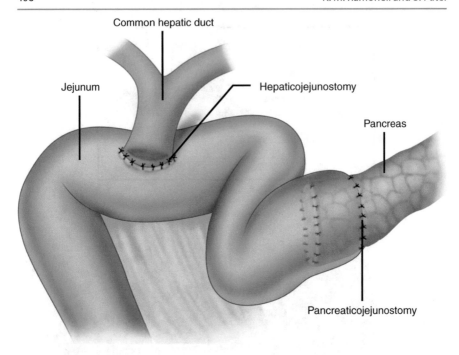

Fig. 9.35 Tacking the jejunum

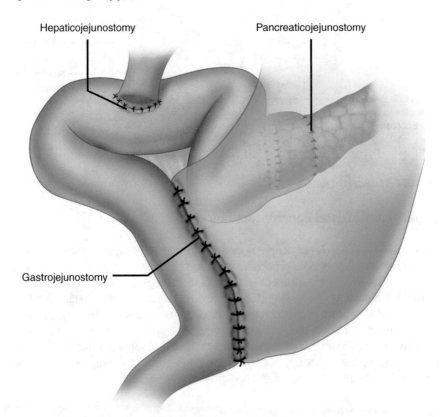

Fig. 9.36 Gastrojejunostomy

In experienced hands, 80% of the body and tail of the pancreas can be safely resected laparoscopically. All benign and premalignant lesions of the body and tail are amenable to LPR. Large malignant lesions of the pancreas, especially those of the pancreatic head, are still better served utilizing an open approach, unless surgery is performed at a center experienced with minimally invasive pancreaticoduodenectomy. Consistent with other advanced laparoscopic techniques, contraindications to LPR include morbid obesity, prior laparotomy with known adhesive disease, and the diagnosis of severe portal hypertension.

Patient positioning for LPR depends on the location of the target lesion. For lesions localized to the distal body and tail of the pancreas, the patient should be positioned in the semi-lateral decubitus position with the left side up. This can be achieved easily with the use of a bean-bag device. For lesions of the body, closer to the head of the pancreas, exposure is often better approached with the patient in the supine position. The following instrumentation is necessary for LPR:

Laparoscopic pancreatic resection instrumentation
0° and 30° laparoscopes
Hand port device
12- and 5-mm trocars
10-mm clip applier
Endovascular GIA stapler (articulating)
EBVS device
Laparoscopic US probe
Laparoscopic fibrin glue applicator

The position of the trocar sites depends on whether a hand-assisted approach is to be used. For most lesions, unless small and of the distal tail, we have found the use of a hand port to be very helpful. Use of the hand cuts down operative time and can aid tremendously in the exposure and mobilization of the pancreas. This is especially useful when attempting splenic preservation, as the hand can be critical for the dissection of the pancreas off of the splenic vessels.

- **Step 1.** Insufflate the abdomen using a Veress needle through the umbilicus.
- **Step 2. Trocar placement**: We utilize (2) 12-mm trocars, (1) 5- or 10-mm trocar, and a hand port in the upper midline location or the right subcostal position depending of the size and location of the lesion. One 12-mm trocar is placed at the infraumbilical position to serve as the main camera port. The other 12-mm trocar serves as the stapler trocar site; it is placed in the right lower abdomen, lateral to the rectus muscle. The other 5-mm trocar serves as the assistant/suction port; it is best placed in the left lower abdomen. All trocars should be placed at a minimum of 8–10 cm apart to minimize "sword fighting" during the dissection. The hand port serves as the site for specimen extraction. As deemed necessary, extra 5- or 10-mm trocars can be added during the progression of the operation to facilitate exposure. Perform diagnostic laparoscopy.
- **Step 3.** If there is no evidence of regional or distant metastatic disease, the operation is commenced by first gaining exposure to the lesser sac. This is facilitated by using the EBVS device to divide the gastrocolic omentum from the pancreatic

head to the splenic flexure. The white line of Toldt should also be taken down to mobilize the splenic flexure. To further mobilize the stomach and to facilitate exposure of the distal pancreas and spleen, the short gastric vessels should be taken down for the entire length of the greater curve. The stomach can be retracted in a cephalad fashion through the assistant port to fully expose the entire pancreas.

- **Step 4.** Mobilization of the pancreas, the next step of the operation, can be the most challenging. If the most delicate of dissection techniques are not followed, untoward bleeding from small peripancreatic and areolar tissue veins can lead to open conversion. Mobilization commences with division of the tissue of the inferior border of the pancreas, utilizing either the ultrasonic dissector or the EBVS device to open the plane of tissue of the peritoneal reflection of the transverse mesocolon. Continue until the splenic vein is visualized. The splenic vein is traced proximally and distally until the inferior mesenteric vein and portal vein/ SMV confluence have been clearly identified.
- **Step 5.** Dissection is continued along the superior border of the pancreas in a similar fashion until the splenic artery is identified. To aid in retraction, a Penrose drain can be used to encircle the pancreas body while dissecting it off of the splenic vessels. Laparoscopic ultrasound can be performed at this time to precisely localize the target lesion and to determine how much pancreas should be mobilized for safe transection of the gland and formation of an adequate margin.
- **Step 6.** At this point in the operation, the decision must be made if the pancreas can be resected with splenic preservation or if tandem splenectomy will be required. Splenic preservation is possible in about 60–80% of cases. Cases where splenic preservation will not be possible include intense inflammatory changes associated with prior episodes of pancreatitis, presence of severe portal hypertension, as well as involvement of the tumor with the splenic vein. All of these clinical scenarios should be determined with preoperative cross-sectional imaging; affected patients should be given prophylactic triple vaccination.
- **Step 7.** For cases where LPR will require splenectomy, it is best to mobilize the spleen and pancreatic tail in a lateral-to-medial fashion prior to gland transection. If splenic preservation is feasible, it can often be helpful to transect the gland first and then mobilize the remainder of the gland in a medial-to-lateral fashion. When pancreas transection is to be performed first (prior to medial-to-lateral mobilization), the peritoneum overlying the splenic artery is opened and the vessel is circumferentially mobilized and isolated. Using a 2.0 mm Endovascular GIA (gray load) stapling device, the artery is transected proximal to the transection line of the pancreas. A relatively avascular plane can then be found between the splenic vein and the pancreas. To facilitate separate transection of the gland with the stapler, the pancreas can be mobilized off the anterosuperior border of the splenic vein with the ultrasonic scalpel. However, if this plane is not accessible due to bleeding from small peripancreatic veins, the pancreas and splenic vein can be stapled en masse with a 3.5 mm (blue load) loaded ENDO GIA stapler. The proximal pancreatic staple line will often ooze after transection. Staple line bleeding can be controlled with clips or low-voltage cautery. Using the ultrasonic dissector, dissection of the distal specimen is continued

medial to lateral below the plane of the vein to include mobilizing the lateral and posterior attachments of the spleen. The entire specimen (pancreas and spleen) is then placed in an endo-catch bag and removed through the hand port incision.
- **Step 8.** The pancreas staple line is again inspected. If an open pancreatic duct is suspected, it should be reenforced by suture ligation with permanent suture. At this time, fibrin glue is used to coat the staple line and peripancreatic tissue. After hemostasis is achieved, a closed suction drain can be brought through one of the trocar sites and placed adjacent to the staple line.

Note
- When performing LPR with splenic preservation, the only significant difference is the meticulous dissection involved in mobilizing the body and tail of the pancreas off of the splenic vessels. Again, opening the peritoneum of the inferior border of the pancreas is often the best approach. Once the splenic vein is identified, the pancreas is retracted with the help of the Penrose drain, and the small venous tributary branches from the pancreas to the splenic vein can be divided with the combination of 5 mm clips and the ultrasonic dissector. Once complete mobilization of the specimen is achieved, the gland is transected as previously described, preserving the splenic vessels and spleen.

LPR is becoming the preferred approach for the management of most benign and premalignant lesions of the body and tail of the pancreas. Outcomes from several large institutional series have shown that this approach is feasible and effective, with decreases in morbidity and length of stay. Perioperative complication rates, specifically pancreatic leak and fistula rates, are similar to those of open pancreatic resection.

For more details, we advise the reader to view the following journal articles:
- Park AE. *Therapeutic Laparoscopy of the Pancreas*. Ann Surg. 2002;236:149
- Lillemoe KD. *Distal Pancreatectomy: Indications and Outcomes in 235 Patients*. Ann Surg. 1999;229:693
- Fernandez-Cruz L. *Outcome of Laparoscopic Pancreatic Surgery: Endocrine and Non-endocrine Tumors*. World J Surg. 2002;26:1057

Robotic-Assisted Distal Pancreatectomy

As surgeon familiarity and access to the daVinci® robot has increased dramatically over the past decade, so has its application in the field of pancreatic surgery. By far the most commonly performed robotic surgery on the pancreas is a robotic-assisted distal pancreatectomy (RDP); additional evolving applications include robotic-assisted pancreaticoduodenectomy, which is beyond the scope of this text. Compared to LDP, RDP provides improved three-dimensional visualization and enhanced operator wrist articulation for meticulous dissection of complex, delicate, and intimately associated structures. There is also data to suggest that RDP has a lower rate of conversion to an open resection compared to LDP. A list of instruments utilized for RDP:

Robotic-assisted distal pancreatectomy instrumentation
Veress needle
12-mm 30° robotic camera
12-mm (1) and 8-mm (3) robotic trocars
12-mm (1) and 5-mm (2) laparoscopic trocars
10-mm clip applier
Triangular liver retractor
60-mm laparoscopic stapler
Robotic instruments: double fenestrated grasper, bipolar fenestrated grasper, monopolar scissors, needle holder
Laparoscopic Ultrasound

Robotic-assisted distal pancreatectomy (RDP) is performed similarly to a LDP with the following differences:

- **Step 1. Patient and equipment positioning:** Patient is placed supine on a split leg operating table with legs securely strapped to allow for steep reverse Trendelenburg positioning. The daVinci® robot is docked over the patient's head and anesthesia personnel, monitors, and tubing are off to patient's left. The assistant surgeon will stand between the patient's legs, while the operating surgeon is at the robotic console.
- **Step 2. Access and port placement:** We obtain intraperitoneal access and insufflation via Veress needle entry at Palmer's point in the left upper quadrant; entry under direct visualization using a 5-mm OptiView port can also be used (with planned upsizing of port to 8-mm robotic trochar). Port placement is depicted in Fig. 9.37.
- **Step 3. Lesser sac entry and pancreatic mobilization:** Entry into the lesser sac and pancreatic mobilization is carried out in a similar fashion to LDP as outlined above in steps 3 through 7 of the preceding section. The robotic vessel sealer (bipolar fenestrated grasper) is utilized for a majority of the dissection. When the pancreas and splenic artery (if applicable) are ready to be divided, the robotic stapler, or laparoscopic stapler, can be used. Depending on the thickness and quality of the pancreatic parenchyma, we divide the pancreas with a 60-mm blue or green load stapler. Occasionally, an additional white load on the stapler may be needed for splenic artery transection. The specimen is then placed in the pelvis for later removal.
- **Step 4. Specimen extraction:** Once hemostasis of the transected pancreatic bed has been assured, the abdomen is irrigated and thoroughly inspected. With insufflation maintained, the 12-mm port sites are closed using a Carter-Thompson laparoscopic suture passer. The abdomen is desufflated, trochars are removed, and the robot is undocked. The patient is returned to a neutral position and a Pfannenstiel incision is made, and the specimen is removed.

For more details, we advise the reader to view the following:

Fig. 9.37 Port placement for robotic-assisted distal pancreatectomy

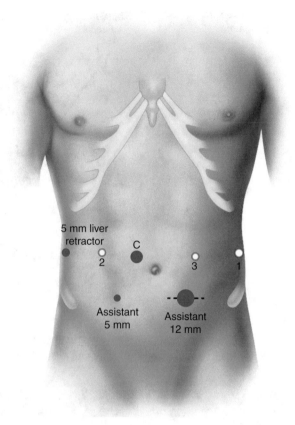

- Suman P, et al. Robotic Distal Pancreatectomy. JSLS (2013)17:627–635
- Bednar F, Hogg ME, Zeh HJ, Zureikat AH. Robotic-assisted distal pancreatectomy. In: Patel A, Oleynikov D (eds). The SAGES Manual of Robotic Surgery. Springer, Cham. 2018:253–264

Transduodenal Pancreatic Biopsy

- **Step 1.** Make a subcostal incision.
- **Step 2.** Mobilize the duodenum by kocherization. Palpate the proximal pancreas for localization of mass (see Fig. 9.29).
- **Step 3.** Place 4–0 silk seromuscular traction sutures anteriorly on the middle part of the descending duodenum. With the traction sutures elevating the anterior duodenal wall, make a small vertical incision by electrocautery.
- **Step 4.** Holding the head of the pancreas with the left hand, insert a Trucut biopsy needle through the posterior duodenal wall into the pancreatic tumor, avoiding the hepatopancreatic ampulla (Fig. 9.38). Send at least two specimens to the lab for frozen section.

Fig. 9.38 Extraction of biopsy specimens

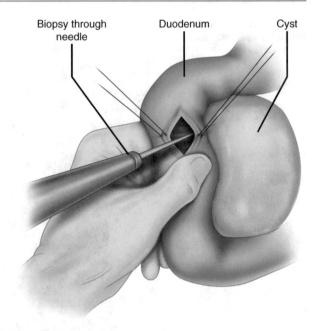

Biopsy through needle   Duodenum   Cyst

- **Step 5.** Close the duodenum in two layers using 4–0 silk in a transverse fashion.
- **Step 6.** Insert a Jackson–Pratt drain and close the wound.

> **Note**
> - Fine-needle aspiration of the head of the pancreas through the duodenum is also acceptable.

Drainage of Pancreatic Pseudocyst

Internal Drainage

There are several procedures: Roux-en-Y, cystogastrostomy, cystoduodenostomy, and cystojejunostomy with Braun jejunojejunostomy.

PRIOR TO SURGERY: (1) Endoscopic retrograde cholangiopancreatography. (2) Sonography. (3) Antibiotics. (4) CT scan. (5) Bowel preparation.

> **Note:**
> - Not all of the preceding are necessary for every patient

POSITION: Supine on operating room X-ray table.

ANESTHESIA: General.

INCISION: Up to the surgeon.

Determine possible location of the cyst and select procedure, keeping in mind the most dependent point for drainage.

Roux-en-Y

- **Step 1.** After elevating the transverse colon, the pancreatic cyst in the lesser sac will present well. For all practical purposes, it is located behind the transverse mesocolon. Identify it by palpation and minimal aspiration. Be sure the cyst is solitary; if in doubt, do an operating room cystogram.
- **Step 2.** Prepare a 40- to 60-cm loop of proximal jejunum, and perform a Roux-en-Y cystojejunostomy in two layers, as described previously (Figs. 9.39 and 9.40).

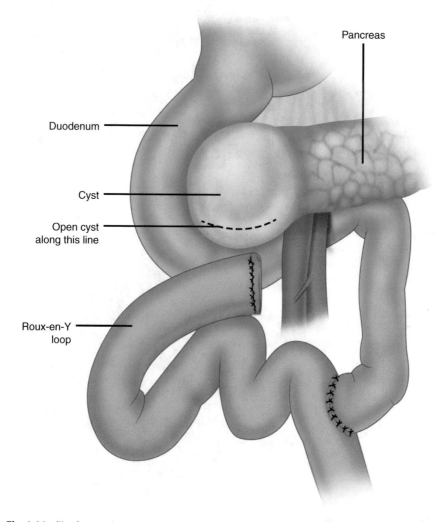

Fig. 9.39 Site for opening the cyst

Fig. 9.40 Roux-en-Y

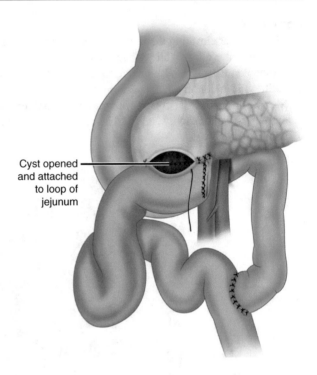

Cyst opened and attached to loop of jejunum

Fig. 9.41 Site of anterior gastrotomy

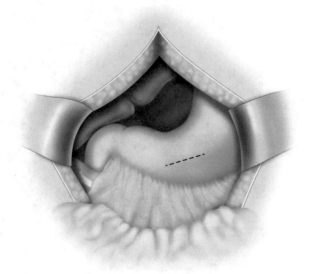

Cystogastrostomy
- **Step 1.** Make an anterior gastric wall incision corresponding to the location of the cyst (Fig. 9.41).
- **Step 2.** Aspirate the cyst (Fig. 9.42).
- **Step 3.** With the needle in situ, perform a posterior gastric wall incision including the cyst wall (Fig. 9.43).

Fig. 9.42 Cyst aspiration

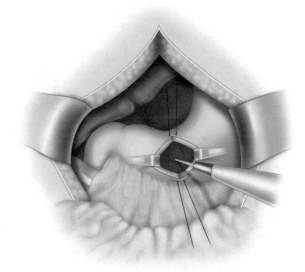

Fig. 9.43 Cystogastrostomy incision

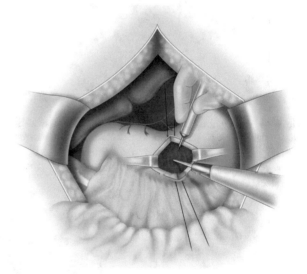

- **Step 4.** Suture the cyst wall to the posterior gastric wall with interrupted 2–0 absorbable synthetic sutures (Fig. 9.44).
- **Step 5.** Suture the anterior gastrotomy (Fig. 9.45).
- **Step 6.** Close the wound.

Note
- Perform cystogastrostomy only when cyst is fixed with the posterior gastric wall.

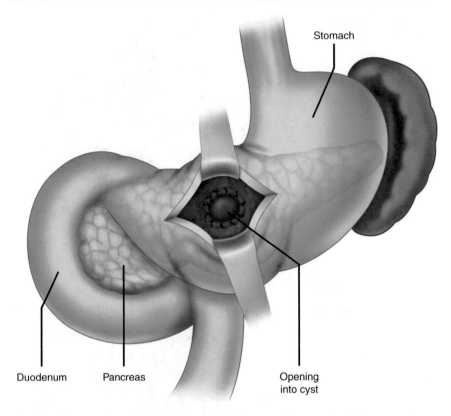

Stomach

Duodenum   Pancreas   Opening
                                               into cyst

Fig. 9.44 Cystogastrostomy. The anterior wall of the stomach is opened, and the pancreatic cyst incised through the posterior wall. The stomach wall and the cyst are sutured to provide drainage

Fig. 9.45 Anterior
gastrotomy closure

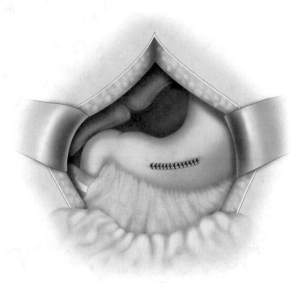

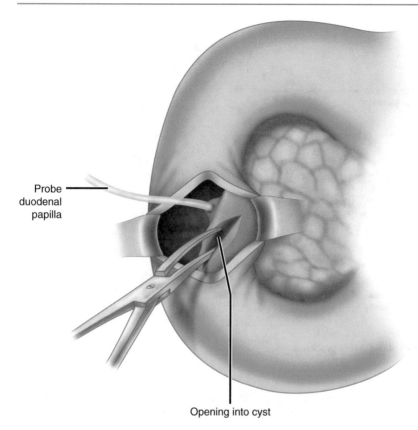

Probe
duodenal
papilla

Opening into cyst

Fig. 9.46 Cystoduodenostomy. A probe is placed in the duodenal papilla to identify and protect the pancreatic duct. The pancreatic cyst is incised through the duodenal wall, and the opening is sutured

Cystoduodenostomy
- **Step 1.** Locate the cyst. Perform a longitudinal duodenotomy.
- **Step 2.** The papilla should be visualized. Pass a small probe or catheter through it to reach the ampulla (Fig. 9.46).
- **Step 3.** Incise the duodenum and cyst. Anastomose with 3–0 absorbable synthetic material (posterior row).
- **Step 4.** Close duodenal wall transversely.
- **Step 5.** Close abdominal wall. Decision whether to insert Jackson–Pratt drain is up to the surgeon.

Note
- Be careful with the duct of Santorini. In 10% of cases, it is the only pancreatic drainage.

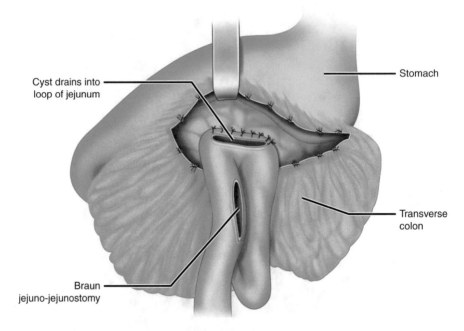

Fig. 9.47 Site of Braun procedure

Cystojejunostomy

Anastomose the cyst with a jejunal loop and perform a Braun enteroenteroanastomosis (Fig. 9.47) or a Roux-en-Y procedure (Fig. 9.48).

External Drainage

External drainage is not recommended except when there is an abscess formation and the patient cannot tolerate a long procedure.

- **Step 1.** Incise gastrocolic ligament.
- **Step 2.** Aspirate cyst for culture and sensitivity.
- **Step 3.** Isolate anterior wall of cyst and incise it. Pack or drain, depending on degree of infection. Occasionally, if the cyst is small, a Foley catheter may be indicated (Fig. 9.49).

Anatomical Complications of the Pancreas Duodenum

- Injury of the left gastric artery and vein during dissection of gastrohepatic ligament.
- Injury to middle colic artery during dissection of gastrocolic ligament.
- Bleeding from pancreaticoduodenal arcades from an aggressive Kocher maneuver.

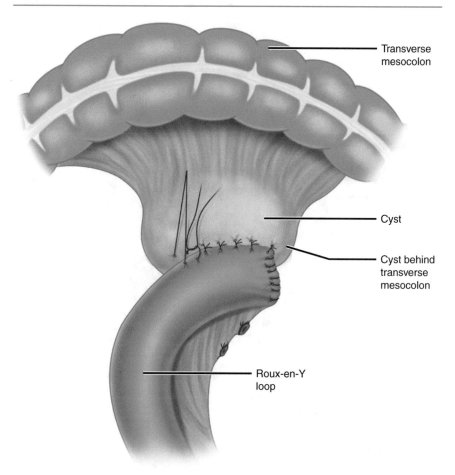

Transverse mesocolon

Cyst

Cyst behind transverse mesocolon

Roux-en-Y loop

Fig. 9.48 Roux-en-Y

- Bleeding from portal vein during exploration of the neck of the pancreas as the surgeon's fingers are passed behind the neck.
- Injury to an aberrant common hepatic artery arising from superior mesenteric artery or one of its branches.
- Injury to an aberrant right hepatic artery arising from the superior mesenteric artery.
- Injury to an aberrant left hepatic artery. This artery presents a problem only when arising from the right side superior mesenteric artery or from the gastroduodenal artery.
- Injury to an aberrant middle colic artery passing through the head of the pancreas or between the head and the duodenum.
- Injury to the cisterna chyli resulting in chylous ascites.

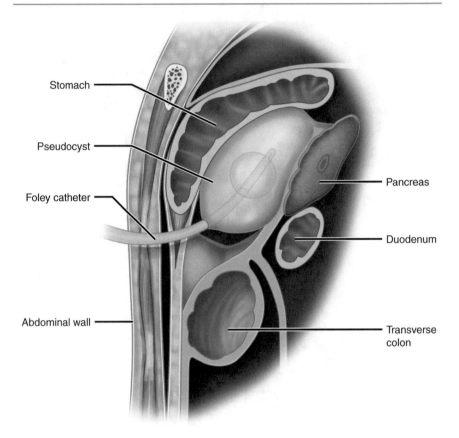

Fig. 9.49 Insertion of Foley catheter

Small Intestine

10

Roger Eduardo

Anatomy

General Description of the Small Intestine

Information about the duodenum has already been presented in detail in Chap. 8. In this chapter, general descriptions of the intestine include the duodenum, but the primary focus is on the jejunum and ileum.

Length of the Intestine

The length of the alimentary tract in humans has proven surprisingly difficult to measure. An average length of 6.0–6.5 m for the small intestine has been widely quoted in textbooks, based mostly on cadaveric measurements. This figure, though, bears an unknown relationship to the length of the intestine in living patients, since at death the intestines elongate; tonus is lost much faster in the longitudinal muscles of the intestine than in the circular muscles. There is also some evidence that intestinal length is greater in obese individuals.

In any case, the surgeon should always be concerned with the length of intestine remaining after any resection, more than the amount resected. Before the intestine is removed, accurate measurements for resection should be made with the least manipulation possible.

R. Eduardo (✉)
Department of Surgery, Beltline Bariatric and Surgical Group, Atlanta, GA, USA
e-mail: reduardomd@bbsg.life

© Springer Nature Switzerland AG 2021
L. J. Skandalakis (ed.), *Surgical Anatomy and Technique*,
https://doi.org/10.1007/978-3-030-51313-9_10

Dimensions of the Mesentery

The mesentery arises from the posterior parietal peritoneum, attached to the posterior abdominal wall, and contains the superior mesenteric artery (SMA) and superior mesenteric vein (SMV). The mesenteric root runs diagonally from the duodenojejunal flexure at ligament of treitz to the ileocecal junction in the right iliac fossa. The length of the mesentery measured between the attachment to the intestine and the root of the mesentery, usually is around 15–20 cm and typically does not exceed 25 cm. The intestinal attachment of the mesentery is the same length as the small intestine itself (around 6 m) and greatly folded.

Layers of the Wall of the Intestine

The intestinal wall is composed of a serosa of visceral peritoneum, longitudinal and circular muscle that perform peristalsis, a submucosa of connective tissue, and a mucosa of connective tissue, smooth muscle, and epithelium (Fig. 10.1). An anastomosis should ideally include all layers, but the integrity of the anastomosis is greater if at least the submucosa, which is collagen laden, is included.

Anatomy of the Ileocecal Valve

The ileocecal valve is a muscular valve and in most patients resembles the cervix protruding into the vagina or the pyloric opening into the duodenum (Fig. 10.2).

The closing mechanism of the papilla is formed by two rings of thickened circular muscle, one at the base of the papilla and one at the free end.

Vascular System of the Small Intestine

Arterial Supply

The intestinal vessels may be appreciated from Fig. 10.3. The superior mesenteric artery (SMA) arises from the aorta below the origin of the celiac trunk.

From the arches of the arcades, numerous arteries (the vasa recta) (Figs. 10.3 and 10.4) arise and pass (without cross-communication) to enter the intestinal wall. They may bifurcate to supply each side or they may pass singly to alternate sides of the intestine. Before piercing the muscularis externa, the vasa recta branch beneath the serosa, but do not anastomose. There is no collateral circulation between the vasa recta or their branches at the surface of the intestines. This configuration provides the best supply of oxygenated blood to the mesenteric side of the intestine and the poorest supply to the antimesenteric border.

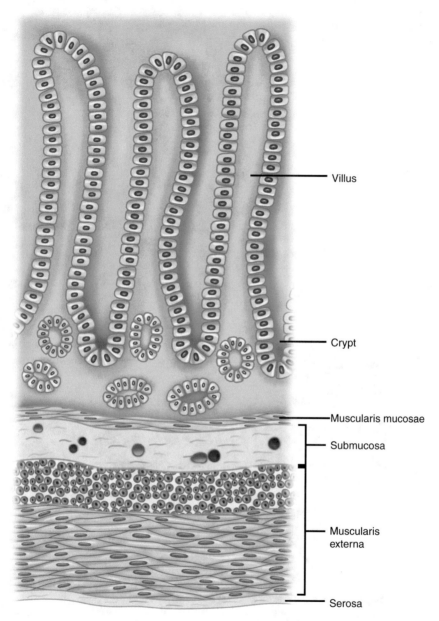

Fig. 10.1 Section through the wall of the small intestine. The submucosa should be included in stitches forming an anastomosis

Fig. 10.2 The papillary
appearance of the ileocecal
valve in the living patient

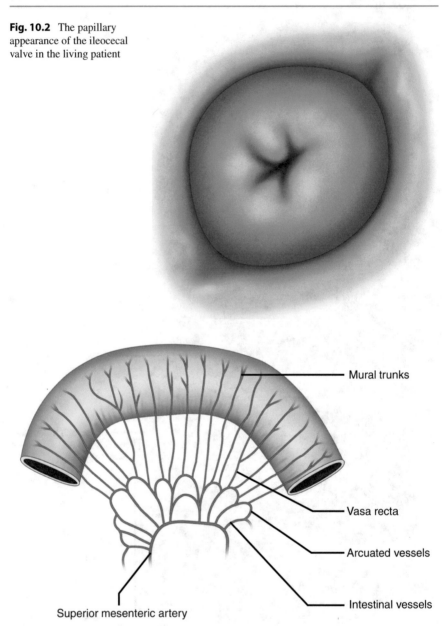

Mural trunks

Vasa recta

Arcuated vessels

Intestinal vessels

Superior mesenteric artery

Fig. 10.3 Arterial supply to the small bowel

Venous Drainage

The veins travel with the arteries in the mesentery and carry blood from the intestinal surface to reach the superior mesenteric vein.

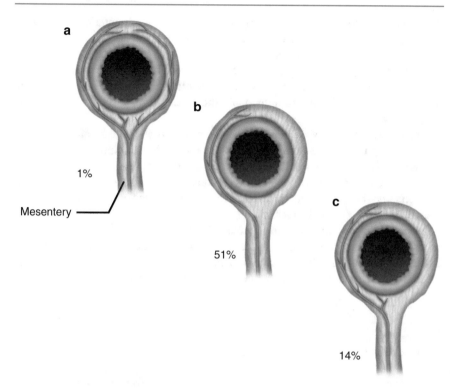

Fig. 10.4 (**a**) The vasa recta may divide into two short vessels to the mesenteric side of the intestine and two long vessels supplying the rest of the intestinal wall. (**b**) More frequently, a single, long vessel supplies one side of the intestine, alternating with a vessel supplying the other side. (**c**) A single long and a single short vessel serving one side only. The remaining 34% are various combinations of paired, single, long, and short vessels

Lymphatic Drainage

The lymphatic flow is via lymphatic channels to lymph nodes lying between the leaves of the mesentery. More than 200 small mesenteric nodes lie near the vasa recta and along the intestinal arteries. Drainage from these ultimately leads to the large superior mesenteric lymph nodes at the root of the mesentery. Efferent channels from these and the celiac nodes form the intestinal lymphatic trunk, which passes beneath the left renal artery and ends in the left lumbar lymphatic trunk (70%) or the cisterna chyli (25%).

Abnormal Development of the Small Intestine

Meckel's Diverticulum

A Meckel's diverticulum is the most common congenital defect of the GI tract and is a result of incomplete obliteration of the vitelline duct of the umbilical cord.

When present, a Meckel's diverticulum arises from the antimesenteric surface of the ileum approximately 40 cm from the ileocecal valve in infants and approximately 50 cm from the valve in adults; it may be less than 15 cm or as much as 167 cm from the valve (Fig. 10.5). Not less than 2 m of ileum should be inspected to ascertain that a diverticulum has not been overlooked. The diverticulum may be as short as 1 cm or as long as 26 cm. In 75% of individuals, the diverticulum will be <5 cm; the rest will be longer.

The diverticulum may be free and mobile, or its tip may still be attached to the anterior body wall at the umbilicus. In a few cases, the structure is patent to the outside (vitelline fistula), a solid cord, or a cystic remnant (Fig. 10.6).

Given the pluripotent cell line of the vitelline duct, the mucosa of the diverticulum can either be native ileal mucosa or heterotopic mucosa (mainly gastric or pancreatic mucosa may also be present).

Meckel's diverticulum is often referred to by the rule of two; Occurs in 2% of the population, 2% are symptomatic, twice as common in males, occurs usually within 2 feet of the ileocecal valve, average of 2 inches in length, two types of heterotopic mucosa (gastric and pancreatic), and symptomatic presentation is often before the age of two.

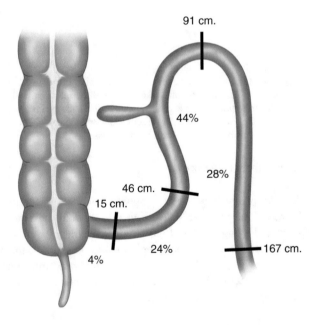

Fig. 10.5 Location on the ileum and frequency of occurrence of Meckel's diverticulum

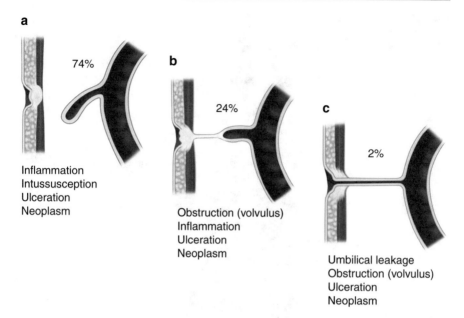

Fig. 10.6 Three major types of Meckel's diverticulum. (**a**) Diverticulum with free end not attached to the body wall. (**b**) Diverticulum connected to the anterior body wall by a fibrous cord. (**c**) Fistula opening through the umbilicus

Surgical Anatomy of Intussusception

An intussusception is created when a proximal segment of intestine invaginates into the portion of intestine immediately distal to it, creating an obstruction that can lead to bowel ischemia and necrosis (Fig. 10.7).

In children, intussusception is the leading cause of bowel obstruction, and Meckel's diverticulum is the most common identifiable cause. Other known causes are intestinal polyps or other tumors (second most common), lymphoid hyperplasia, duplications, and intestinal atresias. However, 75% of intussusceptions in children are idiopathic and cannot be assigned to any specific cause. Reduction of the intussusception may occur spontaneously or require intervention.

In contrast to intussusceptions in children, most adult intussusceptions are caused by a structural or pathologic lesion, and a significant proportion of these lead points are malignant neoplasms. Malignancy accounts for about 66% of colonic intussusceptions and 30% of small bowel intussusceptions. In general, the "2/3 rule" may be applied (all numbers are approximate) – 2/3 of adult intussusceptions are from known causes. Of these, 2/3 are due to neoplasms. Of the neoplasms, 2/3 will be malignant.

Fig. 10.7 Diagram of the
anatomy of an intestinal
intussusception

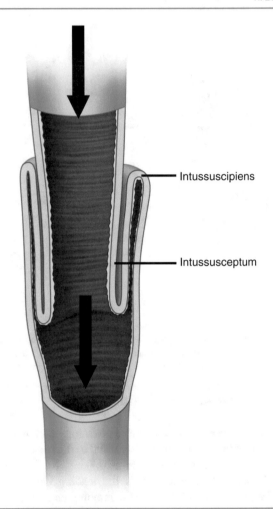

Intussuscipiens

Intussusceptum

Anatomic Guidelines for Surgery

There is no good way to identify an isolated loop of small intestine without follow-ing it in one direction to the duodenojejunal junction at ligament of Treitz or in the other direction to the ileocecal junction.

Exposure and Mobilization

Few organs are more easily exposed and mobilized than are loops of small intestine. Adhesions from previous surgery are generally the chief obstacles to good mobilization.

The only procedures we perform in this part of the gastrointestinal tract are typi-cally resection and anastomosis of the small bowel. In benign disease, we make every effort to save the ileocecal valve, but when malignancy is present, resection is essential. When dealing with resection of the small bowel, the surgeon should always be conservative. The decision in the operating room should be based on pathology, such as tumor (benign or malignant), mesenteric thrombosis of arterial or venous type, and inflammatory processes, such as regional enteritis, tumors of the mesentery causing a desmoplastic reaction, and Meckel's diverticulum.

Technique

Resection of Small Bowel for Tumor

- **Step 1.** In the case of a small bowel tumor, wide local excision with proximal and distal margins of 5–10 cm are appropriate. Create a mesenteric window below the bowel where you intend to divide and score the mesentery of the small bowel with the Bovie toward the root to delineate resection.
- **Step 2.** Using a 60–80 mm gastrointestinal anastomosis (GIA) stapler, transect the small bowel proximally and distally. When applying the GIA stapler, make sure that the stapler end is on the antimesenteric border of the small bowel (Fig. 10.9).
- **Step 3.** The mesentery can be divided either by using electrocautery with a LigaSure, harmonic, bipolar, vessel sealer or similar device, or manually using a hemostat to clamp either end of the vessel and ligating the vessels of the mesentery of the small bowel with 2–0 or 3–0 silk (Figs. 10.8 and 10.9).
- **Step 4.** Remove the specimen and label proximal and distal ends with suture to send to pathology (so that if margins are positive, orientation is known).
- **Step 5.** Align the two remaining segments of small bowel such that the antimesenteric borders abut each other (Fig. 10.10). Using scissors transect the stapled corner of the small bowel at the antimesenteric border and dilate to allow passage of stapler arm.
- **Step 6.** Insert each arm of the GIA stapler into the small bowel through the previously created opening and approximate the stapler such that the antimesenteric portions of the small bowel are in proximity to each other. Fire the stapler. Remove the stapler and briefly inspect the mucosal surface of the anastomosis for bleeding (Fig. 10.11).
- **Step 7.** Re-align the common enterotomy defect so that the staple line ends of the previous stapler firing are oblique to each other and not lined up together. This common enterotomy, can then either either be sutured closed using 2-0 vicryl suture or stapled – using a 60 mm thoracoabdominal (TA) stapler or another GIA stapler, close the enterotomy transversely ensuring all layers of bowel wall are within the stapler. Palpate for patency.
- **Step 8.** Close the mesenteric defect of the small bowel with either a running or interrupted 2–0 or 3–0 suture.
- **Step 9.** Place a supporting 3–0 Vicryl or silk suture in the crotch of the anastomosis.

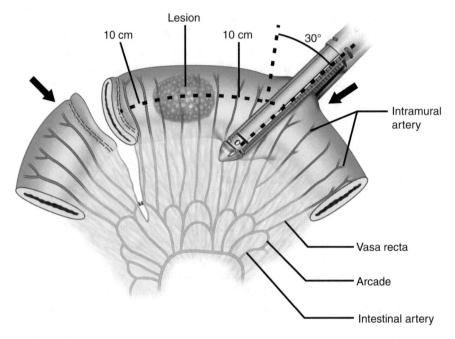

Fig. 10.8 Recommended position of stapler for segmental resection of intestine. The 30° angle from a vertical transection preserves as much of the antimesenteric blood supply as possible (*arrows*) and slightly increases the functional diameter of the anastomosis

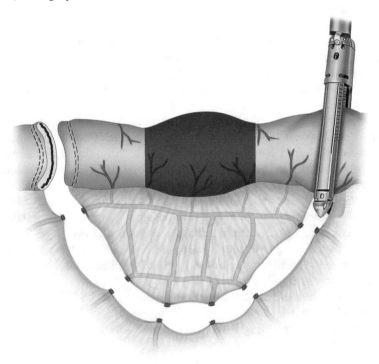

Fig. 10.9 Ligation of vessels

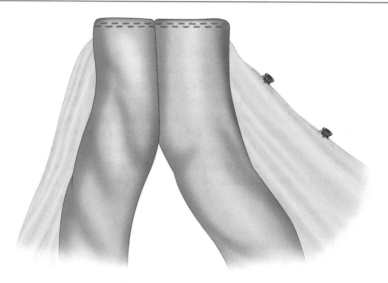

Fig. 10.10 Lining up the antimesenteric borders for stapled anastomosis

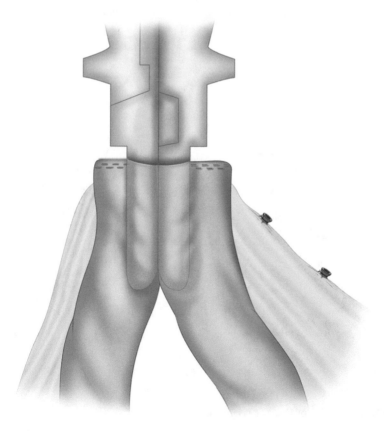

Fig. 10.11 Orientation of GIA stapler

Meckel's Diverticulum (Orientation Fig. 10.5)

An incidentally discovered Meckel's diverticulum does not need to be resected. However, if it is serving as a lead point for intussusception; after reduction of the intussusception, and as long as the bowel does not appear ischemic or necrotic – we prefer a wedge resection of the diverticulum with extension to the mesenteric wall (Fig. 10.12). However, if a patient presents with GI bleeding thought to be secondary to Meckel's diverticulum, the pathology is likely in the ileum adjacent to the diverticulum as a result of acid exposure from heterotopic gastric mucosa within the diverticulum. In these cases, we recommend a segmental resection of the ileum and a stapled functional end-to-end anastomosis (see preceding procedure for resection of small bowel for tumor).

Intussusception (Orientation Fig. 10.7)

The most common type of intussusception in children, accounting for 85% of occurrences, is ileocecal intussusception (Fig. 10.13) – the treatment for which often requires ultrasound-guided or fluoroscopic pneumatic insufflation or hydrostatic enema with normal saline or barium to reduce the invagination. If the patient fails

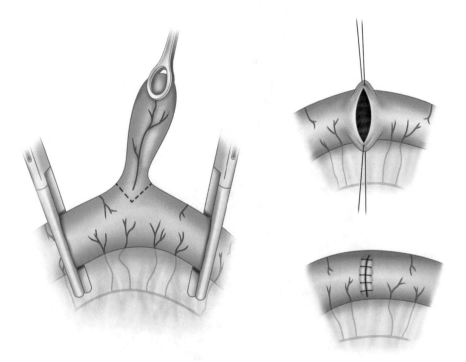

Fig. 10.12 Resection of Meckel's diverticulum

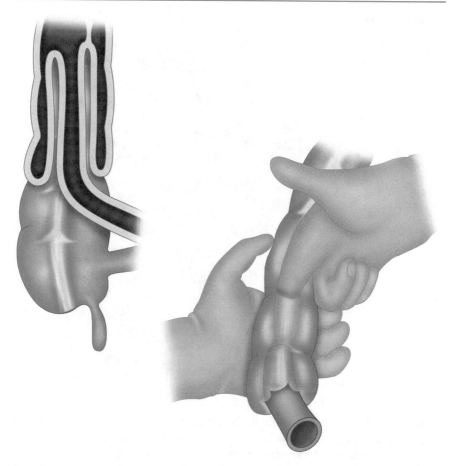

Fig. 10.13 Reduction of intussusception

nonsurgical management and intussusception does not reduce spontaneously or via nonsurgical management as above, perform surgery and reduce (Fig. 10.13). The presence of a pathologic lead point or evidence of bowel necrosis or perforation postreduction are indications for resection and anastomosis.

In adults, given the high association of intussusception with a malignant cause (see "2/3 rule" above), the recommendation for symptomatic adult intussusceptions traditionally involves exploratory laparotomy or diagnostic laparoscopy followed by resection to include lead point masses or areas of ischemia.

Small Bowel Feeding Tubes – Witzel Jejunostomy

- **Step 1.** Select a loop of the proximal jejunum approximately 15–20 cm from the ligament of Treitz (Fig. 10.14) that can easily reach the anterior abdominal wall.
- **Step 2.** Make a stab wound in the abdominal wall and insert a jejunal feeding tube catheter into peritoneum.

Fig. 10.14 Selection of loop

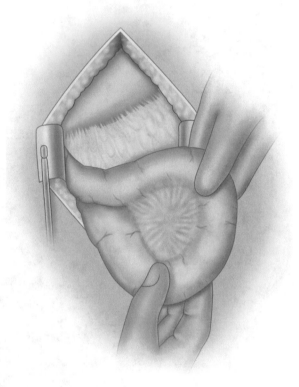

- **Step 3.** Make a small incision on the enteric wall and insert the catheter into intestine ensuring it feeds distally. Place purse–string sutures of 3–0 Vicryl in the intestinal wall around the catheter and tighten them to secure catheter in place (Figs. 10.15 and 10.16).
- **Step 4.** Create a seromuscular tunnel from the point of insertion of intestine and proximally for about 5 cm using 3–0 Vicryl interrupted sutures (Fig. 10.17) invaginated over the tube. Secure in a Stamm position to the anterior abdominal wall using interrupted sutures.
- **Step 5.** Externally, fix the catheter to the skin.

Feeding Jejunostomy

Perform this procedure in the same way as Stamm gastrostomy, except use a small T-tube in a loop of jejunum 15–20 cm distal to the ligament of Treitz. To prevent torsion secure the jejunum to the anterior abdominal wall 5 cm proximal and distal to the Stamm.

Fig. 10.15   Wall is incised

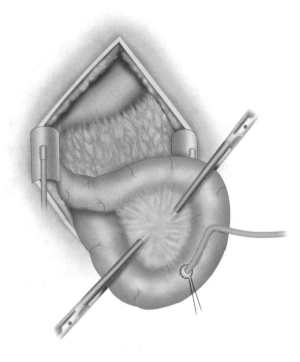

Fig. 10.16   Introduction of catheter

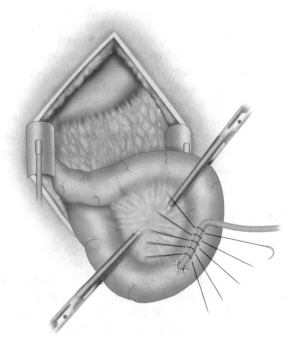

Fig. 10.17 The
seromuscular tunnel

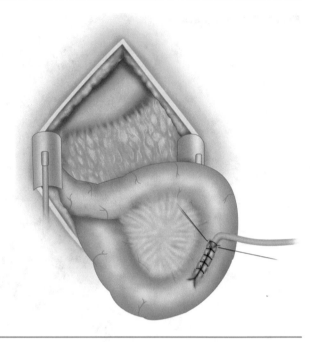

Anatomical Complications

Vascular Injury

- Vascular injury to the superior mesenteric artery must be repaired at once to restore flow. Injury to the mesentery and one or more of the smaller intestinal arteries or vascular arches often requires ligation. This will add to the length of devitalized segment of intestine and hence the length of resection needed. When performing a resection, the aim should be to minimize injury to the blood supply, vascular arches, and vasa recta as best as possible.
- Hematomas at the anastomotic site will cause ischemia, necrosis, and perforation. Hematomas are most common at the junction of the mesentery with the anastomotic site. When this occurs mesenteric vessels can be occluded by the hematoma, producing local ischemia.

Organ Injury

- The abdominal cavity should be well packed before any enterotomy or enterostomy and thoroughly irrigated after to prevent contamination and future infection, which may lead to intraperitoneal or abdominal wall abscess.
- Leakage at the anastomotic suture line is the result of poor technique with inadequate closure or suture line ischemia and may be followed by a fistula (enteroenteric, entero-organ, or enterocutaneous) or free perforation and general

peritonitis. Care in closing the mesentery at the suture line without damage to blood vessels and prevention of tension on the anastomosis reduce the possibility of leakage.

- An inadequate anastomosis will result in stasis of intestinal contents and possible obstruction. A slightly oblique line of resection as described will help enlarge the anastomotic opening and preserve the blood supply to the antimesenteric border.
- Tension and torsion at the anastomosis must be prevented. The surgeon must be sure that any tension or torsion has not been merely transferred to a more distal or proximal site.

Appendix

11

Roger Eduardo

Anatomy

Relations and Positions of the Appendix

The appendix arises from the posteromedial side of the cecum about 2 cm from the end of the ileum. The cecum typically lays anteriorly to the iliopsoas muscle and the lumbar plexus of nerves. Anteriorly, it is often covered by the abdominal wall, the greater omentum, or coils of ileum. The base of the appendix is located at the union of the tenia of the colon. For all practical purposes, the anterior tenia ends at the appendiceal origin.

Five typical locations of the appendix, in order of frequency, are:

- Retrocecal-retrocolic, free or fixed
- Pelvic or descending
- Subcecal, passing downward and laterally
- Ileocecal, passing upward and medially, anterior to the ileum
- Ileocecal, posterior to the ileum

Studies have found that the first two positions are the most common but with significant variations.

Mesentery

The mesentery of the appendix is embryologically derived from the posterior side of the mesentery of the terminal ileum. The mesentery attaches to the cecum, as well as to the proximal appendix, and contains the appendiceal artery.

R. Eduardo (✉)
Department of Surgery, Beltline Bariatric and Surgical Group, Atlanta, GA, USA
e-mail: reduardomd@bbsg.life

© Springer Nature Switzerland AG 2021
L. J. Skandalakis (ed.), *Surgical Anatomy and Technique*,
https://doi.org/10.1007/978-3-030-51313-9_11

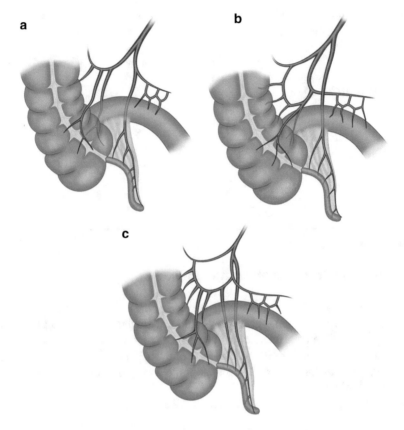

Fig. 11.1 Blood supply to the appendix. (**a**, **b**) Usual type with a single appendicular artery. (**c**) Paired appendicular arteries

Vascular System of the Appendix

Arterial Supply

The appendiceal artery commonly arises from a terminal branch of the ileocolic artery, and less commonly from an ileal artery, or from a posterior cecal artery. Although the appendicular artery is usually singular (Fig. 11.1), duplication is often seen. In addition to the typical appendicular artery, the base of the appendix may also be supplied by a small branch of the anterior or posterior cecal artery.

Venous Supply

The appendicular artery and the appendicular vein are enveloped by the mesentery of the appendix. The vein joins the cecal veins to become the ileocolic vein, which is a tributary of the right colic vein, draining into the superior mesenteric vein (SMV).

Lymphatic Drainage

Lymphatic drainage from the ileocecal region is through a chain of nodes on the appendicular, ileocolic, and superior mesenteric arteries through which the lymph passes to reach the celiac lymph nodes and the cisterna chyli (Fig. 11.2). Some studies describe a secondary drainage (which passes anterior to the pancreas) to subpyloric nodes.

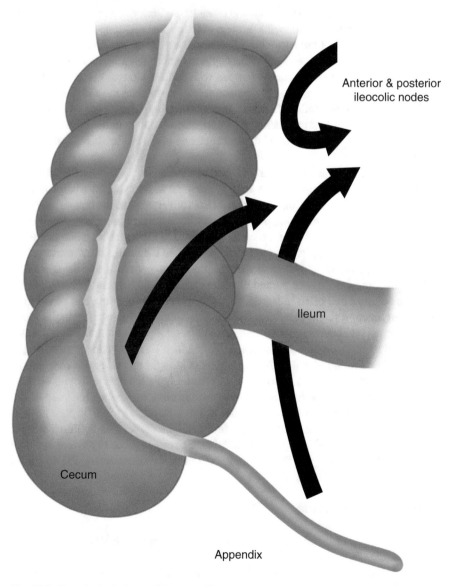

Fig. 11.2 Lymphatic drainage of the appendix

Technique

Appendectomy

The incision for an open appendectomy is usually made over McBurney's point, which is a point about one third of the distance along an imaginary line drawn from the anterior superior iliac spine (ASIS) to the umbilicus. This point correlates to the approximate location of the base of the appendix. The incision should be made through this point perpendicular to the imaginary line (a McBurney-McArthur incision) or horizontally (a Lanz incision) and extended 3–5 cm along skin creases. Bovie electrocautery can be used to incise through both the superficial and the deep fascia, exposing the external oblique aponeurosis. This should be incised along the direction of the muscle fibers, and the muscle fibers split to expose the transversalis fascia and peritoneum. The peritoneum can be grasped with straight clamps, elevated, and subsequently incised carefully using Metzenbaum scissors to enter the abdominal cavity.

The cecum should be identified first. It can be distinguished from the transverse colon by the absence of attachments of the omentum. Though unlikely, if the cecum cannot be located, malrotation of the intestines or undescended cecum should be considered.

When the cecum has been identified, one of the teniae coli can be traced downward to the base of the appendix. In spite of the great mobility of the tip, the base of the appendix always arises from the cecum at the convergence of the teniae. In exposing a deeply buried retrocecal appendix, it may be necessary to incise the posterior peritoneum lateral to the cecum. Congenital absence of the appendix is too rare to be considered seriously, but its apparent absence may be the result of intussusception. In such a case, there should be an obvious dimple at the normal site of the appendix.

Once identified the appendix and mesoappendix should be gently dissected free from the adjacent and often inflamed, tissue. A mesenteric opening can be made at the convergence of the appendiceal base and cecum, and the mesoappendix, containing the appendiceal artery and vein, should be clamped proximally and distally and ligated using 2–0 silk ties. The appendix can then be removed in various ways.

The author's preference is to lift the appendix straight up and attach two clamps to its base. Remove the clamp close to the cecum. Ligate the appendiceal base doubly with #0 absorbable suture. Stump inversion is done only when the base of the appendix is necrotic. When inverting, use a 3–0 silk purse string (Figs. 11.8 and 11.9). Divide the appendix between the clamp and the absorbable ligatures using a knife or electrocautery (Fig. 11.10). Maintain the clamp in place to prevent inadvertent contamination and pass the specimen off the field. Alternatively, the appendix can be divided with a GIA stapler.

Step-by-Step Technique

- **Step 1.** Choice of incision is up to the surgeon. We prefer the McBurney incision (Fig. 11.3).
- **Step 2.** Incise the aponeurosis of the external oblique along the lines of its fibers (Fig. 11.4).

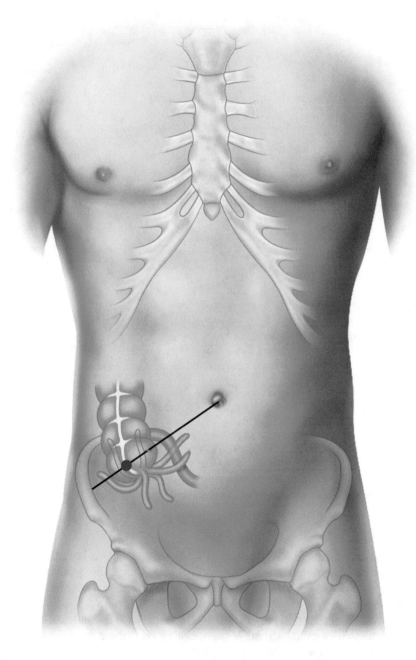

Fig. 11.3 Locating McBurney's point – one third of the distance from ASIS to umbilicus. Note also that although there are multiple locations in which the appendix is found, appendiceal base and insertion point into cecum tend to be fairly consistent, correlating to McBurney's point

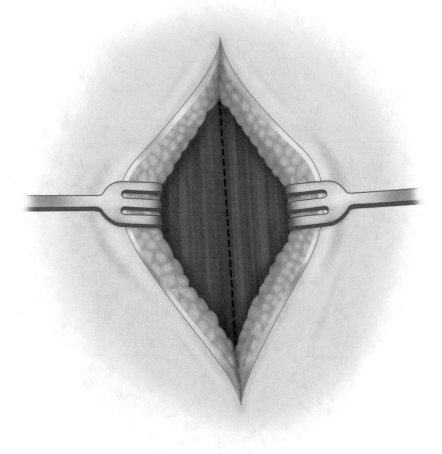

Fig. 11.4 Incision of external oblique follows direction of fibers

- **Step 3.** Use a curved Kelly clamp to make an opening on both the internal oblique and the transversus abdominis muscles. Enlarge the opening with the Kelly clamp and insert two Richardson's retractors to keep the muscle fibers spread.
- **Step 4.** If the transversalis fascia is divided together with the muscles, occasionally there will be a thick stroma of preperitoneal fat that can be pushed laterally or sometimes medially, revealing the peritoneum.

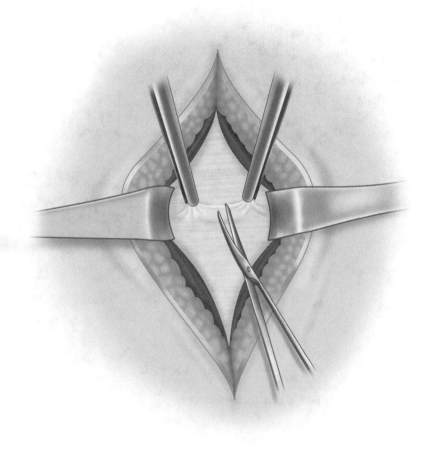

Fig. 11.5 Incising the peritoneum between two straight clamps while ensuring no injury to underlying structures

- **Step 5.** Elevate the peritoneum and, if applicable, the transversalis fascia between two clamps to lift away from underlying structure. Make a small opening in the peritoneum with a knife or Metzenbaum scissors, then enlarge it with both index fingers, and insert the retractors of your choice (Fig. 11.5).
- **Step 6.** Take cultures of the free peritoneal fluid and, using moist gauze, pull the cecum out of the wound and into your field. In most cases, the appendix is delivered with the cecum or can then be found.

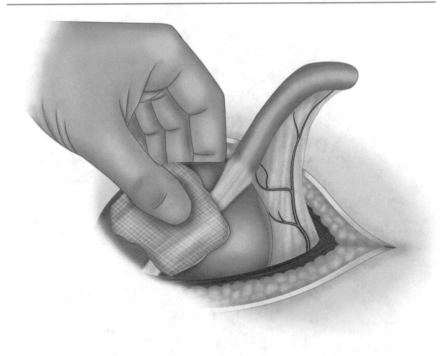

Fig. 11.6 Examining the appendix and its mesentery

- **Step 7.** Grasp and study the mesentery of the appendix and reinsert the cecum into the peritoneal cavity. Divide the mesoappendix between clamps (Fig. 11.6).
- **Step 8.** Ligate the mesoappendix with 2–0 silk (Fig. 11.7).
- **Step 9.** With hemostasis completed, lift the appendix straight up and attach two clamps to its base. Remove the clamp close to the cecum. Ligate the appendiceal base doubly with 0 absorbable suture, such as chromic catgut. Stump inversion is done only when the base of the appendix is necrotic. When inverting, use a 3–0 silk purse string to close the cecal defect around the stump inversion (Figs. 11.8 and 11.9).
- **Step 10.** Divide the appendix between the clamp and the catgut ligatures using a knife or electrocautery (Fig. 11.10). (Alternatively, the appendix can be divided with a GIA stapler.)
- **Step 11.** Irrigate. Close in layers using catgut or absorbable synthetic suture. If peritonitis and frank spillage is present, close the muscle, but not the skin. The authors use iodoform gauze to pack the wound (Figs. 11.11, 11.12, and 11.13).

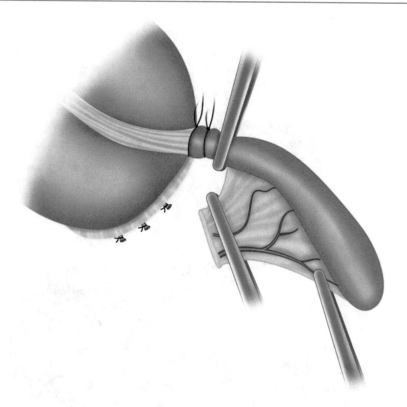

Fig. 11.7 Two ligation sutures placed proximally and clamp distally

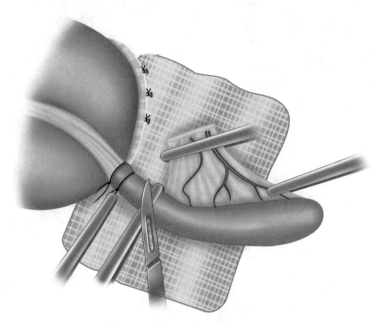

Fig. 11.8 Division of appendix between sutures and clamp

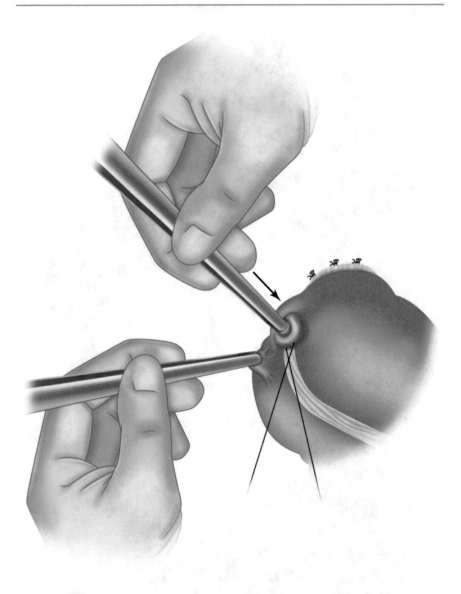

Fig. 11.9 Inversion of appendiceal stump if it is found to be necrotic. Silk purse-string suture is used to close the cecal defect once the stump is inverted

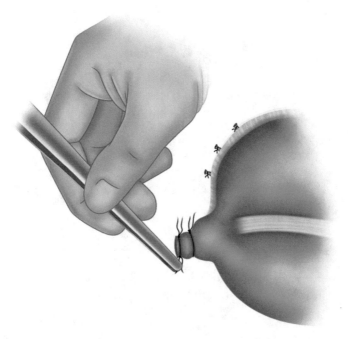

Fig. 11.10 Appendiceal stump with division site distal to second ligature

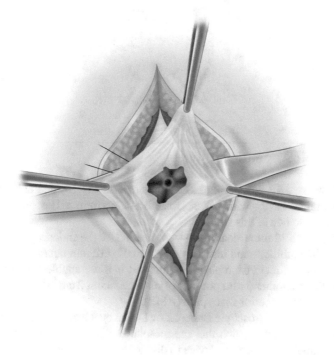

Fig. 11.11 Return cecum to the abdomen and close peritoneum

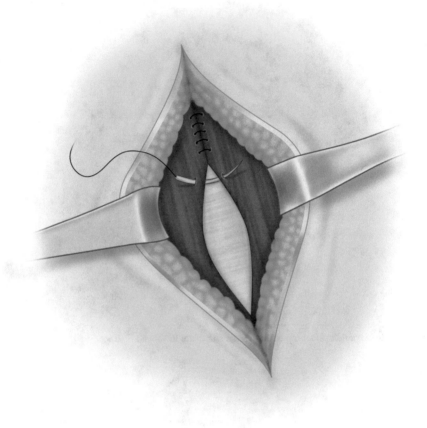

Fig. 11.12 Closing in layers

Laparoscopic Appendectomy

- **Step 1.** Make a 12 mm periumbilical incision (Fig. 11.14) and either insufflate the abdominal cavity with a Veress needle or perform a Hasson technique to enter the abdomen at this site.
- **Step 2.** Place a 12 mm trocar (this size is needed for the endoscopic GIA stapler) through the umbilicus and insert either a 5 mm or 12 mm laparoscope.
- **Step 3.** Under direct vision place a 5 mm port in a suprapubic position.
- **Step 4.** Place another 5 mm port left of midline, about 2 cm above and medial to the left anterior superior iliac spine (ASIS).
- **Step 5.** Using a laparoscopic Babcock or DeBakey, locate and grasp the appendix and apply traction such that the mesoappendix is visualized. Use the harmonic scalpel or a LigaSure device to divide the mesoappendix (Fig. 11.15).

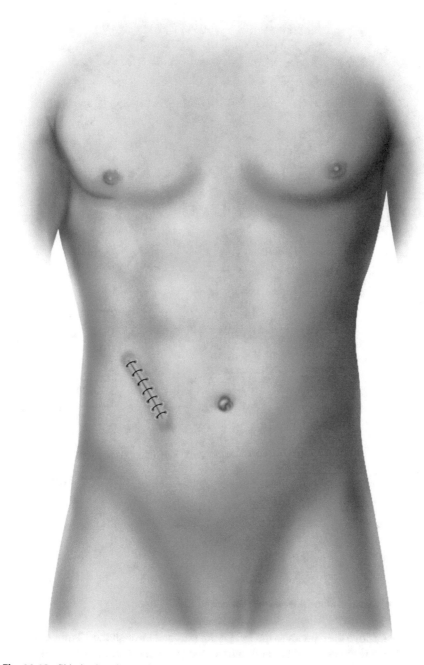

Fig. 11.13 Skin is closed

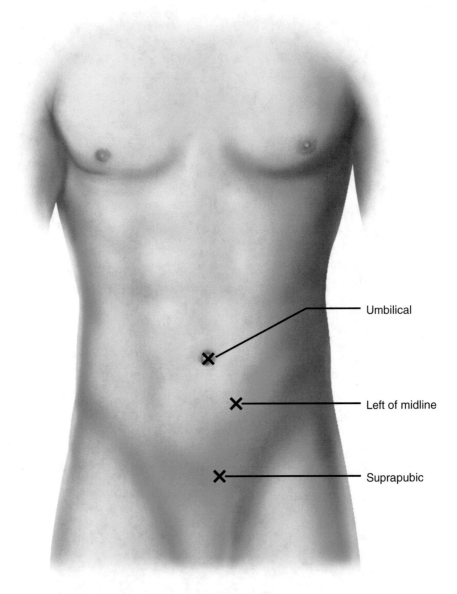

Fig. 11.14 Location of incision and port placement

- **Step 6.** Move the camera to the left lateral port and through the 12 mm umbilical port, insert the GIA stapler, and transect the appendix. Usually one firing is sufficient; however, it may need to be repeated (Fig. 11.16).

  *An alternative method of division – a window can be made in the mesoappendix at the appendiceal base and the appendix transected with stapler as above. Once divided the appendix can be lifted exposing the entire mesoappendix, which can then be divided using a vascular load of the GIA stapler.

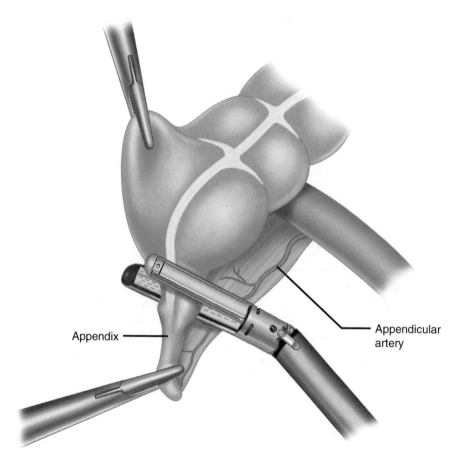

Appendix

Appendicular
artery

Fig. 11.15 Division of the appendix with the Endo GIA stapler

- **Step 7.** Place the appendix into an endoscopic pouch and remove it through the umbilical incision (Fig. 11.16).
- **Step 8.** Close the umbilical fascial defect with a 0 Vicryl suture. Close the skin.

Note
- The patient should have an orogastric tube placed to decompress the stomach, as well as a Foley catheter for bladder decompression. There are instances when the stomach can reach to the level of the umbilicus; decompression will avoid perforation with the Veress needle.
- The Foley catheter will decompress the bladder and keep it from being injured during placement of the suprapubic trocar. However, the trocar should be carefully observed while it is being placed in the suprapubic position. The author has experienced iatrogenic trocar injury to the bladder even though the bladder was decompressed and the insertion was viewed. So, be careful.

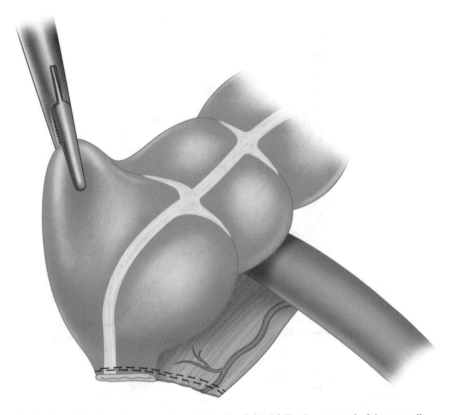

Fig. 11.16 Appendiceal stump and mesoappendix divided following removal of the appendix

Anatomical Complications

Vascular Injury

- Hematoma of the mesentery of the appendix or the ileocecal mesentery.
- Hemoperitoneum due to improper ligation of the appendiceal artery. This can also be due to improper use or failure of an energy device (LigaSure, harmonic scalpel).

Organ Injury

- The cecum or terminal ileum may be injured due to excessive traction or handling.
- The right ureter, fallopian tube, or ovary may be injured.
- A fecal fistula can result due to inadequate ligation of the appendix or failure of the gastrointestinal stapler.

Nerve Injuries

- Injury of the iliohypogastric can occur.

Inadequate Procedure

- Occasionally one may encounter a long appendix some of which may be covered by a peritoneal veil. This could lead one to falsely believe that an adequate appendectomy has been done. Ensure that you visualize the appendiceal insertion into cecum.

Colon and Anorectum

12

Evan N. Feldman

Anatomy

General Description of Colon and Anorectum

The large intestine, or colon, extends from the terminal ileum to the anus. The classic divisions are the cecum, colon proper, rectum, and anal canal. A surgical unit, the right colon, is composed of the cecum, ascending colon, and hepatic flexure. The surgical unit of the left colon consists of the distal transverse colon, splenic flexure, and descending and sigmoid colons.

Cecum

The cecum—the first 5 cm of the large bowel just distal to the ileocecal valve—lies in the right iliac fossa, and in about 60% of living, erect individuals, it lies partly in the true pelvis. In approximately 20%, almost the entire posterior surface of the cecum is attached to the posterior abdominal wall, and, at the other extreme, in approximately 24%, the cecum is wholly unattached. Among the latter are cases of pathologically mobile cecum, in which the lower part of the ascending limb, in addition to the cecum, is unattached.

A fold of peritoneum from the mesentery of the terminal ileum may cross the ileum to attach to the cecum. This fold, the mesentery, and the ileum may form a superior ileocecal fossa. Below are an inferior ileocecal fold and an inferior ileocecal fossa (Fig. 12.1). These folds are inconstant, and the associated fossae can be shallow or absent. Occasionally a retrocecal fossa is present. In some subjects, a fixed terminal ileum may be present and, rarely, a common ileocecal mesentery.

E. N. Feldman (✉)
ATL Colorectal Surgery, P.C, Atlanta, GA, USA

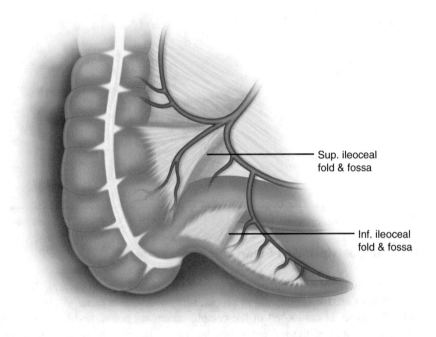

Fig. 12.1 Superior and inferior ileocecal folds forming fossae

Colon Proper

The ascending limb of the colon proper is normally fused to the posterior body wall and covered anteriorly by the peritoneum. There are variations of incomplete fusion ranging from a deep lateral paracolic groove to the persistence of an entire ascending mesocolon (Fig. 12.2). A mesocolon long enough to permit volvulus occurs in approximately 11%. In cadavers, the ascending colon may be mobile in approximately 37% of cases. A mobile cecum, together with a mobile right colon, may be present.

Where the mesocolon is present, the cecum and the proximal ascending colon are unusually mobile. It is this condition that is termed mobile cecum and which can result in volvulus of the cecum and the right colon (Fig. 12.3) as well as cecal bascule.

Two conditions must be present for right colon volvulus to occur: (1) an abnormally mobile segment of colon and (2) a fixed point around which the mobile segment can twist.

The transverse colon begins where the colon turns sharply to the left (the hepatic flexure) just beneath the inferior surface of the right lobe of the liver. It ends at a sharp upward and then downward bend (the splenic flexure) related to the posterolateral surface of the spleen. The tail of the pancreas is above. The anterior surface of the left kidney lies medially.

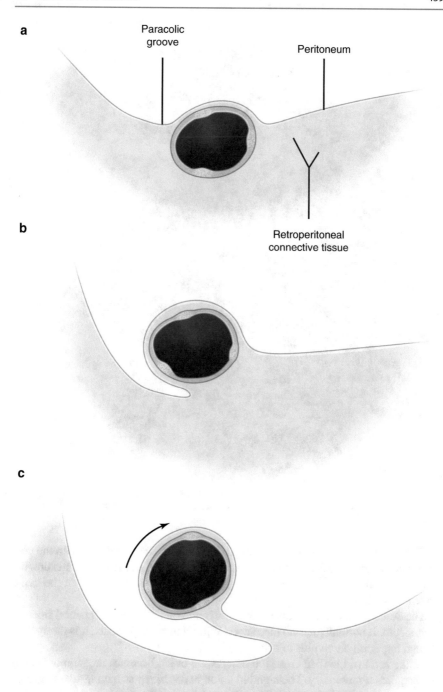

Fig. 12.2 Degrees of attachment of the right colon to the abdominal wall. (**a**) Normal retroperitoneal location of the colon. (**b**) Paracolic gutter. (**c**) Mobile colon with mesentery

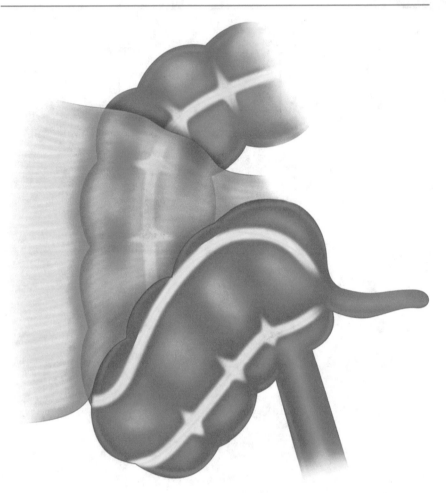

Fig. 12.3 Mobile cecum, distal ileum, and proximal right colon. This configuration is subject to volvulus

The transverse colon has a mesentery which has fused secondarily with the posterior wall of the omental bursa (see Fig. 8.1 in Chap. 8). At the splenic flexure, the colon is supported by the phrenocolic ligament, a part of the left side of the transverse mesocolon.

The descending colon is covered anteriorly and on its medial and lateral sides by peritoneum. It normally has no mesentery. When a mesentery exists, it is rarely long enough to permit a volvulus to occur.

At the level of the iliac crest, the descending colon becomes the sigmoid colon and acquires a mesentery. The sigmoid colon is described as having two portions: iliac (fixed) and pelvic (mobile). The average length of the attachment and the average breadth of the mesentery are shown in Fig. 12.4a. The left ureter passes through the base of the sigmoid mesocolon through the intersigmoid mesenteric recess (Fig. 12.4b).

Fig. 12.4 (a) Average
measurements of the
sigmoid mesocolon. (b)
The relation of the base of
the sigmoid mesocolon to
the left ureter

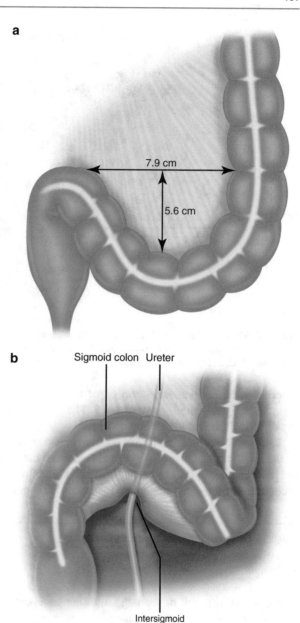

Rectum and Anal Canal

There are many definitions of the junction between the sigmoid colon and the rectum that are inconsistent with each other. Most surgeons consider the rectosigmoid junction to be at the level of the sacral promontory. Anatomists consider the rectosigmoid junction to be located at the level of S3. Others consider the rectosigmoid

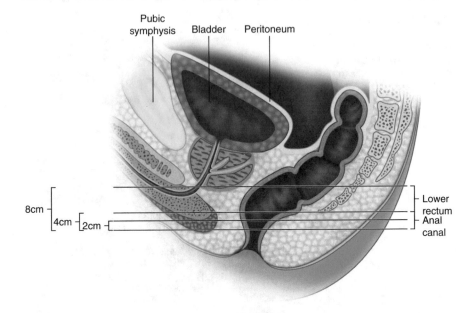

Fig. 12.5 The line of peritoneal reflection on the rectum; lateral view in the male. More of the rectum is covered anteriorly than posteriorly. The measurements of the anal canal and lower rectum from the anal verge are approximate

junction to be the narrowest portion of the large intestine where the teniae fuse together to form a single anterior tenia. The haustra and mesocolon terminate and the diverticula are no longer able to form.

The surgeon considers the anal canal to be the region lying distal to the insertion of the levator ani muscle. The surgical anal canal has a length of 4 cm: 2 cm above the pectinate line and 2 cm below (Fig. 12.5). The functional anal canal extends for 4 cm from the anorectal ring to the intersphincteric groove.

Layers of Wall of Large Intestine

Colon

The layers of the wall of the large intestine are essentially similar to those of the wall of the small intestine. The chief differences are (1) the absence of mucosal villi, (2) longitudinal muscularis externa in three discrete bands (teniae) rather than in a continuous cylinder, (3) the presence of epiploic appendices (appendages), and (4) the presence of haustra or sacculations.

The epiploic appendages are of interest to the surgeon because they may be the sites of diverticula (Fig. 12.6a). Fat may conceal the presence of the diverticulum on inspection, but fecaliths in the diverticula are frequently palpable. The appendages are also subject to infarction and torsion; both produce symptoms of an acute

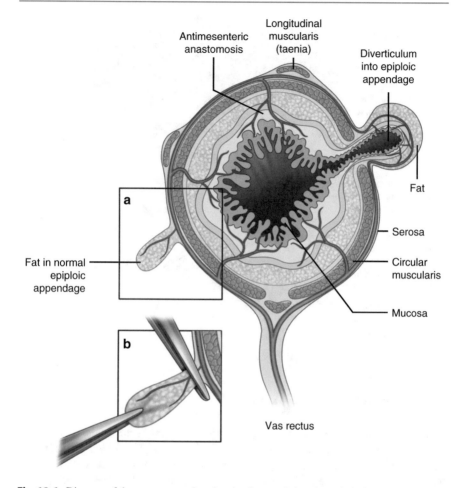

Fig. 12.6 Diagram of the transverse colon showing long and short branches of the vasa recta. On the left is a normal epiploic appendage; on the right, a diverticulum extending into an epiploic appendage. *Inset*: Effect of too much traction on an epiploic appendage resulting in injury to a long branch of a vas rectus followed by antimesenteric ischemia

abdomen. Epiploic appendages should be ligated without traction. This prevents unintentional pulling of a loop of a long colic artery into the appendiceal neck and its accidental inclusion in the ligation (Fig. 12.6b).

Rectum

Grossly, the rectum has no teniae, epiploic appendages, or haustra. The rectum is 12–15 cm in length. It passes through the levator ani to become the anal canal. After surgical mobilization, the rectum can be stretched to 15–20 cm in length. The valves/folds straighten out and contribute to the extra length.

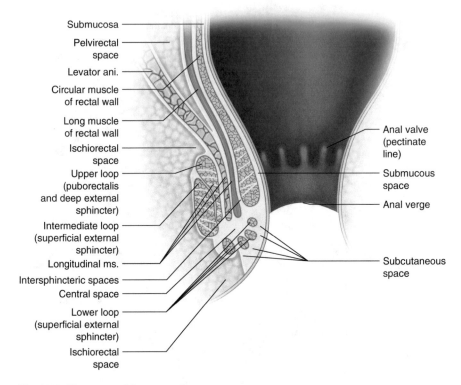

Fig. 12.7 The spaces of the anus and rectum

The rectum contains one to four crescentic plicae, the rectal folds, or valves of Houston. Typically, there are three folds: left superior, right middle, and left inferior. The folds are encountered by the sigmoidoscope at 4–7, 8–10, and 10–12 cm from the anal verge. The middle rectal fold corresponds to the level of the anterior peritoneal reflection.

Anal Canal

The Musculature of the Wall of the Anal Canal

The anorectal ring (palpable as the puborectalis) is located at the junction of the internal anal sphincter and the levator ani complex. The anal canal is approximately 4 cm long.

Two layers of smooth muscle surround the anal canal. The innermost layer is formed by a greatly thickened circular coat which is continuous with the circular muscularis externa of the colon. This is the internal sphincter of the anal canal (Fig. 12.7). The second smooth muscle layer is composed of longitudinal fibers continuous with the fibers of the teniae coli. It descends between the internal and external anal sphincters. The lowest portions traverse the external anal sphincters.

The longitudinal muscle fibers prevent separation of the sphincteric elements from each other and also permit a telescopic movement between internal and

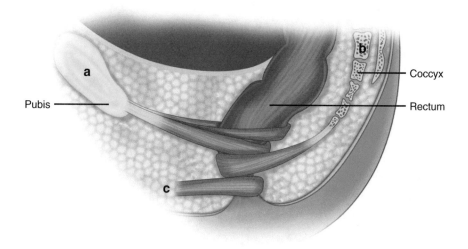

Fig. 12.8 The three loops of the external anal sphincter (**a**, **b**, **c**). Each loop is a separate sphincter with distinct attachments, muscle bundles, and innervations. Continence depends on the preservation of at least one of the three. Some subcutaneous muscle fibers encircle the anus; some attach to the perianal skin anteriorly at (**c**)

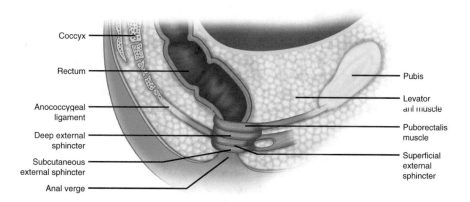

Fig. 12.9 Diagram of the extrinsic muscles of the surgical anal canal

external sphincters. We witness this in the operating room when the external sphincter rolls back and the internal sphincter rolls forward.

Composed of striated muscle, the external sphincter has three separate fiber bundles or loops: subcutaneous, superficial, and deep. It is useful to consider the three parts separately (Figs. 12.8 and 12.9), but the three loops together form an efficient anal closure. Any single one of the loops is capable of maintaining continence to solid stools but not to fluid or gas. The subcutaneous portion surrounds the outlet of the anus, attaching to the perianal skin anteriorly. Some fibers completely encircle the anus.

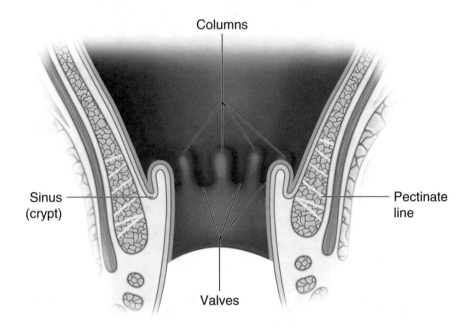

Fig. 12.10 The interior of the anal canal showing the rectal columns, anal valves, and anal sinuses (crypts). They form the pectinate line

The superficial portion surrounds the anus and continues within the anococcygeal ligament, which attaches posteriorly to the coccyx. This creates the small triangular space of Minor behind the anus. Anteriorly, some fibers insert into the transverse perineal muscles at the perineal body, creating a potential space toward which anterior midline fistulas may point. The deep portion surrounds the canal, with no obvious anterior or posterior attachments. In Shafik's view the deep portion and the puborectalis muscle are a single unit.[1]

Lining of the Surgical Anal Canal

There are three histologic regions of the anal canal, which extend from the anal verge to approximately 1 cm above the dentate line. The *cutaneous zone*, up to the anal verge (anocutaneous line), is covered by pigmented skin that has hair follicles and sebaceous glands. Above the anal verge is the *transitional zone*, which consists of modified skin that has sebaceous glands without hair. It extends to the pectinate line defined by the free edges of the anal valves. Above the line begins the *true mucosa of the anal canal* (Fig. 12.10).

The pectinate line is formed by the margins of the anal valves—small mucosal pockets between the five and ten vertical folds of the mucosa known as the anal columns of Morgagni. An anal pit or sinus is located above each valve, draining the

[1] Shafik A. A new concept of the anatomy of the anal sphincter mechanism and the physiology of defecation. The external anal sphincter: a triple-loop system. Invest Urol. 1975;12(5):412–9.

Table 12.1 The pectinate line and changes in the surgical anal canal

	Below the pectinate line	Above the pectinate line
Embryonic origin	Ectoderm	Endoderm
Anatomy		
Lining	Stratified squamous	Simple columnar
Arterial supply	Inferior rectal artery	Superior rectal artery
Venous drainage	Systemic, by way of inferior rectal vein	Portal, by way of superior rectal vein
Lymphatic drainage	To inguinal nodes	To pelvic and lumbar nodes
Nerve supply	Inferior rectal nerves (somatic)	Autonomic fibers (visceral)
Physiology	Excellent sensation	Sensation quickly diminishes
Pathology		
Cancer	Squamous cell carcinoma	Adenocarcinoma
Varices	External hemorrhoids	Internal hemorrhoids

By permission of JE Skandalakis, SW Gray, and JR Rowe. *Anatomical Complications in General Surgery*. New York: McGraw-Hill, 1983

anal glands. These columns extend upward from the pectinate line to the upper end of the surgical anal canal, at the level of the puborectalis sling. They are formed by underlying parallel bundles of the muscularis mucosae. The actual junction of stratified squamous and columnar epithelia is usually just above the pectinate line; hence, the mucocutaneous line is not precisely equivalent to the pectinate line.

The pectinate line is the most important landmark in the anal canal. It marks the transition between the visceral area above and the somatic area below. The arterial supply, the venous and lymphatic drainage, the nerve supply, and the character of the lining all change at or very near the pectinate line (Table 12.1).

Peritoneal Reflections

The entire upper one-third of the rectum is covered by peritoneum (Fig. 12.5). The peritoneum leaves the rectum and passes anteriorly and superiorly over the posterior vaginal fornix and the uterus in females or over the superior ends of the seminal vesicles and the bladder in males. This creates a depression, the rectouterine or rectovesical pouch.

Fascial Relations and Tissue Spaces

Shafik recognized six potential spaces around the rectum. They are important because they may become sites of infection. Knowledge of the spaces will avert injury during surgery. The fascial layers that bound these spaces help limit the spread of both infection and neoplastic disease, although all the spaces are potentially confluent with one another (Figs. 12.7 and 12.11).

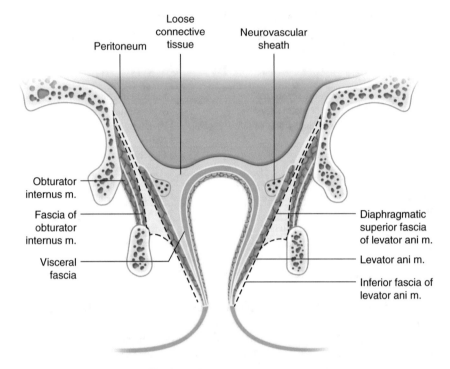

Fig. 12.11 Diagram of some of the fasciae of the pelvis seen in coronal section

The perianal space surrounds the anal canal along the anal verge and is surrounded laterally by fat. The perianal space connects to the superficial postal space, which is the space located below the anococcygeal ligament. The perianal space also communicates with the intersphincteric space, which is located between the anal sphincters. The intersphincteric space contains most of the anal glands. The ischiorectal space is lateral to the perianal space and contains the pudendal nerves and vessels. The apex of the ischiorectal space is formed by the levator and obturator muscles. The ischiorectal space is bound anteriorly by the transverse perineal muscles and bound posteriorly by the gluteal skin. Posteriorly, the ischiorectal space communicates with the deep postanal space, deep to the anococcygeal ligament. An infection communicating in this space is the horseshoe abscess.

Pelvic Diaphragm and Continence

The floor of the pelvis is the pelvic diaphragm (Fig. 12.12), which is composed of two paired muscles: the levator ani and the coccygeus. The levator ani can be considered to be made up of three muscles: the iliococcygeus, the pubococcygeus, and the puborectalis.

The puborectalis, the superficial and deep parts of the external sphincter, and the proximal part of the internal sphincter form the so-called anorectal ring. This

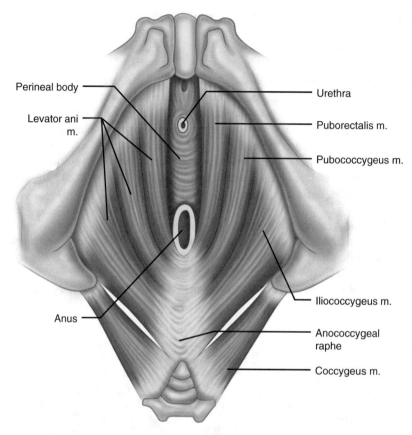

Fig. 12.12 Diagram of the pelvic diaphragm from below. Note that the levator ani is composed of three muscles: puborectalis, pubococcygeus, and iliococcygeus. Some authors would exclude the puborectalis from the levator ani

ring can be palpated; since cutting through it will produce incontinence, it must be identified and protected during surgical procedures. The puborectalis is essential to maintaining rectal continence and is considered by some authors to be part of the external sphincter and not a part of the levator ani. The puborectalis is attached to the lower back surface of the symphysis pubis and the superior layer of the deep perineal pouch (urogenital diaphragm). Fibers from each side of the muscle pass posteriorly and then join posterior to the rectum, forming a well-defined sling (Fig. 12.12). The puborectalis passes adjacent to the vagina where it attaches laterally and is known as the pubovaginalis, supporting the rectum and vagina. It also supports the bladder and the urethra, pulling these anteriorly with contractions. When the puborectalis is lax, the levator sags, the anorectal angle becomes obtuse, and the pelvic floor muscles can relax. Over time, the pelvic floor weakens; a change that can lead to pelvic organ prolapse and incontinence.

Vascular System of the Colon and Rectum

Arteries of the Colon

Superior Mesenteric Artery
The cecum and the ascending colon receive blood from two arterial branches of the superior mesenteric artery: the ileocolic and right colic arteries (Fig. 12.13). These arteries form arcades from which vasa recta pass to the medial colonic wall.

As the vasa recta reach the surface of the colon, they divide into short and long branches, the former serving the medial or mesenteric side of the colon and the latter serving the lateral and antimesenteric side. The long branches send twigs into the epiploic appendages (see Fig. 12.6).

Middle Colic Artery
The transverse colon is similarly supplied by the middle colic artery from the superior mesenteric artery. A study found that in about one-third of cases the splenic flexure was supplied by the middle colic artery; in the remainder, the flexure and the left portion of the transverse colon were supplied by the left colic artery, a branch of the inferior mesenteric artery.

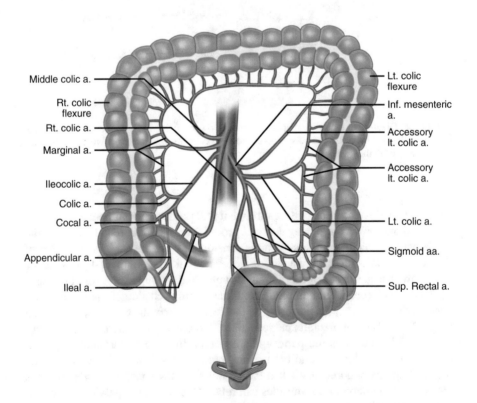

Fig. 12.13 Schema of the blood supply to the large intestine

Inferior Mesenteric Artery

The inferior mesenteric artery arises from the aorta opposite the lower portion of the third lumbar vertebra. The length of the artery prior to its first branch varies from 1.5 to 9.0 cm.

The branches of the inferior mesenteric artery are the left colic artery, with its ascending and descending branches for the descending colon, one to nine sigmoid arteries for the sigmoid colon, and the superior rectal (hemorrhoidal) artery for the rectum (Figs. 12.13 and 12.14c). An accessory middle colic artery is present in roughly 40% of subjects.

Division of the inferior mesenteric artery close to its root has been shown to increase the reach of the colon to the pelvis after proctectomy, leading to less tension on the colorectal or coloanal anastomosis.

Marginal Artery (of Drummond)

The marginal artery is composed of a series of anastomosing arcades between branches of the ileocolic, right colic, middle colic, left colic, and sigmoidal arteries. These form a single, looping vessel. The marginal artery courses roughly parallel with the mesenteric border of the large intestine, from 1 to 8 cm from the intestinal wall (Fig. 12.14a–c). It may or may not terminate at the superior rectal artery (Fig. 12.14c). Occasionally, however, the continuity of this artery is disrupted in one or more points.

Arteries of the Rectum and Anal Canal

The arteries of the rectum and anal canal are the unpaired superior rectal artery, the paired middle and inferior rectal arteries, and median sacral rectal arteries (Fig. 12.15). The superior rectal (hemorrhoidal) artery arises from the inferior mesenteric artery and descends to the posterior wall of the upper rectum. Supplying the posterior wall, it divides and sends right and left branches to the lateral walls of the middle portion of the rectum down to the pectinate (dentate) line.

One study has found that the main trunk of the middle rectal artery was inferior to the rectal stalk and could be endangered when the rectum is separated from the seminal vesicle, prostate, or vagina. In our experience, the middle rectal artery is usually absent in the female. It is probably replaced by the uterine artery. In the male, the chief beneficiaries of the artery are the rectal musculature and the prostate gland.

The inferior rectal (hemorrhoidal) arteries arise from the internal pudendal arteries and proceed ventrally and medially to supply the anal canal distal to the pectinate line.

The median sacral artery arises just above the bifurcation of the aorta and descends beneath the peritoneum on the anterior surface of the lower lumbar vertebrae, the sacrum, and the coccyx. It sends several very small branches to the posterior wall of the rectum.

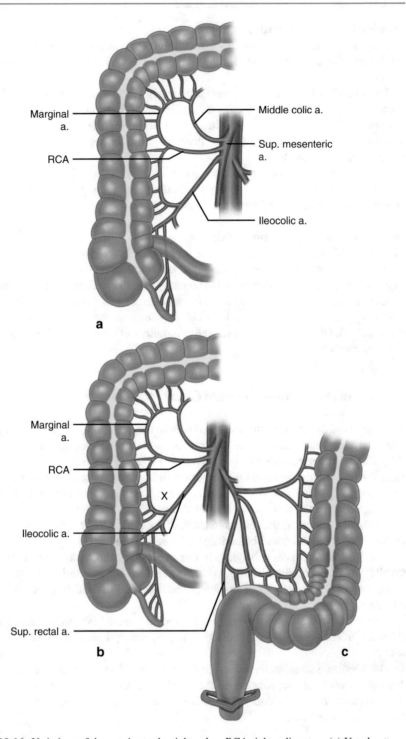

Fig. 12.14 Variations of the arteries to the right colon. RCA right colic artery (**a**) Usual pattern. (**b**) The marginal artery is incomplete at "X." (**c**) Arteries to the left colon. There may be fewer sigmoid arteries than shown here

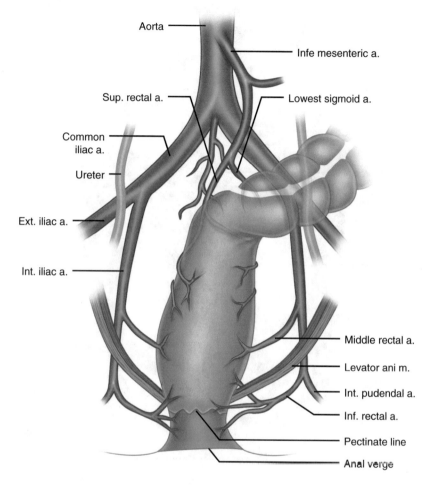

Fig. 12.15 Diagram of the arterial supply to the rectum and anus. The median sacral artery supplying a few small branches to the posterior wall of the rectum is not shown in this figure

Venous Drainage of the Colon, Rectum, and Anus

The veins of the colon follow the arteries. On the right, the veins join to form the superior mesenteric vein. The superior rectal vein drains the descending and sigmoid colon; it passes upward to form the inferior mesenteric veins.

The rectum is drained by the superior rectal veins, which enter the inferior mesenteric veins. This drainage is to the portal system. The middle and inferior rectal veins enter the internal iliac vein and thus drain into the systemic circulation (Fig. 12.16).

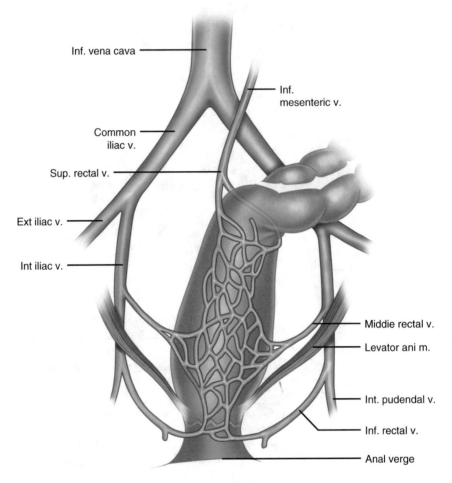

Fig. 12.16 Diagram of the venous drainage of the rectum and anus. The superior rectal vein drains to the portal system, and the middle and inferior rectal veins drain to the systemic veins. The venous plexus between the veins forms a portacaval shunt

Remember:
- Anastomoses occur between the superior rectal vein (portal) and the middle and inferior rectal veins (systemic), constituting a potential portosystemic shunt.

Lymphatic Drainage of the Colon

The lymph nodes of the large intestine have been divided into four groups: epicolic, under the serosa of the wall of the intestine; paracolic, on the marginal artery;

intermediate, along the large arteries (superior and inferior mesenteric arteries); and principal, at the root of the superior and inferior mesenteric arteries (Fig. 12.17). This last group includes mesenteric root nodes (which also receive lymph from the small intestine), aortic nodes, and left lumbar nodes.

Wide resection of the colon should include the entire segment supplied by a major artery. This also will remove most, but not all, of the lymphatic drainage of the segment depending on the level of vascular ligation (Fig. 12.18). A complete mesocolic excision (CME) does maximize the amount of lymphatic tissue that can be removed en bloc with this specimen. A CME involves dissection between the mesenteric plane and the parietal fascia and removal of the mesentery within a complete envelope of fascia and visceral peritoneum that contain all lymph nodes draining the tumor area, combined with a central vascular ligation.

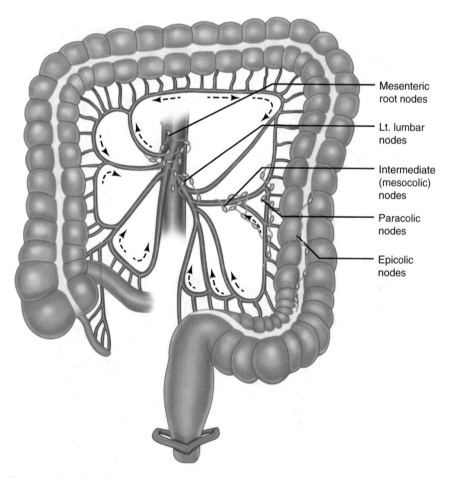

Mesenteric root nodes

Lt. lumbar nodes

Intermediate (mesocolic) nodes

Paracolic nodes

Epicolic nodes

Fig. 12.17 The lymphatics of the colon follow the arteries and drain to the principal nodes at the root of the mesentery. The path is by way of the epiploic, paracolic, and mesocolic lymph nodes

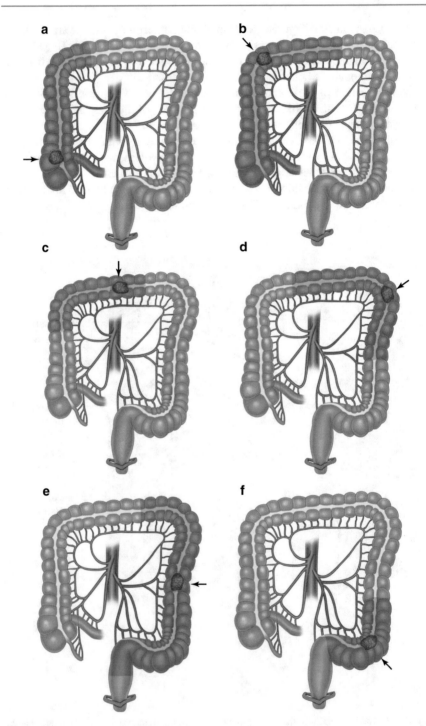

Fig. 12.18 Resection of the colon should include the entire area served by a major artery as well as the lesion itself. Most of the lymphatic drainage will be included. Areas of resection (*shaded*) for lesions in various segments of the colon are shown in (**a–f**). An *arrow* indicates the site of the lesion

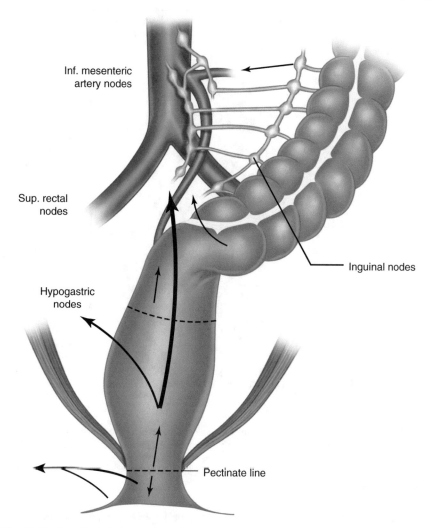

Fig. 12.19 Lymphatic drainage of the sigmoid colon, rectum, and anus. Above the pectinate line, drainage is to the inferior mesenteric nodes. Below the line, drainage is to the inguinal nodes

Lymphatic Drainage of the Rectum and Anal Canal

The lymph channels of the rectum and anal canal form two extramural plexuses, one above and one below the pectinate line. The upper plexus drains through the posterior rectal nodes to a chain of nodes along the superior rectal artery to the pelvic nodes (Fig. 12.19). Some drainage follows the middle and inferior rectal arteries to the hypogastric nodes. Below the pectinate line, the plexus drains to the inguinal nodes.

The "watershed" of the extramural lymphatic vessels is at the pectinate line. The watershed for the intramural lymphatics is higher, at the level of the middle rectal

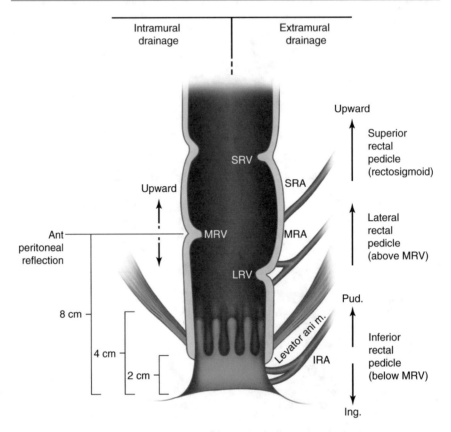

Fig. 12.20 Diagram of lymph drainage of the anus and rectum. The watershed for extramural drainage is at the pectinate line (Fig. 12.19). The watershed for intramural drainage is at the level of the middle rectal valve, about 8 cm above the anal verge. *IRA* inferior rectal artery, *MRA* middle rectal artery, *SRA* superior rectal artery, *LRV* lower rectal valve, *MRV* middle rectal valve, *SRV* superior rectal valve

valve (Fig. 12.20). These two landmarks may be kept in mind by the mnemonic "two, four, eight," meaning:

- 2 cm = anal verge to pectinate line
- 4 cm = surgical anal canal (above and below the pectinate line)
- 8 cm = anal verge to middle rectal valve

Downward spread of lesions of the rectum is rare; perhaps only 2% may spread downward. A margin of 2–3 cm distal to the tumor should be allowed in anterior resection.

Nerve Supply of the Rectum and Anus

Motor innervation of the internal rectal sphincter is supplied by sympathetic fibers that cause contraction and by parasympathetic fibers that inhibit contraction. The parasympathetic fibers are carried by pelvic splanchnic nerves which also convey the afferent nerve fibers that mediate the sensation of rectal distention. The external rectal sphincter is innervated by the inferior rectal branch of the internal pudendal nerve and by the perineal branch of the fourth sacral nerve.

The pelvic splanchnic nerves (parasympathetic and sensory) and the hypogastric nerve (sympathetic) supply the lower rectal wall. These two sources together form the rectal plexus. The levator ani muscles are supplied by the nerve to the levator ani, usually a branch from S4, with variant contributions from S3 and S5.

The inferior rectal branches of the internal pudendal nerve follow the inferior rectal arteries and supply the sensory innervation of the perianal skin.

> **Remember:**
> - The pudendal nerve innervates the external sphincter and possibly the puborectalis muscle. The sympathetic nerves have no influence on the muscular wall of the rectum. Evacuation is accomplished by the pelvic splanchnic nerves; continence is maintained by the pudendal and the pelvic splanchnic nerves.

Technique

Decalogue of Good Colon Surgery

1. Mechanical bowel preparation with oral antibiotics.
2. Administer intravenous antibiotics within 1 h of making your incision. Antibiotics no longer need to be continued for 24 h after.
3. Use orogastric/nasogastric tube only when necessary and remove as soon as possible. Remove Foley catheters on post-op day 1 unless contraindicated.
4. Understand anatomy of blood supply and lymphatics. When performing cancer surgery, ligate vessels at their origins. Consider complete mesocolic excision (CME) for advanced right sided colon cancers and total mesocolic excisions (TME) for rectal cancer.
5. Good technique for performing anastomosis includes:
   (a) Observing whether the cut edges of the intestinal segments to be anastomosed have good texture and color and are bleeding. Avoid formation of hematomata at the anastomotic area. Test the vascular supply with ICG.
   (b) Clearing all fatty tissue from the anastomotic area by removing, without traction, the mesenteric border and the epiploic appendages.
   (c) Leak testing all left sided, sigmoid, and rectal anastomoses.
6. Avoid tension on the anastomosis.
7. Use a headlight and adequate exposure.
8. Be familiar with all surgical procedures and their modifications.
9. Identify the ureters, iliac vasculature, and pelvic nerves to avoid injury.
10. Reapproximate the mesentery to avoid internal hernias if the defect is small. If the defect is large, it is OK to leave them open.

Colostomy

Loop Colostomy

A loop colostomy (Fig. 12.21) is feasible only in the transverse or sigmoid colon because a long mesentery is required. If the transverse mesocolon is short, mobilization of the hepatic and splenic flexures will provide a more mobile loop.

Sigmoid loop colostomy is, for practical purposes, left colon colostomy. The stoma should be located at the junction of the descending and the sigmoid colon so that the peritoneal fixation of the descending colon will protect the proximal stoma from prolapse.

Loop Transverse Colostomy
- **Step 1.** Make a 4- to 6-cm transverse incision at the right, or occasionally left, lateral border of the rectus abdominis muscle (Fig. 12.22).
- **Step 2.** Divide the anterior rectus sheath, rectus abdominis muscle, and posterior sheath.
- **Step 3.** Deliver the transverse colon into the wound outside the peritoneal cavity and form a small hole at the omentum and the mesenteric border of the colon to permit the entrance of a plastic rod (Fig. 12.23).
- **Step 4.** Open the colon as shown and mature to the skin with 3–0 Vicryl sutures (Figs. 12.24 and 12.25).

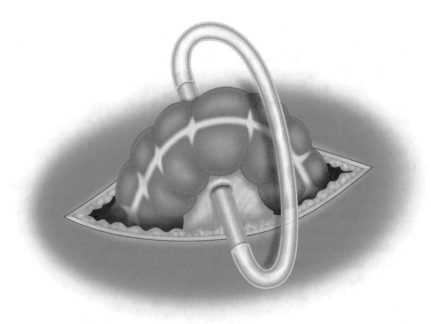

Fig. 12.21 Loop colostomy. The loop of colon has been brought through the incision, held in place by a glass tube with rubber tubing connecting its ends

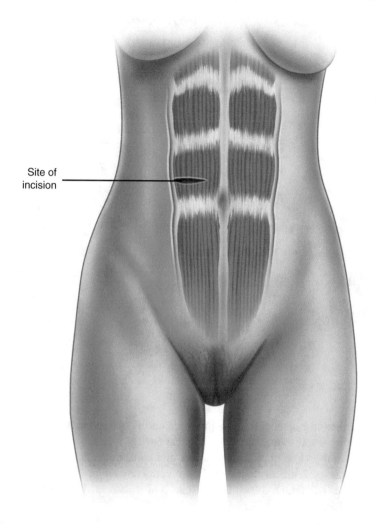

Site of incision

Fig. 12.22 Transverse incision

End Colostomy

The stoma is located along the lower descending colon or along the upper sigmoid colon. Preoperative marking for stoma sites is of utmost importance as it will decrease the number of complications due to poor placement (dermatitis, poor pouching, hernias). Good mobilization of the colon is essential, especially when the stoma is at the lower descending colon or at the iliac part of the sigmoid colon. The mesenteric root should be incised very carefully to avoid bleeding, which would jeopardize the vitality of the bowel. The procedures of end colostomy are the same

Loop of bowel

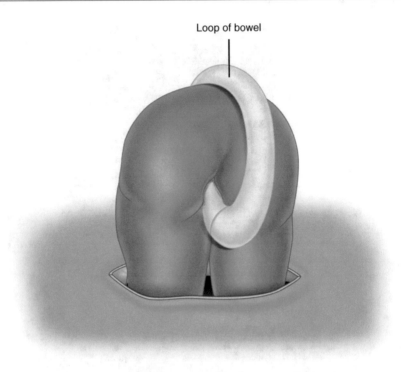

Fig. 12.23 Colon loop

as in left colectomy, except that the proximal end is secured to a skin opening and the distal loop is reinserted into the peritoneal cavity.

- **Step 1.** In the vicinity of the left lower quadrant, excise a round piece of skin approximately 2 cm in diameter. Use electrocoagulation for the division and separation of fat. Expose the fascia and make a longitudinal incision (Fig. 12.26a–d).
- **Step 2.** Separate the rectus muscle fibers longitudinally and expose the peritoneum as in appendectomy (Fig. 12.26e). Direct two fingers from the original incision to the new, round one (Fig. 12.27). Open the peritoneum and insert a Babcock clamp through the skin opening into the peritoneal cavity, and grasp the proximal end of the colon. Gently manipulate the end through the skin. The authors prefer a length of 4–5 cm of proximal colon to hang outside the skin.
- **Step 3.** The full thickness of the colonic wall is sutured with 4–0 Vicryl absorbable sutures to the seromuscular wall and then to the edges of the skin. The tip of the stoma should be located about 1 cm above the skin level to allow for ease of pouching.

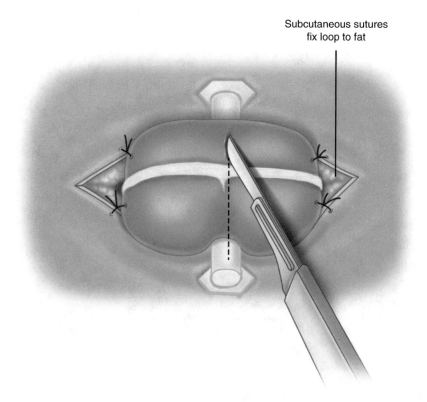

Fig. 12.24 Fixation sutures

Prasad End Loop Colostomy

- **Step 1.** Prior to surgery, place a mark for the stoma close to the obstruction (Fig. 12.28). Note where the patient wears his/her waistband. Avoid folds of fat. Have the patient sit upright to ensure appropriate marking.
- **Step 2.** Using a GIA stapler, perform a typical segmental colectomy appropriate to the disease.
- **Step 3.** Bring the proximal end of the colon through the abdominal wall. Then deliver the antimesenteric corner of the distal colonic staple line through the skin incision (Fig. 12.29).
- **Step 4.** Mature the proximal colon by removing the staple line and suturing the edges to the seromuscular wall and then to the edges of the skin using 4–0 Vicryl absorbable sutures. The tip of the stoma should be located about 1 cm above the

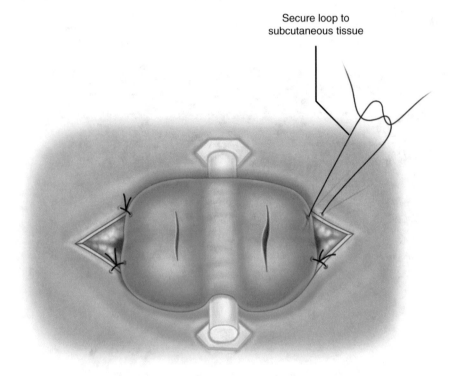

Fig. 12.25 The loop transverse colostomy

skin level to allow for ease of pouching. The distal colon is then matured by removing the stapled corner and fixing it to the proximal colon and to the skin (Figs. 12.30 and 12.31). This allows for distal colonic decompression.

Colon Resection

Figure 12.18 shows the extent of colectomy recommended for cancer at various sites in the colon.

Preoperative Preparation

- Colonoscopy and biopsy, complete oncologic staging as appropriate.
- Mark lesion submucosally with India ink.
- Consider ureteral stent placement, especially if the patient has had prior surgeries, inflammation, or radiation.

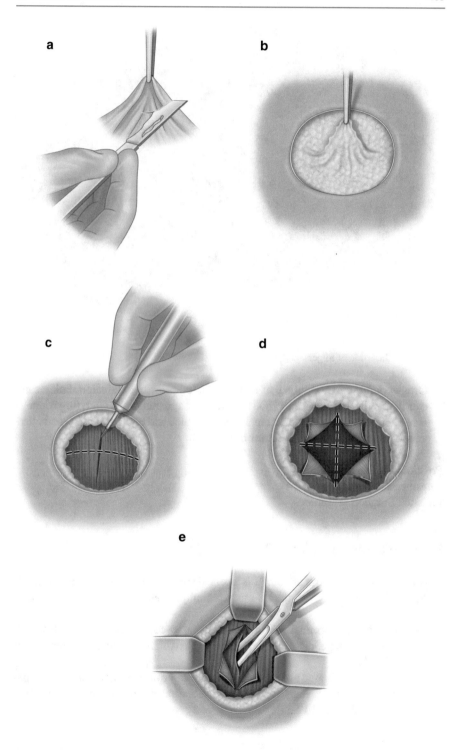

Fig. 12.26 (**a**) Excision, (**b**) separation of fat, (**c**) division of muscles, (**d**) exposure, and (**e**) opening

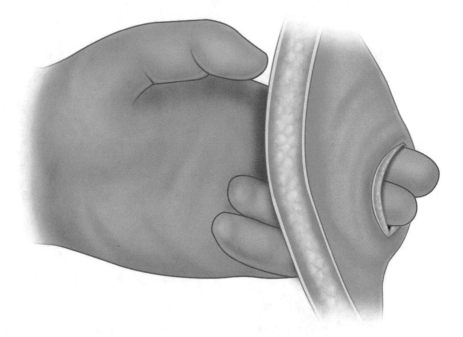

Fig. 12.27 Insertion of fingers

- Orogastric/nasogastric tube that is discontinued prior to extubation, Foley catheter that is discontinued on POD#1, warming elements in the operating room.
- Bowel preparation with mechanical prep of choice and oral antibiotics, and intravenous antibiotics within 1 h prior to incision.

Position: Supine or lithotomy
Anesthesia: General
Incision: Surgeon preference

Right Colectomy (Fig. 12.18a)

- **Step 1.** As soon as the abdomen is open, decide whether to use the routine or no-touch technique. With the no-touch technique that we prefer, we proceed as follows:
  - (a) Lumina of terminal ileum and transverse colon can be occluded with umbilical tape or atraumatic clamps proximal and distal to the tumor (Fig. 12.32).
  - (b) Vessels are ligated at their origin (at the superior mesenteric artery or superior mesenteric vein) for complete isolation of the lymphovascular tree (Figs. 12.32 and 12.33).

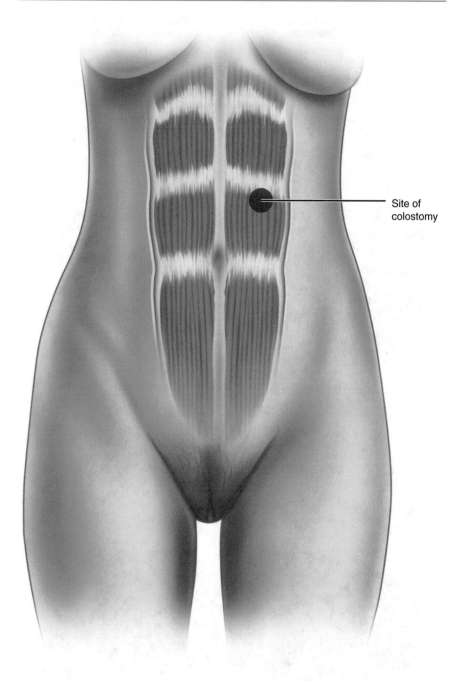

Fig. 12.28 Stoma site

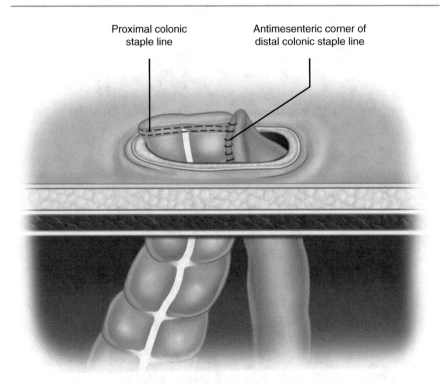

Proximal colonic
staple line

Antimesenteric corner of
distal colonic staple line

Fig. 12.29 Delivering the divided colon

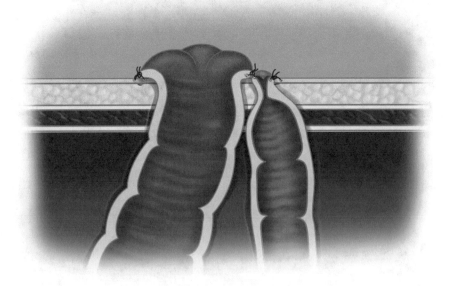

Fig. 12.30 Relation of stoma to skin level

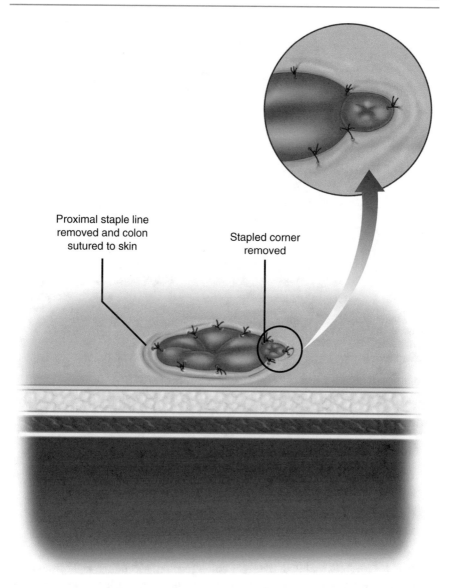

Fig. 12.31 The matured stoma. *Inset*: Fixation of distal colon

Proximal staple line
removed and colon
sutured to skin

Stapled corner
removed

- **Step 2.** Explore the peritoneal cavity looking for metastatic disease, saving until last the vicinity of pathology, i.e., the cecum, ascending colon, or right transverse colon.
- **Step 3.** Make a very superficial incision at the mesentery indicating the line of resection, which should be lateral to the umbilical tape ligatures (Figs. 12.32 and 12.33).

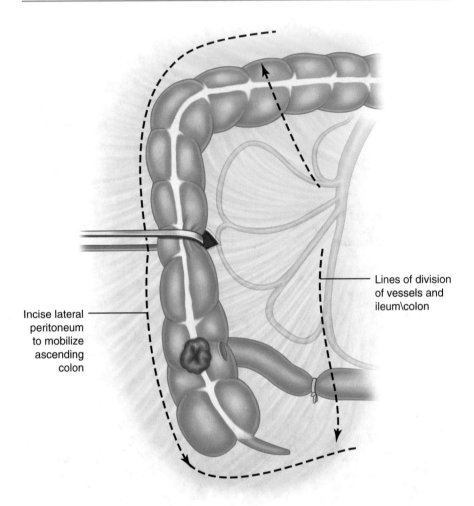

Fig. 12.32 Lines of vascular division. Incision site

- **Step 4.** Carefully mobilize the right colon (cecum, ascending, right transverse) by incising the peritoneal reflection of the paracolic area. Elevate the colon with the index finger, protecting the duodenum, right ureter (over the right common iliac artery), gonadal vessels, and superior mesenteric vessels (Fig. 12.33).
- **Step 5.** Carry out partial omentectomy, removing the right 3/4 of the greater omentum, including the corresponding part of the gastrocolic ligament, if necessary (Fig. 12.34).
- **Step 6.** Ligate the two lymphovascular pedicles (ileocolic and middle colic), keeping in mind that occasionally the right colic artery springs directly from the superior mesenteric artery. These ligations should be done carefully to avoid injury to the superior mesenteric vessels as well as to branches of the middle colic supplying the left transverse colon.

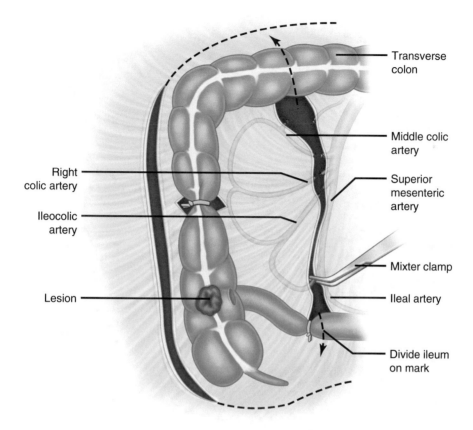

Right colic artery

Ileocolic artery

Lesion

Transverse colon

Middle colic artery

Superior mesenteric artery

Mixter clamp

Ileal artery

Divide ileum on mark

Fig. 12.33 Line of resection

> **Remember:**
> - There are several variations to the anatomy here. Ligate the vessels twice using suture ligatures or a reliable vessel-sealing source.

- **Step 7.** Be sure that both colon and ileum have a good blood supply. This can be confirmed using ICG. We prefer a side-to-side ileotransverse anastomosis using the stapling device. This is done as follows:
  - (a)   Division of the ileum by GIA stapler (Fig. 12.35).
  - (b)   Division of the colon by GIA stapler (Fig. 12.35).
  - (c)   Align colon and ileum side by side with their antimesenteric edges adjacent to each other (Fig. 12.36).

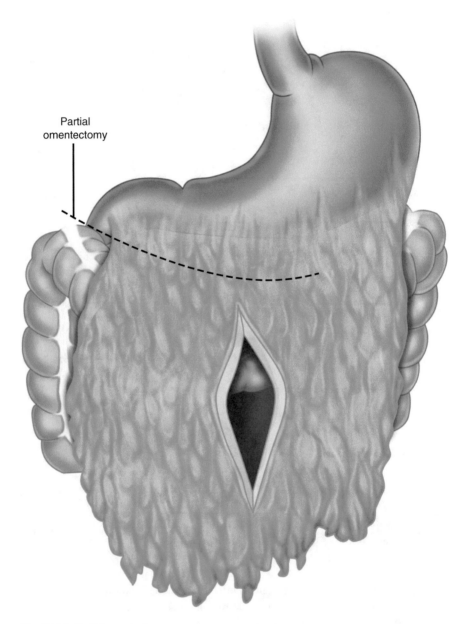

Fig. 12.34 Partial omentectomy

(d) Partial excision of the antimesenteric corner of the stapled ileal and colonic edges.

(e) At the defect, insert the two parts of the GIA stapler, one into the ileal lumen and the other into the colonic lumen. Be sure that the ends of the two parts are at the same point. Fire the instrument. Remove the GIA stapler, inspect the lumina for bleeding, and use the TA stapler to close the triangular areas (Fig. 12.37). The authors like to reinforce the staple line with a few interrupted Lembert sutures.

Note
- Alternatively, a two-layer end-to-end anastomosis can be done using a running 3–0 Vicryl for the mucosal layer and interrupted 3–0 silk Lembert sutures for the seromuscular layer (Fig. 12.38).

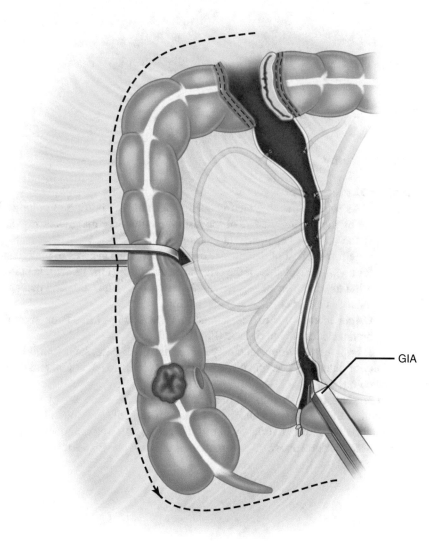

GIA

Fig. 12.35 Colon and ileum divided

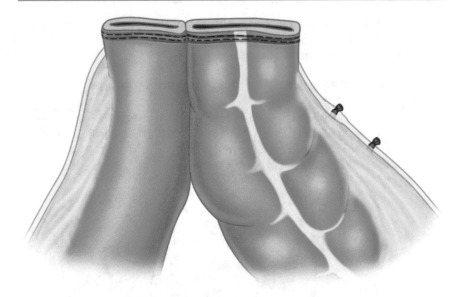

Fig. 12.36 Alignment of colon and ileum

Left Colectomy

Medial to Lateral Approach
- **Step 1.** As soon as the abdomen is open, determine the portion of colon to be removed by identifying the site of the lesion. Evaluate for margins of resection. Identify the vessels to be ligated at their origin:
    - (a) Origin at the root of the inferior mesenteric vessels in cases of malignancy, for complete isolation of the lymphovascular tree (Fig. 12.18e), keeping in mind that in males, the sympathetic nerves live in this area and damage to them can effect erection and ejaculation.
    - (b) Origin at the root of the left colic vessels (Fig. 12.18d) or sigmoidal branches, for benign disease (Fig. 12.18f).
- **Step 2.** Explore the peritoneal cavity for metastatic disease, saving until last the vicinity of pathology, i.e., the distal transverse colon, the left colon, and the sigmoid colon.
- **Step 3.** Retract the left colon at the ligament of Treitz. Make a very superficial incision at the mesentery indicating the line of resection to isolate the inferior mesenteric vein (found at the level of the ligament of Treitz) and artery (found anterior to the aorta above the bifurcation of the common iliac artery). Ligate the pedicles.

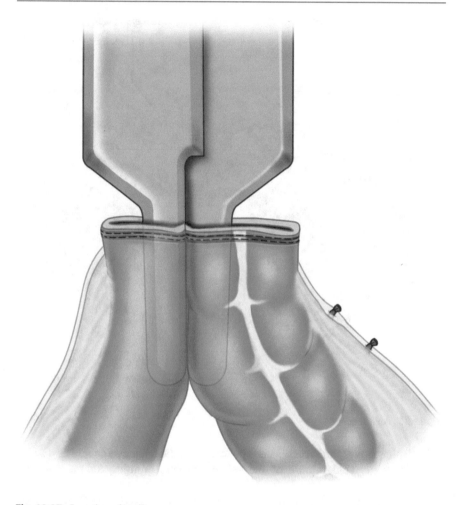

Fig. 12.37 Insertion of stapler

- **Step 4.** Carefully mobilize the left colon (distal transverse colon, descending colon, proximal sigmoid colon) by incising the peritoneal reflection of the paracolic area. Elevate the colon with the index finger, protecting the duodenum, tail of pancreas, and left ureter and gonadal vessels.
- **Step 5.** Carry out partial omentectomy, if necessary.

Many steps for this procedure are similar to the right colectomy. There are three dangerous points, from above downward (from the left upper quadrant to the pelvis):

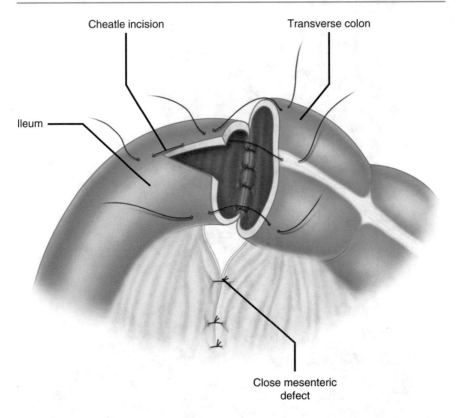

Fig. 12.38 Anastomoses

- The splenocolic, phrenicocolic, and pancreaticocolic ligaments should be divided carefully to avoid rupture of the splenic capsule or injury to the pancreas (Fig. 12.39).
- Avoid injury to the third portion of the duodenum, which almost always covers the origin of the inferior mesenteric artery and its downward continuation, the superior rectal artery. The third part of the duodenum is especially vulnerable if it is located low.
- Identify the left ureter, which may be found crossing the left common iliac vessels. Knowing its location minimizes the possibility it will be injured (Fig. 12.40).

> **Remember**
> - The reverse Trendelenburg position can be helpful to mobilize the splenic flexure.

- **Step 6.** Be sure that both ends of colon have a good blood supply. This can be confirmed using ICG angiography. We prefer a side-to-side colocolic anastomosis using the stapling device.

This is done as follows:

(a) Division of the proximal colon by GIA stapler.
(b) Division of the distal margin of colon by GIA stapler.
(c) Align the two ends of colon side by side with their antimesenteric edges adjacent to each other (Fig. 12.41).
(d) Partial excision of the antimesenteric corners of the two stapled colonic edges.
(e) At the defect, insert the two parts of the GIA stapler, one into the proximal colon lumen and the other into the distal colonic lumen. Be sure that the ends of the two parts are at the same point. Fire the instrument. Remove the GIA stapler, inspect the lumina for bleeding, and use the TA stapler to close the triangular areas. The authors like to reinforce the staple line with a few interrupted 3–0 Lembert sutures.

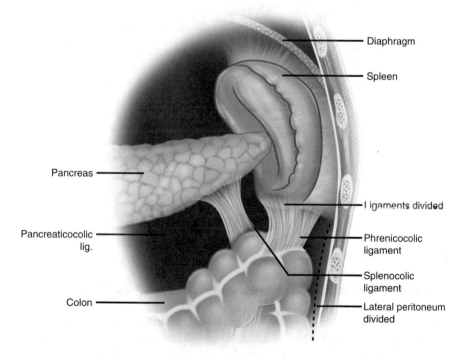

Fig. 12.39 Relation of the pancreatocolic, phrenocolic, and splenocolic ligaments to the transverse mesocolon

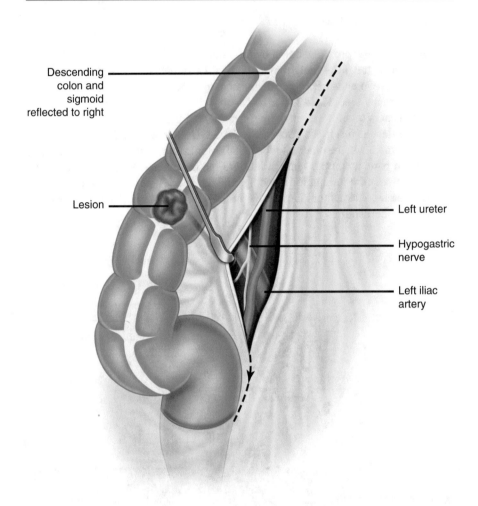

Descending colon and sigmoid reflected to right

Lesion

Left ureter

Hypogastric nerve

Left iliac artery

Fig. 12.40 Location of left ureter

Low Anterior Resection, Triple-Staple Procedure (Fig. 12.18f)

Study the previous information on left colectomy. Mobilize the splenic flexure to avoid tension on your colorectal anastomosis. Dissect under the superior rectal artery to the left colic artery and inferior mesenteric artery. Ligate the vessels (Fig. 12.42).

- **Step 1.** Mobilize the rectosigmoid colon: incise the lateral peritoneal reflection upward to the splenic flexure; incise gently downward to the sacral promontory and the presacral area. Be aware that sympathetic nerve trunks reside in this area and should be identified and preserved. Sharp dissection with electrocautery should be used. Blunt dissection by the surgeon's hand is not advisable (Fig. 12.43).

Remember

- The presacral fascia is part of the endopelvic fascia, without lymphatics, and it is not necessary to remove it (Fig. 12.43).
- Between the fascia and the presacral periosteum, a network of veins drains into the sacral foramina. To avoid bleeding and injury to the fascia, dissect very close to the posterior colonic wall; bleeding is extremely difficult to stop, even with ligation of both hypogastric arteries. Inserting tacks at the bleeding points is helpful (Fig. 12.44). Hemostatic agents can be useful. A small section of rectus muscle or adipose tissue can be excised and cauterized to the bleeding point to seal the site.
- To avoid dysfunction of the urinary bladder, as well as impotence in the male, dissect the left ureter carefully because it travels together with the left hypogastric nerve. Both are located at the posterolateral pelvic wall and hypogastric artery, and the nerve is medial to the ureter (Fig. 12.43).

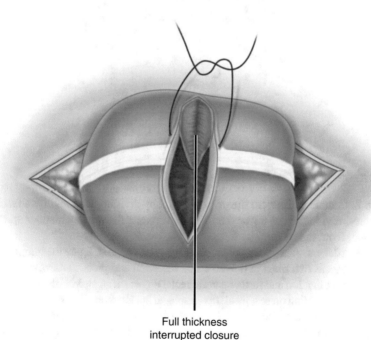

Full thickness
interrupted closure
of bowel wall

Fig. 12.41 Alignment for closure

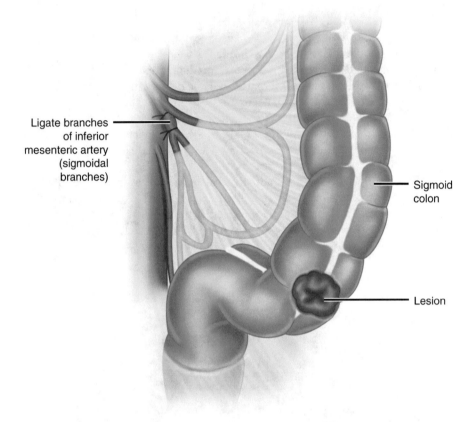

Fig. 12.42 Ligation of vessels

- **Step 2.** In males, dissect at the prostatic area by dividing Denonvilliers fascia. In females, divide the cul-de-sac and further separate the urinary bladder and vaginal wall from the rectum.
- **Step 3.** After satisfactory mobilization of the rectosigmoid, ligate the lymphovascular elements as described in the left colon resection and proceed downward for further vascular ligation and further careful rectal detachment, as described above (steps may vary depending on sex, local topographical anatomy, and obesity of the patient).
- **Step 4. Determine the level of rectal division based on the height of the tumor. A tumor in the upper rectum can be removed with a tumor-specific mesorectal excision.** Place a TA stapler at least 2 cm below the tumor and fire, thus placing a double row of staples across the rectosigmoid. Place an angled bowel clamp proximal to the staple line and divide the colon between the staple line and the bowel clamp (Fig. 12.45). Alternatively, a curved Contour stapler can be used. If the tumor is in the mid to lower rectum, a total mesorectal excision should be performed, with stapling taking placed at the anorectal junction.
- **Step 5.** Place a bowel clamp where the proximal line of excision is to be, divide the colon, and remove the specimen.

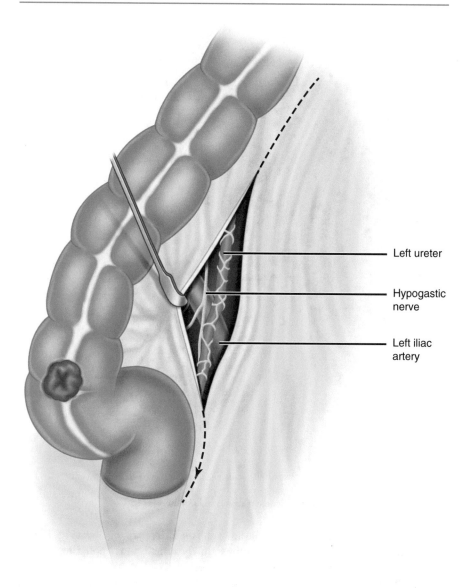

Fig. 12.43 Exposure of presacral fascia

- **Step 6.** *The triple-staple technique.* This is accomplished by inserting the anvil of the EEA into the proximal colon and then stapling the colon closed with the anvil inside (Fig. 12.46). The anvil-connecting end, which is cone shaped and sharp, can then be pushed through the line of staples.
- **Step 7.** Next insert the EEA into the rectum, and when up against the staple line, begin to turn the knob on the device so that the connector end (also sharp and cone shaped) will slide through the TA staple line (Fig. 12.47).

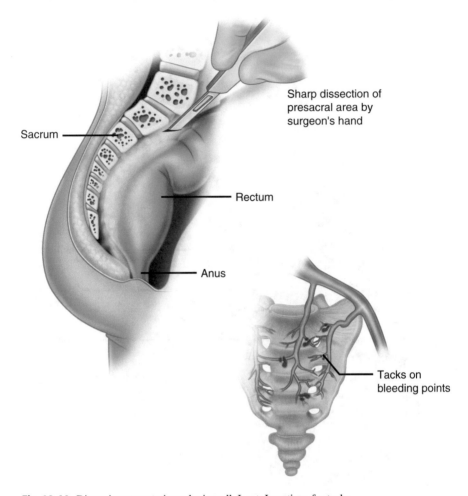

Fig. 12.44 Dissection at posterior colonic wall. Inset: Locations for tacks

- **Step 8.** Next the connectors from the anvil and the EEA snap together (Fig. 12.48). The knob at the end of the EEA is then slowly turned, thus approximating the proximal colon and distal rectum (Fig. 12.49).
- **Step 9.** When they are correctly approximated as indicated on the dial of the EEA, the device can be fired. The knob on the EEA is then opened one turn, and the EEA is then rotated gently and removed from the rectum. In cases involving cancer, send the distal donut as it represents the true distal margin.

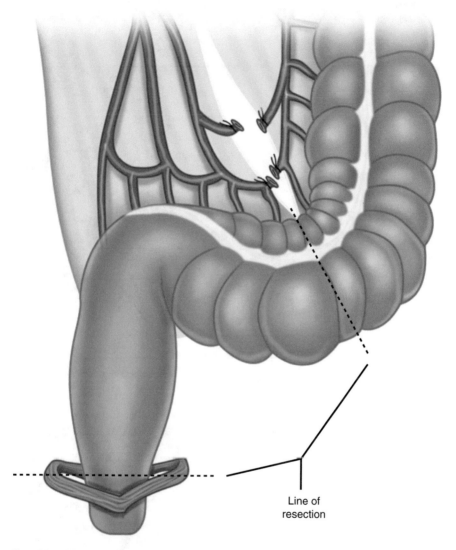

Line of
resection

Fig. 12.45 Resection sites

Note
- There should be two complete doughnuts of tissue present in the EEA indicating a satisfactory anastomosis (if the surgeon has any doubt about the anastomosis, a temporary diverting loop ileostomy can be done. One month following the surgery a low-pressure Gastrografin enema can be done, and if no leakage occurs, the ostomy can be closed).

Fig. 12.46 The triple-
staple technique:
staple line

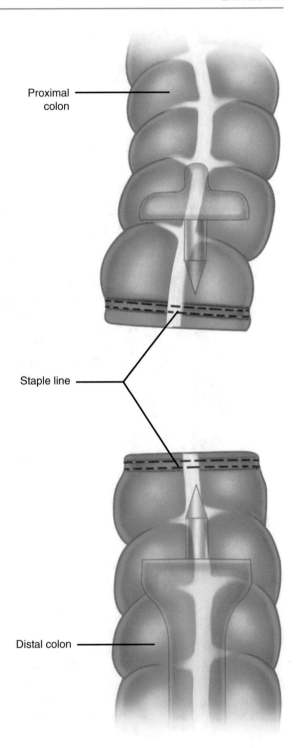

Proximal colon

Staple line

Distal colon

Fig. 12.47 Advancing
through the staple line

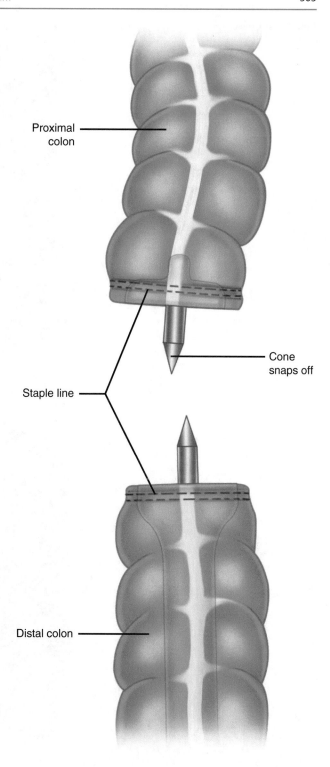

Fig. 12.48 Connectors
snap together

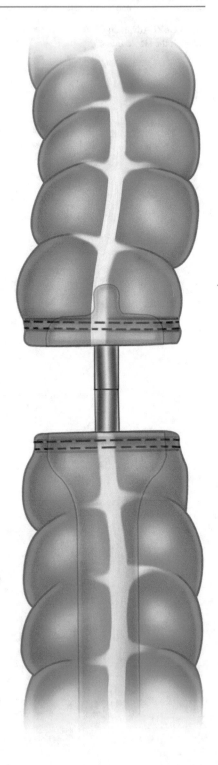

Fig. 12.49 Approximation of proximal colon and distal rectum

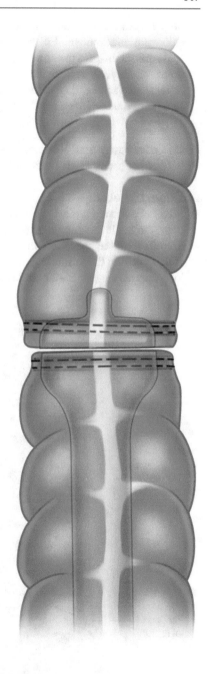

- **Step 10.** Air test the colorectal anastomosis. Occlude the bowel proximal to the colorectal anastomosis. Fill the pelvis with saline irrigation and submerge the anastomosis. Inspect the anastomosis with a rigid proctosigmoidoscope, colonoscope, or simply insufflate air via the anus until the area around the anastomosis is tense. Evacuate the saline irrigation. Placement of closed suction (e.g., Jackson–Pratt) drainage per the surgeon. Close in layers.

Total Colectomy and Ileoanal Anastomosis/Restorative Proctocolectomy with Ileoanal J-Pouch

Position: Lithotomy
- **Step 1.** Perform a typical proctocolectomy from the ileocecal junction (terminal ileum) to the levator ani level (Figs. 12.50. and 12.51).
- **Step 2.** With the specimen out of the peritoneal cavity, prepare a J-pouch construction using the terminal ileum, which may be mobilized carefully. Make the loop approximately 15–20 cm long. Approximate the parts of the loop four or

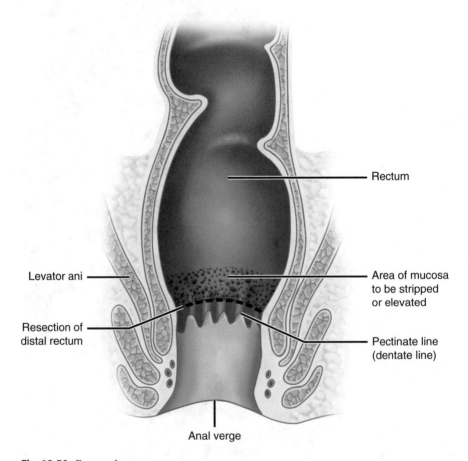

Fig. 12.50 Proctocolectomy

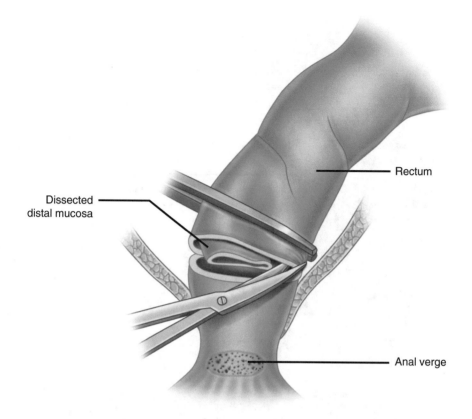

Rectum

Dissected
distal mucosa

Anal verge

Fig. 12.51 Resection site

five times using interrupted sutures. Be sure to have the distal part of the terminal ileum facing upward (Fig. 12.52).

- **Step 3.** Use the GIA stapler to anastomose both limbs, forming a common ileoileal pouch (Fig. 12.53). It will require at least three firings to obtain a pouch of adequate length.
- **Step 4.** Anastomose the apex of the pouch to the vicinity of the dentate line with deep bites of 3–0 Vicryl absorbable suture in an interrupted fashion (Fig. 12.54).
- An alternative procedure is done by performing the J-pouch and anal anastomosis using the double- or triple-staple technique, allowing the anastomosis to be performed almost at the dentate line. The EEA anvil can be placed into the J-pouch with stapling via the anus. Be sure the vagina is not incorporated into the stapler prior to firing the stapler in female patients.
- **Step 5.** Air test the ileoanal anastomosis by occluding the small bowel above the J-pouch. Despite a negative air leak test, the authors advise a diverting ileostomy to protect the anastomosis.
- **Step 6.** Two months postoperatively, a Gastrografin study should be done to check the anastomotic pouch to the last 2 cm of the rectum. If the condition is satisfactory, the ileostomy can be closed.

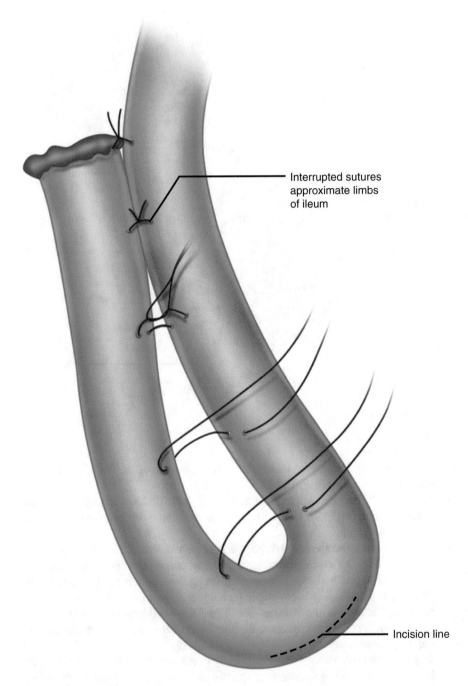

Interrupted sutures
approximate limbs
of ileum

Incision line

Fig. 12.52 J-pouch construction

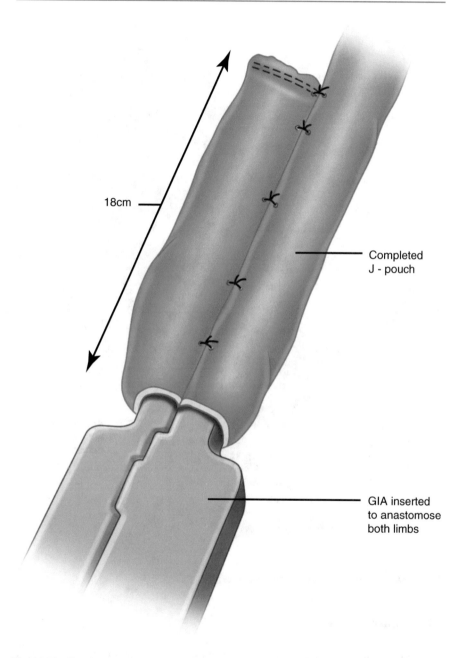

18cm

Completed
J - pouch

GIA inserted
to anastomose
both limbs

Fig. 12.53   Creating the common ileoileal pouch

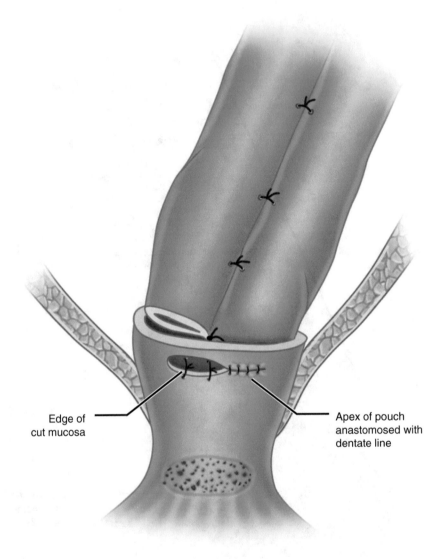

Edge of cut mucosa

Apex of pouch anastomosed with dentate line

Fig. 12.54 Anastomosis with interrupted sutures

Abdominoperineal Resection

An abdominoperineal resection includes removal of the rectum via an abdominal and perineal resection; these two procedures can be performed with two surgical teams synchronously or sequentially by a single team. When performed sequentially, it can be performed starting in the supine lithotomy position and then in the prone jackknife position, or the entire procedure, including the perineal component, can occur in the lithotomy position.

Reassess the tumor via digital rectal exam or rigid proctosigmoidoscopy if performing this surgery for cancer resection. Remember to place ureteral stents to facilitate intraoperative identification of the ureters as needed.

The *abdominal phase* of an abdominoperineal resection includes presacral dissection to mobilize the rectum, which will be removed during the perineal phase. The abdominal portion is simply a proctectomy without creation of an anastomosis and formation of a permanent end colostomy.

An abdominal exploration is first performed to evaluate for metastatic disease. The small bowel is packed into the upper abdomen.

The sigmoid colon is mobilized to the right side and down to the rectovesical or rectouterine fossa by medial and lateral incision of the peritoneal ligaments of the sigmoid colon. To allow for a tension-free colostomy creation, upward mobilization of the distal descending colon along the white line of Toldt is necessary. Mobilization of the splenic flexure is usually not necessary. The left ureter and left gonadal vessels are visualized; the inferior mesenteric artery and its downward continuation as the superior rectal artery are identified. The surgeon is ready to enter the presacral area.

Most of the bleeding is from the presacral veins which lie beneath the endopelvic fascia. As noted earlier, to avoid bleeding and injury to the fascia, dissect very close to the posterior colonic wall; bleeding is extremely difficult to stop, even with ligation of both hypogastric arteries. Inserting tacks at the bleeding points is helpful (Fig. 12.44). Hemostatic agents can be useful. A small section of rectus muscle or adipose tissue can be excised and cauterized to the bleeding point to seal the site.

Use electrocautery for the perirectal tissues and the fascia of Waldeyer, which bridges the sacrum and coccyx to the lower rectum. The St. Mark's or Thorlakson retractor is useful to complete the procedure.

The tip of the prostate, with Denonvilliers' fascia, or the tip of the uterine cervix as well as the tip of the coccyx may now be palpated; the hypogastric nerve and hypogastric (pelvic) plexus must be preserved lest there be problems with ejaculation or a neurogenic bladder.

The ureter (and the lateral ligaments of the rectum) must be traced deep into the pelvis by careful dissection without elevation. Division of the colon and formation of the colostomy may now be performed. The rectum must be mobilized completely to the levator ani muscles to make removal via the perineal dissection easier. Care must be taken to ensure the mesorectal capsule is intact for malignant cases. The rectum can be tucked down into the pelvis. A closed suction drain can be attached to the top of the rectal stump to facilitate palpation of the top of the rectum. The abdomen can be closed, and the colostomy matured.

The *perineal phase* of the abdominoperineal resection encounters the following structures: the pudendal vessels, which should be ligated; the levator sling, which should be excised widely; and the membranous urethra of the male in which a Foley catheter has been placed prior to surgery. Use sharp dissection to separate the prostate from the lower rectum. Important landmarks to use are the coccyx, ischial tuberosities, and perineal body. The rectum is removed, detaching it from the drain. The pelvic peritoneum should be closed to avoid herniation and obstruction of the small bowel. Sometimes, this may require placement of a pedicled muscular flap, such as a rectus or gracilis flap, or an omental flap. The perineum should be closed in layers.

The perineal phase is a separation of the surgical anal canal (the last 4 cm of the anorectum) from the pelvic diaphragm by dissection and sacrifice of the sphincteric apparatus and by removing the specimen and all perineal tissues related to the spaces around the anus (ischiorectal, fossae, retrorectal, etc.)

- **Step 1.** Prep the perineum, vagina, and anus. Close the anal orifice by using a subcutaneous continuous purse-string suture of 0 silk at the skin of the anal verge. Make an elliptical perianal incision approximately 3 cm from the closed anus (Fig. 12.55).
- **Step 2.** Use electrocautery or suture to ligate the inferior and middle rectal vessels and all vessels at the lateral aspect of the wound. Dissection and ligation can also be performed with a tissue sealing device (Ligasure, Enseal, Harmonic Scalpel, etc.). End the procedure with sharp dissection and remove the specimen by division of the pelvic diaphragm with cautery or knife (Figs. 12.56 and 12.57).
- **Step 3.** Remove the rectum. The drain is positioned in the pelvis. If an omental flap was brought down, it is also placed in the pelvis. Hemostasis is checked.
- **Step 4.** Approximate the right and left pelvic diaphragms with synthetic absorbable suture. The tissues are closed in layers with absorbable sutures.
- **Step 5.** Close the perineal wound in layers with Vicryl sutures. The skin may be closed with absorbable sutures.

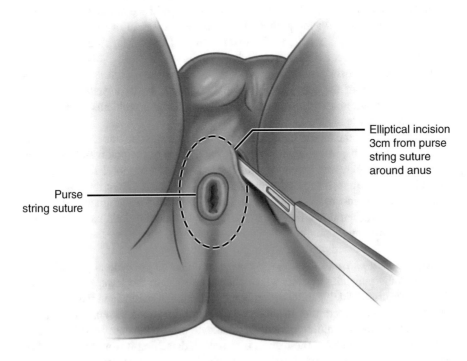

Elliptical incision 3cm from purse string suture around anus

Purse string suture

Fig. 12.55 Perianal incision

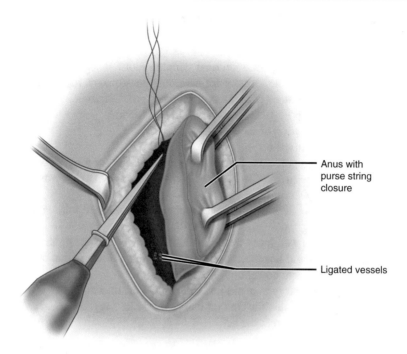

Fig. 12.56 Sharp dissection

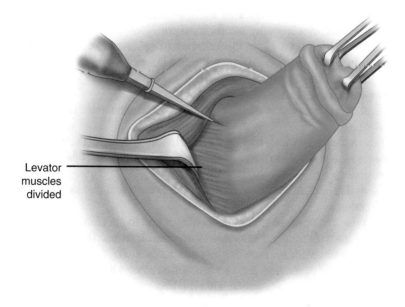

Fig. 12.57 Removal of rectum

General Principles of Laparoscopic Hand-Assisted Colectomy

- Lithotomy position
  - Provides the advantage of additional standing room
  - Provides access to the GI tract for assessing anastomosis in left-sided cases and for intraoperative colonoscopy or rigid proctosigmoidoscopy in some cases where the polyp or lesions is difficult to identify
  - Is ideal for dissection of the flexures
- GelPort/Handport insertion
  - Choose sensible port sites. A low transverse incision for a right colectomy in an obese male is an exercise in futility, while the same in a thin woman can be embarrassingly simple.
  - Use a small incision for maximal efficiency and proceed with simple open dissection.
  - Place all trocars well away from the GelPort to avoid sword fighting.
  - Instruments should be placed through trocars under direct vision or palpation to avoid inadvertent bowel injury.
  - Seat the port properly to avoid loss of pneumoperitoneum.
  - Always remember that the GelPort can be used like a regular trocar by simply placing a trocar through the gel.
- Access
  - Placing the GelPort first allows insufflation under direct vision by placing a port through the gel.
  - All other ports are placed under direct vision to avoid blind insertion and trauma.
  - In particularly elastic abdominal walls, protection can be provided by inserting the hand prior to gently inserting the port.
  - Angled laparoscopes allow identification of epigastric vessels, which helps avoid injury during port insertion. Using a 30- or 45-degree scope facilitates dissection of the flexures and any dissection in the pelvis.
  - Non-bladed trocars minimize trauma at the port site.
  - Small skin incisions allow better seating of trocars and avoid inadvertent pull-out of trocars.
  - Disposable trocars leak less than non-disposable trocars. The use of disposable trocars will help to maintain good pneumoperitoneum, which is essential.
- Dissection
  - The assistant uses both hands: one for the camera and one to assist in tissue dissection.
  - The principle of tissue triangulation allows you to maintain a broad plane of dissection with minimal trauma and maximal traction. Use extra trocars as needed to allow for best traction and countertraction.
  - The principle of traction and countertraction always applies. Traction during dissection facilitates dissection and visualization.
  - Use a tissue sealing device for grasping, division of planes, and ligation of vessels. Current tissue sealing devices can divide vessels 7 mm in diameter. Larger vessels can also be divided with an endovascular stapler.

- Make proper use of gravity. Frequent steep position changes are mandatory; this greatly improves visualization.
- Assess and reassess your plane, dissect in a broad plane, and identify important structures within the plane of dissection before moving to another site.

Laparoscopic Colectomies

Laparoscopic Left Colectomy, Sigmoid Colectomy, and Low Anterior Resection

- **Step 1.** The patient is given general anesthesia and placed in the lithotomy position. Use a Foley catheter to decompress the bladder and an orogastric or nasogastric tube to decompress the stomach (Fig. 12.58).

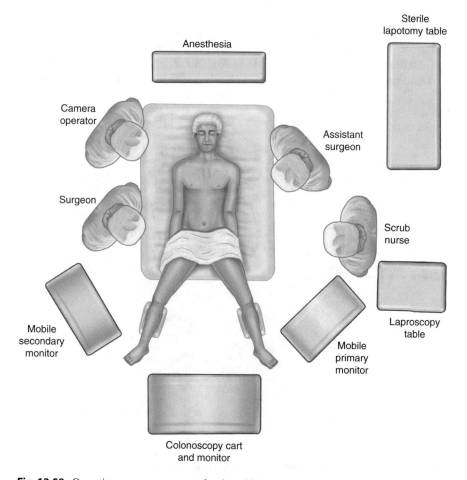

Fig. 12.58 Operating room arrangement for sigmoid resection

- **Step 2.** The surgeon begins on the patient's right. Starting this way gives the surgeon an idea concerning the anatomy of the left and sigmoid colon and redundancy of the sigmoid. This positioning also results in better placement of the trocars or the GelPort. If planning to use hand assistance, create a small incision (periumbilical, lower midline, or Pfannenstiel), and place the GelPort wound protector. This allows initial open dissection of the sigmoid colon and entry by the White line of Toldt. Depending on the patient's body habitus, a great deal of dissection can be done through this open incision, including transection of the mesocolon, lysis of adhesions, and separation of any inflammatory adhesions. Place the GelPort cover, obtain pneumoperitoneum, and place the trocars. Usually trocars are placed in the abdomen as indicated in Fig. 12.59.
- **Step 3.** The patient is in Trendelenburg and the table is rotated so that the patient's right side is down. Place graspers through the trocars to provide traction on the sigmoid colon to bring it medially and superiorly. Begin dissection lateral to the sigmoid colon along the white line of Toldt. Often the tissue sealing device is placed through the right lower quadrant port, and a grasper is placed in the right upper quadrant port to facilitate the dissection with countertraction. Grasp the rectosigmoid and retract toward the right to expose the left mesorectum. Incise the mesorectum. Continue in the left gutter along the white line of Toldt, carrying it all the way up as high as possible to the splenic flexure. This is facilitated by the surgeon placing traction on the sigmoid and left colon and dividing the avas-

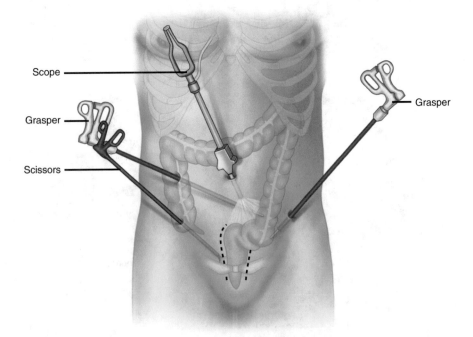

Fig. 12.59 Trocar placement for low anterior and abdominal peritoneal resection

cular plane under the peritoneum in the paracolic gutter. The assistant is in charge of both the camera and of maintaining traction of the colon cephalad for dissection along a broad plane. This allows for easy identification of the left ureter and gonadal vessels.

- The dissection can be taken up to the splenic flexure, and, if necessary, the splenic flexure can be mobilized (Figs. 12.60 and 12.61). We usually mobilize the splenic flexure to avoid tension on our colorectal or colocolic anastomosis.
- **Step 4.** Mobilize the splenic flexure. This is accomplished best with the surgeon between the patient's legs. The LLQ (or LUQ) port is used for dissection from the proximal descending colon around the splenic flexure to the distal transverse colon. The patient is still rotated right side down with leveling of the Trendelenburg from full reverse to flat. The assistant grasps the omentum and retracts it cephalad. The surgeon places gentle traction on the left colon and near the splenic

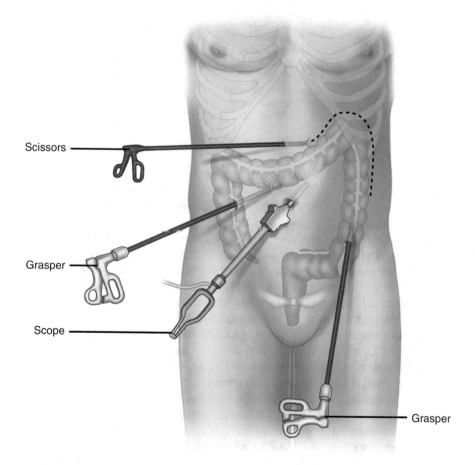

Fig. 12.60 Trocar placement for splenic flexure and left colon

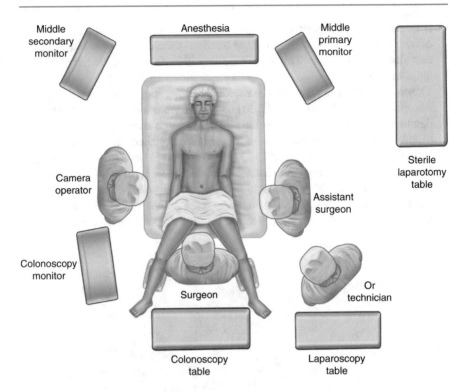

Fig. 12.61 Operating room arrangement for splenic flexure mobilization

flexure. The avascular plane between the omentum and the colon is divided over the distal transverse colon. The attachments of the colon to the spleen (splenocolic ligament) are divided carefully, avoiding the tail of the pancreas and the duodenum.

- **Step 5.** Distally, the dissection is taken down to the peritoneal reflection (for sigmoid colectomy) or to the rectum, as identified by the coalescence of the teniae. For positioning, the surgeon now stands on the patient's left. With the patient in the lithotomy position in steep Trendelenburg, the right side of the mesorectum is divided with the tissue sealing device. Dissection is facilitated by having the surgeon grasp the rectosigmoid and place traction on it toward the left, thus exposing the right mesorectum. Placement of the angled scope in the RLQ or RUQ, with the tissue sealing device in the umbilical port, should facilitate this dissection. Early dissection of the right mesorectum aids later vascular dissection and is more naturally performed from the left of the patient.

- When performing a low anterior resection, the rectal dissection as previously described should progress beyond at least 2 cm further distal than the distal edge of the tumor to allow for adequate resection margins. Attention should be given to locating the left ureter; this can be facilitated by placing ureteral stents preoperatively.

- **Step 6.** The surgeon and the assistant now move back to the same (right) side of the patient. Depending on the surgery, the stapler or tissue sealing device can be introduced through the RLQ port to divide the sigmoidal branches, the left colic vessels, or the inferior mesenteric vessels. Retract the colon laterally. If possible, use the tissue sealing device to score the mesentery of the left/sigmoid colon. Develop a window in the mesocolon and then another window either more proximally or distally. Divide the mesentery, taking care to avoid the left ureter. Repeat division of the mesentery until the segment of colon is mobilized.

- **Step 7.** Distally, divide the colon or rectum by inserting the endoscopic GIA through the right lower quadrant trocar. Once the portion of colon to be removed is freed, it can be extracted via a small abdominal incision or via the GelPort incision site. If only laparoscopic trocars were used, make an incision about 4 cm long in the abdomen to extract the colon. Use of a wound protector can help to compress the anterior abdominal wall fat and has been proven to decrease skin infections. Remove the colon through this site; transect the specimen and remove it from the field.
- **Step 8.**
  (a) For left colectomy, the colocolic anastomosis will be made with a GIA stapler extracorporeally (see "Left Colectomy" described earlier in this chapter). For sigmoid colectomy or low anterior resection, the colorectal anastomosis will be made using an EEA stapler; usually a 28- or 29-mm EEA (depending on the company) is appropriate, but the sizers should always be used to determine the appropriate diameter. Place the anvil of the EEA into the proximal colon, which is then purse-stringed around the anvil-connecting end.
  (b) For sigmoid colectomy and low anterior resection, extracorporeal colorectal anastomoses: the EEA stapler can be placed via the anus and connected to the anvil under direct vision. The anastomosis can be created once the surgeon is satisfied with the orientation of the mesentery and after ensuring all other nearby structures are protected. The colorectal anastomosis should then be air tested with the pelvis filled with saline. Fill the pelvis with saline, and insert a rigid sigmoidoscope or colonoscope into the rectum for a short distance so as to insufflate the colorectal segment and look for air bubbles, which would indicate an incomplete anastomosis. If a leaking site is discovered, there are three options. First and preferably, if there is adequate tissue in reserve, take down the anastomosis and re-do it. Second, but less optimally, suture ligate (Lembert sutures) and retest the anastomosis. Third, create a diverting ostomy and suture ligate the area of leakage. If no air leak is noted, the irrigant is removed. Hemostasis is ensured. The omentum (if still present) is laid back into anatomical position. The fascia can be then be closed.
  (c) For sigmoid colectomy and low anterior resection, intracorporeal colorectal anastomoses: with the anvil in place as described, place the proximal colon back into the abdomen; close fascia using a 0 PDS. Reinsufflate pneumoperitoneum and obtain visualization. Grasp the end of the anvil using an instrument made specifically for that purpose. Next, insert the EEA into the rectum and advance it until it is seen gently pushing up against the rectal stump. Slowly turn the knob at the end of the EEA stapler until the point that attaches to the EEA starts to "tent up" the rectal stump. Then push this sharp,

cone-shaped end of the EEA through the rectal stump just anterior to the rectal stump staple line. Manipulate the anvil until it snaps onto the EEA. Slowly turn the knob at the end of the EEA, thus approximating the proximal colon and rectum. Recheck the mesentery to ensure proper orientation. Check the vagina to ensure it is not incorporated into the stapler prior to firing. When the stapler and anvil head are correctly approximated as indicated on the EEA, fire the device. Remove the EEA from the rectum. One complete doughnut of tissue from the proximal colorectal segment and one from the distal segment should be present in the EEA stapler to indicate a satisfactory anastomosis. In the case of a low anterior resection for cancer, the distal doughnut should be sent as a separate specimen because it represents the true distal margin.

- **Step 9.** The colorectal anastomosis can then be air tested with the pelvis filled with saline as described above in step 8b. If no air leak is noted, the pneumoperitoneum is relieved. Remove all trocars under direct vision and close the fascia at each of the sites >8 mm with a 0 Vicryl suture. The extraction site can be closed with 1 PDS. Close the skin with a subcuticular suture.

Laparoscopic- and Hand-Assisted Right Colectomy

- **Step 1.** After general anesthesia, place the patient in "laparoscopic" lithotomy position and place a nasogastric or orogastric tube and Foley catheter.
- **Step 2.** Make a periumbilical incision for GelPort placement (Fig. 12.62). This allows initial open dissection of the transverse colon and entry to the lesser sac. Depending on the patient's body habitus a great deal of dissection can be done through this open incision, including transection of the mesocolon, lysis of adhesions, and separation of any inflammatory adhesions. Place trocar ports for access.
- **Step 3.** The surgeon stands on the patient's left along with the assistant.
- **Step 4.** With the patient in Trendelenburg position and left side down, the surgeon grasps the cecum and right colon retracting it toward the patient's left. The white line of Toldt is divided caudally and cephalad. Perform this dissection up to and around the hepatic flexure. If using hand assistance, the surgeon's index finger can be strategically placed underneath the lateral attachments of the colon and the hepatocolic ligament for easier dissection and traction. The assistant retracts the omentum cephalad during the hepatic flexure mobilization. The dissection proceeds from lateral to medial. During this phase, all small bowel is manipulated to the left upper quadrant. Carefully identify the ureter and gonadal vessels. This portion of the dissection is complete when the duodenum is visualized, and there is no tension of the transverse colon reaching to the GelPort opening. Continue the dissection toward the patient's lesser sac, dissecting the avascular plane between the omentum and transverse colon.

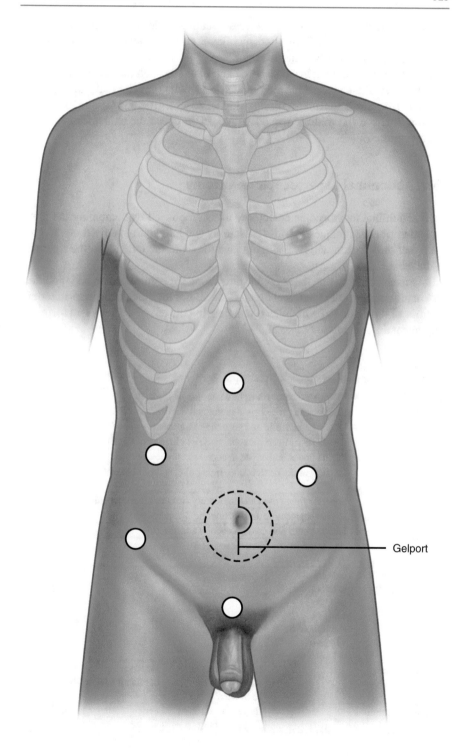

Fig. 12.62 Periumbilical incision

- **Step 5.** Ligate the vessels with the vessel sealing device or the endoscopic GIA, with vascular staples. With good mobilization, the mesocolon can be divided through the periumbilical incision.
- **Step 6.** Bring out the transverse colon and ileum through the periumbilical incision. During this phase, the GelPort acts as a wound retractor and wound protector. Perform a stapled anastomosis using an 80-mm GIA and 60-mm TA.
- **Step 7.** Close the midline wound with 1 PDS. Close the skin with subcuticular suture.

Total Abdominal Laparoscopic Colectomy

Total abdominal laparoscopic colectomy is accomplished by combining the previously described techniques for right colectomy and left/sigmoid colectomy. Keep in mind that the surgeon will be changing position from the left side to the right side of the table.

It is recommended that the surgeon starts along the sigmoid colon and mobilizes proximally, ending at the terminal ileum. This allows for the most redundant mobile portions of the colon to be mobilized first, leaving the terminal ileum and rectum to help maintain orientation (Table 12.2).

Table 12.2 Synopsis of laparoscopic colectomies

Right colectomy lateral to medial	Mobilize cecum and right white line of Toldt			
	Identify and protect right ureter and duodenum			
	Divide hepatocolic and gastrocolic ligaments			
	Divide ileocolic, right colic, and right branch of middle colic vessels			
	Divide bowel and create ileocolic anastomosis			
Right colectomy medial to lateral	Isolate and divide ileocolic, right colic, and right branch of middle colic vessels			
	Separate right colon and mesentery from retroperitoneum			
	Divide hepatocolic and gastrocolic ligaments			
	Divide bowel and create ileocolic anastomosis			
	Port location	Patient position	Surgeon position	Monitor location
Number of ports: 4 or 5	Umbilical (camera) 12 LLQ 5 LUQ or subxiphoid 5 RLQ or suprapubic 5			
Hepatic flexure mobilization		Right side elevated Reverse Trendelenburg	Between legs or patient's left	Right shoulder
Ascending colon dissection		Right side elevated Trendelenburg	Patient's left	Right hip

Table 12.2 (continued)

Left colectomy lateral to medial	Mobilize sigmoid colon and white line of Toldt
	Identify and protect left ureter, tail of pancreas, and duodenum
	Divide lienocolic and gastrocolic ligaments
	Divide inferior mesenteric vessels and left branch of middle colic vessels
	Divide bowel and create colocolic anastomosis
Left colectomy medial to lateral	Isolate and divide inferior mesenteric vessels and left branch of middle colic vessels
	Separate left colon and mesentery from retroperitoneum
	Divide lienocolic and gastrocolic ligaments
	Divide bowel and create colocolic anastomosis
Low anterior resection	Mobilize sigmoid colon and white line of Toldt
	Identify and protect left ureter, tail of pancreas, and duodenum
	Divide lienocolic and gastrocolic ligaments
	Divide inferior mesenteric vessels and left branch of middle colic vessels
	Dissect beneath superior rectal vessels behind rectum
	Divide bowel and create colorectal anastomosis

	Port location	Patient position	Surgeon position	Monitor location
Number of ports: 4 or 5	Umbilical (camera) 12 RLQ 5 RUQ or subxiphoid 5 LLQ or suprapubic 5/12			
Splenic flexure mobilization		Left side elevated Reverse Trendelenburg	Between legs or patient's right	Left shoulder
Descending colon dissection		Left side elevated Neutral	Patient's right	Left hip
Rectal dissection		Pelvis elevated Trendelenburg	Patient's right	Left hip or between legs

Procedures of the Surgical Anal Canal and Perianal Regions

No anorectal procedure should be undertaken without digital and proctoscopic examination. The following section details the anatomy as encountered by the examiner's finger or as seen in the anoscope or sigmoidoscope. Digital examination should always precede anoscopy or sigmoidoscopy. It relaxes the sphincters and reveals any obstruction that might be injured by the anoscope or sigmoidoscope.

The anal verge separates the pigmented perianal skin from the pink transition zone. The verge is the reference line for the position of all other structures encountered (Fig. 12.63).

When the gloved and lubricated index finger is inserted so that the distal interphalangeal joint is at the anal verge, the subcutaneous portion of the external

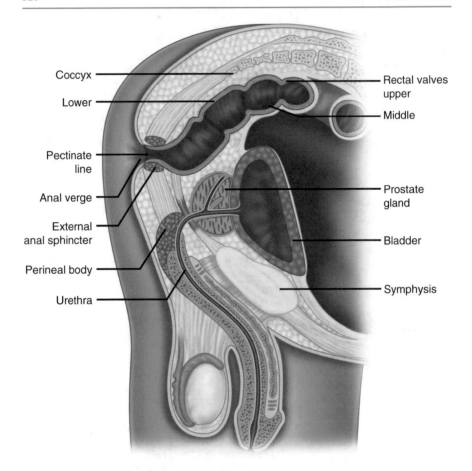

Fig. 12.63 Diagram of anorectal landmarks for sigmoidoscopic examination: patient in knee/chest or knee/elbow position

(voluntary) sphincter is felt as a tight ring around the distal half of the distal phalanx (Fig. 12.64a). The fingertip should detect the pectinate line of anal valves that lies about 2 cm above the anal verge. The anal columns (Morgagni) above the valves also may be felt. External hemorrhoids, polyps, and hypertrophied anal papillae in this region are readily detected. Good palpation of the prostate in males is paramount.

Further insertion of the finger to the level of the middle interphalangeal joint brings the first joint to the anorectal ring formed by the deep component of the external sphincter, the puborectalis loop, and the upper margin of the internal sphincter. The ring is felt posteriorly and laterally, but not anteriorly (Fig. 12.64b).

Still further penetration of the finger to the level of the metacarpophalangeal joint allows the distal phalanx to enter the rectum. The left lower rectal fold may often be touched. At this point the pelvirectal space lays lateral and the rectovesical or rectovaginal space lies anterior. Further anterior to the rectum one can palpate the prostate gland in men (Fig. 12.64c) and the upper vagina and cervix in women.

Fig. 12.64 Digital examination. (**a**) Distal interphalangeal joint at the anal verge. Hemorrhoids can be detected at this stage. (**b**) Middle interphalangeal joint at the anal verge. (**c**) Metacarpophalangeal joint at the anal verge. The tip of the finger is at or just above the inferior rectal valve

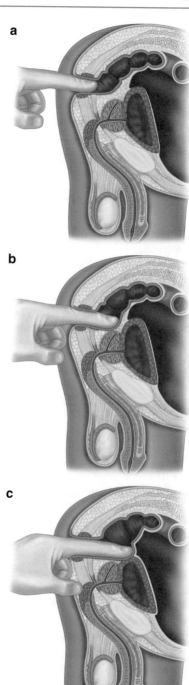

The anoscope should be inserted, aimed at the patient's umbilicus. At 5 cm from the anal verge, the tip will be at the anorectal ring (Fig. 12.65a). With the obturator removed, the left lower rectal fold might be visible. With a sigmoidoscope, at about 8 cm from the verge, the middle rectal fold may be seen. This is the level of the peritoneal reflection. The superior rectal fold is reached at 10–12 cm, and beyond this, passage of the instrument is easy (Fig. 12.65b).

For the surgeon, the most dangerous area is between the middle and superior rectal folds, just above the peritoneal reflection. This is the area in which perforation by the sigmoidoscope may occur.

Ischiorectal Abscess: Incision and Drainage

Position: Prone jackknife with buttocks retracted laterally with tape for maximal effacement.

Anesthesia: Local; in most cases, as an office procedure, particularly if a fluctuant area is palpable around the anus.

Procedure: Make an incision (elliptical or cruciate shape, extending radially and long enough to drain the cavity) as close to the anus as possible, depending, of course, on the localized maximum swelling and tenderness (Fig. 12.66). Perform intracavital digital examination to break possible septa (Fig. 12.67). Irrigate with normal saline. If used, light packing with gauze should be removed in 24 h (Fig. 12.68).

> **Remember**
> • Later, if fistulas requiring surgical treatment develop, they will be close to the anal verge and easier to treat.

Anal Fistulotomy (Figs. 12.69, 12.70, 12.71, and 12.72)

Identify the primary internal opening of the tract. Identify the relation of the tract to the anal sphincters and, in particular, to the puborectalis muscle. To maintain continence, minimize the amount of sphincter muscle to be divided.

Fistulectomy is the complete removal of the fistula tract. Fistulotomy is the laying open of the tract with the tract curetted. They are functionally equivalent, but fistulotomy is less destructive to the surrounding tissue, so it is generally preferred over fistulectomy.

Preoperative preparation: 1–2 enemas.

Position: Prone jackknife with buttocks retracted laterally with tape for maximal effacement.

Anesthesia: General, spinal, or MAC w local.

a

b

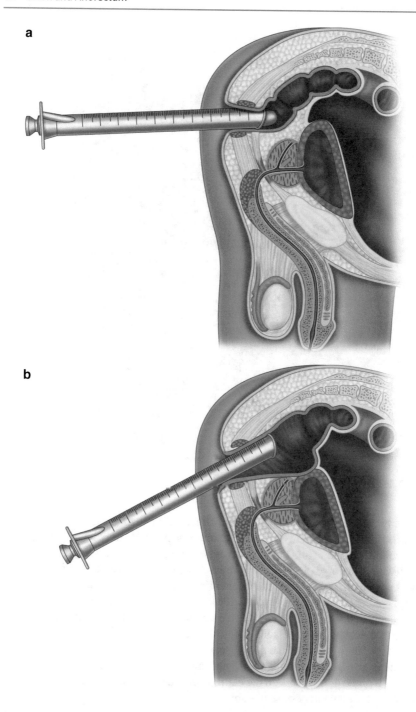

Fig. 12.65 Sigmoidoscopic examination (**a**). The instrument is directed toward the umbilicus. The tip is just past the anorectal ring (**b**). With obturator removed, the instrument is passed by direct observation. The *tip* shown here is almost up to the middle rectal valve

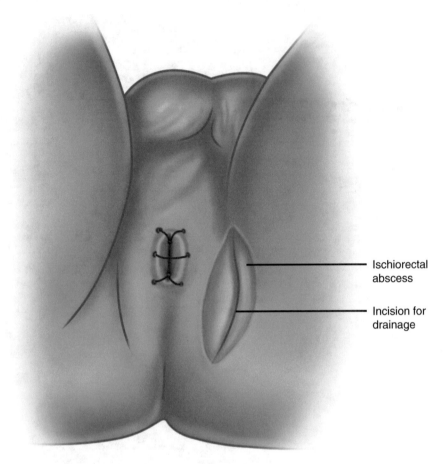

Fig. 12.66 Incision at swelling

Examination: Digital, dilatation, retractor of choice, and very careful external and internal probing. Methylene blue staining or peroxide may be of great help to localize the internal fistula opening. Avoid creating a false tract with probing while identifying the course of the primary tract. If the tract is palpable along the surface, it is likely superficial. Supralevator induration may be a sign of deeper involvement or cephalad extension of the abscess. Identify any secondary tracts or extensions.

Procedure: If the fistula is simple and not deep, excise the fistulous tract in toto, leaving the wound open. Fistulectomy involves pulling the tract and dissecting around it to "core" it out of the tissue, separating the tract out from surrounding tissue; this is particularly useful for suprasphincteric fistulas. Fistulotomy involves inserting a probe gently through the entire tract and cutting the tissue "roof" over the tract using electrocautery or scalpel blade.

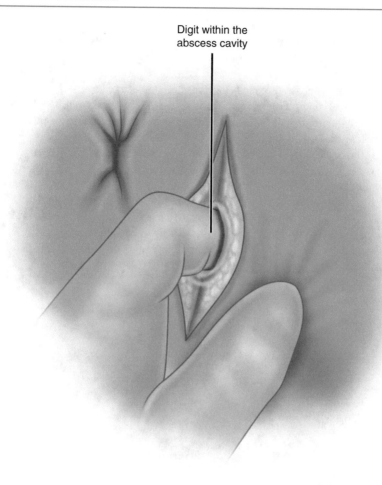

Fig. 12.67 Intracavital digital examination

Note
- The subcutaneous and superficial external sphincters can be divided with impunity in patients with normal continence at baseline, but be very careful with the deep external sphincter and the puborectalis.
- If the fistula is deep or if there is concern that there is too much muscle within the fistula (a high fistula), the seton procedure is the treatment of choice. The seton (thin silastic vessel loop) may be tied around the probe and threaded through the tract (Fig. 12.71).
- Most of the fistulas in ano are midline posterior.

- Learn Goodsall–Salmon's rule of fistulas (Fig. 12.72), which relates the internal location of the fistula to its external opening:
  - If the external opening of the fistula is anterior to an imaginary transverse line across the anus, the most probable tract of the fistula is a straight line terminating into the anal canal. If the external opening is located more than 3 cm anterior to the line, the tract may curve posteriorly, terminating in the posterior midline.
  - If the external opening of the fistula is posterior to the imaginary transverse line, the most likely tract is a curve, terminating into the posterior midline wall of the anal canal.
- Horseshoe fistula is a U-shaped connection of multiple external openings around the anus, with an internal opening usually found in the posterior midline. The fistula can be intersphincteric or trans-sphincteric. The internal opening is excised, while the external openings debrided for adequate drainage.

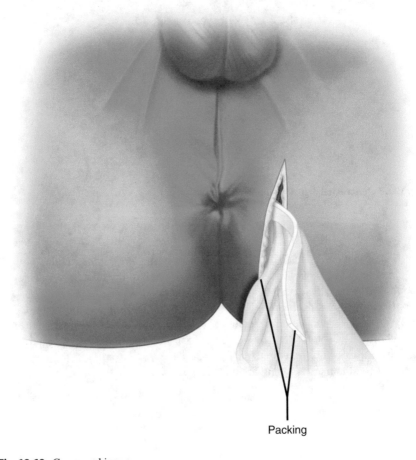

Packing

Fig. 12.68 Gauze packing

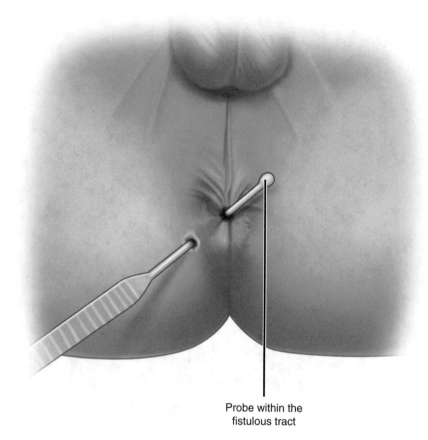

Probe within the
fistulous tract

Fig. 12.69   Probing internal fistula opening

Ligation of Intersphincteric Fistula Tract (LIFT)

Identify the intersphincteric or trans-sphincteric fistula tract to divide and ligate the tract in the intersphincteric groove. This avoids division of any sphincter muscle.

Preoperative preparation: 1–2 enemas; seton already in place for at least 6 weeks prior to surgery to mature the fistula tract.

Position: Prone jackknife.

Anesthesia: General or spinal.

Procedure: As described above in anal /fistulotomy, identify the fistula tract. Use an anoscope to place the anal sphincter on tension. Leave the fistula probe in the fistula (Fig. 12.73a). Palpate the intersphincteric groove and create a curvilinear incision over the groove above the fistula tract. A Lone Star retractor can be very

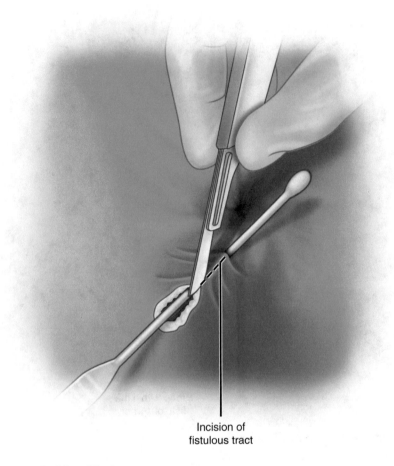

Incision of
fistulous tract

Fig. 12.70 Excision of fistulous tract

useful in obtaining proper exposure. Dissect in the intersphincteric groove to dissect out the fistula tract, which lies perpendicular to the groove (Fig. 12.73b). Place 2–0 Vicryl ties on both sides of the tract (next to the internal and external sphincter). Divide the tract (with or without removing excess tract). Suture ligate each side in the intersphincteric groove to ensure complete closure (Fig. 12.73c, d). Test with peroxide from the external and internal openings of the fistula. Irrigate, and close the cavity with absorbable sutures (Fig. 12.73e, f). Both external and internal openings are gently curetted to remove any granulation tissue and then left open for drainage.

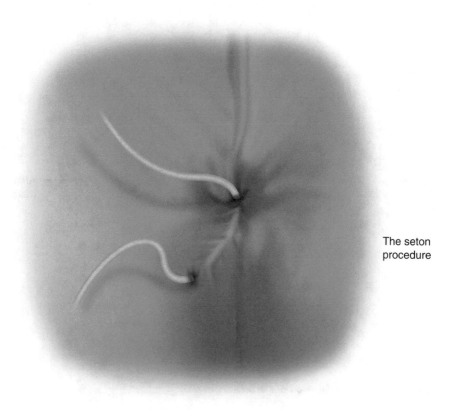

The seton
procedure

Fig. 12.71   Seton placement

Anal Fissure

Preparation: Enemas as tolerated.

Position: Prone jackknife.

Anesthesia: General or MAC with local block. Block with bupivacaine with epinephrine is recommended to relax the sphincter and for postoperative analgesia.

Procedure: Lateral internal sphincterotomy.

Note
- Anterior or posterior midline sphincterotomy can lead to a "keyhole" deformity and should be avoided at all costs.

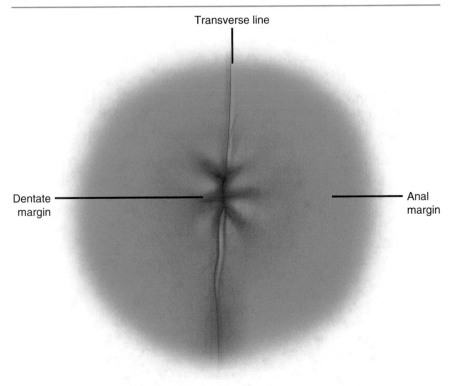

Fig. 12.72 Goodsall–Salmon's rule of fistulas (see text)

The anal fissure is examined with an anoscope to determine its length into the anal canal and its relation to the dentate line. With the anal sphincter on tension using a Pratt bivalve or Hill-Ferguson retractor, the surgeon palpates the intersphincteric groove with the finger and the top of the anal sphincter is also palpated. Along the lateral position, the internal anal sphincter is dissected in the intersphincteric groove and in the submucosal plane. To prevent fistula formation, care is taken to avoid disrupting the mucosa. Under direct vision, the distal portion of the internal anal sphincter is transected perpendicularly for the length of the fissure less than 1 cm in total length. The wound is irrigated, and the mucosa checked for any holes. The wound is then closed loosely with absorbable suture.

Note
- Hypertrophied edges of the anal fissure and the base of the fissure can be debrided to facilitate fissure healing. Sentinel anal tags can be excised.

Hemorrhoidectomy (Figs. 12.74, 12.75, 12.76, and 12.77)

Preparation: 1–2 enemas.
Position: Lithotomy or prone jackknife.

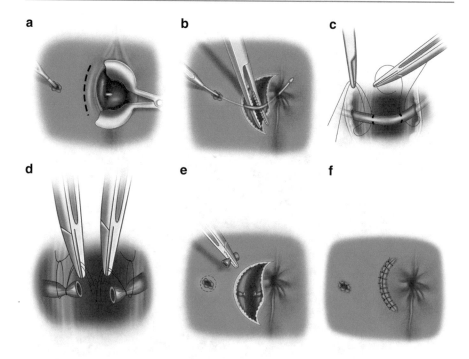

Fig. 12.73 (**a**) Introduction of fistula probe through the tract. (**b**) Dissection of intersphincteric groove and identification of fibrotic fistula tract. (**c**) Suture ligation of fistula tract proximally, distally. (**d**) Additional ligature reinforcing tract closure. (**e**) Division of fistula tract; if tract is quite long, a segment of the tract is excised. (**f**) LIFT wound is closed loosely, and external opening of the tract is enlarged to facilitate drainage

Anesthesia: General. Local block with bupivacaine with epinephrine is recommended to relax the sphincter and for postoperative analgesia.

- **Step 1.** Perform digital rectal examination, anal dilatation, and anoscopic evaluation.
- **Step 2.** Insert a gauze sponge into the lower rectum to prevent downward fecal leakage. Withdraw sponge and identify the prolapsing hemorrhoids (Fig. 12.74).
- **Step 3.** Use a medium or large Hill-Ferguson anoscope. With a clamp of your choice, gently grasp the prolapsing hemorrhoid. Minimize the width of anoderm to be excised to avoid stenosis.
- **Step 4.** Make an elliptical-shaped incision, including the skin of the anal verge up to the base of the hemorrhoid. Avoid the anal sphincters by elevating the hemorrhoidal tissue and pushing the sphincter muscles downward and away. Excision of the hemorrhoid can also be performed with the Harmonic scalpel or bipolar cautery device (see below).
- **Step 5.** Clamp the dissected hemorrhoid and apply tension to visualize the mucocutaneous junction. Excise it using a scalpel (Fig. 12.75), scissor, or monopolar electrocautery. Suture ligate the apex of the hemorrhoidal bundle. Close the

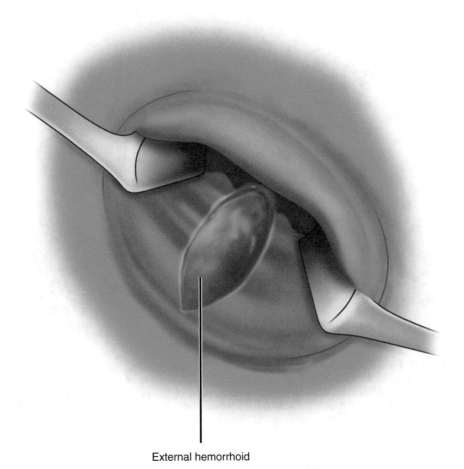

External hemorrhoid

Fig. 12.74 Prolapsing hemorrhoid

mucosal wound with absorbable suture (0 chromic, 2–0 Vicryl) to the anal verge in a running locking fashion. If the external wound is large, it can be loosely reapproximated with interrupted absorbable sutures. The external skin can be left open for drainage to heal by secondary intention. Be sure to save enough mucosa and anoderm between the excised hemorrhoids to prevent anal stenosis (Fig. 12.76).

- **Step 6.** Occasionally an internal hemorrhoid has a polyp-like formation and may be excised in toto. The floor should be sutured with continuous absorbable suture (Fig. 12.77).

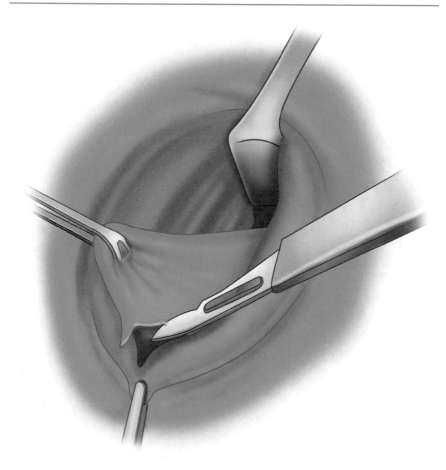

Fig. 12.75 Grasping the prolapsing hemorrhoid

Note
- Alternatively, the Harmonic scalpel or a bipolar cautery device (Ligasure, Enseal) can be used to excise the hemorrhoidal tissue. Typically, these devices divide and coagulate tissue simultaneously. In comparison with monopolar electrocautery, use of bipolar devices leads to faster operating times and less postoperative pain, due to decreased thermal injury. Absorbable sutures can be used to oversew the excision sites as needed.

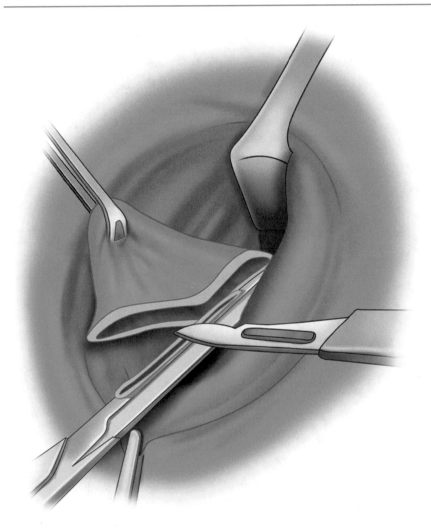

Fig. 12.76 Excision of hemorrhoid

Procedure for Prolapse and Hemorrhoids (PPH) Stapled Hemorrhoidopexy

Preparation: 1–2 enemas.

Position: Prone jackknife.

Anesthesia: General. Local block with bupivacaine with epinephrine is recommended to relax the sphincter and for postoperative analgesia.

- **Step 1.** Perform digital rectal examination, anal dilatation, and anoscopic evaluation.
- **Step 2.** Gradual digital anal dilation to allow placement of the circular anal dilator (CAD) and obturator. With four 2–0 silk sutures, secure the CAD to the peri-

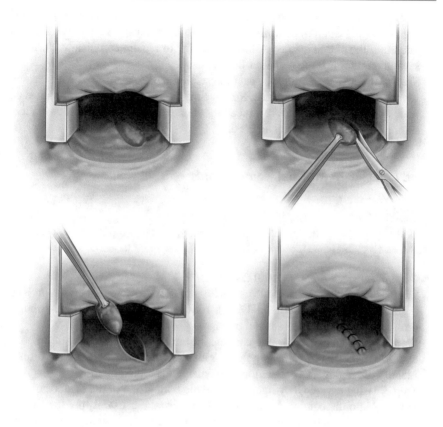

Fig. 12.77   In toto excision of internal hemorrhoid

anal skin. Remove the obturator. The dentate line should be visible through the CAD.

- **Step 3.** Insert the open-sided anoscope and place a running 2–0 monofilament submucosal purse-string suture 3–4 cm from the anal verge, staying superficial to the rectal muscle. Placing the purse-string too close to the dentate line increases postoperative pain and can impair sensation. Placing the purse-string too high above the hemorrhoids may not reduce the hemorrhoids. Involving the rectal muscle can lead to sepsis or incontinence.
- **Step 4.** Remove the anoscope. Insert the stapler with the anvil head through the purse-string suture using the CAD as a guide. Tie the purse-string around the anvil head. If using the Ethicon PPH stapler, bring the monofilament suture ends through the stapler. Tie a loose knot in the suture outside the stapler. If using the Covidien stapler, the anvil is placed through the purse-string. The purse-string is tied around the anvil head with the suture ends brought through the holes of the anvil spike, and then the stapler mechanism is attached to the anvil spike.

- **Step 5.** Apply traction on the suture and close the stapler. In females, perform a digital vaginal exam to confirm that the rectovaginal wall has not been incorporated into the closed stapler. Allow the stapler to remain completely closed for several minutes prior to and after firing.
- **Step 6.** Remove the stapler. Inspect the staple line for hemostasis with the anoscope while the CAD is in place. Remove the CAD and reinspect for hemostasis with the anoscope alone. Any bleeding should be oversewn with 3–0 Vicryl suture. Electrocautery is not advised.

Band Ligation of Internal Hemorrhoids

Important Note
- Avoid banding patients who may require anticoagulation within 2 weeks.

Position: Prone jackknife or lateral decubitus.
- **Step 1.** Digitally examine the anus for masses and to reduce any prolapse (Figs. 12.78, 12.79, 12.80 and 12.81). Ensure that there is only hemorrhoidal prolapse (not full thickness rectal prolapse).
- **Step 2.** Insert an anoscope and examine the entire lower rectum for thrombosis, hypertrophied anal papillae, polyps, radiation proctitis, or Crohn's disease. Identify the major areas of hemorrhoid enlargement and prolapse.
- **Step 3.** Using a McGivney ligator, clamp the midportion of the hemorrhoid and retract it into the bander. Avoid the sensitive distal mucosa. Apply the band. If using a McGowan band ligator, apply suction to the hemorrhoid. If there is sensation, release and suction more proximally. Apply the band.
- **Step 4.** The hemorrhoidal tissue within the band may be infiltrated with lidocaine or dibucaine in small amounts to decrease slippage of the band and for local analgesia.

Thrombosed External Hemorrhoids

Position and preparation: As described for hemorrhoids.

Anesthesia: Local anesthetic around the base of the thrombosed external hemorrhoid (TEH).

Procedure: Incision and drainage.

Incise at the hemorrhoidal apex and evacuate the thrombus by pressure at the base of the hemorrhoid or by instrument (curette or curved hemostat).

Procedure: excision.

Using sharp scissors or a scalpel, create an elliptical incision closely around the base of the thrombosed external hemorrhoid. Start distally and elevate TEH away from the base, removing the thrombus in toto up to the anal verge. Achieve hemostasis with direct pressure, silver nitrate, or electrocautery. If the wound is very

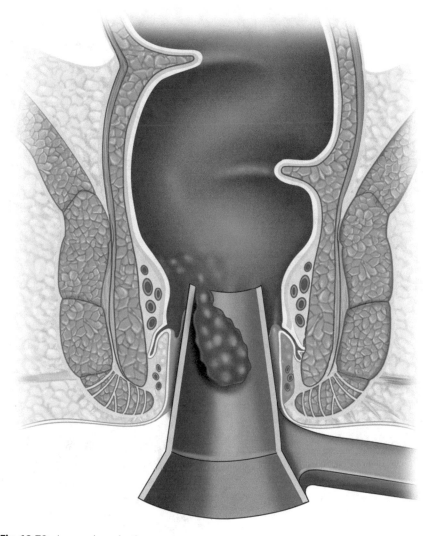

Fig. 12.78 Anoscopic evaluation

large, loosely reapproximate the wound with 3–0 absorbable suture, leaving enough of the wound open for drainage.

Excision of Pilonidal Cyst

Position: Jackknife.

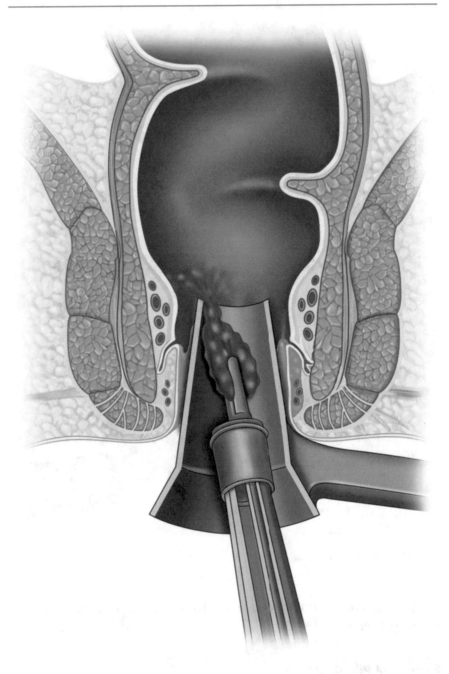

Fig. 12.79 Examination of lower rectum

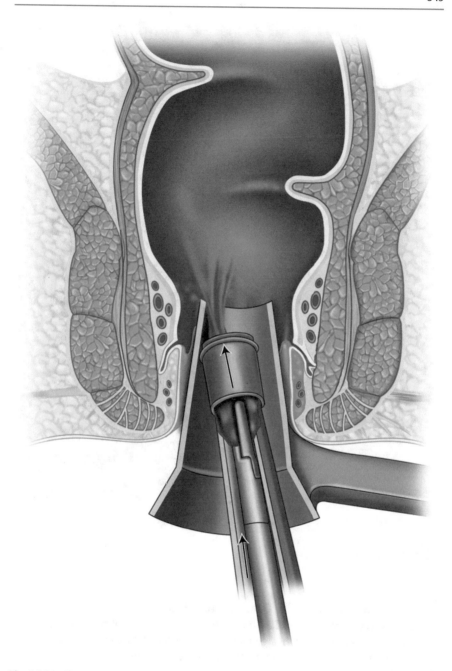

Fig. 12.80 Hemorrhoid is clamped

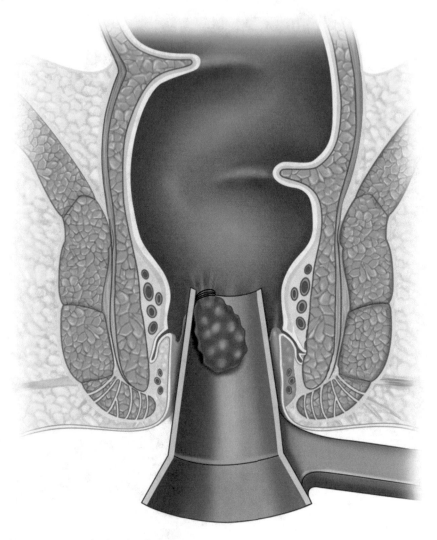

Fig. 12.81 Retraction into bander

Preparation and anesthesia: General. Local block with bupivacaine with epinephrine is recommended to relax the sphincter and for postoperative analgesia.

- **Step 1.** Fix extra-large adhesive tape to both lower gluteal areas and perineum. Anchor the tape to the operating room table, separating the intergluteal fold (Fig. 12.82).
- **Step 2.** Probe the sinus gently, since occasionally it may travel laterally (Fig. 12.83). With an ovoid incision down to the fascia (Fig. 12.84), remove the cyst and the sinuses en bloc and in toto, including subcutaneous tissue. Injecting

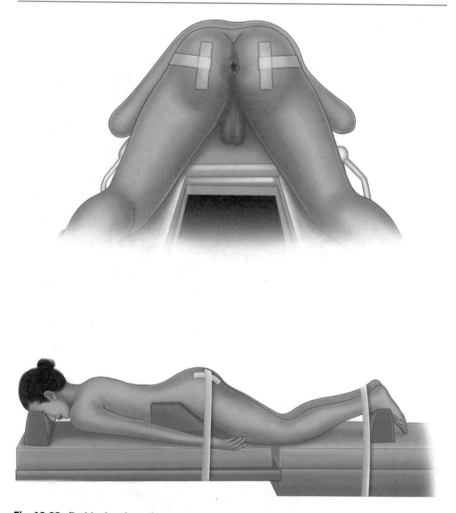

Fig. 12.82   Positioning the patient

methylene blue into the pilonidal cyst can aid with excision of the entirety of the cyst and all associated sinuses.

- **Step 3.** After good hemostasis is established, the skin edges of the wound can be marsupialized with a running locking suture or interrupted sutures. Pack the wound with iodoform gauze to heal by secondary intention. If there is no infection, the wound can be closed in one layer using 3–0 nylon with interrupted vertical mattress sutures, including the fascia, as demonstrated in Fig. 12.85. Alternatively, there are several flap closures described for tension-free tissue approximation in cases of larger excised pilonidal cysts.

Fig. 12.83 Probing the sinus. Incising the cyst

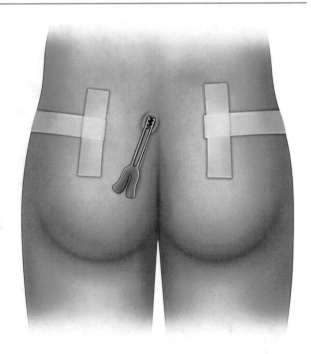

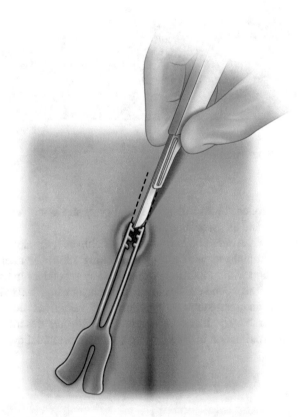

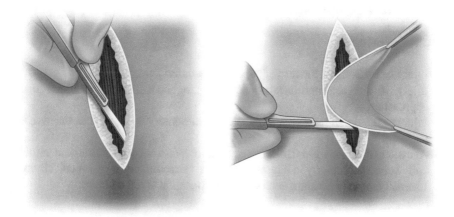

Fig. 12.84 Cyst is incised and removed

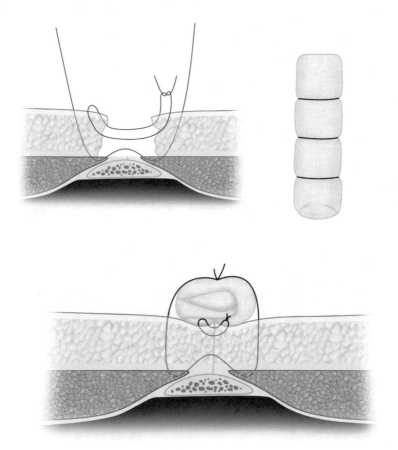

Fig. 12.85 Marsupialization and packing of wound

Anatomical Complications

Right Colectomy

- Injury or inadvertent ligature of superior mesenteric vessels.
- Injury to the retroperitoneal duodenum, for both laparoscopic and open approaches.
- Injury to the right ureter if dissection of the mesentery is deeper than the avascular plain.
- Avulsion of venous branch between inferior pancreaticoduodenal and middle colic veins, particularly in aggressive medial retraction during open colectomy.
- Lateral colon mobilization enters retroperitoneal fat and the kidney.

Left Colectomy

- Excessive traction on the descending colon before dividing the lienocolic ligaments can cause splenic capsule laceration.
- Inadequate mobilization of colon length creates tension at an anastomosis and increases the risk of leakage.
- Injury to the left ureter if dissection is carried deeper than the avascular plain.
- Laparoscopic dissection deep into lumbar vessels.

Rectosigmoid Colectomy

- Presacral hemorrhage.
- Injury to ureters as they cross over the ileac vessels.
- Anastomotic tension from failure to mobilize splenic flexure.
- Exact location of the level of rectal tumor and assessment of its mobility allow use of the resection procedure with least morbidity.
- Injury to the hypogastric nerves diminishes sexual function.
- Failure to resect the mesorectum and achieve full radial clearance increases the likelihood of local recurrence of tumor.
- Resection of the presacral fascia increases the risk for bleeding from sacral veins.
- Incorrect positioning in lithotomy or poor placement of rigid retractors can result in neuropathies in the legs.

Liver

13

Marty T. Sellers

Anatomy

The current anatomical terminology alluded to above is known as the Brisbane
Liver Terminology and was adopted in 2000 in order to standardize descriptions of
liver resections in the international literature. The liver is primarily divided into
right and left hemilivers. "Hemiliver" is technically a misnomer, however, in that
the right hemiliver is larger, generally comprising approximately 60% of the entire
liver volume. This terminology, including references to the 8 Couinaud segments
(which are defined by the distribution and branching pattern of the intraparenchymal arteries, portal veins, and bile ducts), is illustrated in Figs. 13.1, 13.2, 13.3, and
13.4 and will be used throughout this chapter; the caudate (segment 1) is a separate
region divided into right and left subsegments. A more complete description of the
Brisbane Liver Terminology can be found at http://www.ahpba.org and http://www.
ihpba.org and in the article by Strasberg referenced at the end of the chapter. Briefly,
the right hemiliver consists of Couinaud segments 5, 6, 7, and 8; and the left hemili
ver consists of segments 2, 3, 4A, and 4B. The respective hemilivers are subdivided
into "sections" (or "sectors"): right anterior and posterior sections and left medial
and lateral sections. The sections subdivide into the Couinaud segments: segments
2 and 3 comprise the left lateral section; segments 4a and 4b, the left medial section;
segments 5 and 8, the right anterior section; and segments 6 and 7, the right posterior section. For historical context, the right anterior section is the former anterior
segment of the right lobe; the right posterior section is the former posterior segment
of the right lobe; the left lateral section is the former left lateral segment; and the left
medial section is the former left medial segment.

M. T. Sellers (✉)
Department of Surgery, Emory University, Atlanta, GA, USA
e-mail: mtselle@emory.edu

© Springer Nature Switzerland AG 2021
L. J. Skandalakis (ed.), *Surgical Anatomy and Technique*,
https://doi.org/10.1007/978-3-030-51313-9_13

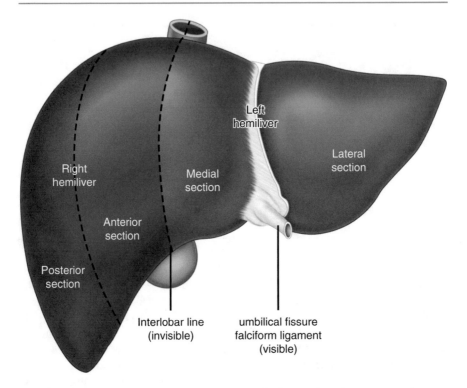

Fig. 13.1 Current anatomical description of the liver: diaphragmatic surface

Topographic Anatomy of the Liver

Diaphragmatic Surface Relations

For descriptive purposes, the diaphragmatic surface of the liver is divided into superior, posterior, anterior, and right portions:

- The superior portion is related to the diaphragm and, from right to left, right pleura and lung, pericardium and heart (cardiac impression), and left pleura and lung.
- The posterior portion is related to the diaphragm and lower ribs. It contains the greater part of the bare area and the sulcus of the inferior vena cava (IVC).
- The anterior part is related to the diaphragm and costal margin, xiphoid process, the abdominal wall, and the sixth to tenth ribs on the right.
- The right portion is related to the diaphragm and the seventh to eleventh ribs. It is a lateral continuation of the posterior portion.

Anteriorly, the inferior border of the liver is marked by two notches. These are a deep notch accommodating the ligamentum teres and a shallow notch allowing space for the gallbladder.

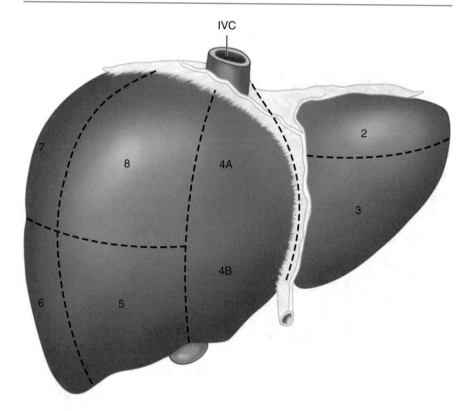

Fig. 13.2 Segments of the liver. Terminology of Couinaud

Visceral Surface Relations

The visceral surface of the liver is related to the following organs from right to left·
- The hepatic flexure of the colon and part of the right transverse colon are related to the anterior one-third of the visceral surface of the right hemiliver, passing behind the normally sharp, anterior inferior margin of the liver.
- Behind the colic impression is the renal impression, produced by the right kidney and right adrenal gland. Fat, connective tissue, and peritoneum intervene between these organs and the liver. The right adrenal gland is in contact with the bare area of the liver.
- The gallbladder lies in a fossa just beneath the anterior inferior border of the liver.
- To the left of the gallbladder is a depression for the first and second portions of the duodenum. Posterior to the gallbladder fossa is the fossa for the IVC.
- Posteriorly and to the left of the ligamentum venosum, one can see a small impression for the abdominal esophagus.
- Almost the entire visceral surface of the left hemiliver is in contact with the stomach, forming the gastric impression.

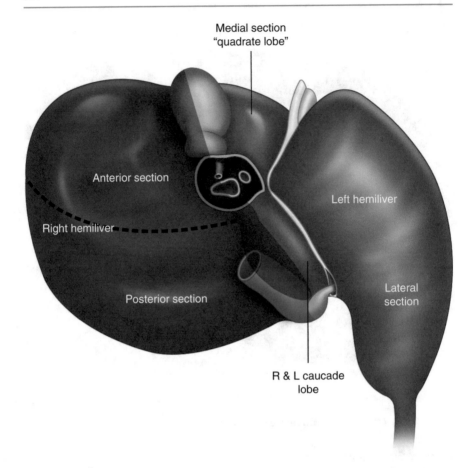

Fig. 13.3 Visceral surface of the liver. The plane between the left medial and left lateral sections is variously referred to as the umbilical fissure, the fissure of the ligamentum teres, or the fissure of the falciform ligament

Peritoneal Reflections and Ligaments of the Liver

The liver is attached to the anterior abdominal wall and the inferior surface of the diaphragm by the falciform, round, and coronary ligaments. The peritoneum covering the liver is reflected onto the diaphragm as two separate leaves – the anterior and posterior coronary ligaments. Between these is an area in which the diaphragm and the liver are in contact without peritoneum. This is the "bare area." On the left, the two leaves of the coronary ligament approach and join to form the left triangular ligament; on the right, their apposition forms the right triangular ligament (Fig. 13.5).

Anteriorly, the anterior layer of the coronary ligament forms a fold that extends over the superior surface of the liver and is reflected over the anterior abdominal wall. This fold is the falciform ligament. Between the two layers of the fold, the remnant of the embryonic left umbilical vein forms the round ligament (ligamentum teres) of the liver. The falciform and round ligaments extend into the liver to form the obvious fissure that separates the medial (segments 4A and 4B) and lateral (segments 2 and 3) sections of the left hemiliver. On the visceral surface, the fissure for the round ligament extends posteriorly on the fissure for the ligamentum venosum. Between the fissure and the bed of the gallbladder lies the quadrate "lobe," which is seen on the visceral surface of the left medial section. It is separated from the more posterior caudate process (segment 1) by the transverse fissure or porta hepatis (Fig. 13.3).

At the porta hepatis, the peritoneum of the liver forms the lesser omentum, which extends to the lesser curvature of the stomach as the hepatogastric ligament and to the first inch (2.54 cm) of the duodenum as the hepatoduodenal ligament (Fig. 13.6). The right margin of the lesser omentum contains the hepatic artery, the portal vein, and the common bile duct. The bile duct is usually on the right, in the free edge of the omentum.

The surgeon should remember the approximate rib levels of the liver, lungs, and pleurae, as shown in Table 13.1.

Morphology of the Liver

Injection and corrosion preparations of the bile ducts, hepatic arteries, and portal veins have shown conclusively that there are distinct right and left sides of the liver (Fig. 13.1). The hepatic veins do not follow this division.

First-order division			
Anatomical term	**Couinad segments referred to**	**Term for surgical resection**	**Diagram (pertinent area is in red)**
Right hemiliver OR Right liver	Sg 5–8 (+/–Sgl)	Right hepatectomy OR Right hemihepatectomy (stipulate +/-segment I)	
Left hemiliver OR Left liver	Sg 2–4 (+/–Sgl)	Left hepatectomy OR Left hemihepatectomy (stipulate +/–segment I)	

Border or watershed: The border or watershed of the first order division which seperates the two hemilivers is plane which intersects the gallbladder fossa and the fossa for the IVC and is called the midplane of the liver.

Fig. 13.4 Brisbane liver terminology based on (a) first-, (b) second-, and (c) third-order divisions of hepatic arteries, bile ducts, and portal veins

	Second-order division		
	(second-order division based on bile ducts and hepatic artery)		
Anatomical term	**Couinad segments referred to**	**Term for surgical resection**	**Diagram** (pertinent area is in red)
Right anterior section	*Sg 5,8*	Add (-ectomy) to any of the anatomical terms as in *Right anterior sectionectomy*	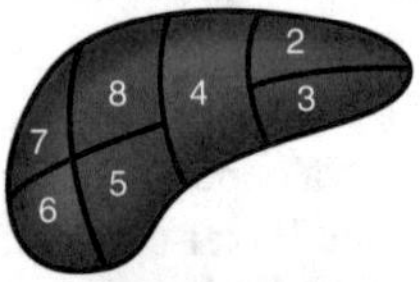
Right posterior section	*Sg 6,7*	Right posterior sectionectomy	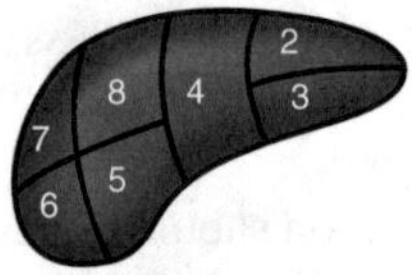
Left medial section	*Sg 4*	Left medial sectionectomy **OR** **Resection segment 4** (also see Third order) **OR** **Segmentctomy 4** (also see Third order)	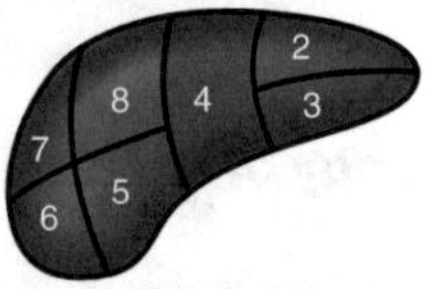
Left lateral section	*Sg 2,3*	Left lateral sectionectomy **OR** **Bisegmentectomy 2,3** (also see third order)	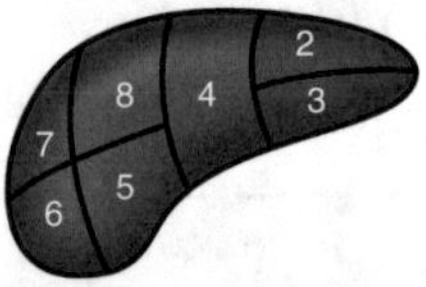
	Other "sectional" liver resections		
	Sg 4–8 (+/-SgI)	**Right trisectionectomy** (preferred term) or **Extended right hepatectomy** or **Extended right hemihepatectomy** (stipulate +/–segment I)	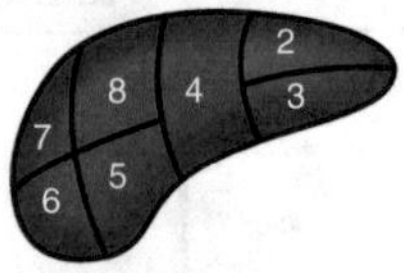
	Sg 2,3,4,5,8	**Left trisectionectomy** (preferred term) or **Extended left hepatectomy** or **Extended left hemihepatectomy** (stipulate +/–segment I)	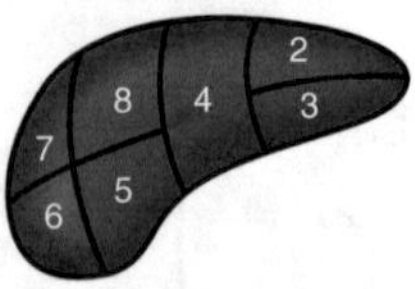

Border or watershed: The border or watershed of the sections are planes reffered to as the right and left interesctional planes. The left intersectional plane passes though the umbilical fissure and attachment of the falciform ligament. There is no surface marking of the right intersectional plane.

Fig. 13.4 (continued)

Third-order division			
Anatomical term	**Couinad segments referred to**	**Term for surgical resection**	**Diagram** (pertinent area is in red)
Segments 1–9	Any one of Sg 1 to 9	Segmentectomy (e.g. segmentectomy 6)	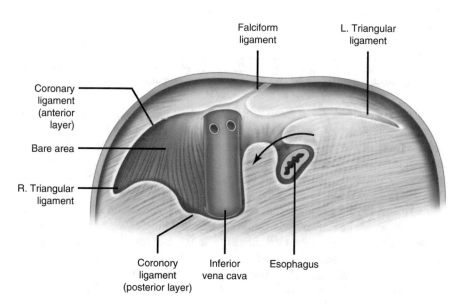
2 contiguous segments	Any two of Sg 1 to Sg 9 in continuity	Bisegmentectomy (e.g. bisegmentectomy 5,6)	

For clarity Sg. 1 to 9 are not shown. It is also acceptable to refer to ANY resection by its third-order segments, eg. right hemihepatectomy can also be called resection sg 5–8.

Border or watershed: The border or watershed of the segments are planes reffered to as intersegmental planes.

Fig. 13.4 (continued)

Fig. 13.5 The inferior surface of the diaphragm showing the peritoneal attachments of the liver (*broken lines*). Within the boundaries of these attachments is the "bare area" of the liver and the diaphragm. The *arrow* passes through the posterior layer of the coronary ligament

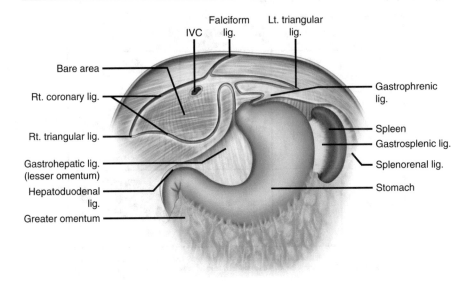

Fig. 13.6 Peritoneal reflections of the liver: the lesser omentum (hepatogastric and hepatoduode-nal ligaments) and its relation to the coronary ligament of the liver and diaphragm

Table 13.1 Approximate rib levels of liver, lungs, and pleura

	At the lateral sternal line	At the midaxillary line	At the vertebral spine line
Liver	5	6	8
Lung	6	8	10
Pleura	7	10	12

From Lockhart RD, Hamilton GF, Fyfe FW. *Anatomy of the Human Body*. Philadelphia: JB Lippincott, 1959, p. 549. Reprinted with permission from John Wiley and Sons

On the visceral surface of the liver, the plane separating the right and left hemili-vers (the "midplane" of the liver) passes through the bed of the gallbladder below and the fossa of the IVC above. On the diaphragmatic surface, there is no visible external mark. The midplane is an imaginary line that passes from the notch of the gallbladder anteriorly, parallel to the fissure of the round ligament, to the IVC above (Fig. 13.2).

As before, the left hemiliver thus consists of medial and lateral sections. Each of these sections can be further divided into superior and inferior segments on the basis of the distribution of the bile ducts, hepatic arteries, and portal veins. The superior segments are 4A (medial section) and 2 (lateral section); the inferior segments are 4B (medial section) and 3 (lateral section). The locations of these segments are deter-mined on CT and MRI scans based on the cephalocaudal location of the portal vein.

The right hemiliver is divided by the right fissure into anterior and posterior sec-tions. The plane of this fissure corresponds to the line of the eighth intercostal space. Similar to the left side, each section of the right hemiliver can be subdivided into superior and inferior segments on the basis of the distribution of the bile ducts, hepatic arteries, and portal veins. The superior segments are 7 (posterior section) and 8 (anterior section), and the inferior segments are 6 (posterior section) and 5 (anterior section). Again, these segments are determined on CT and MRI scans based on the cephalocaudal location of the portal vein.

Segment 1 (the caudate) is a separate region divided by the midplane into right and left subsegments. Its bile ducts, arteries, and portal veins arise from both right and left main branches. Segment 1 is drained by two small, fairly constant hepatic veins that enter the left side of the IVC. The historical "quadrate lobe" is contained within segments 4A and 4B and has little to no relevance to current surgical practice.

At the present time, we believe there are interlobar anastomoses between the right and left hemilivers. In other words, there is communication between the right and left arteries, veins, and ducts.

Clinically, hepatic artery ligation can be safe and is sometimes necessary, and interruption of the right or left hepatic duct may produce only transitory jaundice. In spite of these findings, we must remember Michel's dictum that "the blood supply of the liver is always unpredictable." *Possible* collateral pathways are not always *actual*.

Intrahepatic Duct System

The usual pattern of intrahepatic ducts is shown in Figs. 13.7 and 13.8. The most frequent variations are those in which the right anterior or posterior duct crosses the midplane to enter the left hepatic duct (Fig. 13.9).

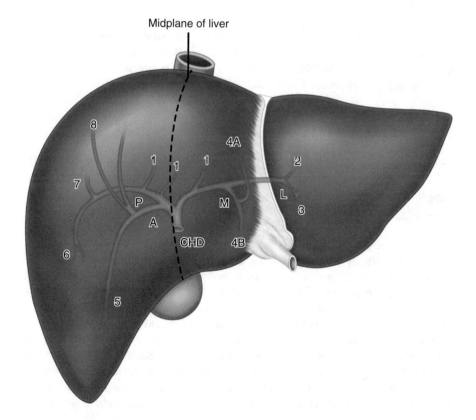

Fig. 13.7 Diagram of the intrahepatic distribution of the bile ducts. The segmental branches are labeled numerically. *A*, anterior; *C*, caudate; *L*, lateral; *M*, medial; *P*, posterior; *CHD*, common hepatic duct

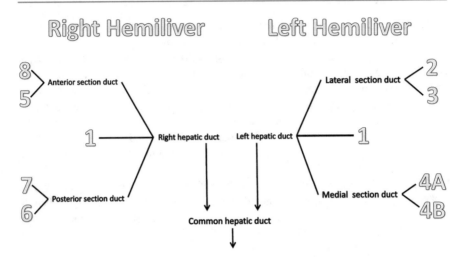

Fig. 13.8 Terminology and pattern of intrahepatic bile ducts; numbers refer to Couinaud's segments

Anomalies

The most common hepatic anomaly is diminished size of the left hemiliver. Small accessory "lobes" attached to the liver or to a mesentery are often reported. The most striking of these is "Riedel's lobe," an elongated tongue of liver extending from the right hemiliver to or below the umbilicus (Fig. 13.10).

Vascular System of the Liver

The liver receives blood from two sources: the hepatic artery and the portal vein. The hepatic artery provides about 25% of the hepatic blood supply and 50% of the oxygen. The hepatic portal vein contributes about 75% of the blood flow and 50% of the oxygen.

Hepatic Artery

In the usual pattern, the common hepatic artery arises from the celiac trunk. After giving origin to the gastroduodenal artery, the hepatic artery continues as the proper hepatic artery in the hepatoduodenal ligament. In this ligament, the proper hepatic artery lies to the left of the common bile and hepatic ducts and anterior to the portal vein. It divides into right and left hepatic arteries before entering the porta.

An aberrant hepatic artery is one that arises from some vessel other than the celiac trunk and reaches the liver by an abnormal course. Such an aberrant artery is *accessory* if it supplies a segment of the liver that also receives blood from a normal hepatic artery (Fig. 13.11a). It is *replacing* if it is the only blood supply to such a segment (Fig. 13.11b). A replaced/accessory right hepatic artery, present in

Fig. 13.9 Intrahepatic
section ducts. (**a**) Usual
pattern. (**b**) Anomalous
origin of right anterior
duct. (**c**) Anomalous origin
of right posterior duct.
Both ducts cross the
midplane to reach their
destinations

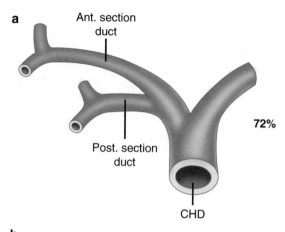

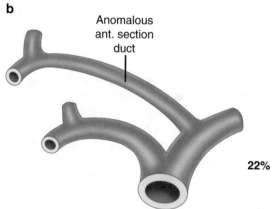

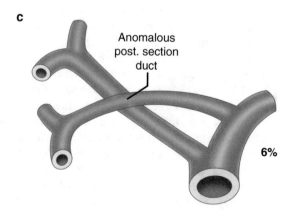

Fig. 13.10 Riedel's lobe
of the liver. This
anomalous lobe is found
usually in middle-aged
women and presents as an
asymptomatic but
unexplained mass

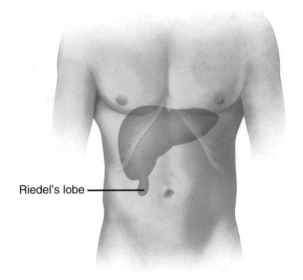

Riedel's lobe ————

approximately 10% of patients, most commonly arises from the superior mesenteric artery, and courses along the pancreatic uncinate process and posterior to the bile duct before entering the liver; therefore, it is at risk of inadvertent injury if the surgeon operating in this area is not aware of its presence. A replaced/accessory left hepatic artery, also present in approximately 10% of patients, most commonly arises from the left gastric artery and courses through the lesser omentum before entering the liver. Other origins of replaced/accessory left and right hepatic arteries also exist; awareness of this possibility is helpful, especially in the field of liver transplantation.

At the porta hepatis, the right hepatic artery passes to the right of and usually (85%) posterior to the hepatic duct – but occasionally (15%) anterior to it. The cystic artery generally arises from the right hepatic in the hepatocystic triangle located between the cystic duct and the common hepatic duct. The left hepatic artery usually supplies the entire left hemiliver (Fig. 13.12a). However, in some individuals the left hepatic artery supplies only the left lateral section, with the left medial section being supplied by a branch of the right hepatic artery that crosses the midplane (Fig. 13.12b) or as a third branch of a trifurcating proper hepatic artery. This medial section artery is also referred to as the "middle hepatic artery" (Fig. 13.13).

Within the liver, the arteries follow the course of the bile ducts and portal veins, dividing into anterior and posterior branches in the right hemiliver and into lateral and medial branches in the left hemiliver (Fig. 13.14); these are the second-order divisions and further subdivide into third-order (segmental) divisions (Fig. 13.4).

Ligation of the right or left hepatic artery results in ischemia for about 24 h, after which intraparenchymal collateral vessels restore arterial blood to the deprived portion. With arteriography in patients, the existence of an arterial collateral network following ligation of one hepatic artery has been appreciated. Of note, splenic artery ligation has been shown to increase flow in the hepatic artery by approximately 30%.

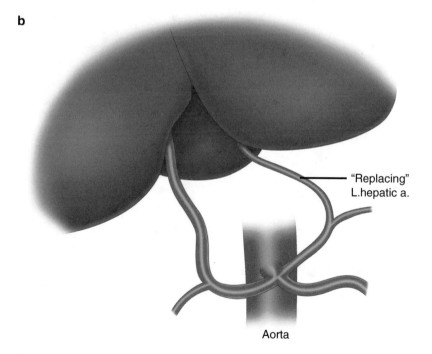

Fig. 13.11 Aberrant hepatic arteries. (**a**) Accessory type. (**b**) Replacing type

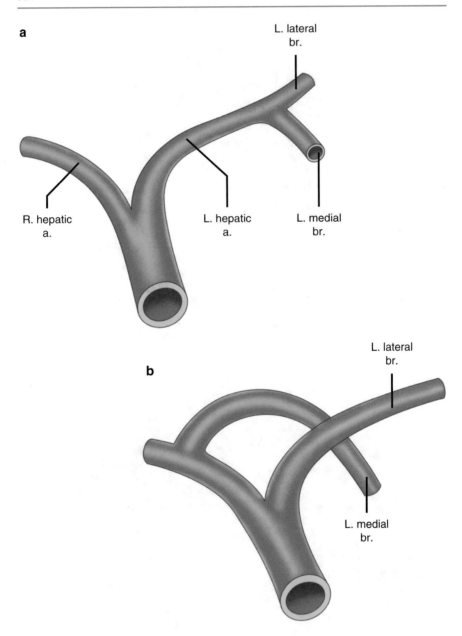

Fig. 13.12 Hepatic arteries. (**a**) Usual pattern of segmental hepatic arteries. (**b**) Anomalous origin of the left medial segmental artery from the right hepatic artery, crossing the midplane to reach the medial segment of the left lobe. This may be encountered in 25% of individuals

Remember

- Hepatic arteries are not end arteries in vivo; ligation of the right or left hepatic artery results in intraparenchymal and subcapsular collateral circulation within 24 h.
- After ligation of the common hepatic artery, the right gastric and gastroduodenal arteries will maintain hepatic blood flow.
- Right or left hepatic artery ligation is generally well tolerated. Death following such ligation does not usually result.
- Cholecystectomy must always accompany right hepatic artery ligation.

Portal Vein

The portal vein originates with the confluence of the superior mesenteric and splenic veins behind the pancreas. In about one-third of individuals, the inferior mesenteric vein enters at this confluence; in the rest, it enters either the superior mesenteric vein or the splenic vein below the junction.

In its upward course, the portal vein receives the left gastric and several smaller veins before dividing into right and left branches at the porta hepatis. Here it lies posterior to the hepatic duct and the hepatic artery (Fig. 13.13).

Portal vessels follow the pattern of the hepatic arteries and the bile ducts. The right portal vein divides into anterior and posterior (second-order) vessels, each

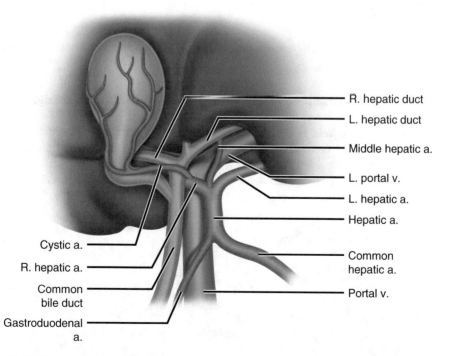

Fig. 13.13 Relationship of the hepatic ducts, the hepatic artery, and the portal vein at the porta hepatis

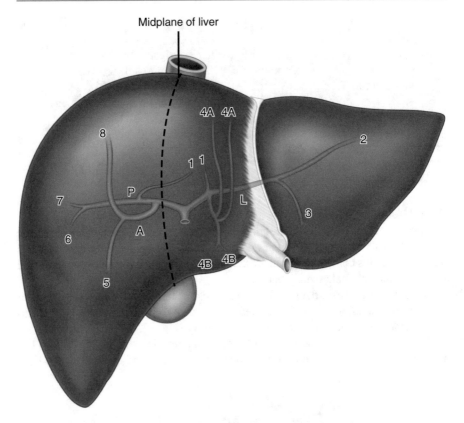

Fig. 13.14 Diagram of the intrahepatic distribution of the hepatic artery. Numbers refer to Couinaud's segments

dividing further into third-order (segmental) branches. Near its origin, the right portal vein sends a branch to the right side of segment 1.

The left portal vein is longer and smaller than the right vein. It divides into medial and lateral (second-order) vessels, each dividing further into third-order (segmental) branches. It also it gives a branch to the left side of segment 1. The medial vessel (to segment 4) contains a dilatation, the pars umbilicus, which represents the orifice of the obliterated embryonic ductus venosus (Fig. 13.15).

Remember
- Right or left portal vein ligation leads to atrophy of the ipsilateral hemiliver and hypertrophy of the contralateral hemiliver.
- Reduction in portal blood flow increases hepatic artery blood flow. The reverse is not true.
- Following a radical pancreaticoduodenal resection, the main portal vein should not be ligated. Portal blood flow must be restored by a shunt or a replacement graft.

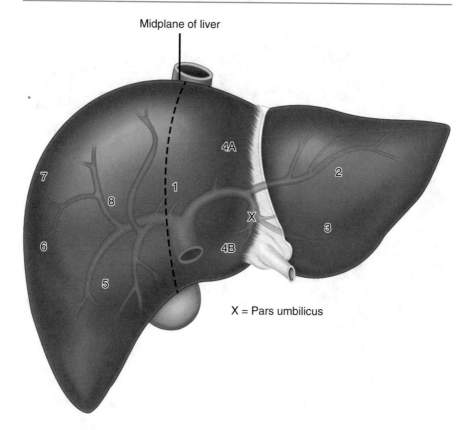

Fig. 13.15 Diagram of the intrahepatic distribution of the portal vein. Numbers refer to Couinaud's segments

Hepatic Veins

As before, the branching patterns of the bile ducts, hepatic arteries, and portal veins define the segmental anatomy of the liver. Alternatively, the hepatic veins lie in the planes between the sections. Therefore, if the middle hepatic vein is to be preserved in a right hemihepatectomy, the transection line in which must be just to the right of the midplane; similarly, for a left hemihepatectomy, the transection line should be just to the left of the midplane. Fortunately, overlap of venous drainage is present, allowing ligation of one outflow from a portion of the liver without requiring resection of that portion. The usual pattern of the hepatic veins is as follows (Fig. 13.16):

- The right hepatic vein (RHV) primarily drains segments 6, 7, and 8. It is located between the right anterior and posterior sections (in the right fissure) and is the easiest vein to ligate due to a longer extrahepatic portion before entering the IVC.
- The middle hepatic vein (MHV) drains portions of the right and left hemiliver and provides the primary drainage of segments 4B and 5. It is located in the midplane of the liver.
- The left hepatic vein (LHV) drains the ductus venosus (in the fetus) and is the primary drainage of segments 2, 3, and 4A. It courses between segments 2 and 3.

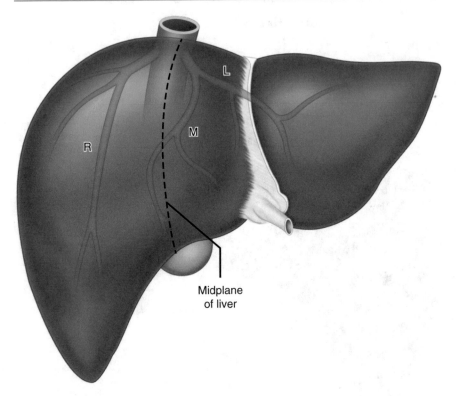

Fig. 13.16 Diagram of the intrahepatic distribution of the hepatic veins. Note that they are inter-lobular rather than lobular. *L*, left; *M*, medial; *R*, right

- The MHVs and LHVs approach one another and usually (approximately 60%) form a common trunk as they enter the IVC less than 1 cm below the diaphragm. In addition to three major veins, there are 1 or 2 substantial segment 1 veins draining directly into the IVC and as many as 50 (usually much less) smaller veins (dorsal hepatic veins), most of which are of insignificant size – but can still be the source of or lead to substantial bleeding if not controlled prior to division. Occasionally, an accessory inferior right hepatic vein draining segments 5 and 6 is present; this vein enters the IVC at approximately the same level as the right adrenal vein and can be appreciated on contrast imaging. It can be ligated with impunity except in the rare circumstance that it will provide the major drainage of the liver remnant following resection.

Remember
- Hepatic resection following ligation of a hepatic vein is not necessary.
- Because of its longer extrahepatic component, ligation of the RHV is usually possible prior to right hepatectomy. The use of vascular staplers has significantly simplified this and also makes it easier to ligate the LHV extrahepatically as well.

Fig. 13.17 Diagram of
the superficial lymphatic
drainage of the liver:
frontal and sagittal views

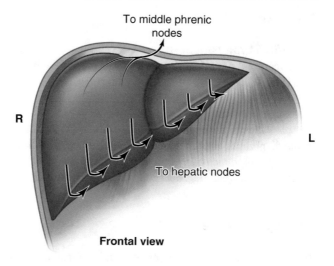

To middle phrenic
nodes

R

L

To hepatic nodes

Frontal view

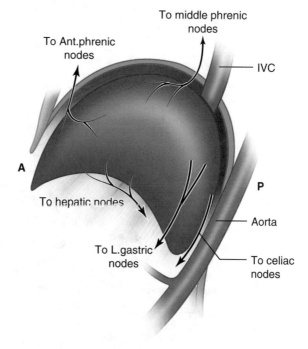

To Ant.phrenic
nodes

To middle phrenic
nodes

IVC

A

P

To hepatic nodes

Aorta

To L.gastric
nodes

To celiac
nodes

Sagittal view

Lymphatic Drainage

Superficial Lymphatics
The superficial lymphatics lie near the surface of the liver within the Glisson's capsule (Fig. 13.17).

Deep Lymphatics
The pathways of the deep lymphatics drain to (1) the middle (lateral) phrenic nodes of the diaphragm and (2) nodes of the porta hepatis following portal vein branches. The deep lymphatics carry the greater part of lymphatic outflow. There is free communication between the superficial and deep lymphatic systems.

Perihepatic Spaces

The perihepatic spaces (subphrenic and subhepatic) and the collection of fluid within may be appreciated surgicoanatomically from Figs. 13.18, 13.19, 13.20, 13.21, 13.22, 13.23, 13.24, and 13.25.

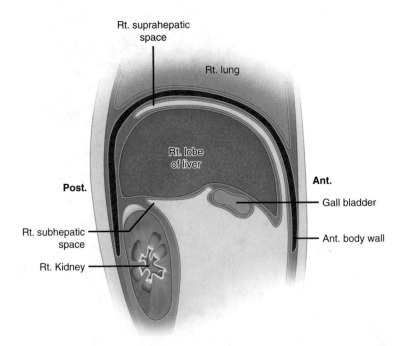

Fig. 13.18 Diagrammatic parasagittal section through the upper abdomen showing the potential right suprahepatic and subhepatic spaces. The thick black line represents the diaphragm

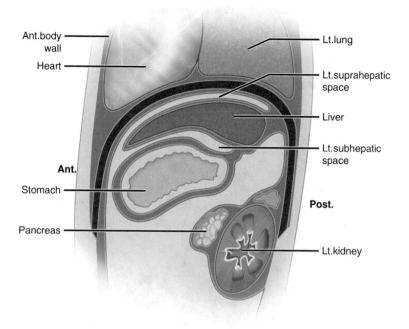

Fig. 13.19 Diagrammatic parasagittal section through the trunk showing the potential left suprahepatic and subhepatic spaces

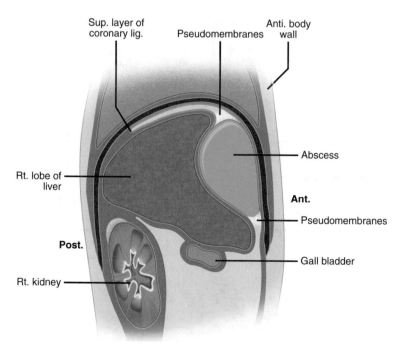

Fig. 13.20 Relations of an abscess in the anterior portion of the right suprahepatic space

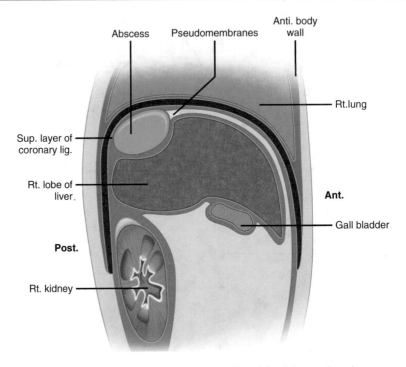

Fig. 13.21 Relations of an abscess in the posterior portion of the right suprahepatic space

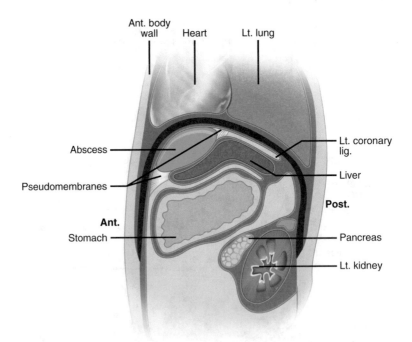

Fig. 13.22 Relations of an abscess in the anterior portion of the left suprahepatic space

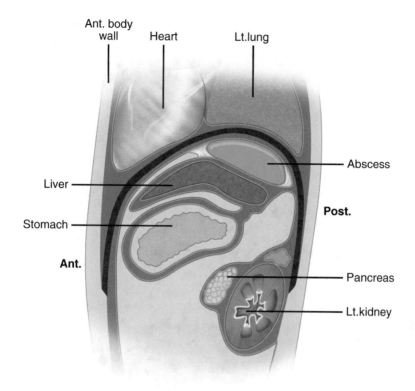

Fig. 13.23 Relations of an abscess in the posterior portion of the left suprahepatic space

Technique

Needle Biopsy

Use a Tru-Cut needle, then Bovie the liver capsule where it is bleeding.

Excisional Biopsy

There are two excisional biopsy procedures: wedge type and nonwedge type (circumferential type).

Wedge-Type Biopsy
- **Step 1.** With 0 chromic catgut or synthetic absorbable, place mattress sutures 1½–2 cm from the periphery of the lesion (Fig. 13.26).
- **Step 2.** Using electrocautery, remove the lesion with at least 1 cm healthy liver tissue. Depending on the size of the specimen to be removed, using vascular

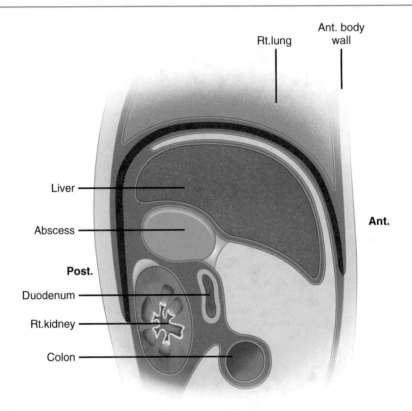

Fig. 13.24 Relations of an abscess in the right subhepatic space

staplers to divide the parenchyma is potentially very helpful in maintaining better hemostasis.
- **Step 3.** Obtain hemostasis along the cut edge with electrocautery, argon beam coagulator, Gelfoam, and/or tissue sealants. It is not necessary to close the cavity, but it is important to leave a drain if there is any bile staining.

Nonwedge- or Circumferential-Type Biopsy
- **Step 1.** Depending on the deepest component of the lesion, place deep hemostatic sutures, as in step 1 of wedge-type excisional biopsy, at least 1½–2 cm from the periphery of the lesion (Fig. 13.27). If the deepest portion is no more than 1½–2 cm from the capsule, these sutures are likely not necessary.
- **Step 2.** Remove lesion by electrocautery. Suction cautery or argon laser might be very helpful for controlling bleeding of liver parenchyma.
- **Step 3.** Obtain hemostasis along the cut edge with electrocautery, argon beam coagulator, Gelfoam, and/or tissue sealants. It is not necessary to close the cavity, but it is important to leave a drain if there is any bile staining.

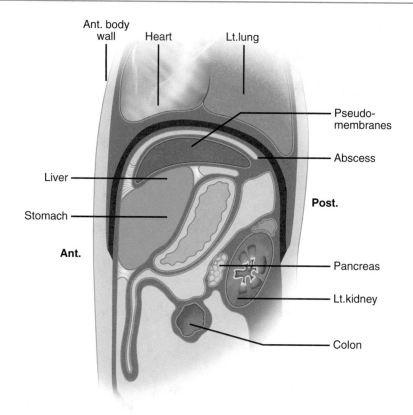

Fig. 13.25 Relations of an abscess in the left subhepatic space

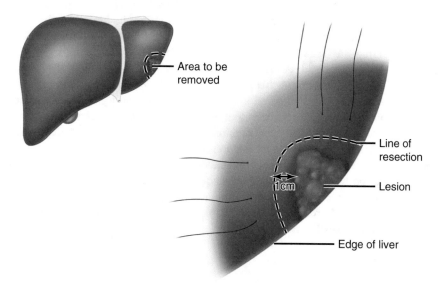

Fig. 13.26 Wedge biopsy. Placement of sutures. *Inset*: resection site

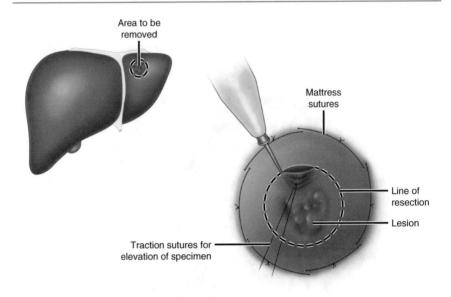

Fig. 13.27 Circumferential (nonwedge) biopsy. Placement of sutures. *Inset*: resection site

Hepatic Resections

Anatomical Landmarks for Liver Resection

Except for the falciform ligament, which delineates the plane between the left medial and lateral sections (Figs. 13.1 and 13.2), the surface of the liver gives little indication of its anatomical segmental boundaries, which are defined by the intraparenchymal distribution and branching pattern of the arteries, bile ducts, and portal veins. Therefore, anatomic resections require interrupting the blood supply to the targeted specimen while leaving the blood flow to the future liver remnant (FLR) intact, creating an ischemic demarcation and identifying the boundary of the segment(s) to be removed. For right and left hepatectomies, ligation of the respective inflow vessels and draining hepatic ducts can be done extrahepatically and individually or intrahepatically and en masse via the Glissonian technique (described below). Since second-order branching of the vessels and biliary ducts occurs intrahepatically, a Glissonian approach is required for all other less-than-hemihepatectomy true anatomic resections whose transection line is not guided by the location of the falciform ligament. Advances in instrumentation (e.g., staplers) have allowed results of nonanatomic resections to replace anatomic resections without compromising outcomes in many circumstances; in particular, these nonanatomic resections are the usual approach in robotic or laparoscopic liver resections, especially if the targeted specimen is smaller than a hemiliver.

General Principles

As detailed earlier, in order to internationally standardize terminology for the reporting of hepatic resections, the Brisbane Liver Terminology was adopted in 2000. This terminology, including references to Couinaud segments, is depicted in Figs. 13.2 and 13.4, and we will adhere to it in in the describing various resections; note will be made where historical terminology would apply. An unambiguous description of a resection will specify the segments removed (e.g., bisegmentectomy 2,3 denotes removal of segments 2 and 3). As long as the size of the future liver remnant (FLR) is adequate, each Couinaud segment can be safely resected individually or in any combination with other segments. In general, a FLR consisting of at least 2 healthy contiguous segments is considered adequate; a more accurate assessment can be made with CT- or MRI-volumetric assessment of the FLR, whereby a 25% residual volume of a healthy liver will suffice.

Primary malignant liver tumors often arise in the setting of chronic liver disease/cirrhosis and are often multifocal. Metastatic tumors are often multifocal and involve multiple segments. Segment-oriented resection permits expansion of historic resectability criteria while still adhering to the principles of parenchymal preservation and tumor clearance. Combined with the increased effectiveness of systemic therapy for micrometastatic disease (especially in colorectal carcinoma), the ability to resect individual liver segments provides hope for patients with multifocal malignant liver tumors. Most benign liver tumors do not require resection, but there are circumstances where their removal is also clearly indicated. Knowledge of segment-oriented liver resection is a must for a liver surgeon's armamentarium to be complete.

To define the boundary of resection, the author's preferred intraoperative technique is referred to as the *Glissonian approach, more details of which can be found in references 2 and 3 at the end of this chapter.* The Glissonian approach takes advantage of the fact that the hepatic artery, portal vein, and bile duct divisions within the substance of the liver are maintained in a sheath of fibrous tissue (pedicle) that is palpably distinct from softer surrounding parenchyma. This sheath is the internal extension of Glisson's capsule, and the distinction is apparent even in fibrotic/cirrhotic livers. Identifying, clamping, and ligating these pedicles within the liver, while leaving the blood flow to the rest of the liver intact, will delineate the segment(s) supplied by that pedicle and, thus, the transection plane to be used in removing the segment(s). While the Glissonian approach is optimal for resections that require true delineation of segmental boundaries, a more common approach in the USA for hemihepatectomy is to ligate the right or left hepatic artery, portal vein, and hepatic duct extrahepatically, providing ischemic demarcation of the midplane of the liver and, thus, the transection plane for this operation. Because of the simplicity of dissection, the author's usual preference for these major operations is to still use the Glissonian approach even for hemihepatectomy. The experience and comfort level of the surgeon, along with lesion characteristics, should dictate the chosen method.

With knowledge of the intraparenchymal branching pattern of the main pedicle into right and left pedicles and their further branching into second- and third-order divisions, the Glissonian approach allows identification of separate segment-specific pedicles. In the right hemiliver, clamping third-order pedicles while allowing blood flow to the rest of the liver makes possible the surface delineation of the segment supplied by that pedicle. If a second-order pedicle in the right hemiliver is clamped, the demarcation encompasses two contiguous segments (e.g., clamping the right anterior pedicle demarcates both segments 5 and 8).

All liver resections, opened and minimally invasive, should balance the principle of maximum preservation of non-tumorous parenchyma with the necessity of obtaining adequate tumor clearance. While these goals can be met with nonanatomic resections, they are more consistently achieved through segment-oriented (anatomic) resection than by nonanatomic resection. Even for benign lesions where margins are less critical, segment-oriented resection has been associated with less blood loss. Because of the complexity of applying strict anatomic principle to minimally invasive liver resections, however, most robotic and laparoscopic liver resections are nonanatomic. This approach is associated with excellent, sometimes superior, outcomes and has been made possible with increasing experience and by the advancement of instrumentation (e.g., surgical staplers). These improvements have also led to increased utilization of the nonanatomic approach and open resections. As long as oncologic principles and blood loss can be kept in line with anatomic resections, there is no practical disadvantage to the nonanatomic approach. Still, the ability to do a true segment-oriented liver resection via the Glissonian approach enhances a liver surgeon's armamentarium and in some situations is clearly advantageous.

After the abdomen is entered, liver resections begin with visual, palpable, and/or sonographic assessment of the extent of disease (including the possibility of extrahepatic disease) and of the size and quality of the future liver remnant. This assessment will help determine if proceeding with resection is advisable from a risk/benefit perspective. Depending on the planned resection, the falciform, left triangular, hepatogastric, and/or right triangular ligaments are divided. The gallbladder, if present, is removed. Beginning caudad and proceeding cephalad, the liver is mobilized off the retrohepatic IVC by ligation and division of several small venous tributaries until the major hepatic veins (right, middle, left) are encountered. Occasionally, a large accessory right inferior hepatic vein (draining segments 6 and/or 7) is encountered. This accessory vein can be ligated with impunity unless it is expected to be the primary drainage of a remnant segment(s). If segment 1 (caudate) is to be resected, its venous drainage to the IVC is also carefully sacrificed. Because these veins are broad-based and have almost no extraparenchymal component, sacrificing them is more involved than sacrificing other direct IVC tributaries (dorsal hepatic veins). While some resections do not require full mobilization of the liver, the importance of adequate mobilization cannot be overemphasized. It helps the surgeon avoid and get out of trouble. Surgeon experience will dictate what extent is appropriate in an individual patient.

Parenchymal Transection Technique

Ongoing communication is maintained with the anesthesia staff to maintain a low (0–5 mmHg) central venous pressure (CVP), which minimizes blood loss during the parenchymal transection; this does not require formal CVP monitoring, though some surgeons prefer this. Suffice to say, restriction of intravenous fluids is a useful strategy. In addition to maintenance of a low CVP, Pringle maneuvers can minimize blood loss during parenchymal transection. Most resections can be performed with less than 20 min of total Pringle clamping by experienced surgeons. If parenchymal transection is expected to exceed 20 min, intermittent clamping lasting 10–15 min alternating with 5 min of unclamping is an effective strategy. Patients with well-compensated cirrhosis and patients with moderately steatotic livers are able to tolerate intermittent ischemia, as long as the cumulative clamp time is not excessive. If the segment(s) to be removed are rendered ischemic prior to parenchymal transection (by inflow ligation), a Pringle maneuver is arguably not necessary.

A detailed analysis of techniques and devices commonly employed during segment-oriented liver dissection is beyond the scope of this chapter. An incomplete list of transection techniques includes hydrojet or ultrasonic dissection, clamp-crushing technique, and precoagulation of the transection plane. Instrumentation includes ultrasonic aspirators, vessel sealing devices, and vascular staplers. Even if not used during the parenchymal transection, vascular staplers are useful devices for ligating/dividing pedicles and hepatic veins. To summarize, all the abovementioned techniques and devices are effective; the experience of the surgeon with each modality dictates the appropriate method.

Operations on the Right Hemiliver

Right Hemihepatectomy

This was formerly known as "right hepatic lobectomy." The liver is mobilized as described above and the gallbladder removed. For a Glissonian approach, a Pringle maneuver is performed. Hepatotomies are made anterior (incision #3, Fig. 13.28) and posterior (incision #4, Fig. 13.28) to the porta hepatis, taking care to avoid any recently ligated venous tributaries. Alternatively, hepatotomies in the gallbladder fossa (incision #2, Fig. 13.28) and in the caudate process parallel to and immediately to the right of the IVC (incision #1, Fig. 13.28) also provide good access to the right main pedicle and its branches. Glisson's capsule is incised immediately anterior to the hepatoduodenal ligament (lowering of the hilar plate). This step allows the parenchyma immediately anterosuperior to the plate to be gently pushed away, exposing the portal triad bifurcation into right and left main pedicles. With the surgeon on the patient's right side, the right index finger is inserted into the posterior hepatotomy and the right thumb into the anterior hepatotomy until they meet around the right main pedicle sheath (Figs. 13.29 and 13.30), around which an umbilical tape is passed (Fig. 13.31). Leftward traction on this tape protects the left-sided structures when the right main pedicle is clamped and stapled. (Note: placement of tapes around both main sheaths allows retraction of them into an almost extrahepatic location, facilitating further dissection.) Stapling the right main pedicle and

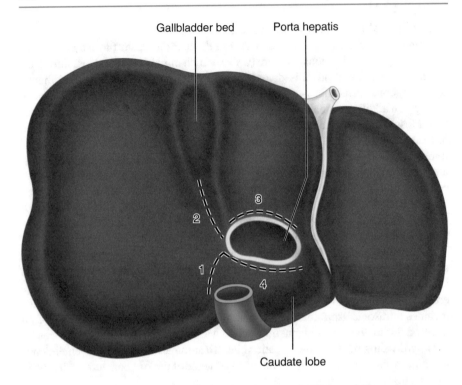

Fig. 13.28 Incisions used for the posterior intrahepatic approach: (*1*) through the caudate process, (*2*) through the gallbladder bed, (*3*) in front of the porta hepatis, (*4*) behind the porta hepatis

Fig. 13.29 The index finger passes behind the hilar structures and emerges above the confluence of the right and left Glissonian sheaths

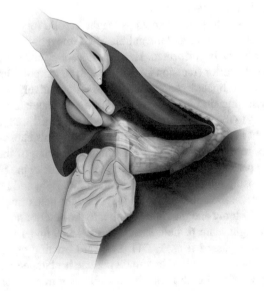

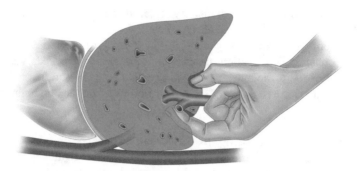

Fig. 13.30 Sagittal view of the posterior approach

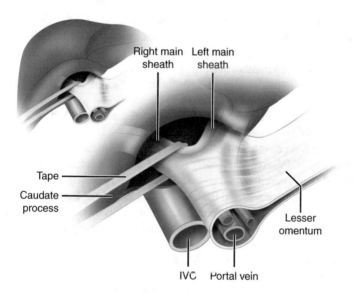

Fig. 13.31 Posterior approach for hemihepatectomy, showing tape around the confluence of the right main Glissonian sheath. Traction on this tape to the right (as shown) protects the right main pedicle and its contents from injury during stapling of the left main pedicle. Using the tape to place traction to the left will protect the left main pedicle during stapling of the right main pedicle

releasing the Pringle maneuver show the ischemic demarcation along the midplane of the liver; parenchymal transection will proceed immediately to the right of this demarcation.

Since the right hepatic artery, portal vein, and hepatic duct are amenable to extra-hepatic isolation, an alternate option to the Glissonian technique is to individually ligate them in the porta hepatis, resulting in the ischemic demarcation along the midplane. This is preferred by many surgeons in the USA, but the author's experience is that this dissection takes longer than isolating and clamping them en masse via the Glissonian technique, which can be done within 2–5 min. The Glissonian technique also avoids the need to identify replaced/accessory vessels and ducts, as these are also confined within the fibrous sheath.

After stapling the right main pedicle, the liver surface is scored with diathermy along the ischemic demarcation, parenchymal transection proceeds via one or a combination of the techniques mentioned above. The RHV can be encircled and ligated/divided prior to beginning the transection or as the last component of the resection.

Right Hemihepatectomy Using the Glissonian Approach

- **Step 1.** Divide the falciform and right triangular/coronary ligaments (Fig. 13.32); (dividing the hepatogastric and left triangular/coronary ligaments is sometimes useful as well to enhance mobilization).
- **Step 2.** Perform cholecystectomy.
- **Step 3.** Perform hepatic ultrasound (if applicable).
- **Step 4.** Mobilize the liver off the IVC; include segment 1 mobilization as appropriate. Depending on the circumstances, full mobilization might not be necessary.
- **Step 5.*** Apply Pringle maneuver.
- **Step 6.*** Make hepatotomies in appropriate locations (incisions #1 and #2, Fig. 13.28).
- **Step 7.*** Isolate and clamp/ligate right main pedicle (Figs. 13.29 and 13.30) and release Pringle.
- **Step 8.** Score liver along ischemic demarcation (midplane of liver).
- **Step 9.** Ligate RHV extrahepatically (Fig. 13.33); alternatively, the RHV can be ligated during the parenchymal transection.
- **Step 10.** Perform parenchymal transection, use Pringle as necessary.
- **Step 11.** Place drain if appropriate (i.e., biliary anastomosis, diaphragm resection, bile staining). These three occasions mandate placing a drain and are the only times one is indicated.
- **Step 12.** Reattach falciform and/or left triangular ligaments, if previously divided, to prevent torsion of liver remnant.
- **Step 13.** Close the incision according to general surgical principles.
  *For the non-Glissonian technique, replace steps 5–7 with individually dissecting and ligating the right hepatic artery, portal vein, and hepatic duct, as in Fig. 13.34.

Segmental Resections of the Right Hemiliver

The right main pedicle is isolated as described above. The sheaths surrounding the right anterior and posterior pedicles are identified by dissecting distally along the right main sheath. Clamping of selective pedicles delineates surface boundaries of corresponding sections and segments, allowing their individual removal. Although some surgeons utilize intraoperative ultrasound to facilitate identifying segmental boundaries, we have not found this step to be necessary.

If segment 6 only is to be removed, its pedicle is easily identified by performing hepatotomies through the caudate process and through the gallbladder bed (incisions #1 and #2, Fig. 13.28). The segment 6 pedicle is found approximately 2 cm deep to the gallbladder fossa.

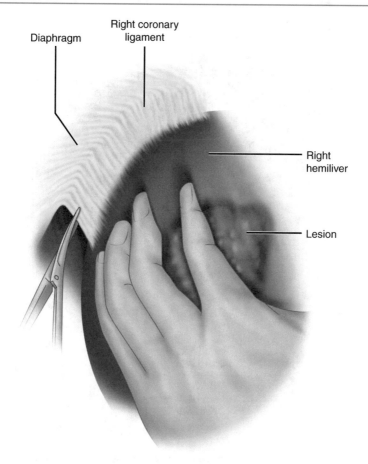

Fig. 13.32 Incising the right coronary ligament. Scissors are being used here; the electrocautery is more commonly used

As seen in Fig. 13.35, the segment 7 pedicle is deeper and directed superoposteriorly; therefore, it is more difficult to isolate singly. In the author's experience, the surface boundary of segment 7 is more easily identified by temporarily clamping the segment 6 pedicle. The inferior boundary of segment 7 is identical to the superior boundary of segment 6; its medial boundary is always the RHV. Therefore, a straight line from the visible extrahepatic (superior) aspect of the RHV to the medial boundary of segment 6 practically identifies the medial boundary of segment 7.

The (second-order) right anterior pedicle shortly divides into (third-order) pedicles to segments 5 and 8, with the segment 5 pedicle being easier to isolate singly. Clamping of the entire anterior sheath or either third-order sheath delineates segments 5 and/or 8 from the rest of the liver, allowing their removal together or separately. For the sake of surgical simplicity, segment 8 often is not removed alone; segment 5 is usually removed with it. However, adoption of the Glissonian approach allows segment 8-only resections to be performed when advisable.

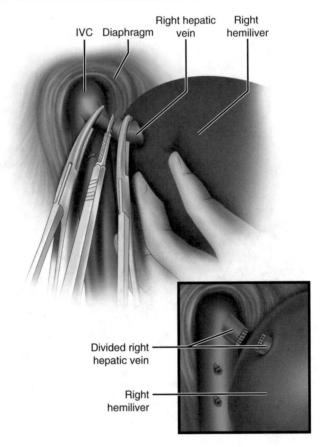

Fig. 13.33 IVC and its branches. *Inset*: RHV. The RHV is now more frequently divided with a vascular stapler

It is noteworthy that the inferior aspect of segment 5 is occasionally V-shaped and, therefore, may not extend far (if at all) to the right of the gallbladder fossa. This finding is relevant in anatomic resections done for gallbladder cancer (which minimally include segments 4B and 5) and indicates that segment 6 will also need to be included in the resection.

Unless an accessory inferior hepatic vein is first encountered and preserved, the RHV must be preserved during a right anterior sectionectomy (bisegmentecomy 5,8). Because the right anterior section is also drained by tributaries to the MHV, the RHV can be sacrificed in a right posterior sectionectomy (bisegmentectomy 6,7). Our routine practice is to preserve the RHV in right-sided resections other than hemihepatectomies. If preservation of the vein compromises oncologic clearance, then a right hemihepatectomy is likely more advisable than attempting to spare the RHV by a less comprehensive resection.

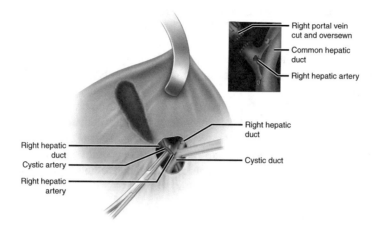

Fig. 13.34 Contents of right portal pedicle ligated individually. This is not done with the Glissonian technique; it requires more time but is sometimes necessary (e.g., centrally located tumors, living-donor liver transplantation)

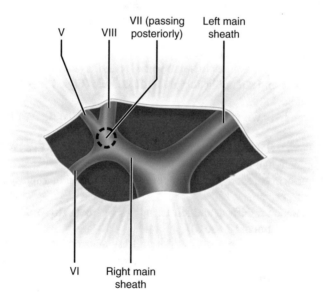

Fig. 13.35 Posterior approach showing the sheaths that are usually exposed on the right side

Right-Sided Segment-Oriented Resections Using the Glissonian Approach

- **Step 1.** Divide the falciform and right triangular/coronary ligaments (dividing the hepatogastric and left triangular/coronary ligaments is sometimes useful as well).
- **Step 2.** Perform cholecystectomy.

- **Step 3.** Perform hepatic ultrasound (if applicable).
- **Step 4.** Mobilize the liver off the IVC; include segment 1 mobilization as appropriate.
- **Step 5.** Apply Pringle maneuver.
- **Step 6.** Make hepatotomies in appropriate locations (incisions #1 and #2, Fig. 13.28).
- **Step 7.** Isolate and clamp/ligate pedicle(s) to segments to be resected.
- **Step 8.** Release Pringle and score liver along ischemic demarcation.
- **Step 9.** Perform parenchymal transection, use Pringle as necessary.
- **Step 10.** Place drain if appropriate (i.e., biliary anastomosis, diaphragm resection, bile staining). These three occasions mandate placing a drain and are the only times one is indicated.
- **Step 11.** Close the incision.

Right Trisectionectomy (Removal of Segments 4, 5, 6, 7, and 8 [and Sometimes 1]; Formerly Known as "Right Trisegmentectomy")

- **Step 1.** Divide the falciform and right and left triangular/coronary ligaments.
- **Step 2.** Perform cholecystectomy.
- **Step 3.** Perform hepatic ultrasound (if applicable).
- **Step 4.** Mobilize the liver off the IVC; include segment 1 mobilization as appropriate.
- **Step 5.*** Apply Pringle maneuver.
- **Step 6.*** Make hepatotomies in appropriate locations (Fig. 13.28).
- **Step 7.*** Isolate and clamp/ligate right main pedicle (Figs. 13.29 and 13.30) and release Pringle.
- **Step 8.** Score liver with electrocautery immediately to the right of the falciform ligament.
- **Step 9.** Ligate RHV extrahepatically; alternatively, the RHV can be ligated during the parenchymal transection.
- **Step 10.** Perform parenchymal transection, carefully avoiding injury to the LHV, use Pringle as necessary.
- **Step 11.** Reattach falciform and left triangular ligaments to avoid torsion of the liver remnant (segments 2 and 3).
- **Step 12.** Place drain if appropriate (i.e., biliary anastomosis, diaphragm resection, bile staining). These three occasions mandate placing a drain and are the only times one is indicated.
- **Step 13.** Reattach falciform and left triangular ligaments to prevent torsion of liver remnant (segments 2 and 3).
- **Step 14.** Close the incision.
  *For the non-Glissonian technique, replace steps 5–7 with individually dissecting and ligating the right hepatic artery, portal vein, and hepatic duct, as in Fig. 13.34.

Operations on the Left Hemiliver

The left main pedicle extends leftward and anteriorly into the umbilical fissure. It can be isolated, and an umbilical tape can be passed around it as described above, using hepatotomies in front of and behind the porta hepatis (incisions #3 and #4, Fig. 13.28). Rightward traction on the tape protects right-sided vessels/ducts upon clamping/stapling of the left main pedicle (Fig. 13.31).

The (second-order) pedicles to segments 2, 3, 4A, and 4B originate within the umbilical fissure. Segments 2 and 3 pedicles pass leftward, and 4A/4B pedicles pass rightward; therefore, the umbilical fissure and falciform ligament mark the boundary between segments 2 and 3 (left lateral section) and segment 4. A bridge of tissue of varying size usually spans superficial to and across the ligamentum teres within the umbilical fissure. The tissue bridge (if present) can be divided with impunity to access the second-order pedicles or to facilitate any left-sided resection where segments 2, 3, and 4 are not removed in unison.

Left Hemihepatectomy

This was formerly known as "left hepatic lobectomy." The liver is mobilized as described above and the gallbladder removed. A Pringle maneuver is performed. Hepatotomies are made anterior (incision #3 in Fig. 13.28) and posterior (incision #4 in Fig. 13.28) to the porta hepatis. The left main pedicle is isolated intrahepatically and clamped/ligated, resulting in ischemic demarcation of the midplane of the liver. Since the MHVs and LHVs usually converge and have a shorter extrahepatic component, extrahepatic isolation of either or both is not as easy as isolation of the RHV; therefore, these veins usually are sacrificed intrahepatically during the transection. The liver surface is scored along the ischemic line, followed by parenchymal transection utilizing one or a combination of the abovementioned techniques. For reasons noted above, the LHV and/or MHV is usually sacrificed within the parenchyma during the parenchymal transection.

- **Step 1.** Divide the falciform, left triangular/coronary, and hepatogastric ligaments (Fig. 13.36). Dividing the right triangular ligament is sometimes useful as well to enhance mobilization.
- **Step 2.** Perform cholecystectomy.
- **Step 3.** Perform hepatic ultrasound (if applicable).
- **Step 4.** Mobilize the liver off the IVC; include segment 1 mobilization as appropriate. Depending on the circumstances, full mobilization of the liver off the IVC might not be necessary.
- **Step 5.*** Apply Pringle maneuver.
- **Step 6.*** Make hepatotomies in appropriate locations (incisions #3 and #4, Fig. 13.28).
- **Step 7.*** Isolate and clamp/ligate left main pedicle (Figs. 13.29 and 13.30) and release Pringle.
- **Step 8.** Score liver along ischemic demarcation (midplane of liver).

- **Step 9.** The LHV and MHV are usually not ligated extrahepatically and will be divided during the parenchymal transection. Vascular staplers are excellent tools for this.
- **Step 10.** Perform parenchymal transection, use Pringle as necessary.
- **Step 11.** Place drain if appropriate (i.e., biliary anastomosis, diaphragm resection, bile staining). These three occasions mandate placing a drain and are the only times one is indicated.
- **Step 12.** Reattach falciform ligament if it and the right triangular ligament were divided, to prevent torsion of liver remnant.
- **Step 13.** Close the incision according to general surgical principles.
  *For the non-Glissonian technique, replace steps 5–7 with individually dissecting and ligating the left hepatic artery, portal vein, and hepatic duct (Fig. 13.37).

Removal of Segments 2 and 3

This is also called left lateral sectionectomy or sectorectomy and was formerly known as "left lateral segmentectomy." Mobilization of the liver off the IVC is not necessary for removal of segments 2 and 3 (left lateral sectionectomy) or either segment separately; a Pringle maneuver is not always necessary. To perform a bisegmentectomy 2,3, Glisson's capsule is scored with diathermy immediately to the left of the falciform ligament. The pedicles to segments 2 and/or 3 can be taken during

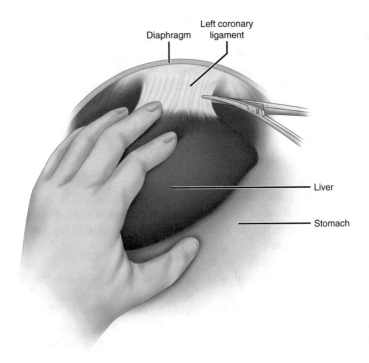

Fig. 13.36 Division of left triangular/coronary ligaments. Scissors are being used here; the electrocautery is more commonly used.

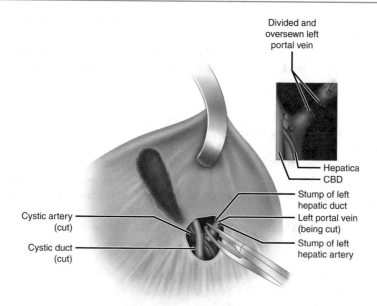

Fig. 13.37 Division of left portal vein. *Inset*: detailed view. Also, a vascular stapler is a useful tool for dividing the left portal vein

(standard technique) or before (Glissonian approach) the parenchymal transection, depending on the ease of access. If either segment 2 or 3 only is to be removed, clamping the appropriate pedicle and scoring the liver along the ischemic demarcation precedes the parenchymal transection.

- **Step 1.** Divide the falciform, left triangular, and hepatogastric ligaments.
- **Step 2.** Perform hepatic ultrasound (if applicable).
- **Step 3.** Score liver immediately to the left of the falciform ligament.
- **Step 4.** Isolate and ligate pedicles to segments 2 and 3; or (more commonly) they can be taken during the parenchymal transection.
- **Step 5.** The LHV is usually not ligated extrahepatically and will be divided during the parenchymal transection. Vascular staplers are excellent tools for this.
- **Step 6.** Perform parenchymal transection. Pringle is usually not necessary.
- **Step 7.** Place drain if appropriate (i.e., biliary anastomosis, diaphragm resection, bile staining). These three occasions mandate placing a drain and are the only times one is indicated.
- **Step 8.** Close incision.

(Mono)segmentectomy 2 or 3 Using the Glissonian Approach

Step 1. Divide the falciform, left triangular, and hepatogastric ligaments.
Step 2. Perform hepatic ultrasound (if applicable).
Step 3. Apply Pringle maneuver.
Step 4. Isolate and clamp/ligate appropriate pedicle.

Step 5. Release Pringle and score liver along line of ischemic demarcation.

Step 6. Perform parenchymal transection.

Step 7. Place drain if appropriate (i.e., biliary anastomosis, diaphragm resection, bile staining). These three occasions mandate placing a drain and are the only times one is indicated.

Step 8. Close incision.

Segmentectomy 4A and/or 4B

It is unusual to remove segments 4A and/or 4B only. The midplane of the liver and the falciform ligament will mark the right and left resection boundaries, respectively. Following the procedures described above, the pedicles to segments 4A and/or 4B can be taken during or before the parenchymal transection, depending on the ease of access.

- **Step 1.** Divide falciform, left triangular, right triangular, and hepatogastric ligaments.
- **Step 2.** Perform cholecystectomy.
- **Step 3.** Perform hepatic ultrasound (if applicable).
- **Step 4.** Mobilize liver off IVC; include segment 1 mobilization as appropriate.
- **Step 5.** Isolate and ligate pedicles to 4A and/or 4B, depending on targeted specimen.
- **Step 6.** Score liver immediately to the right of the falciform ligament and along ischemic demarcation.
- **Step 7.** Perform parenchymal transection, during which the MHV will be sacrificed.
- **Step 8.** Place drain if appropriate (i.e., biliary anastomosis, diaphragm resection, bile staining). These three occasions mandate placing a drain and are the only times one is indicated.
- **Step 9.** Close incision.

Left Trisectionectomy (Removal of Segments 2, 3, 4, 5, 8 [and Sometimes 1]; Formerly "Left Trisegmentectomy")

- **Step 1.** Divide falciform, left triangular/coronary, right triangular/coronary, and hepatogastric ligaments.
- **Step 2.** Perform cholecystectomy.
- **Step 3.** Perform hepatic ultrasound (if applicable).
- **Step 4.** Mobilize liver off IVC; include segment 1 mobilization.
- **Step 5.*** Apply Pringle maneuver.
- **Step 6.*** Make hepatotomies in appropriate locations (incisions #3 and #4, Fig. 13.28).
- **Step 7.*** Isolate and clamp/ligate right anterior section pedicle (to segment 5 and 8; Figs. 13.29 and 13.30). From the right side of the table, identifying this pedicle can simply be done by placing the right index finger into the incision #3 and sweeping toward the right along the right main sheath.
- **Step 8.** Release Pringle.

- **Step 9.** Core liver along ischemic demarcation (between right anterior and posterior sections, along the course of the RHV).
- **Step 10.** Perform parenchymal transection, carefully preserving the RHV.
- **Step 11.** Place drain if appropriate (i.e., biliary anastomosis, diaphragm resection, bile staining). These three occasions mandate placing a drain and are the only times one is indicated.
- **Step 12.** Close incision.

Segment 1 (Caudate) Resection

Caudate resection is rarely indicated but deserves special mention due to its complexity. Segment 1 is not solely part of the right hemiliver or left hemiliver; it receives blood supply from and drains bile into both sides. The short and broad-based nature of its venous drainage requires special care to avoid injury and major hemorrhage during mobilization of segment 1 off the IVC. Once this segment is disconnected from the IVC, the parenchyma overlying the plane (dorsal fissure, denoted by the insertion of the hepatogastric ligament) between segment 1 posteriorly and segments 4 and 8 anteriorly is scored. The pedicles supplying segment 1 are sacrificed during the ensuing parenchymal transection.

Central Liver Resections

Central liver resections involve removal of segments 4A, 4B, 5, and/or 8. The details as outlined above will allow the surgeon to combine all of these segments in a single resection ("mesohepatectomy" or, more appropriately, trisegmentectomy 4,5,8) or in any combination. Therefore, with knowledge of intrahepatic segmental anatomy, tumors in the central portion of the liver can be removed without unnecessarily sacrificing the parenchyma in a right or left trisectionectomy. The ability to perform these types of resections is crucial during operations on patients with chronic fibrotic liver disease or with evidence of chemotherapy-induced steatosis. During these operations, adherence to the principle of non-tumorous parenchymal preservation lessens the chances of postoperative liver failure.

Intrahepatic isolation and clamping of the appropriate pedicles through the techniques outlined in steps above delineates the surface boundaries of the resection to be performed, thereby allowing parenchymal transection to be performed in a segmental fashion. The MHV usually joins the LHV before entering the IVC as a common orifice; thus, isolating it extrahepatically is not usually feasible or safe. Therefore, the MHV is sacrificed when it is encountered during the parenchymal transection.

Minimally Invasive Hepatic Resection

Laparoscopic and, more recently, robotic liver resections have gained favor due to inherent advantages of minimally invasive surgery (MIS). Because of logistical and practical reasons, most of these approaches are nonanatomic and take advantage of advances in surgical instrumentation, particularly the use of vessel sealers and staplers in parenchymal transection. Despite the historical advantages inherent in open anatomic resections, these advances have made nonanatomic MIS resections practical, sometimes even superior, alternatives to open resection. Anatomic MIS resections are also increasingly being done. Coupled with the inherent MIS advantages in surgical morbidity, MIS resection by experienced surgeons is the more appropriate approach in a majority of patients today. A full step-by-step illustration of MIS hepatic resection is beyond the scope of this chapter, but several excellent textbooks singly devoted to this topic are available and recommended (e.g., reference 4 at the end of this chapter). Appropriate oncologic principles remain sovereign, and MIS resection should not be attempted if these principles would be expectedly compromised.

Anatomical Complications

- Bleeding from a hepatic vein, portal vein, or inferior vena cava
- Air embolism from an inadvertent injury to the hepatic vein
- Budd Chiari syndrome from thrombosis of a hepatic vein postoperatively
- Hepatic ischemia from arterial or portal vein thrombosis
- Biliary fistulas from ductal damage during portal dissection or from inadequate ligation of ducts during parenchymal transection
- Hepatic insufficiency from ischemia after extended hepatectomy
- Injury to the right hepatic artery originating from the superior mesenteric artery during dissection of the hepatoduodenal ligament
- Anastomotic leak of hepaticojejunostomy
- Portal vein thrombosis
- Adjacent organ injury: duodenum, colon, or diaphragm

References

References are suggested reading for anyone desiring a more thorough description of segment-oriented and minimally invasive liver resections.

1. Asbun H, Geller D. ACS multimedia atlas of surgery: liver surgery volume. Chicago: American College of Surgeons; 2014.
2. Launois B, Jamieson GG. The posterior intrahepatic approach for hepatectomy or removal of segments of the liver. Surg Gynecol Obstet. 1992;174:155.
3. Launois B, Jamieson GG. The posterior intrahepatic approach in liver surgery. New York: Landes Bioscience/Springer; 2013.
4. Strasberg SM. Nomenclature of hepatic anatomy and resections: a review of the Brisbane 2000 system. J Hepato-Biliary-Pancreat Surg. 2005;12:351.

Extrahepatic Biliary Tract

14

Mohammad Raheel Jajja and Snehal Patel

Anatomy

Right, Left, and Common Hepatic Ducts

The right and left hepatic ducts join soon after emerging from the liver to form the common hepatic duct (Fig. 14.1b). The junction lies 0.25–2.5 cm from the surface of the liver. The left duct is longer (1.7 cm, average) and has a longer extrahepatic course than the right duct (0.9 cm, average). In some cases, intrahepatic junction of the hepatic ducts is the result of liver enlargement (Fig. 14.1a); retraction of the liver may then be necessary to expose the junction.

Measurements of the common hepatic duct are highly variable. The duct is said to be absent if the cystic duct enters at the junction of the right and left hepatic ducts (Fig. 14.1c). In most individuals, the duct is between 1.5 and 3.5 cm long.

Three types of cystohepatic junction have been described: angular (Fig. 14.1a, b), parallel (Fig. 14.2a), and spiral (Fig. 14.2b, c).

M. R. Jajja
Department of Surgery, Winship Cancer Institute, Emory University, Atlanta, GA, USA

S. Patel (✉)
Department of Surgery, Emory University, Atlanta, GA, USA
e-mail: snehal.patel@emory.edu

© Springer Nature Switzerland AG 2021
L. J. Skandalakis (ed.), *Surgical Anatomy and Technique*,
https://doi.org/10.1007/978-3-030-51313-9_14

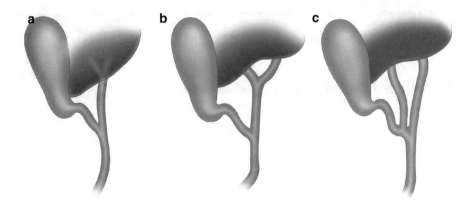

Fig. 14.1 Variations of the hepatic ducts. (**a**) Intrahepatic union of left and right hepatic ducts; (**b**) usual extrahepatic union of left and right hepatic ducts; (**c**) distal union of hepatic ducts producing absence of the common hepatic duct

Anomalous Hepatic Ducts: Surgically Significant Sources of Bile Leakage (Fig. 14.3)

An aberrant hepatic duct is a normal segmental duct that joins the biliary tract just outside the liver instead of just within; it drains a normal portion of the liver. Such a duct passing through the hepatocystic triangle is important because it is subject to inadvertent section with subsequent bile leakage (Fig. 14.3).

Subvesicular bile ducts, found in approximately 35% of individuals, are small blind ducts emerging from the right lobe of the liver and lying in the bed of the gallbladder. They do not communicate with the gallbladder.

Hepatocystic ducts drain bile from the liver directly into the body of the gallbladder or into the cystic duct.

Occasionally, the right, left, or even both hepatic ducts enter the gallbladder. This is an argument in favor of removing the gallbladder at the fundus, from above downward.

Cystic Duct

The cystic duct is about 3 mm in diameter and about 2–4 cm long. If surgeons are unprepared for a short duct (Fig. 14.2e), they may find themselves inadvertently entering the common bile duct. If they underestimate the length, they may leave too long a stump, predisposing to the cystic duct remnant syndrome.

Very rarely, the cystic duct is absent, and the gallbladder opens directly into the common bile duct. In such a case, the common bile duct might be mistaken for the cystic duct.

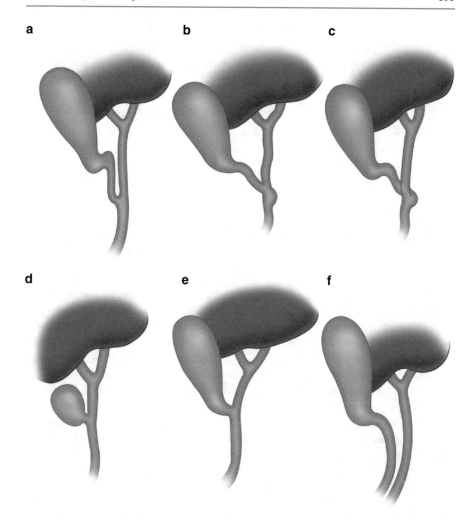

Fig. 14.2 Types of cystohepatic junction. (**a**) Parallel type. (**b, c**) Spiral types. (**d, e**) Short cystic ducts. (**f**) A long cystic duct ending in the duodenum. This may also be called "absence of the common bile duct"

Gallbladder

The gallbladder is located on the visceral surface of the liver in a shallow fossa at the plane dividing the right lobe from the medial segment of the left lobe (the GB-IVC line). The gallbladder is separated from the liver by the connective tissue of Glisson's capsule. Anteriorly, the peritoneum of the gallbladder is continuous with that of the liver, and the fundus is completely covered with peritoneum.

a   b   c

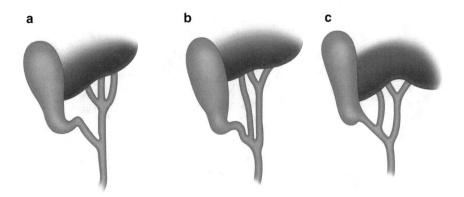

Fig. 14.3 Accessory hepatic ducts. (**a**) Accessory duct joins the common duct along with the usual left and right hepatic ducts. (**b**) Accessory duct joins at the intersection of the cystic duct. (**c**) Accessory duct enters the cystic duct directly. Additional, minute hepatic ducts are not unusual

The body of the gallbladder is in contact with the first and second portions of the duodenum. The body is also related to the transverse colon. Only in the rare presence of a mesentery (wandering gallbladder), a prerequisite for acute torsion, is the body completely covered by peritoneum. Several other anomalous peritoneal folds connected with the body of the gallbladder – cholecystogastric, cholecystoduodenal, and cholecystocolic – are redundancies of the lesser omentum.

The infundibulum is the angulated posterior portion of the body between the neck and the point of entrance to the cystic artery. When this portion is dilated, with eccentric bulging of its medial aspect, it is called a Hartmann's pouch. When this pouch achieves considerable size, the cystic duct arises from its upper left aspect rather than from what appears to be the apex of the gallbladder. The pouch is often associated with chronic or acute inflammation due to lithiasis and often accompanies a stone impacted in the infundibulum.

The neck of the gallbladder is S-shaped and lies in the free border of the hepatoduodenal ligament. The mucosa lining the neck is a spiral ridge said to be a spiral valve, but not to be confused with the spiral valve of the cystic duct (the valve of Heister).

A deformity of the gallbladder seen in 2–6% of individuals is the Phrygian cap (Fig. 14.4a). Hartmann's pouch (Fig. 14.4b) is probably a normal variation rather than a true deformity.

Common Bile Duct

The length of the common bile duct begins at the union of the cystic and common hepatic ducts and ends at the papilla of Vater in the second part of the duodenum. It varies from 5 to 16 cm depending on the actual position of the ductal union. The duct can be divided into four portions (Fig. 14.5): supraduodenal, retroduodenal, pancreatic, and intramural (intraduodenal).

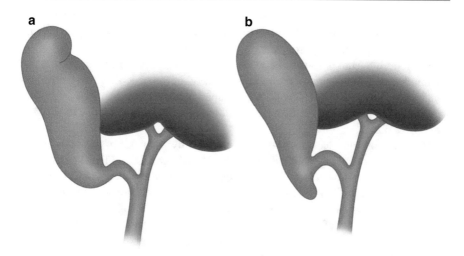

Fig. 14.4 Deformities of the gallbladder. (**a**) "Phrygian cap" deformity; (**b**) Hartmann's pouch

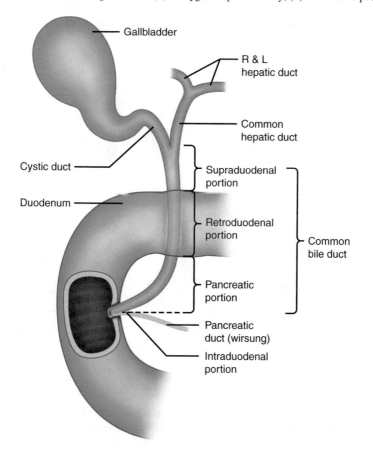

Fig. 14.5 The extrahepatic biliary tract and the four portions of the common bile duct

The supraduodenal portion lies between the layers of the hepatoduodenal ligament in front of the epiploic foramen of Winslow, to the right or left of the hepatic artery, and anterior to the portal vein.

The retroduodenal portion is between the superior margin of the first portion of the duodenum and the superior margin of the head of the pancreas. The gastroduodenal artery lies to the left. The posterior superior pancreaticoduodenal artery lies anterior to the common bile duct. The middle colic artery lies anterior to the duct and other arteries.

The common bile duct may be partly covered by a tongue of pancreas (44%) (Fig. 14.6a, b); completely within the pancreatic substance (30%) (Fig. 14.6c); uncovered on the pancreatic surface (16.5%) (Fig. 14.6d); or completely covered by two tongues of pancreas (9%) (Fig. 14.6e). Even when completely covered, the groove or tunnel occupied by the duct may be palpated by passing the fingers of the left hand behind the second part of the duodenum after mobilization with the Kocher maneuver.

The normal outside diameter of the first three regions of the common bile duct is variable, but a common bile duct more than 8 mm in diameter is considered enlarged and, therefore, pathological. Radiological studies in asymptomatic patients demonstrate an increase 0.3 mm increase in CBD diameter for every decade of life after age 20 with average CBD diameter being 4 mm (based on end-expiration MRCP images).

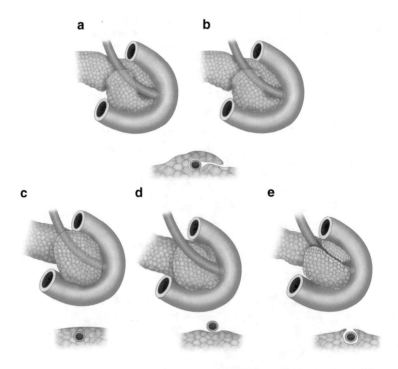

Fig. 14.6 Relation of the pancreas and the common bile duct. (**a, b**) The duct is partially covered by a tongue of pancreas (44%). (**c**) The duct is completely covered by the pancreas (30%). (**d**) The duct lies free on the surface of the pancreas (16.5%). (**e**) The duct is covered by two tongues of pancreas with a cleavage plane between

The fourth, or intramural (sometimes called intraduodenal), portion of the common bile duct (see Fig. 9.9) passes obliquely through the duodenal wall together with the main pancreatic duct. Within the wall, the length averages 15 mm. As it enters the wall, the common duct decreases in diameter. The two ducts usually lie side by side with a common adventitia for several millimeters. The septum between the ducts reduces to a thin mucosal membrane before the ducts become confluent (see Chap. 9).

Hepatocystic Triangle and Triangle of Calot

The hepatocystic triangle is formed by the proximal part of the gallbladder and cystic duct to the right, the common hepatic duct to the left, and the margin of the right lobe of the liver superiorly (Fig. 14.7). The triangle originally described by Calot defined the upper boundary as the cystic artery. The area included in the triangle has enlarged over the years to include the lower edge of the right lobe as the superior, the common hepatic duct as the medial, and the cystic duct as the inferior-lateral boundaries. Within the boundaries of the triangle as it is now defined are several structures that must be identified before they are ligated or sectioned.

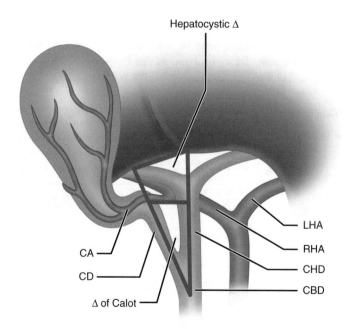

Fig. 14.7 The hepatocystic triangle and the triangle of Calot. The upper boundary of the hepatocystic triangle is the margin of the liver; that of the triangle of Calot is the cystic artery; the triangle of Calot is stippled. *CA* cystic artery, *CD* cystic duct, *CBD* common bile duct, *RHA* right hepatic artery, *LHA* left hepatic artery, *CHD* common hepatic duct

The hepatocystic triangle contains the right hepatic artery (and sometimes an aberrant right hepatic artery), the cystic artery, and sometimes an aberrant (accessory) bile duct.

In 87% of individuals, the right hepatic artery enters the triangle posterior to the common hepatic duct, and in 13% it enters anterior to it. In one study of cadavers, the right hepatic artery could have been mistaken for the cystic artery 20% of the time. As a rule of thumb, any artery more than 3 mm in diameter within the triangle will probably not be a cystic artery.

In 18%, there was an aberrant right hepatic artery. In 83% of these specimens, the cystic artery arose from the aberrant artery within the triangle. In 4%, the aberrant artery was accessory to a normal right hepatic artery, and in 14%, it was a replacing artery, the only blood supply to the right lobe of the liver (see Fig. 13.8).

The cystic artery usually arises from the right hepatic artery or an aberrant right hepatic artery within the hepatocystic triangle. At the neck of the gallbladder, the cystic artery divides into a superficial and a deep branch (Table 14.1).

In 16%, there were aberrant (accessory) bile ducts within the hepatocystic triangle that may cause bile to leak into the abdominal cavity.

Vascular System of the Extrahepatic Biliary Tract

Arterial Supply
In general, the major blood vessels to the extrahepatic biliary tree are posterior to the ducts, but in several cases they may lie anteriorly. The surgeon must recognize and preserve these arteries. Table 14.2 shows the frequency with which specific arteries are found anterior to segments of the biliary tract.

Table 14.1 Origin of the cystic artery

Origin	Percent
Right hepatic artery	
Normal	61.4
Aberrant (accessory)	10.2
Aberrant (replacing)	3.1
Left hepatic artery	5.9
Bifurcation of common hepatic artery	11.5
	92.1
Common hepatic artery	3.8
	95.9
Gastroduodenal artery	2.5
Superior pancreaticoduodenal artery	0.15
Right gastric artery	0.15
Celiac trunk	0.3
Superior mesenteric artery	0.9
Right gastroepiploic artery	Rare
Aorta	Rare
	99.9

Data from BJ Anson. Anatomical considerations in surgery of gallbladder. *Q Bull Northwest Univ Med School.* 1956;30:250

The gallbladder is supplied by the cystic artery. The bile ducts are supplied by branches of the posterior superior pancreaticoduodenal, retroduodenal, and right and left hepatic arteries. Do not devascularize more than 2–3 cm of the upper surface of the duct (Fig. 14.8).

Table 14.2 Segments of the biliary tract and the frequency of arteries lying anterior to them

Segment	Artery anterior	Percent frequency
Right and left hepatic ducts	Right hepatic artery	12–15
	Cystic artery	<5
Common hepatic duct	Cystic artery	15–24
	Right hepatic artery	11–19
	Common hepatic artery	<5
Supraduodenal common bile duct	Anterior artery to common bile duct	50
	Posterior superior pancreaticoduodenal artery	12.5
	Gastroduodenal artery	5.7–20[a]
	Right gastric artery	<5
	Common hepatic artery	<5
	Cystic artery	<5
	Right hepatic artery	<5
Retroduodenal common bile duct	Posterior superior pancreaticoduodenal artery	76–87.5
	Supraduodenal artery	11.4

Data from Johnson and Anson. *Surg Gynecol Obstet* 1952;94:669 and Maingot (ed.), *Abdominal Operations*, 6th ed. Norwalk, CT: Appleton & Lange, 1974
[a]In another 36%, the gastroduodenal artery lay on the left border of the common bile duct

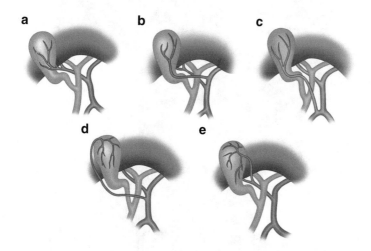

Fig. 14.8 Some possible origins of the cystic artery. (**a**) Usual pattern (74.7%) from the right normal or aberrant hepatic artery. (**b**) Origin from the common hepatic artery, its bifurcation, or from the left hepatic artery and crossing in front of the common hepatic duct (20.5%). (**c**) Origin from the gastroduodenal artery (2.5%). The remainder arises from a variety of sources. (**d, e**) Very rarely the cystic artery reaches the gallbladder at the fundus or body ("recurrent" cystic artery)

The blood supply of the supraduodenal common bile duct is essentially axial. The major supply comes from below (60% from the retroduodenal artery), and 38% comes from above (from the right hepatic artery). The bile ducts in the hilum and the retropancreatic bile duct have an excellent blood supply.

Ischemia of the bile duct can be avoided with a high or low transection, but bleeding of the edges should be checked prior to anastomosis.

Venous Drainage
Several cystic veins, rather than one, enter the hepatic parenchyma (Fig. 14.9).

An epicholodochal venous plexus helps the surgeon identify the common bile duct. Remember that stripping of the common bile duct is not permissible.

Lymphatic Drainage
Collecting lymphatic trunks from the gallbladder drain into the cystic node in the crotch of the junction of the cystic and common hepatic ducts to the "node of the hiatus" and posterior pancreaticoduodenal nodes (Fig. 14.10).

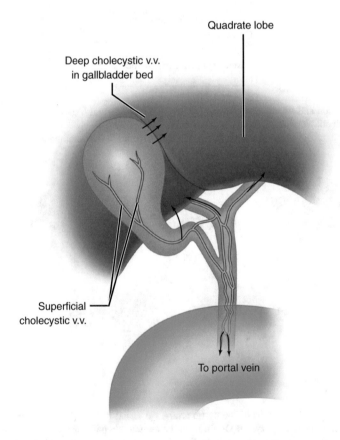

Fig. 14.9 Venous drainage of the biliary tract. Most of the drainage is from the gallbladder bed into the quadrate lobe of the liver. Veins of the duct system drain upward to the liver and downward to the portal vein

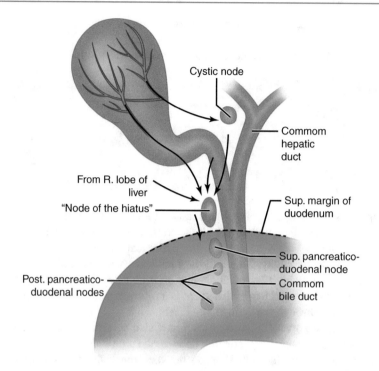

Fig. 14.10 Lymphatic drainage of the biliary tract. The cystic node and the node of the hiatus are relatively constant. Drainage from the gallbladder, the cystic duct, and the right lobe of the liver reaches the posterior pancreaticoduodenal nodes

The pericholedochal nodes receive lymphatics from the extrahepatic bile ducts and from the right lobe of the liver.

Technique

Cholecystectomy

Three procedures for cholecystectomy are presented: (1) laparoscopic (robotic) cholecystectomy, (2) removal of the gallbladder from above downward, and (3) removal of the gallbladder from below upward

Laparoscopic and Robotic Cholecystectomy

Figure 14.11 shows port placement. Functions of each port follow (Table 14.3):

Procedure

Position: Supine on X-ray operating room table
    Anesthesia: General
    Other: Knee-high pneumatic apparatus. Foley catheter and nasogastric tube placement is not routinely recommended and should be tailored to expected level of case difficulty and operative time.

- **Step 1.** Using a No. 10 scalpel blade, make a longitudinal 5-mm incision in the umbilical area long enough to permit the entrance of a 5-mm trocar.
- **Step 2.** Insert a Veress needle into the peritoneal cavity at a 45-degree angle toward the pelvic cavity. This may be facilitated with upward traction of the abdominal wall using two towel clamps on each side of the incision. Aspirate with a 10–20-cm³ syringe, and if there is no return with the aspiration, inject normal saline through the syringe.
    Alternatively an open Hasson approach may also be utilized for gaining access to the peritoneal cavity by dissecting down to the rectus sheath and lifting it with Kocher clamps. An incision is made between the clamps and 10-mm trocar inserted under direct visualization.

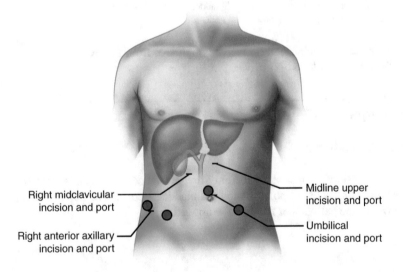

Fig. 14.11 Sites of incisions and ports. For robotic cholecystectomy, we recommend moving the right midclavicular port to the midpoint of the line between the umbilical port and the right anterior axillary line port. The midline upper port can be moved to the left abdomen to mirror the contralateral midclavicular port. The closed blue circles represent one iteration of the working ports for a robotic cholecystectomy

Table 14.3 Laproscopic cholecystectomy port placement

Umbilical	Laparoscopic examination of the peritoneal cavity; gallbladder localization; removal of the gallbladder
Upper midline	Surgical dissection of the gallbladder and partially of the hepatic triad at the hilum; clips may be accommodated through this port
Right anterior axillary line	Retraction of the gallbladder
Right midclavicular line	Retraction of the gallbladder

- **Step 3.** If normal saline is easily injected, insufflate CO_2.

Remember
- During insufflation, the intraperitoneal pressure should be 0–5 mm, except when the Veress needle is not well placed. With obesity, initial pressure may be a little higher.

- **Step 4.** If abdominal distention is satisfactory, proceed with the following "trocar steps," for robotic cholecystectomy see Fig. 14.11 for the suggested port placement.
  - (a) Insert a 5-mm trocar at the umbilical area at a 45-degree angle cephalad.
  - (b) Insert the laparoscope with the attached camera.
  - (c) erform laparoscopic inspection and begin exploration for any gross pathology.
  - (d) Visualize the gallbladder.
  - (e) Under direct vision, insert a 5-mm trocar through the incision at the upper midline or to the right of the midline or a similar incision. The need for narrow or wide costal margins and the patient's length of trunk should be considered because low placement will clash with the laparoscope, while in high placement the liver will interfere with dissection.
  - (f) Also under direct vision, place the remaining two 5-mm trocars at the right anterior axillary line and the right midclavicular line.
  - (g) Set the table in reverse Trendelenburg with rolling to the left.
- **Step 5.** Retract the dome of the gallbladder anteriorly and upward by grasping the fundus with the port of the anterior axillary line. Grasp Hartmann's pouch with the port at the midclavicular line and retract laterally (Fig. 14.12).
- **Step 6.** Dissect and visualize the cystic duct and common bile duct. Begin dissection by incising the peritoneal reflections both medially and laterally to the gallbladder. If a cholangiogram is required, it may be done through the cystic duct prior to its ligation.
- **Step 7.** Make sure to visualize the critical view of safety. The three components needed to achieve CVS are (1) the hepatocystic triangle is cleared of fat and fibrous tissue. (2) The lower one third of the gallbladder is separated from the liver to expose the cystic plate. (3) Two and only two structures should be seen

Fig. 14.12 Gallbladder is
raised. Hartman's pouch is
retracted laterally

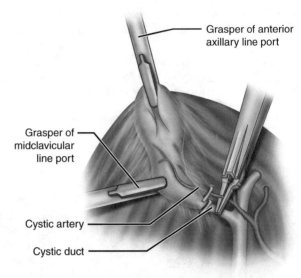

Grasper of anterior
axillary line port

Grasper of
midclavicular
line port

Cystic artery

Cystic duct

Fig. 14.13 Ligation
and division of cystic
artery and cystic duct

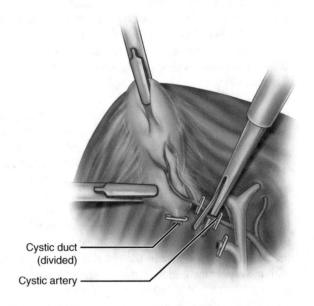

Cystic duct
(divided)

Cystic artery

entering the gallbladder. The doublet view (anterior and posterior visualization
should be utilized to demonstrate the CVS).

- **Step 8.** Carefully ligate the cystic artery and cystic duct by proximal and distal
  clipping. Divide both entities (Figs. 14.12 and 14.13).
- **Step 9.** Dissect the gallbladder from the liver using the "hook" electrocautery
  (Fig. 14.14).

- **Step 10.** Slowly and carefully separate the gallbladder from its bed. Obtain hemostasis. Perform repeated irrigations (Fig. 14.15).
- **Step 11.** Remove the gallbladder through the umbilical port. The umbilical incision may be enlarged to permit the cholecystic exodus.

Fig. 14.14 Dissection of gallbladder from the liver

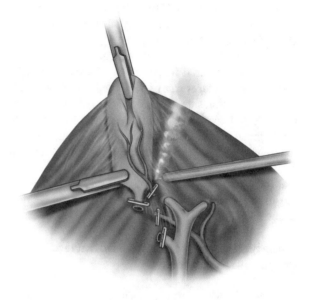

Fig. 14.15 Separating gallbladder from its bed

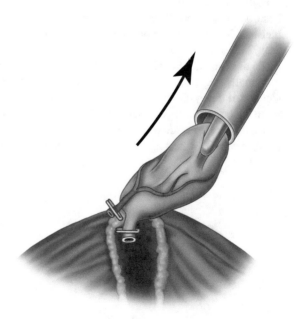

- **Step 12.** After ascertaining that there is no bleeding, remove all trocars under direct vision.
- **Step 13.** Close the umbilical incision by suturing the fascia and the skin. Close the skin of the other ports.

Fluorescent Visualizations of Biliary Structures Using Near-Infrared Imaging Capability of New Camera Systems

Patients are administered 2.5 mg of indocyanine green (ICG) intravenously at the start of the procedure. Indocyanine green (ICG) is an FDA-approved hydrophilic anionic dye and has an excellent safety profile. During or after cystic plate dissection, the near-infrared functionality of such equipped cameras can be switched on and biliary structures can be very well visualized using this technique. The use of ICG visualization should be considered on every laparoscopic (robotic) case where near-infrared camera capability is available. The biliary structures will appear as bright green (or other colored depending upon manufacturer camera settings) structures against a dark background. Extrahepatic biliary anatomy can be visualized for assisting in safe performance of cholecystectomy. It is extremely important to note that the use of fluorescence imaging does not obviate the need for visualization of the critical view of safety, which needs to be done for each procedure and documented.

Cholecystectomy from Above Downward

Preoperative preparation:

- Prior to incision, intravenous antibiotic of choice
  Anesthesia: General
  Position: Supine on a special X-ray operating room table
  Incision: Right subcostal or other incision of choice
- **Step 1.** Dissect the area of the cystic duct and the common duct. Identify the cystic duct and double pass a 2–0 silk around it. Identify the cystic artery. Ligate proximally and distally with 2–0 silk and divide. If there is any doubt about the identity of the cystic artery, do not divide yet.
- **Step 2.** Using the Bovie, carefully dissect the gallbladder from the liver from above downward until you reach the hepatoduodenal ligament. Inspect the gallbladder fossa for leakage of bile or bleeding and treat using electrocautery (Fig. 14.16).

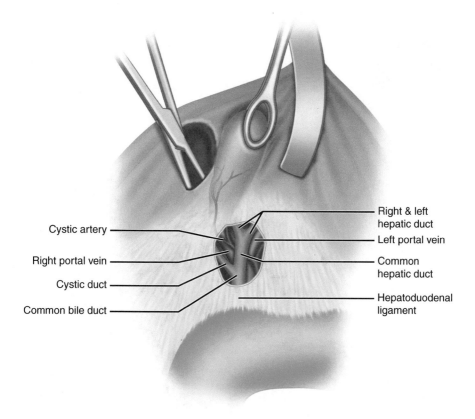

Fig. 14.16   Area of cystic duct and cystic artery is dissected

- **Step 3.** If the cystic artery has not yet been divided, divide it. It should be located near and parallel to the cystic duct (Fig. 14.17).
- **Step 4.** Isolate the cystic duct. Decide whether to perform a cholangiogram. If not, carefully clamp the cystic duct proximally and distally between two clamps. Divide the cystic duct between the clamps and ligate (Fig. 14.18).
- **Step 5.** Remove the specimen and irrigate the gallbladder fossa and right upper quadrant.
- **Step 6.** Decide whether to drain the area. If so, use a Jackson-Pratt drain, bringing it out through a stab wound. Close in layers.

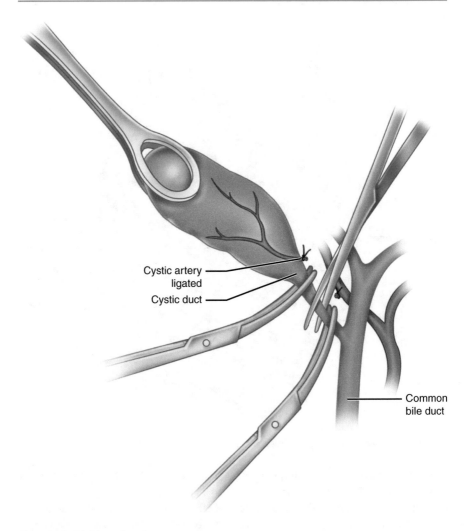

Fig. 14.17 Division of cystic artery

Cholecystectomy from Below Upward

- **Step 1.** Dissect the area of the cystic and common ducts and identify these structures as well as the cystic arteries (Figs. 14.19 and 14.20).
- **Step 2.** Doubly ligate the cystic duct and cystic artery with 2–0 silk. Incise all
  around the serosa of the gallbladder approximately 1–1½ cm from the liver edge.
  Using the Bovie and right-angle clamp, dissect the gallbladder from the liver.
  Upward traction by placing a clamp near the cystic duct (on the gallbladder) is
  helpful.

Fig. 14.18 Division of cystic duct

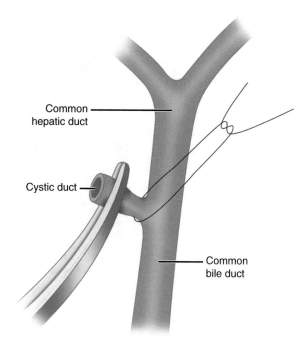

Common hepatic duct

Cystic duct

Common bile duct

Fig. 14.19 Dissecting area of cystic and common ducts

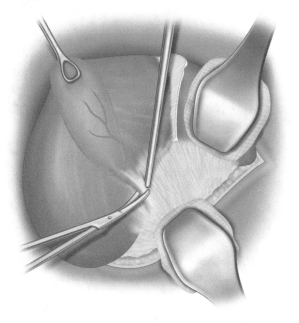

Fig. 14.20 Bed of
cystic arteries

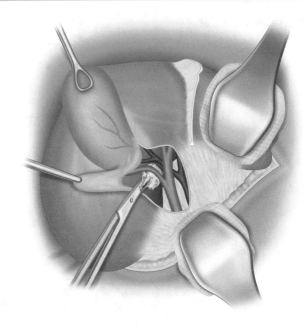

Fig. 14.21
Electrocoagulation of
gallbladder fossa

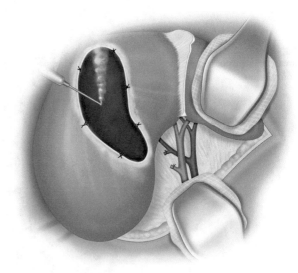

- **Step 3.** Remove the gallbladder and electrocoagulate the gallbladder fossa to
  stop bleeding or bile leakage (Fig. 14.21).

Operating Room Cholangiogram

To perform an adequate operative cholangiogram, the volume of the biliary tract is
more important than the length or the diameter. The capacity is between 12 and
20 ml. Obviously, the presence of stones will markedly reduce the capacity.

Note

- The anterior leaf of the hepatoduodenal ligament is routinely incised over the hepatocystic triangle and the underlying structures are revealed. In more difficult cases, where adhesions from inflammation or previous surgery have obscured normal relationships, greater efforts are required:
  - The hepatic flexure of the colon and the duodenum may be mobilized to the left.
  - The liver may be retracted to the right. This will put slight tension on the biliary ducts and open the epiploic foramen (Winslow's foramen), providing better orientation of the field.
  - In dissecting the gallbladder away from the liver bed, the cystic artery may be exposed by the rotation of the gallbladder to the left. This will also expose the common hepatic duct, the right and left hepatic ducts, and the cystic duct. Being able to perform this maneuver is one of the advantages of removing the gallbladder from the fundus downward.
  - Use suction and Bovie for the bleeding bed. The gallbladder bed may be filled with omentum and a drain placed over the omentum (not between the bed and the omentum).
  - The subserous excision of the gallbladder uses the lamina propria of loose connective tissue as the plane of dissection.
  - Another approach is to identify the cystic artery and duct and then ligate and transect them. The gallbladder may then be dissected from its bed from below upward.
  - Another option is to begin at the fundus of the gallbladder and dissect downward toward the neck with the following steps: (1) dissection of the gallbladder, (2) exposure of the cystic duct and its union with the common bile duct, (3) an operating room cholangiogram, and (4) dissection and ligation of the cystic duct and removal of the gallbladder.
  - Regardless of the direction of the procedure, the junction of the cystic and common hepatic ducts should be identified.

If a cholangiogram is performed, the patient should be rotated slightly to the right so that the common bile duct is rotated off the spine and becomes clearly visible.

An operative cholangiogram will be of great assistance to the surgeon passing a probe through the common bile duct. There is a potential danger if the surgeon passes a probe and expects it to take a straight line to the ampulla and encounters instead a 90-degree turn as the duct enters the duodenum. If the duct is fixed by disease or prior surgery, and if the surgeon is a little too rough, perforation can result.

- **Step 1.** For traction, use mild tension on the proximal ligation of the cystic duct (which, though ligated, is still connected to the gallbladder). Make a minute opening into the anterior wall of the cystic duct with a No. 11 blade (Fig. 14.22). Through this opening, insert a Reddick balloon catheter. It is secured by inflating the balloon.
- **Step 2.** Take two X-rays: the first after injecting 7 cm³ of 30% Renografin and the second using 14 cm³ of contrast. Have the anesthesiologist stop ventilating the patient during exposure.

Fig. 14.22 Cystic duct
is entered

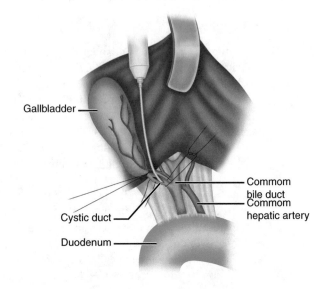

Gallbladder

Commom
bile duct
Commom
hepatic artery

Cystic duct

Duodenum

Fig. 14.23 T-tube
drainage. Inset: T-tube

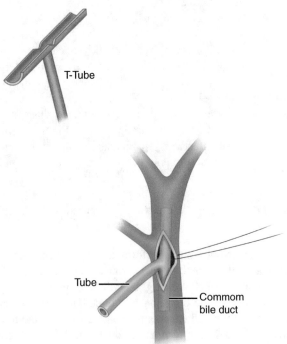

T-Tube

Tube

Commom
bile duct

- **Step 3.** If there is no pathology, remove the catheter and doubly ligate the cystic
  duct. If choledocholithiasis or other pathology is found, proceed with common
  duct exploration. Occasionally, choledochoscopy is helpful.
- **Step 4.** T-tube draining is essential (Fig. 14.23).

Note
- If the common bile duct is not completely filled, the patient can be placed in a slight Trendelenburg position and 20 cm³ of 30 percent Renografin used.

Common Bile Duct Exploration

- **Step 1.** Perform duodenal kocherization by careful incision of the lateral peritoneum and palpation of the duodenum, head of the pancreas, and distal common bile duct (Figs. 14.24 and 14.25).
- **Step 2.** Dissect tissue overlying the common bile duct no more than 1–2 cm distal to the cystic stump. Skeletonization of more than 2½ to 3 cm can result in ischemia to the duct.

Fig. 14.24 Dissecting the lateral peritoneum

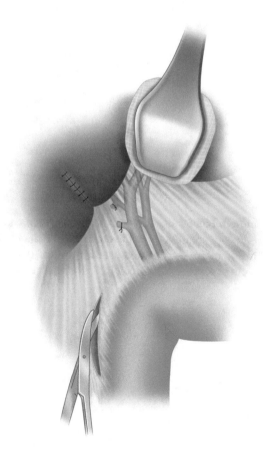

Fig. 14.25 Palpation

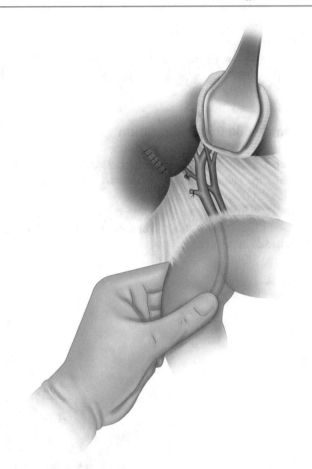

- **Step 3.** Place 4–0 Vicryl stay sutures medial and lateral to the cleaned common bile duct area. Aspirate the common bile duct to make sure you are in the right place. Incise the elevated anterior wall of the common bile duct to a length of 1 cm or less (Figs. 14.26, 14.27, 14.28, and 14.29).

Fig. 14.26 Stay sutures

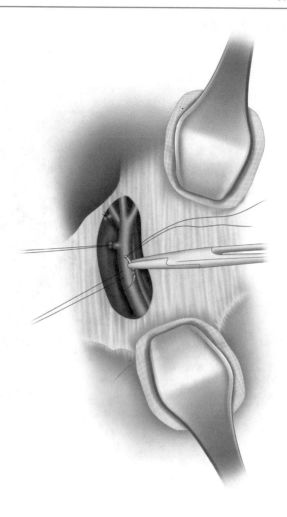

Fig. 14.27 Incision site

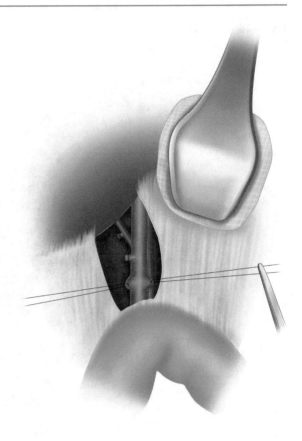

Fig. 14.28 Incision

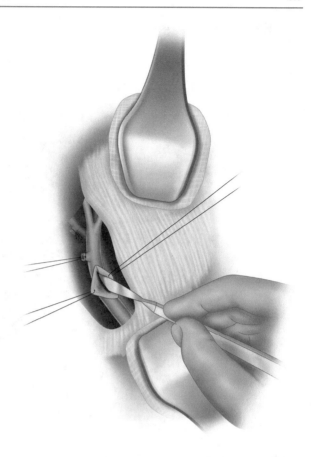

Fig. 14.29 Opening for
stone removal

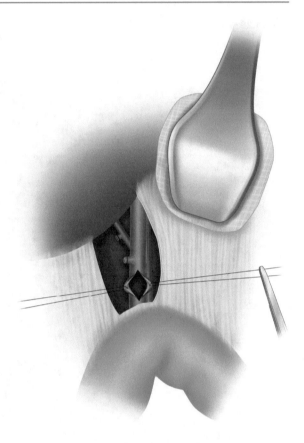

- **Step 4.** Remove stones by instrumentation (Randall stones forceps, scoops of several types and sizes, irrigation catheter, biliary Fogarty catheter) or extrinsic pressure by milking the stones to the upward choledochotomy (Figs. 14.30 and 14.31).

Fig. 14.30   "Milking" the stones

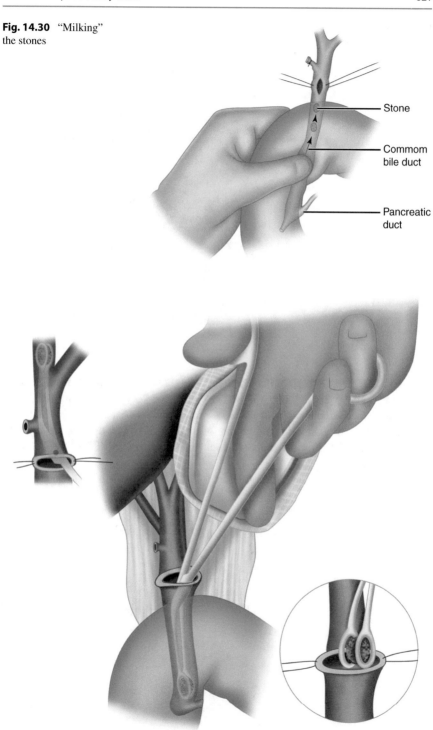

Fig. 14.31   Stones removed by instrumentation. Left inset: forceps grasps stone. Right inset: stone is extracted

Fig. 14.32
Demonstrating patency

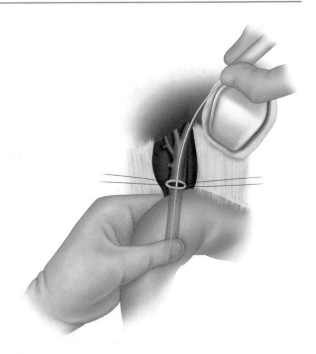

- **Step 5.** Demonstrate ampullary patency using a small French catheter. If doubt about patency remains, use a Bakes No. 3 dilator very carefully to avoid false passage. Choledochoscopy may be helpful. Conduct repeated irrigation of the biliary ducts to remove small stones or sludge. If stones are impacted in the ampulla, papillotomy for their removal will be necessary (Figs. 14.32, 14.33, 14.34, and 14.35).

Fig. 14.33 Incision site
for duodenotomy

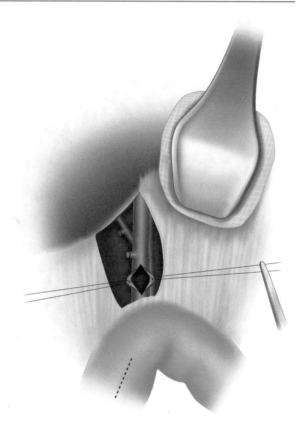

Fig. 14.34 Perform the duodenotomy only if it is necessary

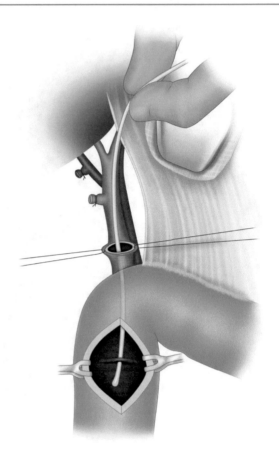

Fig. 14.35 Papillotomy

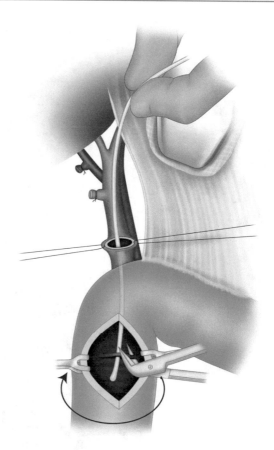

- **Step 6**. Insert a T-tube and close the common bile duct with 4–0 interrupted Vicryl (Figs. 14.36 and 14.37).
- **Step 7.** Carry out T-tube cholangiography and bring T-tube straight out through the abdominal wall by a minute stab wound. Secure to skin with 2–0 silk.
- **Step 8.** Close abdominal wall.

Remember These Indications for Exploration of the Common Bile Duct
- Presence of a palpable stone in common bile duct.
- Failure of stone extraction by ERCP.
- Positive intraoperative cholangiogram.
- Jaundice in absence of ERCP.
- Cholangitis.
- When in doubt, explore! Exposure and mobilization of 2–5 cm in length may be obtained by mobilizing the distal common bile duct from the undersurface of the pancreas. Because the duct may be intrapancreatic (Fig. 14.6c), the pancreas and duodenum should be mobilized (Fig. 14.6b, d, e).

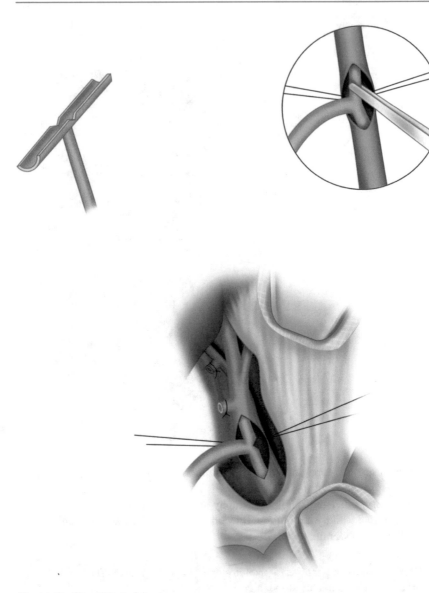

Fig. 14.36 Site of T-tube insertion

Fig. 14.37 Closure

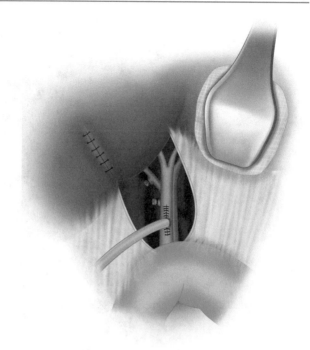

Sphincteroplasty

- **Step 1.** Perform cholecystectomy and operating room cholangiogram.
- **Step 2.** Carry out duodenal kocherization (Fig. 14.38) and choledochotomy. Insert balloon catheter all the way down through the ampulla. Place stay sutures of 4–0 silk at the duodenal wall in the area of the palpable balloon. Perform duodenotomy using electrocautery (Fig. 14.39).

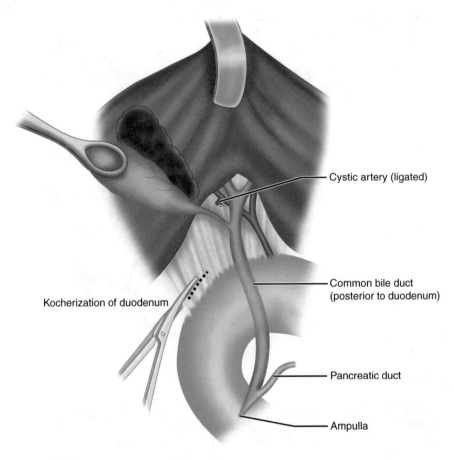

Fig. 14.38 Duodenal Kocherization

Fig. 14.39 Duodenotomy
with electrocautery

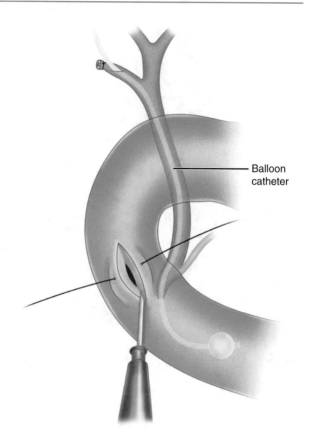

Balloon
catheter

- **Step 3.** Localize the ampulla.
- **Step 4.** At the 3 and 9 o'clock positions in the periampullary area, place 5–0 silk
  stay sutures (Fig. 14.40).

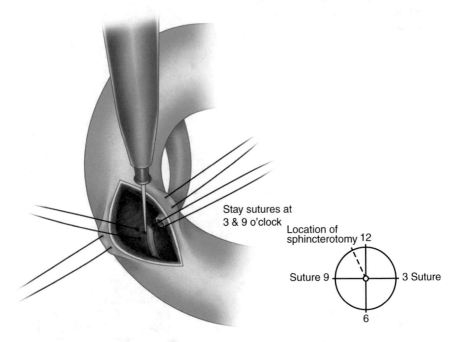

Fig. 14.40 Placement of stay sutures. Inset: schema

- **Step 5.** Perform a sphincterotomy between the 10 and 11 o'clock positions to a depth of 2–3 mm using electrocautery (Fig. 14.41).
- **Step 6.** Approximate the ductal and duodenal mucosa with interrupted 5–0 synthetic absorbable sutures (Figs. 14.41 and 14.42).

Fig. 14.41 Above: sphincterotomy. Below: mucosa is approximated

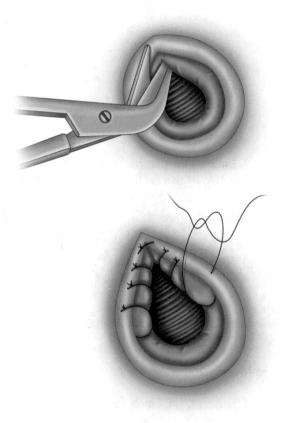

Fig. 14.42 Septotomy site

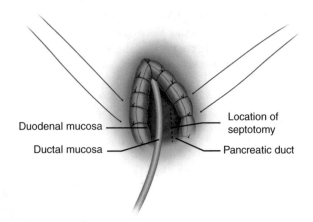

Duodenal mucosa

Ductal mucosa

Location of septotomy

Pancreatic duct

- **Step 7.** Localize the pancreatic duct opening, insert a probe, and carefully perform a septotomy to a depth of 2–4 mm by knife or Pott's scissors.

Note
- Wirsung's ductoplasty by interrupted sutures, as in step 6, is optional. If the ductal orifice is not found, secretin injection will be very helpful: one unit per kilogram of body weight.

- **Step 8.** Execute duodenorrhaphy in two layers. Place a T-tube into the common bile duct and insert a Jackson-Pratt drain (Fig. 14.43).

Choledochoduodenostomy

- **Step 1.** Establish good mobilization of the common bile duct and duodenum to avoid anastomotic tension. Anchor the duodenum to the common bile duct by placing a row of 4–0 Vicryl sutures posteriorly (Fig. 14.44).
- **Step 2.** Make a 1.5- to 2-cm transverse incision of the duodenum just below the suture line and a vertical or transverse incision of the common bile duct just above the suture line (Fig. 14.45).

Fig. 14.43
Duodenorrhaphy. Drain
and T-tube placed

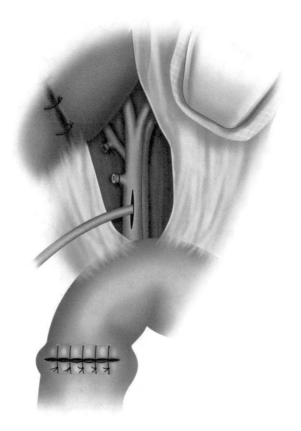

Fig. 14.44 Duodenum
is anchored

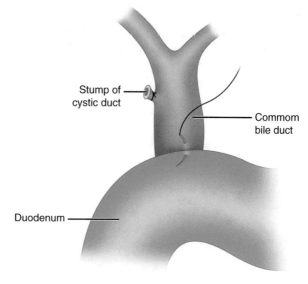

Stump of
cystic duct

Commom
bile duct

Duodenum

Fig. 14.45 Duodenum
and common bile duct
are incised

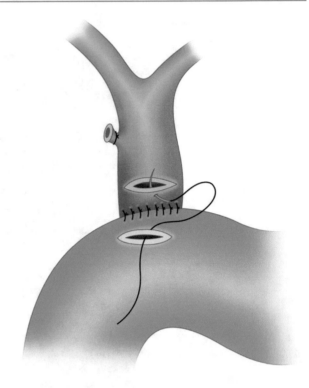

- **Step 3.** Perform the anastomosis in a single layer using interrupted 4–0 Vicryl sutures, full thickness, to the common bile duct and duodenum (Figs. 14.45, 14.46, and 14.47).

Note
- Alternatively, a side-to-side anastomosis can be performed.

Fig. 14.46 Placement
of sutures

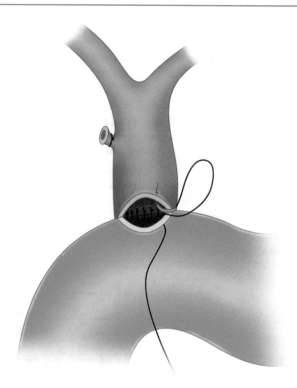

Fig. 14.47 Anastomosis
of common bile duct and
duodenum

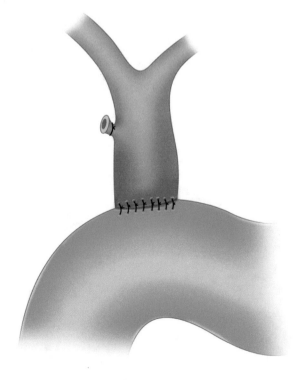

Choledochocystectomy

- **Step 1.** Evaluate the extent of the cyst (Fig. 14.48).
- **Step 2.** Execute lysis of pericystic adhesions (Fig. 14.48).
- **Step 3.** Perform cholecystectomy and choledochocystectomy (Fig. 14.49).
- **Step 4.** Perform internal drainage by a 60-cm Roux-en-Y jejunal loop.
  - (a) Jejunal interruption at approximately 60 cm using GIA.
  - (b) Small opening in transverse mesocolon.
  - (c) Distal jejunal Roux-en-Y loop up through the transverse mesocolon opening.
  - (d) End-to-side hepaticojejunal anastomosis in one layer with interrupted 4–0 absorbable sutures (Fig. 14.50).
  - (e) Secure the jejunum to the transverse mesocolon opening.

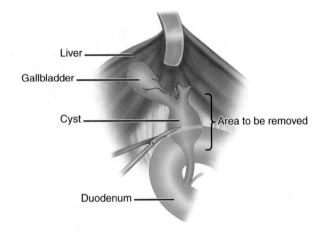

Fig. 14.48 Evaluation and lysis

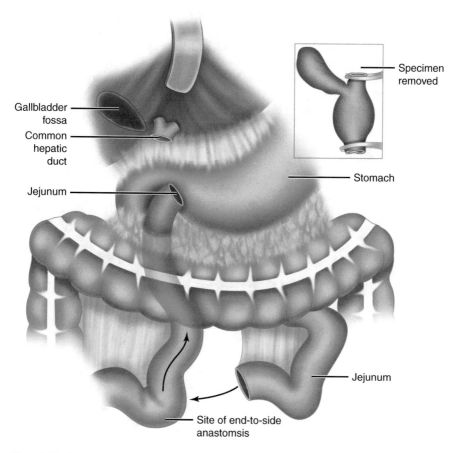

Fig. 14.49 Creation of Roux-en-Y. Inset: the specimen

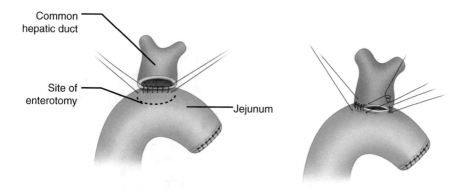

Fig. 14.50 Hepaticojejunal anastomosis

(f) End-to-side jejunojejunal anastomosis in two layers (Figs. 14.51 and 14.52).

(g) Be sure to secure the Roux-en-Y loop to the vicinity of the gallbladder fossa with two or three interrupted 3–0 silk sutures to avoid possible herniation as well as weight tension.

(h) If there is room, it is advisable to insert a T-tube into the common hepatic duct (Fig. 14.53).

- **Step 5.** Insert Jackson-Pratt drain and close abdominal wall.

Fig. 14.51 Site of end-to-side jejunojejunal anastomosis

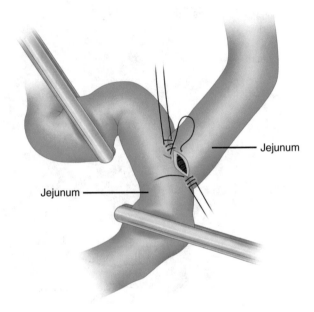

Fig. 14.52 Completed two-layer anastomosis

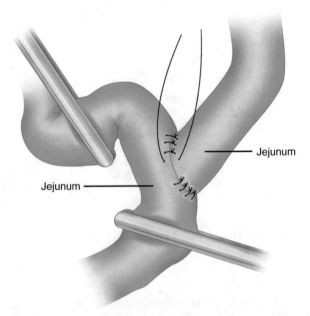

Fig. 14.53 The completed hepaticojejunostomy and jejunojejunostomy anastomosis

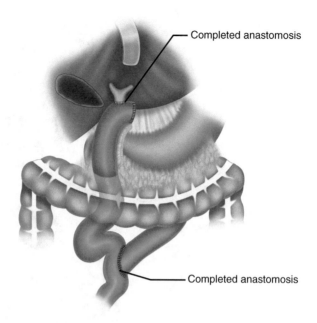

Completed anastomosis

Completed anastomosis

Hepp-Couinaud Procedure

The Hepp-Couinaud procedure is an alternative method for secondary repair of bile duct injuries. It allows the surgeon to avoid the inflamed lower CBD and utilizes virgin territory in the hilum for ease of anastomosis. This procedure is also extremely useful when sufficient proximal trunk is not available. Additionally, this procedure allows the surgeon to perform a long patent biliary-enteric anastomosis regardless of the caliber of the bile duct.

Preoperative preparation:

- Prior to incision, intravenous antibiotic of choice
  Anesthesia: General
  Position: Supine on a special X-ray operating room table
  Incision: Right subcostal or upper midline
- **Step 1.** The patient is placed in a position slightly slanted to the left decubitus. A long italic S-shaped subcostal incision provides wide and easy access to the region and allows for easy rotation of the liver.
- **Step 2.** The liver parenchyma is separated from the thickened capsule with a spatula or a surgical cotton ball. This zone bleeds little (some small venous elements) and hemostasis is easy, either by electrocoagulation or by hemostatic pads (Fig. 14.54).
- **Step 3.** Once the left hepatic duct has been exposed (Fig. 14.55), it may be incised to the right, the incision may extend to the anterior aspect of the convergence, or even onto the visible part of the right hepatic duct. To the left, the inci-

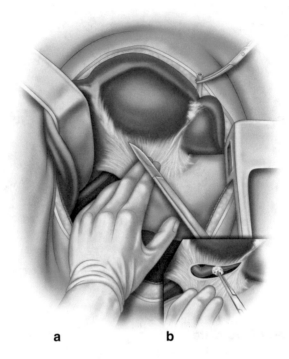

a   **b**

Fig. 14.54 (**a**) Glissonian capsule dissection off liver parenchyma. (**b**) Exposure of left hepatic duct. (Technique from Hepp J. Hepaticojejunostomy using the left biliary trunk for iatrogenic biliary lesions: the French connection. World J Surg. 1985;9:507–11)

Fig. 14.55 Exposure of left hepatic duct. (Technique from Hepp J. Hepaticojejunostomy using the left biliary trunk for iatrogenic biliary lesions: the French connection. World J Surg. 1985;9:507–11)

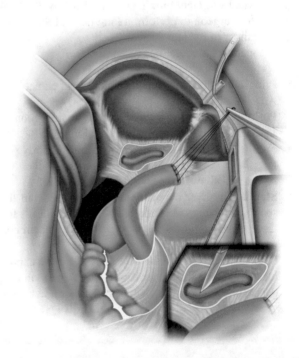

sion may be extended as needed in order to obtain an ideal minimum of 3 cm (Fig. 14.56).

One must remember that the arteries running to the left and quadrate lobes are superficial and close to the round ligament. They, of course, must be respected. This may be accomplished by separating them from the biliary wall and retracting them to the left.

- **Step 4.** Prior to anastomosis, the biliary tract must be cleared of all stones. Stones may be extracted in either duct by using either Dormia's probe or by washing them out. Fiber-optic endoscopy is usually impossible because of the small caliber of the ducts.
- **Step 5.** A 60-cm Roux loop, with the end closed, is then brought up retrocolically and an equivalently sized opening is made on its antimesenteric border.
- **Step 6.** From about 2 cm from the closed intestinal end, the jejunal loop is then opened on its free convex border for a distance equal to that of the intrahepatic duct incision.
- **Step 7.** The anastomosis is fashioned side-to-side with interrupted fine monofilament sutures. Six points are usually needed for each line of suture, the knots being tied on the inside for the posterior line, and on the outside for the anterior line (Fig. 14.57). Routine use of transanastomotic tubes is not recommended. If the apposition is imperfect or there is concern for anastomotic stricture a transient transanastomotic tube could be considered.

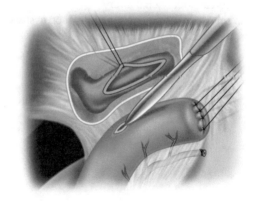

Fig. 14.56 Incision of left hepatic duct and jejunal loop. (Technique from Hepp J. Hepaticojejunostomy using the left biliary trunk for iatrogenic biliary lesions: the French connection. World J Surg. 1985;9:507–11)

Fig. 14.57 Side-to-side anastomosis accomplished via interrupted monofilament sutures. (Technique from Hepp J. Hepaticojejunostomy using the left biliary trunk for iatrogenic biliary lesions: the French connection. World J Surg. 1985;9:507–11)

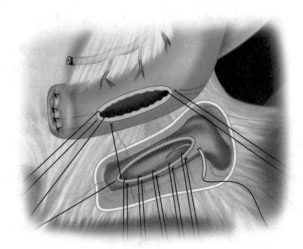

Anatomical Complications

- Vascular injury resulting in hemorrhage from the cystic artery, right hepatic artery, gastroduodenal artery veins in the gallbladder bed, inferior vena cava, and portal vein
- Ischemia from ligation of normal or aberrant right hepatic artery
- Overzealous skeletonization of common bile duct, supraduodenal artery, posterior pancreaticoduodenal artery
- Organ injury: injury to common bile duct, cystic duct, stomach, duodenum, pancreas, liver, and colon

Spleen

15

Lee J. Skandalakis

Anatomy

General Description of the Spleen

The spleen is concealed at the left hypochondrium and is not palpable under normal conditions. It is associated with the posterior portions of the left 9th, 10th, and 11th ribs – separated from them by the diaphragm and the costodiaphragmatic recess (Fig. 15.1).

Fig. 15.1 Location of the spleen

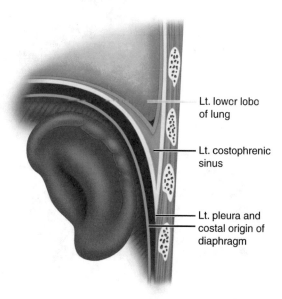

Lt. lower lobe of lung

Lt. costophrenic sinus

Lt. pleura and costal origin of diaphragm

L. J. Skandalakis (✉)
Department of Surgery, Piedmont Hospital, Atlanta, GA, USA

© Springer Nature Switzerland AG 2021
L. J. Skandalakis (ed.), *Surgical Anatomy and Technique*,
https://doi.org/10.1007/978-3-030-51313-9_15

If one divides the spleen into three parts, the upper third is related to the lower lobe of the left lung, the middle third to the left costodiaphragmatic recess, and the lower third to the left pleura and costal origin of the diaphragm.

For all practical purposes, the spleen has two surfaces: parietal and visceral (Fig. 15.2). The convex parietal surface is related to the diaphragm, and the concave visceral surface is related to the surfaces of the stomach, kidney, colon, and tail of the pancreas. On the concave hilar surface, the entrance and exit of the splenic vessels at the splenic portals in most specimens form the letter S, which is evident if one connects the upper polar, hilar, and lower polar vessels.

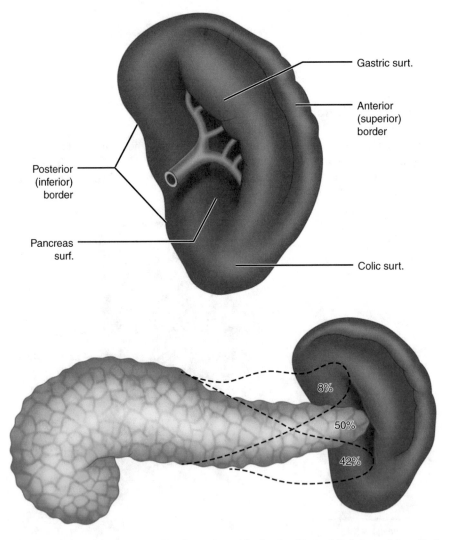

Fig. 15.2 Splenic borders. (*Top*) Anterior and posterior border. (*Bottom*) Relations of the tail of the pancreas to the spleen

A double layer of peritoneum covers the entire spleen, except for the hilum (Fig. 15.3).

Chief Splenic Ligaments

At the hilum, the visceral peritoneum joins the right layer of the greater omentum and forms the gastrosplenic and splenorenal ligaments, the two chief ligaments of the spleen (Figs. 15.4 and 15.5). These two ligaments form the splenic pedicle. The splenic capsule is formed by the visceral peritoneum; it is as friable as the spleen itself and as easily injured (Fig. 15.4).

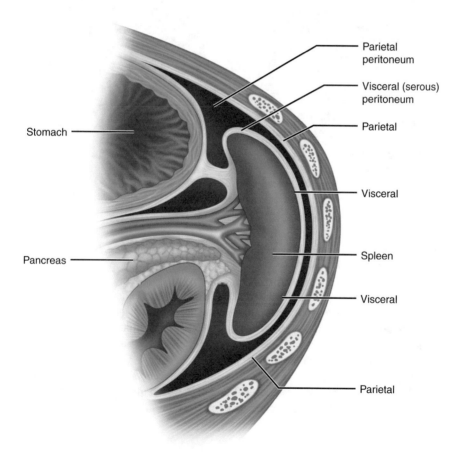

Fig. 15.3 Sagittal view of peritoneum covering the spleen

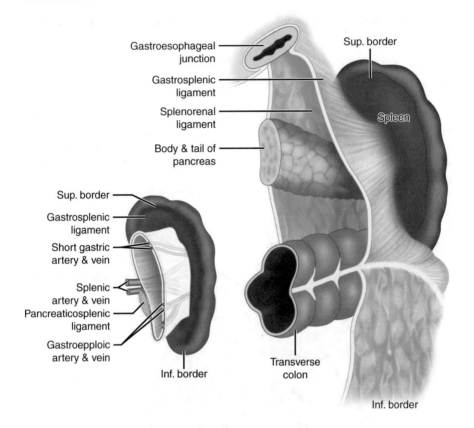

Fig. 15.4 The peritoneal attachments of the spleen. (*Inset*) The hilum of the spleen showing the short gastric and gastroepiploic vessels in the gastrosplenic ligament

The superior pole of the spleen lies close to the stomach and may be fixed to it. The inferior pole lies 5–7 cm from the stomach. The gastrosplenic ligament contains the short gastric arteries above and the left gastroepiploic vessels below; it should be incised only between clamps or preferably after the vessels are ligated one by one. Transfixion sutures may be used.

The splenorenal ligament envelops the splenic vessels and the tail of the pancreas. The outer layer of the splenorenal ligament forms the posterior layer of the gastrosplenic ligament. Careless division of the former may injure the short gastric

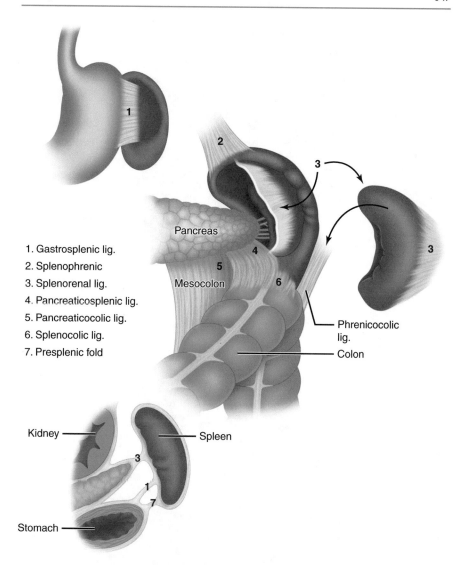

1. Gastrosplenic lig.
2. Splenophrenic
3. Splenorenal lig.
4. Pancreaticosplenic lig.
5. Pancreaticocolic lig.
6. Splenocolic lig.
7. Presplenic fold

Pancreas

Mesocolon

Phrenicocolic lig.

Colon

Kidney — Spleen

Stomach

Fig. 15.5 Chief and minor splenic ligaments

vessels. Bleeding from these vessels may be the result of too-enthusiastic deep posterior excavation by the index and middle fingers of an operator seeking to mobilize and retract the spleen to the right. The splenorenal ligament itself is nearly avascular and may be incised, but the fingers should stop at the pedicle (Fig. 15.6).

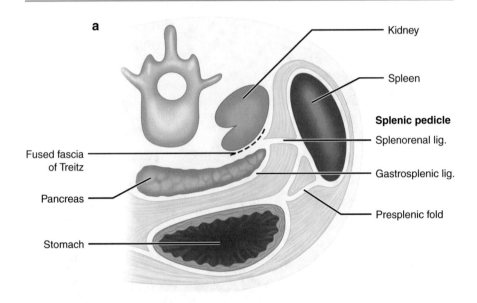

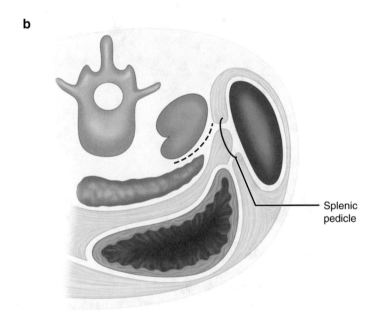

Fig. 15.6 The splenic pedicle. (**a**) Long pedicle with a presplenic fold. (**b**) Short pedicle

Minor Splenic Ligaments

The spleen has several minor ligaments, and their names indicate their connections (Fig. 15.5): the splenophrenic, splenocolic, pancreaticosplenic, pancreaticocolic, and phrenicocolic ligaments and the presplenic fold. The splenophrenic ligament (Fig. 15.5) is the reflection of the leaves of the mesentery to the posterior body wall and to the inferior surface of the diaphragm at the area of the upper pole of the spleen close to the stomach. It is usually avascular, but it should be inspected for possible bleeding after section.

Tortuous or aberrant inferior polar vessels of the spleen or a left gastroepiploic artery can lie close enough to the splenocolic ligament to be injured by careless incision of the ligament, possibly resulting in massive bleeding. The ligament should be incised between clamps.

The pancreaticosplenic ligament (Fig. 15.5) is said to be present when the tail of the pancreas does not touch the spleen.

The pancreaticocolic ligament (Fig. 15.5) is the upper extension of the transverse mesocolon and is somewhat of a bridge from the tail or body of the pancreas to the splenic flexure of the colon (Fig. 15.7).

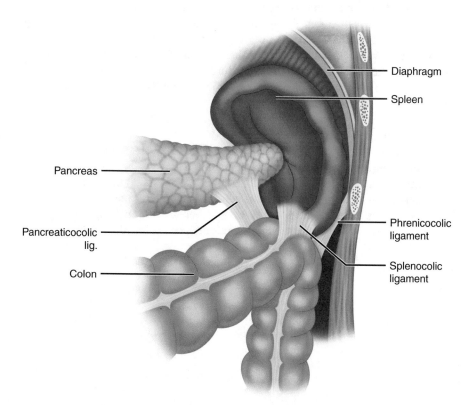

Fig. 15.7 Relation of the pancreaticocolic, phrenicocolic, and splenocolic ligaments to the transverse mesocolon

The "phrenicocolic ligament" is not a splenic ligament, i.e., it is not connected to the spleen, but the spleen rests upon it. It extends between the splenic flexure of the colon and the diaphragm and constitutes the "splenic floor" (Fig. 15.5).

The presplenic fold is a peritoneal fold anterior to the gastrosplenic ligament (Fig. 15.5), often containing the left gastroepiploic vessels. Excessive traction on this fold during upper abdominal operations can result in a tear in the splenic capsule.

Vascular System of the Spleen

Splenic Artery and Its Branches

The splenic artery, in most people, is a branch of the celiac trunk, arising together with the common hepatic and left gastric arteries. The splenic artery varies in length from 8 to 32 cm and in diameter from 0.5 to 1.2 cm. The normal course of the splenic artery crosses the left side of the aorta, passes along the upper border of the pancreas reaching the tail in front, and then crosses the upper pole of the left kidney.

The left gastroepiploic artery arises most often from the splenic trunk. Less often it arises from the inferior terminal splenic branch or its branches and rarely from the middle splenic trunk or the superior terminal branch.

There is no question that the spleen can tolerate ligation of the splenic artery because of the available collateral circulation. Therefore, the spleen can be saved if necessary. Surgeons should remember that ligation of the splenic artery near its origin can result in hyperamylasemia resulting from deterioration of the pancreatic blood supply. Preoperative splenic arterial embolization as an adjunct to high-risk splenectomy has been advised.

Splenic Vein and Its Branches

The splenic vein travels with the splenic artery (Fig. 15.8), sometimes crossing over or under it. The anatomy of the splenic vein is summarized in Fig. 15.9. The patterns are highly variable, and as in the arteries, no one vein resembles the next. The single characteristic of most of the short gastric veins is that they communicate directly with the spleen, entering at its upper part, rather than through the extrasplenic venous vessels. The left gastroepiploic venous drainage is into the splenic veins.

a

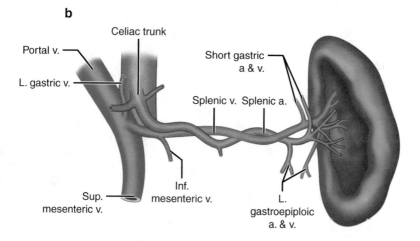

b

c

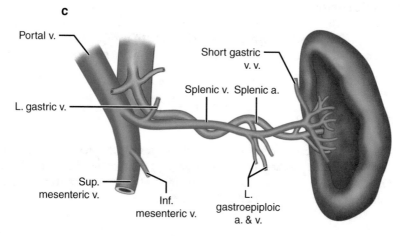

Fig. 15.8 Relation of splenic artery and splenic vein. (**a**) Artery anterior to vein (usual pattern). (**b**) Artery both anterior and posterior to vein. (**c**) Artery posterior to vein (least common configuration)

Fig. 15.9 Anatomy of the splenic vein

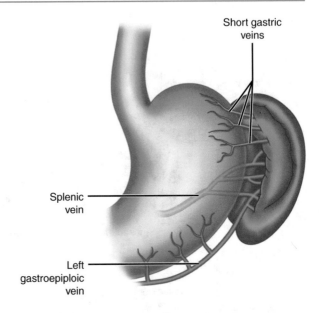

Short gastric veins

Splenic vein

Left gastroepiploic vein

Fig. 15.10 Lymphatic drainage of the spleen

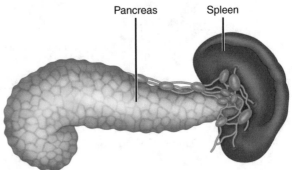

Pancreas   Spleen

Lymphatic Drainage

One of the peculiarities of the spleen is the lack of provision for lymphatics for the splenic pulp. The splenic lymphatic chain (Fig. 15.10) is reported to be formed by suprapancreatic nodes, infrapancreatic nodes, and afferent and efferent lymph vessels.

Segmental Anatomy

We propose that the term *segments* be used when referring to splenic parts separated by avascular planes, elsewhere called *lobes*. Studies indicate that the majority of the population has two splenic segments – superior and inferior. However, three and more segments have been reported in the literature.

Accessory Spleens

The reported incidence of accessory spleens in autopsies varies from approximately 20% to 30%. In approximately 60% of affected patients, only one accessory spleen is present. In 20%, two such spleens are present, and in 17%, there are three or more splenic structures. Two-thirds to three-fourths of accessory spleens are located at or near the hilum of the normal organ, and about 20% are embedded in the tail of the pancreas. The remainder is distributed along the splenic artery, in the omentum, in the mesentery, or beneath the peritoneum (Fig. 15.11). They range from 0.2 to 10 cm in size, resembling lymph nodes or miniature spleens.

Fig. 15.11 Sites of accessory spleens in order of frequency: (*1*) near the splenic hilum; (2) tail of the pancreas (these contain 86–95% of all accessory spleens); (*3*) omentum; (4) along the splenic artery; (*5*) splenocolic ligament; (*6*) mesentery; and (7) testis or ovary (3–7 are unusual locations)

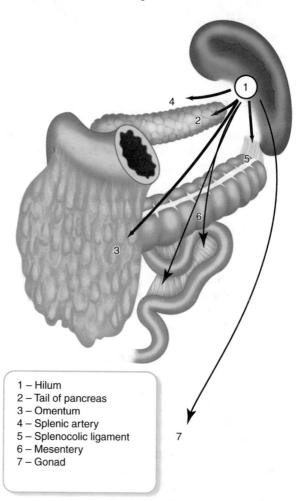

1 – Hilum
2 – Tail of pancreas
3 – Omentum
4 – Splenic artery
5 – Splenocolic ligament
6 – Mesentery
7 – Gonad

Note

- Patients with fractures of the left 9–11th ribs should be observed closely for splenic rupture.
- In splenomegaly, the spleen is always located in front of the splenic flexure of the colon. Adhesions are almost always present and sometimes vascular. Often an enlarged spleen has extensive adhesions to the colon.
- In elective splenectomies if splenomegaly is present, intestinal preparation is essential.
- After radiologic evaluation of the topography of both the upper splenic pole and the left costodiaphragmatic recess, a left thoracotomy tube should be introduced above the upper pole of the spleen.

Technique

Splenectomy

A splenectomy is usually performed for one of the following four reasons: hemorrhage, hypersplenism, Hodgkin's disease staging (diagnostic laparotomy), or a problem such as an abscess, cyst, or tumor.

Splenectomy Due to Hemorrhage Secondary to Trauma

- **Step 1.** Make an incision.
- **Step 2.** Mobilize the spleen.
- **Step 3.** Ligate the vessels.
- **Step 4.** Divide the hilum.
- **Step 5.** Obtain hemostasis.
- **Step 6.** Provide drainage.
- **Step 7.** Close the wound.

Splenectomy Due to Hematological Disorders (Hypersplenism)

- **Step 1.** Make an incision.
- **Step 2.** Ligate the arteries.
- **Step 3.** Mobilize the spleen.
- **Step 4.** Divide the hilum.
- **Step 5.** Obtain hemostasis.
- **Step 6.** Search for accessory spleens.
- **Step 7.** Provide drainage.
- **Step 8.** Close the wound.

Ligation of the Splenic Pedicle: Anterior Approach

- **Step 1.** Incision (Fig. 15.12).
- **Step 2.** Clamp, incise, and ligate the left part of the gastrocolic ligament and the gastroepiploic artery and vein. This will provide access to the lesser sac (Fig. 15.12).
- **Step 3.** Locate the splenic artery at the superior border of the body of the pancreas. Carefully ligate the artery in continuity and doubly, with ligatures being placed as distally as possible (Fig. 15.13).
- **Step 4.** Clamp, divide, and ligate the short gastric arteries and veins, one at a time (Fig. 15.13).

Fig. 15.12 Incision for total splenectomy by the anterior approach and access to the lesser sac. (*1*) subcostal; (*2*) Kehr subcostal; (*3*) bilateral subcostal; (*4*) midline

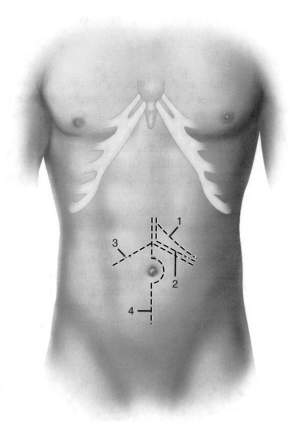

Fig. 15.13 Ligation of the splenic artery and the short gastric arteries and vein

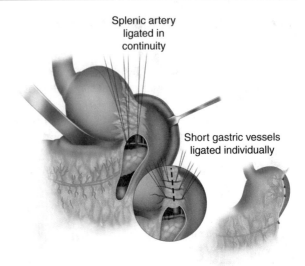

Splenic artery ligated in continuity

Short gastric vessels ligated individually

- **Step 5.** Mobilize the spleen by dividing the several ligaments with scissors. Insert the index finger deeply to separate the spleen from the renal covering. With the use of sharp and blunt dissection, clamp, divide, and ligate the splenocolic and splenophrenic ligaments.
- **Step 6.** Elevate the spleen, tail, and part of the body of the pancreas, being particularly careful with the tail of the pancreas. The spleen is now outside the peritoneal cavity and is attached only by one of the branches of the splenic arteries and veins.
- **Step 7.** Close to the hilum, clamp, divide, and ligate all branches of the splenic artery. The splenic vein and its branches are easily torn and should not be clamped. Ligate and divide the splenic vein and branches in continuity with 2–0 silk. The spleen is now free and should be removed (Figs. 15.14 and 15.15). All of the above can be accomplished with the endoscopic GIA with vascular loads.
- **Step 8.** Inspect the site for bleeding, beginning with the diaphragm and continuing to the greater curvature of the stomach, pancreatic tail, gastrosplenic ligament, splenorenal ligament, splenocolic ligament, and splenic bed and other ligaments.

Remember
- Complete hemostasis is essential. After complete inspection for bleeding, search for accessory spleens.

Fig. 15.14 Division of the
ligaments and delivery of
the spleen to the outside of
the peritoneal cavity

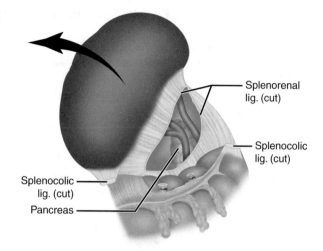

Splenorenal
lig. (cut)

Splenocolic
lig. (cut)

Splenocolic
lig. (cut)

Pancreas

Fig. 15.15 Ligation of the
splenic vein

Splenic vein
ligated in continuity

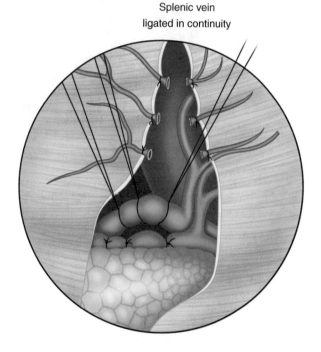

Ligation of the Splenic Pedicle: Posterior Approach

- **Step 1.** Hold the spleen medially (Fig. 15.16).
- **Step 2.** Divide the splenorenal, splenophrenic, and splenocolic ligaments (Fig. 15.16).
- **Step 3.** Lift the spleen outside the peritoneal cavity, being particularly careful with the tail of the pancreas.
- **Step 4.** Dissect rapidly and mobilize the bleeding spleen immediately. Bleeding can be controlled by manually compressing the splenic artery and vein and the tail of the pancreas between the thumb and index finger or with a noncrushing clamp (Fig. 15.17).

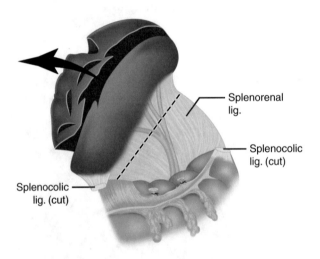

Fig. 15.16 Medial position of the spleen during the posterior approach to splenectomy, showing division of the splenocolic ligaments

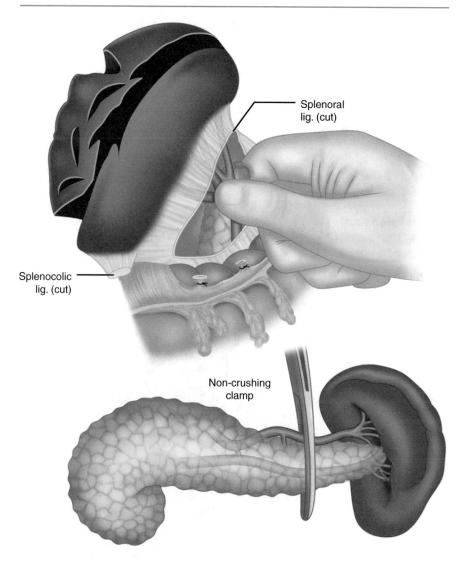

Fig. 15.17 Compression of the splenic artery and vein

- **Step 5.** Ligate the arterial and venous branches close to the hilum using 2–0 and 3–0 ligatures. Doubly ligate the splenic artery (Fig. 15.18).
- **Step 6.** Ligate the short gastric vessels.
- **Step 7.** Remove the spleen and secure any bleeding points.
- **Step 8.** Close the abdominal wall.

Note
- A GIA stapler with a vascular load can be used to divide the splenic artery and vein together at the hilum. The harmonic scalpel can be used to divide the short gastric vessels.

Partial Splenectomy

The major indication for partial splenectomy is trauma to the spleen; it is sometimes performed for nonparasitic splenic cysts, in Gaucher's disease, etc. An effort to save the spleen is paramount. However, it is our opinion that, if there is any doubt, the spleen should be removed. Detailed evaluation of the trauma must be done. Decisions must be made about the procedure of choice:

Fig. 15.18 Ligation of the splenic artery

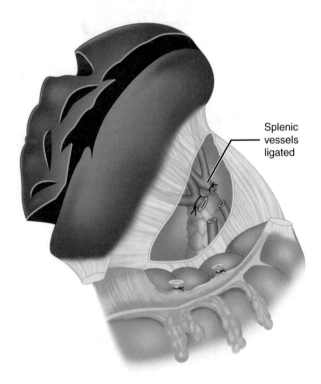

Splenic vessels ligated

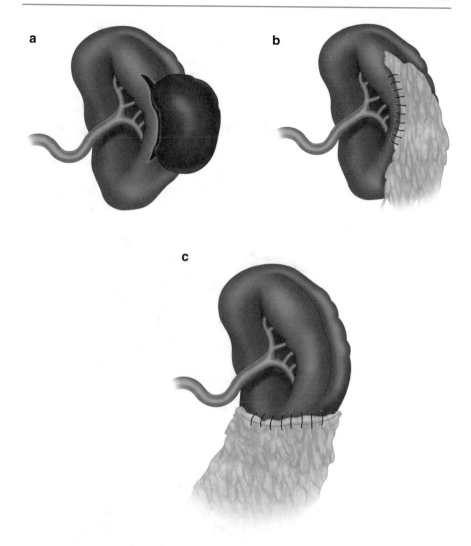

Fig. 15.19 (**a**) Splenic rupture with hematoma. (**b**) Splenorrhaphy with omental fixation. (**c**) Partial splenectomy with omental fixation

- Splenorrhaphy
- Splenorrhaphy with omental fixation (Fig. 15.19)
- Debridement, perhaps with partial splenectomy and omental fixation
- Splenic mesh wrap (Fig. 15.20)
- Autotransplantation (Fig. 15.21)

Technique of Intrasplenic Dissection

With scalpel (not cautery), make a superficial anterior incision (not circumferential) of the splenic capsule on the viable side of the line of demarcation. Using the scalpel handle, gradually deepen the incision until the entire spleen has been divided.

Fig. 15.20 Splenic mesh wrap. (*Top*) Passage of injured spleen through hole in center of mesh. (*Middle*) Wrapping spleen in mesh. (*Bottom*) Sewing opposite edges of mesh to each other to create tamponade

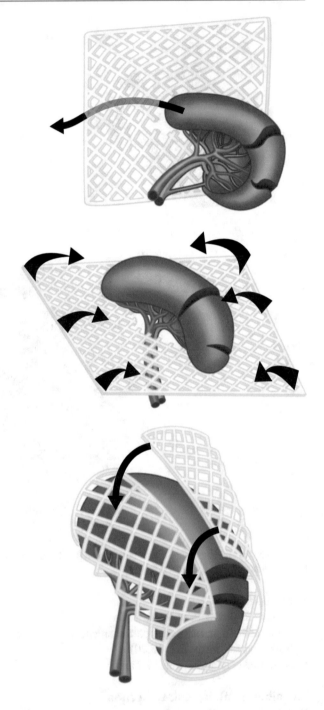

Fig. 15.21
Autotransplantation

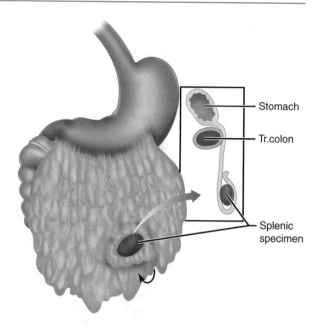

Stomach

Tr.colon

Splenic
specimen

Ligate all vessels with hemoclips or with figure-of-eight 4–0 silk. If oozing occurs, apply a hemostatic substance.

An alternative technique for treating the raw splenic remnant is placement of interlocking mattress sutures of 2–0 chromic catgut, 0.5–1 cm from the divided edge, compressing the splenic parenchyma for hemostasis. Tie these over pledgets of Gelfoam (absorbable gelatin sponge) or Surgicel (oxidized regenerated cellulose). A topical hemostatic agent may be applied for capsular avulsions or to arrest hemorrhage of very superficial lacerations.

Both an ultrasonic surgical aspirator (Cavitron) and an argon laser (which produces heat coagulation of blood vessels) have been used for identification and control of the intrasplenic vessels.

In partial splenectomy or a deeply lacerated spleen, use absorbable mesh. Observe the splenic remnant for 10 min to ascertain the completeness of hemostasis. The surgeon should determine whether drainage is required.

Occlusion of the Splenic Artery

- **Step 1.** Perform temporary occlusion of the main splenic artery.
- **Step 2.** Remember that the splenic vasculature is segmental and highly variable; isolate the segmental branches. The superior polar artery is, however, quite constant, generally arising approximately 1–3 cm from the splenic hilum. At or near the splenic hilum, the splenic artery branches further into three to five major branches and into several large and small branches. The splenic veins follow the pattern of the arterial distribution more consistently in the smaller branches than in the larger ones.

Once the segment chosen for preservation is delineated, begin a systematic, stepwise ligation and division of the branches to the segment to be removed. As the ligation proceeds, evidence of the devascularization of the spleen will become increasingly obvious as segment after segment undergoes a color change ranging from dark bluish-purple to bluish-black.

Remove the devascularized splenic parenchyma. The remnant should be of normal color, size, and consistency, indicating adequate arterial inflow and venous outflow.

Remember
- The splenorenal ligament is almost avascular, but small veins can cause problems.
- Perisplenic adhesions are vascular.
- The terminal splenic vessels are fragile and easily torn.
- The splenic capsule also is friable.
- Dissection of the splenic artery close to the celiac artery through the gastrocolic omentum can be done if moderate splenomegaly and adhesions are present. However, to avoid sudden, large loss of blood, the surgeon must be aware of the highly fragile splenic vein, which can coil around the artery.
- For huge spleens with multiple vascular adhesions, the artery can be ligated along the upper pancreatic border after the gastrocolic ligament is opened.
- A healthy ruptured spleen can be delivered easily from the abdomen.
- A large, diseased spleen requires careful dissection of the pre-hilar area and ligation of the vessels.
- In thrombocytopenic purpura, the abdomen should be explored after the spleen is removed to avert unnecessary bleeding.
- In idiopathic thrombocytopenic purpura, the splenic artery should be ligated as soon as possible.
- In the presence of hemolytic anemia, transfusions should not be given before the operation. Platelets should be transfused after splenic artery ligation.
- The splenic artery is the most unpredictable artery of the human body. If it is ligated proximally, it should also be ligated distally close to the hilum.
- The pancreatic tail should be handled gently at the hilum, especially when it is located posterior to the pedicle.
- Handle the renocolosplenic area gently to avoid bleeding and/or injury to the spleen, kidney, or colon.
- If the splenic pedicle is ligated en masse, the hilar vessels should be religated. The pedicle should be ligated twice with heavy silk.
- The pancreas should be separated from the spleen by division of the splenic artery and vein distal to the tip of the pancreas. The spleen survives on the short gastric vessels, if carefully preserved.

- When there is splenomegaly, heavy adhesions are present between the spleen and the diaphragm above and laterally, the stomach medially, and the splenic flexure below.
- Adhesions associated with splenomegaly may contain large neoplastic vessels, which can produce tremendous bleeding if not ligated and secured before their division.
- If a patient has a hemorrhagic disorder, a nasogastric tube should be inserted in the operating room, not in the patient's room, by an anesthesiologist.
- In elective splenectomy with a large spleen, intravenous preoperative antibiotics and occlusion of the splenic artery are advisable. Preoperative splenic embolization should be considered. With such a procedure, the surgeon is committing to a total splenectomy.
- Monitor the patient closely for 24 h.
- Perform repeated hematocrit readings.
- If splenorrhaphy or splenic preservation has been performed, the patient should avoid sports for 3 months.
- If the patient has been on steroids, give a dose on induction.

Laparoscopic Splenectomy

Splenectomy has traditionally been performed through a left subcostal or upper midline incision. More recently, splenectomy is performed using minimally invasive techniques. Because of the spleen's unique anatomical feature of possessing both anterior and posterior peritoneal attachments (Fig. 15.3), the laparoscopic approach to splenectomy uses lateral patient positioning (Fig. 15.22) to allow performance of both anterior and posterior approaches (previously described in this

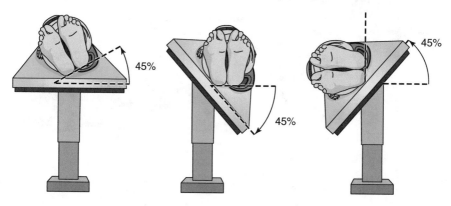

Fig. 15.22 Patient positioning for lateral approach laparoscopic splenectomy. A rotating table that allows the patient's position to be changed from supine to true lateral facilitates a combined anterior/posterior approach to splenectomy

chapter). The supine position provides an anterior approach for safe visualization, exposure, and control of the short gastrics and the splenic artery through the lesser sac, while the lateral position facilitates a posterior approach for mobilization and final excision of the spleen. This minimally invasive procedure has been termed the "leaning spleen" technique of laparoscopic splenectomy.

Preoperative: Administration of polyvalent pneumococcal vaccine at least 2 weeks before operation; mild laxative evening before surgery (e.g., one bottle of magnesium citrate orally).

> **Note**
> - Patients with ITP and critically low platelet counts (<20,000 U/dl) should receive preoperative IgG to raise the immediate preoperative platelet levels to a safe range.
> - Several units of packed red cells are cross-matched. In patients with ITP, platelets are crossed for administration after the splenic artery has been ligated intraoperatively.
> - Patients who have been receiving corticosteroids within 6 months of surgery are given stress doses of intravenous corticosteroids.

Position: Modified left lateral decubitus; iliac crest at table break; kidney rest elevated (Fig. 15.23)

Anesthesia: General

Other: Foley catheter, orogastric tube, pneumatic compression hose; all pressure points well padded

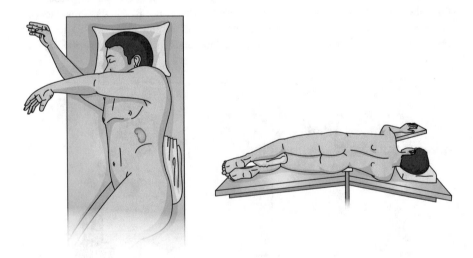

Fig. 15.23 Modified left lateral decubitus positioning with iliac crest at table break and kidney rest elevated

- **Step 1.** Prep and drape the patient so that either laparoscopy or open surgery can be performed.
- **Step 2.** Establish carbon dioxide pneumoperitoneum to 15 mmHg with a Veress needle inserted at either the umbilicus or the midclavicular line below the left costal margin (cannula site for the camera).
- **Step 3.** Insert cannulas as shown in Fig. 15.24.
- **Step 4.** Visually explore for accessory splenic tissue (Fig. 15.11).
- **Step 5.** Tilt the operating table to place the patient in the supine position. Enter the lesser sac by isolating and dividing the short gastrics.

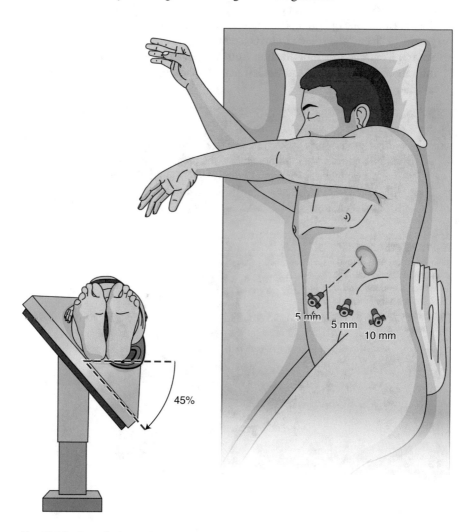

Fig. 15.24 Cannula sites and their uses for laparoscopic splenectomy

- **Step 6.** Using the harmonic scalpel, carefully divide the gastrosplenic and sple-nocolic ligaments (Fig. 15.25).

Note
- If indicated, platelets are transfused after splenic artery ligation.

- **Step 7.** The tail of the pancreas and splenic hilum will begin to come into view. Carefully isolate the hilum of the spleen with blunt dissection using a combina-tion of dissection with a Kittner (peanut) and a blunt-tipped dissector.
- **Step 8.** Rotate the operating table into the near-lateral position, thereby allowing gravity to "hang" the spleen from its lateral and posterior peritoneal attachments.
- **Step 9.** Continue this mobilization from caudad to cephalad until the spleen is fully mobilized laterally, and the left hemidiaphragm is visualized from behind and above the spleen.

Note
- The gravity-facilitated dissection allows the spleen to fall medially, provid-ing complete visualization of the tail of the pancreas and the splenic hilum.
- Use great care when manipulating the spleen. This will avoid capsular dis-ruption which could lead to splenosis and recurrent hematologic disease.

Fig. 15.25 The short gastric vessels are divided with an energy device. The lesser sac is entered, and the splenic artery isolated with a blunt-tipped right angle

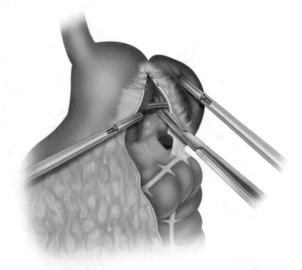

- **Step 10.** The splenic artery and vein are now easily ligated and divided using a vascular linear cutting stapler (Fig. 15.26).

Note
- Care should be taken to identify and avoid the tail of the pancreas during this final hilar dissection and division.

- **Step 11.** Splenorenal ligament is divided (Fig. 15.27).
- **Step 12.** Gently push the disconnected spleen medially and out of the left upper quadrant. Position a nylon-reinforced specimen retrieval sac in the left upper quadrant. With the help of gravity, gently push the spleen into the sac using peri-splenic attachments or the hilar pedicle (Fig. 15.28).

Note
- The bag must be stout enough not to rupture during extraction; a ruptured bag could cause splenosis.

Fig. 15.26 The splenic hilum is the only remaining attachment of the spleen. This is easily controlled and divided with a vascular stapler

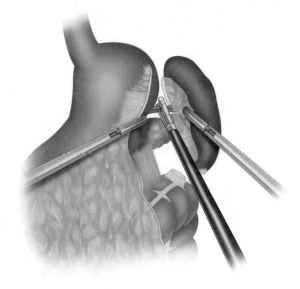

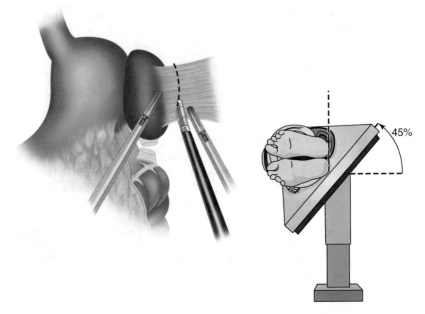

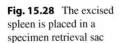

Fig. 15.27 By rotating the operating table, the patient is placed in a true lateral position. The suspended spleen is mobilized by dividing the splenocolic and splenorenal ligaments

Fig. 15.28 The excised spleen is placed in a specimen retrieval sac

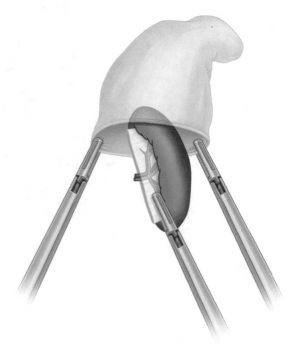

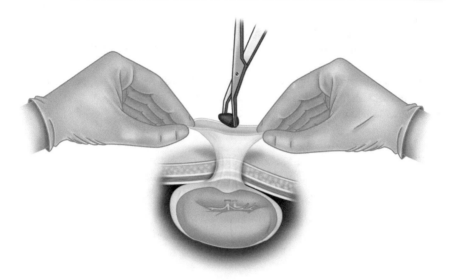

Fig. 15.29 The mouth of the retrieval sac is pulled through one of the 10 mm cannula sites. The spleen is morcellated within the sac with ringed forceps until the sac can be removed

- **Step 13.** Pull the mouth of the specimen retrieval sac out through the midclavicular cannula site. Enter the sac extracorporeally and morcellate the spleen, removing it piecemeal from the sac with ring forceps until the sac can be extracted (Fig. 15.29).
- **Step 14.** Inspect the operative site for hemostasis.
- **Step 15.** Remove cannulas and allow carbon dioxide insufflation to entirely escape the abdominal cavity.
- **Step 16.** Close the fascia of the 10 mm incision with an absorbable 0 suture and the skin with a subcuticular 4–0 absorbable suture.

Anatomical Complications

Hemorrhage
- Bleeding can result from polar arteries arising proximal to the ligated or stapled splenic artery.
- A superior polar artery may arise from the third segment of the splenic artery.
- Retrograde bleeding from splenic arteries distal to the ligation (short gastric, tidal pancreatic and left gastroepiploic arteries may arise from terminal branches of the splenic artery beyond the point of ligation). Whenever possible ligate distal to the origin of the left gastroepiploic.
- Short gastric veins are another source of bleeding.
- Bleeding may occur from the preserved splenic remnant after a partial splenectomy.
- Mobilization of the spleen with excessive traction may result in an avulsion of the splenic capsule resulting in bleeding.

Organ Injury
- Though unusual the diaphragm may be injured.
- The most commonly injured organ is the pancreas because of the proximity of the tail to the splenic.
- AD vascular is an injury to the stomach, although rare, can happen. This may result from ligation of the short gastric arteries.
- Gastric cutaneous fistulas may occur.

Inadequate Procedures
- If a splenectomy is required for ITP or other hemolytic disease and accessory spleens are left in the body, the procedure is in adequate.

Adrenal Glands

16

Bruce J. Feigelson

Anatomy

General Description of the Adrenal Glands

Each adrenal gland, together with the associated kidney, is enclosed in the renal fascia (of Gerota) and surrounded by fat.

The glands are firmly attached to the fascia, which is in turn attached firmly to the abdominal wall and the diaphragm. A layer of loose connective tissue separates the capsule of the adrenal gland from that of the kidney. Because the kidney and the adrenal gland are thus separated, the kidney can be ectopic or ptotic without a corresponding displacement of the gland. Fusion of the kidneys, however, is often accompanied by fusion of the adrenal glands.

Occasionally the adrenal gland is fused with the kidney so that separation is almost impossible. If individuals with such a fusion need a partial or total nephrectomy, they also require a coincidental adrenalectomy.

The medial borders of the right and left adrenal glands are about 4.5 cm apart. In this space, from right to left, are the inferior vena cava, the right crus of the diaphragm, part of the celiac ganglion, the celiac trunk, the superior mesenteric artery, part of the celiac ganglion, and the left crus of the diaphragm.

Relations of the Adrenal Glands

Each adrenal gland has only an anterior and a posterior surface. Some of the relationships to other structures can be seen in Fig. 16.1.

B. J. Feigelson (✉)
Department of General Surgery, Colorado Permanente Medical Group, Denver, CO, USA
e-mail: Bruce.X.Feigelson@kp.org

© Springer Nature Switzerland AG 2021
L. J. Skandalakis (ed.), *Surgical Anatomy and Technique*,
https://doi.org/10.1007/978-3-030-51313-9_16

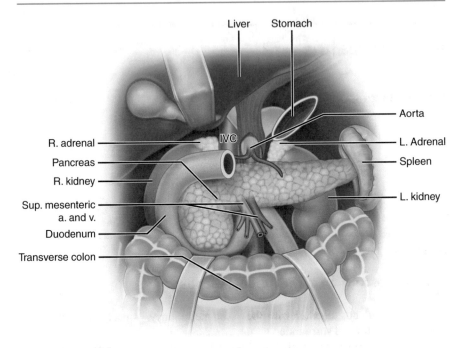

Fig. 16.1 The relations of the adrenal glands from the anterior approach

Right Adrenal Gland

- Anterior surface:

    (a) Superior – "bare area" of liver
    (b) Medial – inferior vena cava
    (c) Lateral – "bare area" of right lobe of liver
    (d) Inferior – peritoneum (very rarely, if ever) and first part of the duodenum (occasionally)

- Posterior surface:

    (a) Superior – diaphragm
    (b) Inferior – anteromedial aspect of right kidney

Left Adrenal Gland
- Anterior surface:

    (a) Superior – peritoneum (posterior wall of omental bursa) and stomach
    (b) Inferior – body of the pancreas

- Posterior surface:

(a) Medial – left crus of diaphragm
(b) Lateral – medial aspect of left kidney

Vascular System of the Adrenal Glands

Arterial Supply

The arterial supply of the adrenal glands (Fig. 16.2) arises, in most cases, from three sources:

- The superior adrenal arteries. A group of six to eight arteries arises separately from the inferior phrenic arteries.
- The middle adrenal artery arises from the aorta just proximal to the origin of the renal artery. It can be single, multiple, or absent. It supplies the perirenal fat only.
- One or more inferior adrenal arteries arise from the renal artery, an accessory renal artery, or a superior polar artery. Small twigs may arise from the upper ureteric artery.

All these arteries branch freely before entering the adrenal gland, so 50–60 arteries penetrate the capsule over the entire surface.

Venous Drainage

The adrenal venous drainage does not accompany the arterial supply and is much simpler (Fig. 16.2). A single vein drains the adrenal gland, emerging at the hilum. The left adrenal vein passes downward over the anterior surface of the left adrenal gland. This vein is joined by the left inferior phrenic vein before entering the left

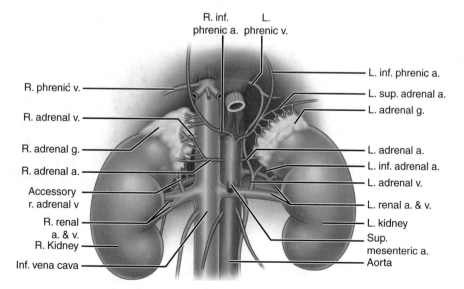

Fig. 16.2 The arterial supply and venous drainage of the adrenal glands. As many as 60 arterial twigs may enter the adrenal gland. One or, occasionally, two veins drain the adrenal gland

renal vein. From the right adrenal gland, the right adrenal vein passes obliquely to open into the inferior vena cava posteriorly.

Occasionally an adrenal gland has two veins, one following a normal course and the other being an accessory vein that enters the inferior phrenic vein.

When the posterior approach to the adrenal gland is used, the left adrenal vein is found on the anterior surface of the gland. The right adrenal vein is found between the inferior vena cava and the gland. Careful mobilization of the gland is necessary for good ligation of the vein.

> **Remember**
> - The adrenal glands vie with the thyroid gland for having the greatest blood supply per gram of tissue.

Lymphatic Drainage

The lymphatics of the adrenal gland are usually said to consist of a profuse subcapsular plexus that drains with the arteries and a medullary plexus that drains with the adrenal veins. Drainage is to renal hilar nodes, lateral aortic nodes, and nodes of the posterior mediastinum above the diaphragm by way of the diaphragmatic orifices for the splanchnic nerves (Fig. 16.3). Lymphatics from the upper pole of the right

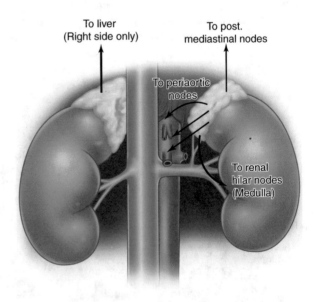

Fig. 16.3 The lymphatics of the adrenal glands

Fig. 16.4 Incisions for anterior exposure of the adrenal glands. The chevron transabdominal incision provides excellent bilateral exposure

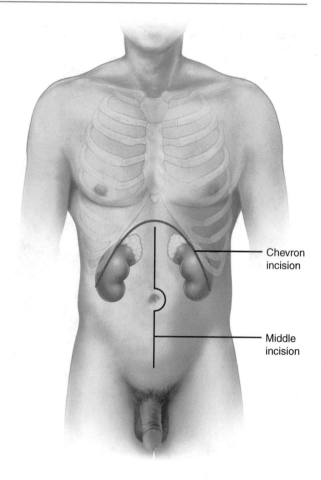

Chevron incision

Middle incision

adrenal gland may enter the liver. The majority of capsular lymphatic vessels pass directly to the thoracic duct without the intervention of lymph nodes (Fig. 16.4).

Technique

Adrenalectomies

Exposure and Mobilization of Left Adrenal Gland General Discussion

Exposure of the left adrenal gland begins with the incision of the posterior parietal peritoneum lateral to the left colon. The incision is carried upward, dividing the splenorenal ligament (Fig. 16.5). Avoid injury to the spleen, splenic capsule, splenic vessels, and the tail of the pancreas, which are enveloped by the splenorenal ligament.

Fig. 16.5 Incision of the parietal peritoneum lateral to the left colon. The incision divides the splenorenal ligament

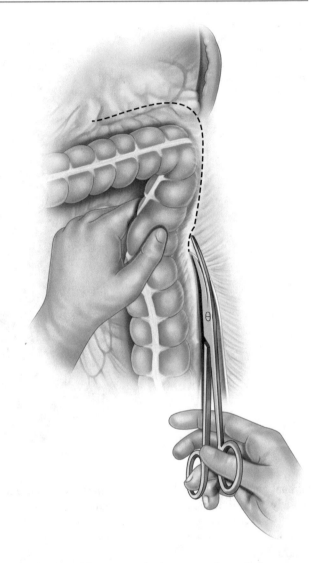

Another approach to the left adrenal is to open the lesser sac through the gastro-colic omentum. The incision should be longitudinal outside the gastroepiploic arcade (Fig. 16.6). Care must be taken to avoid traction on the spleen or the spleno-colic ligament. The ligament may contain tortuous or aberrant inferior polar renal vessels or a left gastroepiploic artery.

In both approaches, the peritoneum under the lower border of the pancreas should be incised halfway along the tail and the incision extended laterally for about 10 cm. By gently retracting the pancreas upward, the left adrenal gland on the superior pole of the left kidney will be exposed. Both the kidney and the gland are covered with renal fascia (of Gerota). The gland will be lateral to the aorta, about 2 cm cranial to the left renal vein. By incising the renal fascia, the adrenal gland is completely exposed and the adrenal vein is accessible.

If the operation is for pheochromocytoma, the adrenal vein should be ligated at once to prevent the release of catecholamines into the circulation during subsequent manipulation of the gland. If it is impossible to refrain from using retractors in this area, place them gently to avoid tearing the inferior mesenteric vein from the splenic vein.

In patients whose left adrenal lesion is anterior, a third approach is useful. The gland is exposed by an oblique incision of the left mesocolon (Fig. 16.7). The arcuate vessels may be divided, but the major branches of the middle and left colic

Fig. 16.6 Approach to the left adrenal through the gastrocolic omentum opening the lesser sac

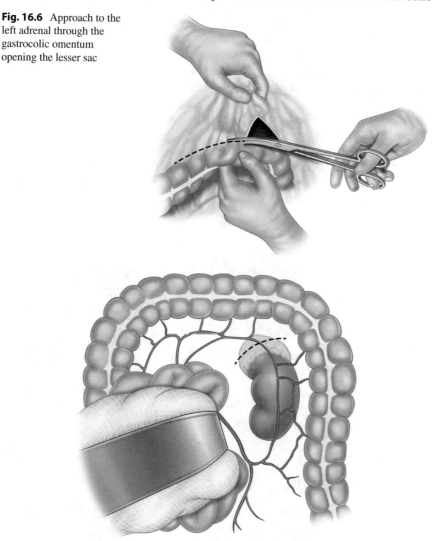

Fig. 16.7 Approach to the left adrenal by incision of the left mesocolon near the splenic flexure. The major branches of the middle and left colic arteries must be spared, but the marginal artery may be sectioned

arteries must be preserved. Injury to the wall of the left colon can be avoided by minimizing retraction.

Use part of the adjacent periadrenal fascia to handle the gland, and for manipulation use only fine forceps. The numerous arteries can be clipped or electrocoagulated to maintain hemostasis.

The dissection starts at the inferolateral aspect of the left adrenal gland and proceeds superiorly (Fig. 16.8). Remaining alert to the possible presence of a superior renal polar artery, the surgeon should retract the gland superiorly. Remember that the left adrenal gland extends downward, close to the left renal artery and vein.

After the adrenal gland has been removed, inspect its bed for bleeding points. Check surrounding organs, especially the spleen and pancreas, for injury. If injuries exist, they may be repaired with sutures over a piece of retroperitoneal fat, Gelfoam, or Avitene, and if the pancreas is injured, drain placement. More severe splenic injuries may require partial or even total splenectomy.

Exposure and Mobilization of Right Adrenal Gland
General Discussion
The anterior approach to the right adrenal gland begins with the mobilization of the hepatic flexure of the colon. Posterior adhesions of the liver to the peritoneum are divided by sharp dissection. Keep in mind that medial attachments may contain hepatic veins.

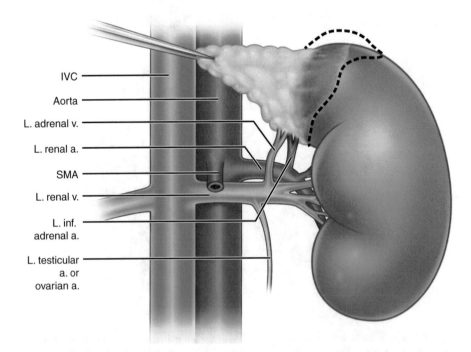

Fig. 16.8 Direction of dissection of the left adrenal gland. Note the position of the left adrenal vein

The duodenum is exposed by mobilizing the colon. The duodenum's second portion is freed by incision of its lateral, avascular peritoneal reflection. After separating it from retroperitoneal structures, reflect it forward and to the left (Kocher maneuver) (Fig. 16.9). The vena cava, right adrenal gland, and upper pole of the right kidney are now exposed (Fig. 16.10). The surgeon must remember that the common bile duct and the gastroduodenal artery are in this area.

Unlike the left adrenal gland, the right adrenal gland rarely extends downward to the renal pedicle. Usually the right adrenal vein leaves the gland on its anterior surface close to the cranial margin and enters the vena cava on its posterior surface (Fig. 16.10). To prevent release of catecholamines and to avoid stretching the vein, place hemostatic clips as soon as both borders of the vein are visible. Hemorrhage from the vena cava may follow if the vein is stretched and avulsed.

Fig. 16.9 Path of midline incision

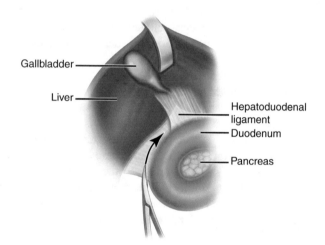

Fig. 16.10 Dividing the medial blood supply for the right adrenal gland

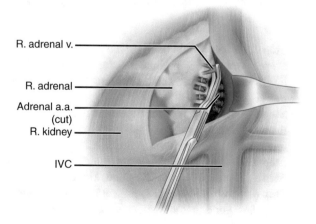

Open Anterior Approach

The anterior approach is considered when: (1) the adrenal disease is bilateral (10 percent), (2) the tumor is over 10 cm in size, or (3) the tumor has invaded surrounding structures. Using the anterior approach, both glands can be inspected, palpated, or biopsied. (In spite of this advantage, the use of the *posterior approach* has increased because of improvements in preoperative diagnosis, such as CT and selective adrenal angiography.)

The incision for an anterior approach may be vertical midline or chevron (Fig. 16.4).

Left Adrenalectomy

Begin dissection of the left adrenal gland on the medial aspect, clipping the arteries encountered. Remember that the pancreas lies just anterior to the gland and is easily injured. Identify the left adrenal vein, which usually emerges from the medial aspect of the gland and courses obliquely downward to enter the left renal vein. Avoid undue traction on the gland, so the renal vein will not be torn.

Right Adrenalectomy

Approach the right adrenal gland by retracting the superior pole of the right kidney inferiorly; the posterior surface of the adrenal gland can then be dissected free from fatty tissue. When the apex of the gland is reached, retract the liver upward. After freeing the lateral borders, the only attachments are the medial margins.

Retract the right adrenal gland laterally, and ligate the arterial branches from the aorta and the right renal artery to the gland. Also ligate the right adrenal vein. Because of the possibility of hemorrhage from the vena cava or the adrenal vein, we recommend freeing up the vena cava far enough to ensure room for an angle clamp. After removing the gland and inspecting for air leaks and bleeding, the incision is closed.

Open Right Adrenalectomy Step-by-Step Technique
Right Anterior

- **Step 1.** Patient should be in supine position.
- **Step 2.** Make a long midline incision from the xiphoid process to the lower midline or bilateral subcostal. If exploring for pheochromocytoma, use a longer midline (Fig. 16.4).
- **Step 3.** Perform lysis of the hepatocolic, hepatoduodenal, and hepatogastric ligaments with downward and left mobilization of the hepatic flexure and upward retraction of the right lobe of the liver.
- **Step 4.** Kocherize the duodenum, which is retracted medially (Fig. 16.9).
- **Step 5.** Visualize the adrenal gland, kidney, and inferior vena cava (Fig. 16.10).
- **Step 6.** Gently and carefully dissect the adrenal gland downward with the finger. Maintain good hemostasis, and apply downward retraction to the kidney (Fig. 16.11).

Fig. 16.11 Downward
retraction

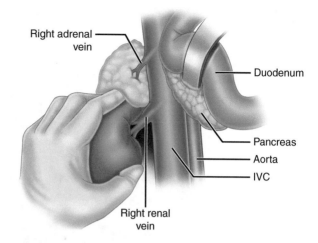

Right adrenal
vein

Duodenum

Pancreas

Aorta

IVC

Right renal
vein

Step 7. Remember
- The right adrenal vein empties into the lateral surface of the inferior vena cava, is usually short, and should be clipped or ligated carefully.
- The arterial supply, from branches of the inferior phrenic artery superiorly, renal artery inferiorly, and aorta medially, is very rich. Perform careful ligation and lysis of any adhesions (Fig. 16.10).

- **Step 8.** The surgeon decides whether a Jackson-Pratt drain is required. Close in layers.

Right or Left Posterior Approach
This approach is seldom used. Use the posterior approach for any adrenalectomy that precludes a laparoscopic or anterior approach. This may occur if the patient has had multiple abdominal operations and has been deemed to have a hostile abdomen.

Posterior Unilateral or Bilateral Adrenalectomy

- **Step 1.** Place patient in prone position with flexion of hips and shoulders and rolls underneath.
- **Step 2.** Incise skin and subcutaneous fat along the length of the 11th rib, using knife or electrocautery (Fig. 16.12).
- **Step 3.** Divide the latissimus dorsi and serratus posterior muscles with electrocautery (Fig. 16.13).
- **Step 4.** Perform subperiosteal resection of the 11th rib (Fig. 16.14).
- **Step 5.** Carefully push the pleura upward, or, if necessary, incise the pleura and the diaphragm.

Fig. 16.12 Incisions for a
posterior approach to the
adrenal glands

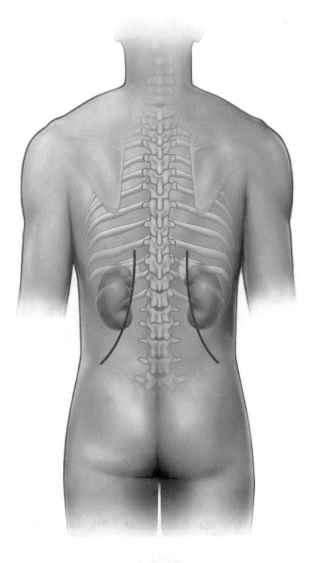

Fig. 16.13 Dividing
latissimus dorsi and
serratus posterior muscles

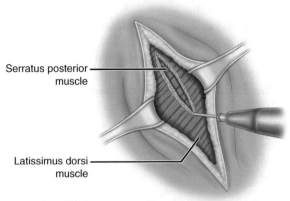

Serratus posterior
muscle

Latissimus dorsi
muscle

Fig. 16.14 Resecting
11th rib

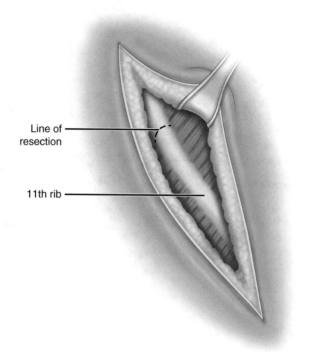

Line of resection

11th rib

- **Step 6.** Incise Gerota's fascia and carefully push the kidney downward (Fig. 16.15).
- **Step 7.** Perform very careful finger dissection of the adrenal gland. Any palpated cordlike formation should be clipped (Fig. 16.16).
- **Step 8.** After good mobilization, divide the adrenal vein between clips (Fig. 16.17).

Remember
- The adrenal vein on the right is very short and, in most cases, drains into the inferior vena cava; but on the left side the adrenal vein is, in most cases, long and drains into the left renal vein.

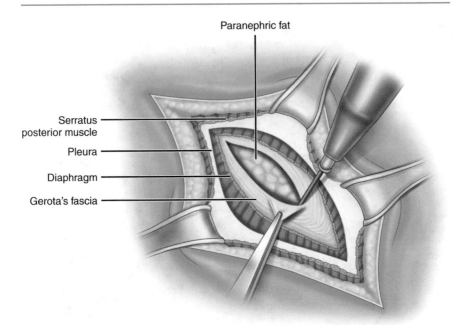

Fig. 16.15 Incising Gerota's fascia

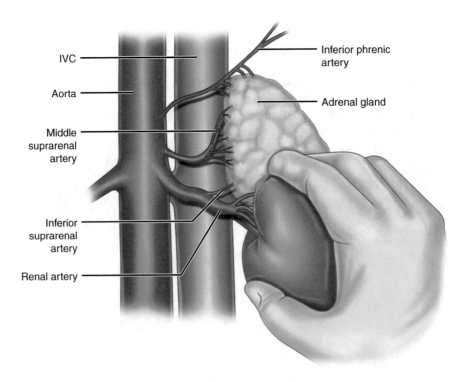

Fig. 16.16 Finger dissection

Fig. 16.17 Dividing adrenal vein

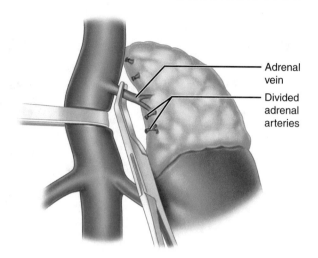

Adrenal vein

Divided adrenal arteries

- **Step 9.** If pleura and diaphragm are incised, close diaphragm with interrupted nonabsorbable sutures. Use a thoracotomy tube through a stab wound and close the wound in layers. The surgeon determines whether a Jackson-Pratt drain is required.

Thoracoabdominal Approach

Better exposure for large tumors of a single adrenal gland is achieved through the thoracoabdominal approach. On the left, it facilitates removal of the spleen and distal pancreas should they be involved with the adrenal tumor. Splenectomy is to be avoided whenever possible.

Start the incision at the angle of the eighth to the tenth ribs and extend it across the midline to the midpoint of the contralateral rectus muscle just above the umbilicus (Fig. 16.18). Remove the tenth rib, open the pleura, and incise the diaphragm from above. Follow the anterior approach procedure to complete the surgery.

Laparoscopic Adrenalectomy

Laparoscopic adrenalectomy results in enhanced recovery and shorter hospital stay when compared to open adrenalectomy. In most patients, laparoscopic adrenalectomy has become the gold standard for adrenalectomy.

Reviewing the discussions above for open exposure and mobilization is very useful in preparing for and executing successful laparoscopic adrenalectomy.

Fig. 16.18 Incision for a thoracolumbar approach to the adrenal gland

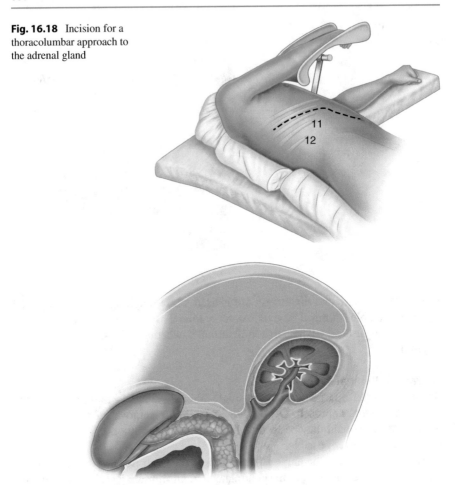

Fig. 16.19 Cross section of patient in left lateral decubitus position demonstrating gravity-facilitated mobilization of spleen and distal pancreas to expose the left adrenal

The transabdominal approaches continue to provide the best overall view of the areas of dissection and surrounding structures. Of the transabdominal approaches, the lateral approach offers many advantages over the anterior approach and has been the technique of choice for most surgeons performing laparoscopic adrenalectomy. The transabdominal *lateral* approach to adrenalectomy places the patient in lateral decubitus position to allow a gravity-facilitated exposure of the adrenals (Fig. 16.19).

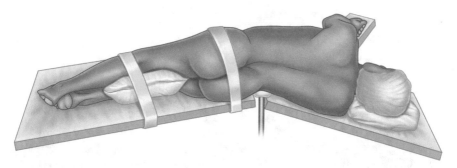

Fig. 16.20 Patient positioning in left lateral decubitus position with kidney rest and table break at iliac crest

In this way, tissue and organs overlying the adrenals do not need to be manipulated with laparoscopic instruments, and the complications and bleeding associated with such manipulation are avoided.

Laparoscopic Left Adrenalectomy

Preoperative: Consider mild laxative evening before surgery (e.g., one bottle of magnesium citrate orally)

Position: Left lateral decubitus, iliac crest at table break, and kidney rest elevated (Fig. 16.20)

Anesthesia: General

Other: Consider Foley catheter, orogastric tube, place pneumatic compression hose, all pressure points well padded, and utilize an energy-based laparoscopic dissector

- **Step 1.** Prep and drape the patient so that either laparoscopy or open surgery can be performed (Fig. 16.21).
- **Step 2.** Access the peritoneal cavity at the midclavicular line below the right costal margin (cannula site for the camera) with open approach, Optiview or Veress needle. Establish pneumoperitoneum to 15 mmHg.
- **Step 3.** Insert cannulas as shown in Fig. 16.22.

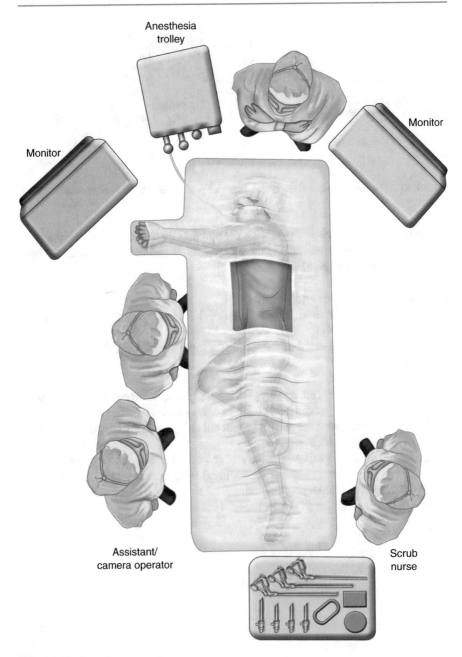

Fig. 16.21 Operating room setup

Fig. 16.22 Cannula sites
and uses

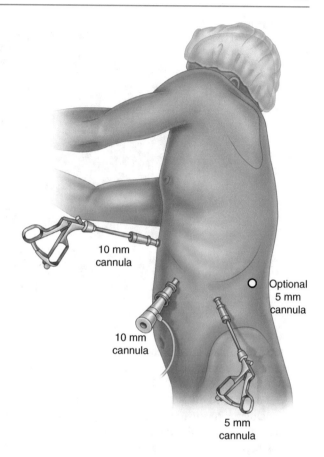

10 mm
cannula

○ Optional
5 mm
cannula

10 mm
cannula

5 mm
cannula

- **Step 4.** Using a laparoscopic dissector and shears, incise the splenorenal ligament and mobilize the spleen laterally (Fig. 16.23). The decubitus positioning
  facilitates this dissection and mobilization. With gravity pulling the spleen medially and away from the anterior surface of the kidney, dissect the spleen and tail
  of the pancreas away from the retroperitoneum as the superior pole of the kidney
  and the adrenal are exposed.

Note
- This dissection plane is relatively avascular. If excessive bleeding is
  encountered, the wrong plane of dissection may be created.

Fig. 16.23 Initial incision along splenorenal and splenocolic ligaments

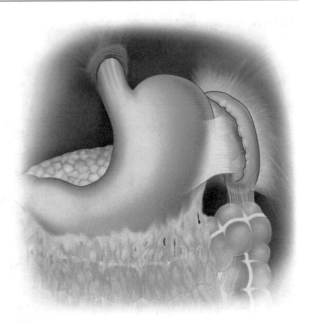

- **Step 5.** Continue the dissection along the anterior surface of the kidney and adrenal until the inferior pole and medial border of the adrenal are exposed. It is important to continue this mobilization up to the diaphragm and close to the greater curve of the stomach and short gastric vessels. In this way, the exposure is analogous to opening a book, with the pages of the book being the spleen/pancreatic tail and the anterior surface of the kidney/adrenal, and the spine of the book being a line just beyond the medial edge of the adrenal gland (Fig. 16.24).

Note
- DO NOT mobilize the adrenal gland along its lateral edge too early in the exposure. If this mistake is made, gravity will allow the mobilized adrenal to fall medially and prevent visualization and access to the medial and inferior edges of the gland, where the left adrenal vein is most likely encountered.

- **Step 6.** Isolate and clip the left adrenal vein (Fig. 16.25)

Note
- Risk of injuring the left renal vein is minimized by staying close to the adrenal gland during this dissection. A right angle dissector greatly facilitates this exposure and isolation.

Fig. 16.24 "Opening the Book." Mobilized spleen and tail of pancreas rotated off of the kidney and adrenal

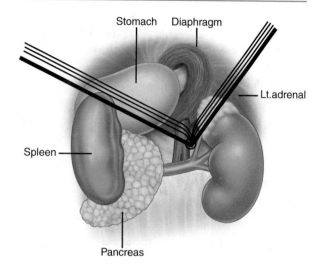

Fig. 16.25 Isolation and control of left adrenal vein

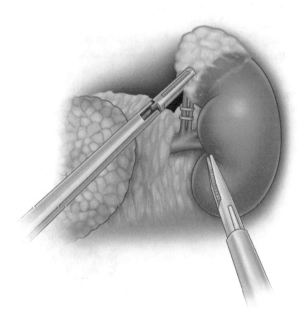

- **Step 7.** Transect the adrenal vein.
- **Step 8.** Excise the adrenal gland from inferior and medial to superior and lateral following the anterior surface of the kidney. Clip small feeding vessels as they are encountered.
- **Step 9.** Place the adrenal in a specimen retrieval sac and remove (Fig. 16.26).

Note
- The bag must be stout enough not to rupture during extraction (Fig. 16.27).
- The fascia of the cannula site of extraction may need to be stretched with a Kelly clamp to facilitate removal.
- For large tumors, the entire incision may need to be extended.
- The adrenal should not be morcellated.

- **Step 10.** Irrigate and suction the operative field dry, and carefully inspect for hemostasis.
- **Step 11.** Remove cannulas and allow carbon dioxide insufflation to entirely escape the abdominal cavity.
- **Step 12.** Close the fascia of the 10 mm incisions with an absorbable 0 suture and the skin with a subcuticular 4–0 absorbable suture.

Fig. 16.26 The excised adrenal gland is placed in specimen retrieval sac

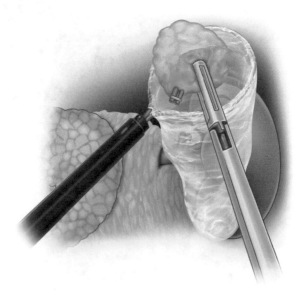

Fig. 16.27 Specimen
retrieval sac is extracted
from abdomen through
10 mm cannula site

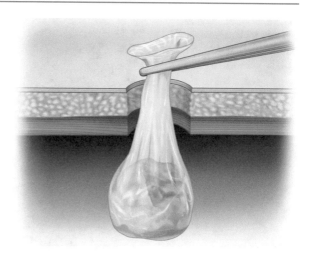

Laparoscopic Right Adrenalectomy

Preoperative: Consider mild laxative evening before surgery (e.g., one bottle of magnesium citrate orally).

Position: Right lateral decubitus, iliac crest at table break and kidney rest elevated (Fig. 16.20).

Anesthesia: General.

Other: Consider Foley catheter, orogastric tube, place pneumatic compression hose, all pressure points well padded, and utilize an energy-based laparoscopic dissector.

- **Step 1.** Prep and drape the patient so that either laparoscopy or open surgery can be performed.
- **Step 2.** Access the peritoneal cavity at the midclavicular line below the left costal margin (cannula site for the camera) with open approach, Optiview or Veress needle. Establish pneumoperitoneum to 15 mmHg.
- **Step 3.** Insert cannulas as shown in Fig. 16.28.

Note
- A fourth cannula in the epigastrium is necessary for a retractor to elevate the right lobe of the liver.

Fig. 16.28 Cannula sites and uses for laparoscopic right adrenalectomy

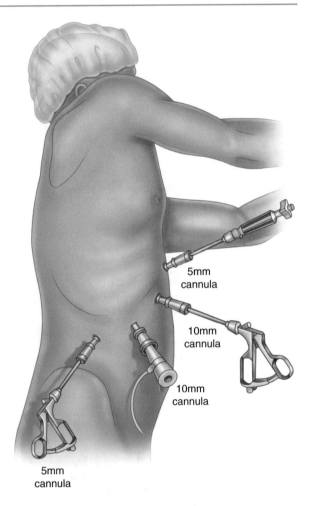

5mm
cannula

10mm
cannula

10mm
cannula

5mm
cannula

- **Step 4.** With the liver retractor positioned, fully mobilize the right lobe of the liver, the anterior surface of the right kidney and the lateral edge of the inferior vena cava can be clearly seen. Begin dissection by creating a hockey stick-shaped incision along the retroperitoneal attachment of the right lobe of the liver and the medial border of inferior vena cava (Fig. 16.29).

Note
- This mobilizes the right lobe of the liver posteriorly and allows exposure of the anterior surface of the adrenal as the liver is pushed cephalad.
- The lateral positioning of the patient facilitates exposure of this area. Gravity holds the hepatic flexure of the colon and the omentum away from the operative field.
- It is rarely necessary to dissect the hepatic flexure or perform a Kocher maneuver to complete the dissection of the right adrenal.

Fig. 16.29 Hockey stick incision for initial dissection of right adrenal

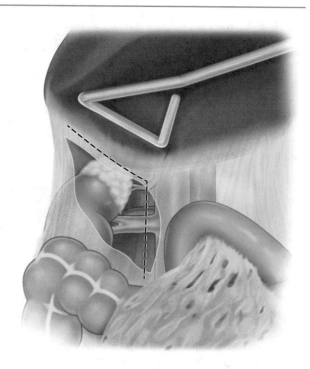

- **Step 5.** Carefully dissect the medial border of the right adrenal, which will either be in close proximity to or immediate next to the lateral margin of the inferior vena cava, looking for the right adrenal vein (Fig. 16.30).

Note
- The right adrenal vein is typically broad, short and enters the vena cava slightly posteriorly.
- It is commonly found cephalad to the initial retroperitoneal incision along the right lobe of the liver.
- A blunt-tipped right angle dissector is best for isolating the adrenal vein.

Fig. 16.30 Exposure and
isolation of vena cava and
right adrenal vein using
blunt-tipped right angle
dissector

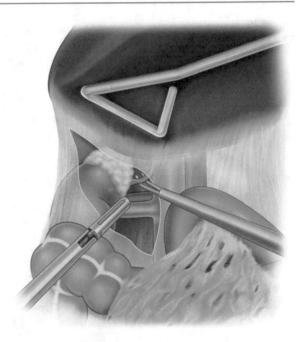

- **Step 6.** Ligate the adrenal vein with three medium-large Ligaclips proximally and two distally (Fig. 16.31).

Note
- Because of the short length of this vein, the proximal-most clip should be immediately at the edge of the cava.

- **Step 7.** Transect the adrenal vein.
- **Step 8.** Excise and remove the adrenal gland as described for left adrenalectomy.

Laparoscopic Bilateral Adrenalectomy

Bilateral laparoscopic adrenalectomies are performed in the manner already described for each individual side. Because right adrenalectomy has a higher risk of conversion to open adrenalectomy as a result of the immediate consequences of an adrenal vein/caval injury, left adrenalectomy should be performed first. In this way, the patient will have the greatest likelihood of benefiting from a laparoscopic approach. Before repositioning for right adrenalectomy the entire left adrenalectomy is completed, including wound closure and abdominal desufflation (minimizing duration of CO_2 pneumoperitoneum).

Fig. 16.31 Ligation of
right adrenal vein with
Ligaclips

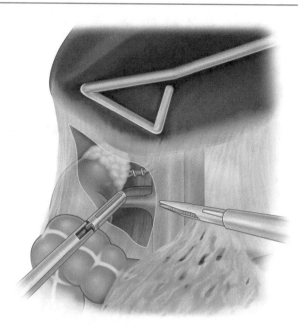

Anatomical Complications

The inferior mesenteric vein may be avulsed by excessive traction at its junction
with the splenic vein. The middle and left colic arteries may be severed by dissection through the left mesocolon. The left adrenal gland extends downward almost to
the hilum of the kidney. It is therefore possible to injure the renal vessels while
mobilizing the gland. Lateral retraction of the right adrenal gland can avulse the
right adrenal vein leading to a rupture of the vena cava. Be aware of the accessory
right adrenal vein coming off of the right renal vein. Though uncommon, injury to
the gastroduodenal artery can occur. If injured, ligate it.

Traction on the spleen may result in avulsion of the splenic capsule. Pancreatic
parenchyma can be injured if it is necessary to mobilize the gland cephalad. The
capsule of the kidney may be injured during dissection of the inferior medial margin
of the left adrenal gland. The left colon could be injured during its mobilization
while incising the left mesocolon. Injury to the liver may occur from excessive
retraction. A catastrophic postoperative duodenal fistula may occur after an unrecognized injury to the duodenum during its mobilization. During a posterior approach
the plural may be injured resulting in a pneumothorax. Be aware during a posterior
approach of the 12th intercostal nerve. Injury to this nerve could result in a postoperative hypesthesia.

Vascular System

17

Andrew Walter Unzeitig and Lee J. Skandalakis

Anatomy

Anatomy for Carotid Endarterectomy

The vagus nerve descends from the jugular foramen posteriorly between the internal jugular vein and the internal carotid artery. The ansa hypoglossi comes off hypoglossal nerve anteriorly and supplies the strap muscles. The facial vein enters the internal jugular vein. To expose the carotid bifurcation, division and ligation of the ansa hypoglossi and facial vein may be required. The hypoglossal nerve is often encountered as it descends from the jugular foramen in the carotid sheath traveling over the internal carotid artery and anterior to the external carotid artery toward the tongue.

Anatomy for Abdominal Aortic Aneurysm Repair

The abdominal portion of the aorta extends from the diaphragmatic hiatus to the level of the fourth lumbar vertebra (Fig. 17.1). It terminates as the left and right common iliac arteries and the middle sacral artery. The abdominal aorta gives off visceral branches as the celiac, superior, and inferior mesenteric arteries and the suprarenal, spermatic, and renal arteries. Originating anteriorly from the aorta are the celiac, superior mesenteric, and inferior mesenteric arteries. The parietal

A. W. Unzeitig (✉)
Department of Vascular Surgery, Piedmont Atlanta Hospital, Atlanta, GA, USA
e-mail: Andrew.Unzeitig@piedmont.org

L. J. Skandalakis
Department of Surgery, Piedmont Hospital, Atlanta, GA, USA

© Springer Nature Switzerland AG 2021
L. J. Skandalakis (ed.), *Surgical Anatomy and Technique*,
https://doi.org/10.1007/978-3-030-51313-9_17

Fig. 17.1 The abdominal aorta as it extends from the diaphragmatic hiatus to the common iliac bifurcation

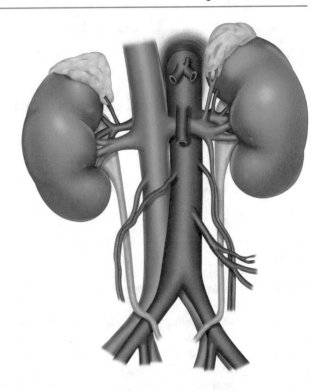

branches off the abdominal aorta include the paired inferior phrenic arteries arising near the aortic hiatus and the multiple lumbar arteries, which divide into ventral and dorsal branches at the border of the psoas muscle.

Anatomy for Lower Extremity Bypass

The infrainguinal region is bounded medially by the pectineus muscle and laterally by the tensor fascia lata muscle. Its superior border is the inguinal ligament, which is a strong, fibrous band that stretches from the anterior superior iliac spine to the pubic tubercle.

The external iliac artery becomes the common femoral artery as it emanates from a point under the middle of the inguinal ligament. The artery is relatively superficial proximally, but somewhat deeper where it terminates. Approximately 5 cm below the inguinal ligament, the profunda femoral branch takes origin from the common femoral artery, usually arising posterolaterally.

The femoral artery continues down the thigh as the superficial femoral artery (Fig. 17.2). The profunda femoris artery passes beneath the adductor longus muscle, while the superficial femoral artery remains above it. The profunda femoris tends to remain patent in patients with superficial femoral artery occlusive disease and thus provides a source of collateral circulation. It has several important branches: lateral

Fig. 17.2 Vascular anatomy of the lower extremity.
Note occlusion of the distal superficial femoral artery

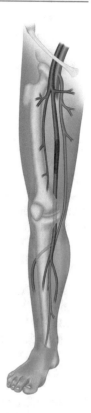

and medial circumflex femoral arteries (though they may occasionally arise from the common femoral artery) and the supreme geniculate artery. Distally, the superficial femoral artery courses under the sartorius muscle and into the adductor (Hunter's) canal.

From superficial to deep, the adductor canal is composed of the following muscles: adductor longus, adductor brevis, and adductor magnus. The superficial femoral artery becomes the popliteal artery as it emerges anterior to the adductor magnus. The popliteal artery then courses anterior to the semimembranosus, gastrocnemius, plantaris, and soleus muscles; this depth often makes palpating a popliteal pulse difficult.

Distal to the popliteus muscle, the popliteal artery bifurcates into the anterior tibial artery and the tibioperoneal trunk. The anterior tibial continues down the leg, anterior to the tibia, and becomes the dorsalis pedis artery in the foot. The peroneal and posterior tibial arteries arise from the tibioperoneal trunk, approximately 2 cm below the tendon of the soleus muscle. The peroneal artery divides into calcaneal branches as it passes behind the inferior tibiofibular articulation. The posterior tibial artery travels along the medial aspect of the leg and posterior to the medial malleolus.

The great saphenous vein starts on the medial side of the foot, just anterior to the medial malleolus. It continues along the medial aspect of the calf and thigh and courses anteriorly as it enters the femoral vein just below the inguinal ligament. The great saphenous vein is an ideal conduit for use in bypass surgery because of its convenient location next to the femoral artery and its superficial course in the subcutaneous tissue exterior to the investing fascia.

Technique

Carotid Endarterectomy

PRIOR TO SURGERY: On preoperative imaging, locate the carotid bifurcation to assist in correct placement of the incision. If there is a history of neck surgery, perform preoperative laryngoscopy to ascertain and document status of vocal cords; the recurrent laryngeal nerve may have been injured during the past procedure.

POSITION: Patient's head turned away from the operative side; neck extended.
ANESTHESIA: General or local (Fig. 17.3).

- **Step 1.** Make an incision along the anterior border of the sternocleidomastoid muscle (SCM). Incise the platysma.
- **Step 2.** Locate the external jugular vein and greater auricular nerve, which rest atop the SCM. Divide the vein to facilitate exposure, but preserve the nerve intact.
- **Step 3.** Dissect around the relatively avascular anterior border of the SCM until the internal jugular vein is identified within the carotid sheath. Take care not to injure the vagus nerve.
- **Step 4.** Divide and ligate the ansa hypoglossi and facial vein to expose the carotid bifurcation (Fig. 17.4).

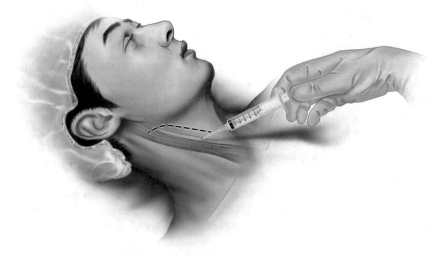

Fig. 17.3 Infiltration of local anesthesia along the planned line of incision

Fig. 17.4 Exposure of the
carotid bifurcation and
adjacent nerves

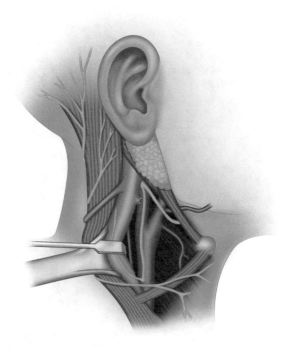

- **Step 5.** Dissect the carotid sufficiently to identify the internal and external carotid branches. Proximal arterial control is accomplished by encircling the common carotid artery in an area relatively free of atherosclerosis. Distal arterial control is achieved by encircling the internal carotid artery at the most superior aspect of the wound where normal, non-atherosclerotic artery is encountered.
- **Step 6.** If an additional 1–2 cm of distal exposure is needed, divide the posterior belly of the digastric muscle. Be alert for the hypoglossal nerve.
- **Step 7.** Free the external carotid artery and facilitate vascular control of the three arterial trunks with Rummel's tourniquets (Fig. 17.5).
- **Step 8.** Identify and isolate the superior thyroid artery.
- **Step 9.** Systemically anticoagulate the patient with heparin.
- **Step 10.** Clamp the distal internal carotid artery and then the common carotid artery and the external carotid artery.
- **Step 11.** Control the superior thyroid artery by the loose application of a metallic clip or silk tie (which is removed at the end of the procedure).

Fig. 17.5 Arterial control of common carotid, internal carotid, and external carotid arteries with umbilical tape. Arterial control of superior thyroid artery with 3–0 silk tie

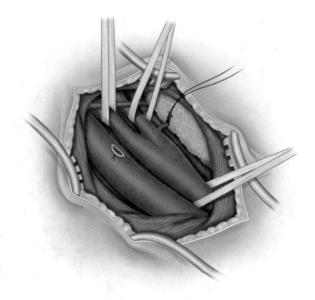

Fig. 17.6 An arteriotomy is made with a scalpel and extended with Potts scissors

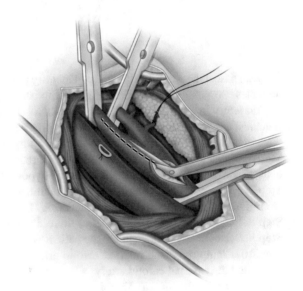

- **Step 12.** With a sharp knife and Potts scissors, perform an arteriotomy from the distal common carotid artery to the proximal internal carotid artery (Fig. 17.6).
- **Step 13.** To maintain adequate blood flow, place an indwelling shunt first into the internal carotid artery and then into the common carotid artery (Fig. 17.7).
- **Step 14.** Begin the endarterectomy in a deep plane between the plaque and the adventitia using a spatula (Fig. 17.8). Proceed proximally down the common carotid artery until the plaque thins; at this point sharply transect it.

Fig. 17.7 Placement of an indwelling shunt from the internal carotid artery to the common carotid artery

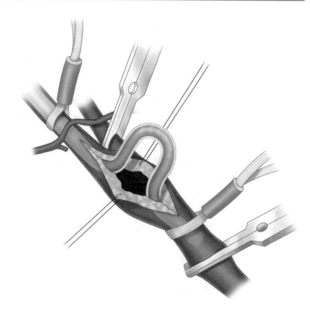

Fig. 17.8 An endarterectomy spatula is used to lift plaque off the adventitia

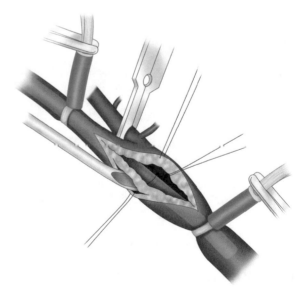

- **Step 15.** Tease the plaque from the external carotid artery using the endarterectomy spatula or a fine hemostat.
- **Step 16.** As the atheromatous plaque thins distally in the internal carotid, there is transition to a more superficial plane at which point it usually feathers away from the very thin normal intima.
- **Step 17.** Flush the inside of the artery with heparinized saline. Inspect.
- **Step 18.** If the end-points of the dissection are not adequately visualized, extend the arteriotomy.
- **Step 19.** If the distal end-point requires tacking, use simple sutures with the knots outside the artery to make the intima adherent.
- **Step 20.** Flush with heparinized saline to detect loose tags of circumferentially oriented media. Grasp with fine forceps and remove.
- **Step 21.** Close the arteriotomy by applying a collagen-impregnated polyester patch or bovine patch using a continuous layer of 6–0 monofilament suture (Fig. 17.9). Prior to completing the closure, remove the shunt and then vent the artery so that clot, debris, and air escape completely.
- **Step 22.** Remove clamps first from the external carotid artery, followed by the common carotid artery, and then the internal carotid artery.
- **Step 23.** Place a suction drain through a stab wound low in the neck (Fig. 17.10).
- **Step 24.** Close the platysma with a running absorbable suture; close the skin with a monofilament suture.

Remember
- The diseased artery is not dissected from the patient, but rather the patient is dissected away from the artery. In other words, during maneuvers near the carotid, the artery should be minimally disturbed. This is based on the premise that undue manipulation of the vessel increases the risk of embolization of stroke-producing thrombus.
- Beware of the nonrecurrent laryngeal nerve in patients with an abnormal aortic arch, because the nerve may leave the carotid sheath in the neck.
- Avoid damage to cranial nerves during dissection by properly placing retractors or vascular clamps and by precise use of electrocoagulation current.

Elective Infrarenal Abdominal Aortic Aneurysm Repair

PRIOR TO SURGERY: Document lower extremity pulse examination.
    POSITION: Supine.
    ANESTHESIA: General.

- **Step 1.** Make a midline incision from the xiphoid process to the symphysis pubis to provide excellent exposure.
- **Step 2.** Reflect upward the transverse colon and mesocolon; reflect the small bowel to the right and upward.

Fig. 17.9 Closure of arteriotomy with a bovine patch using 6–0 monofilament suture

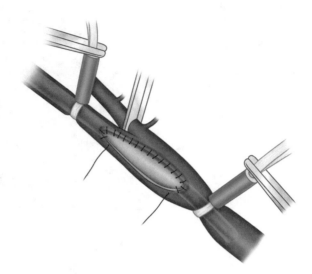

Fig. 17.10 Placement of a Jackson–Pratt drain through a separate incision and skin closure

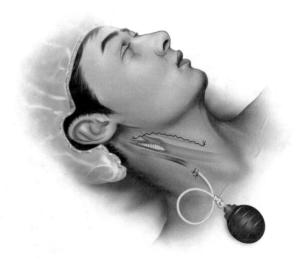

- **Step 3.** Incise the ligament of Treitz and the superior and medial duodenal attachments.
- **Step 4.** If the inferior mesenteric vein cannot be laterally displaced, divide it to facilitate exposure.
- **Step 5.** Open the retroperitoneum distally to expose the common iliac artery bifurcations (Fig. 17.11).
- **Step 6.** Superiorly, perform retroperitoneal dissection to expose and encircle the infrarenal aortic wall.
- **Step 7.** Assess patency and flow status of the inferior mesenteric artery by palpation and Doppler probe interrogation (Fig. 17.12).

Fig. 17.11 A vertical incision is made in the posterior parietal peritoneum to provide exposure from the infrarenal aorta to the common iliac arteries

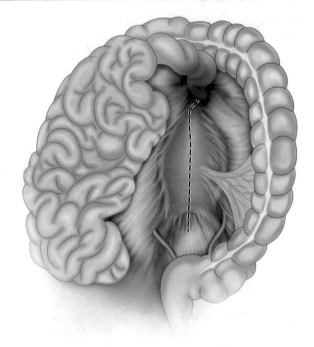

Fig. 17.12 Doppler ultrasound interrogation of the inferior mesenteric artery

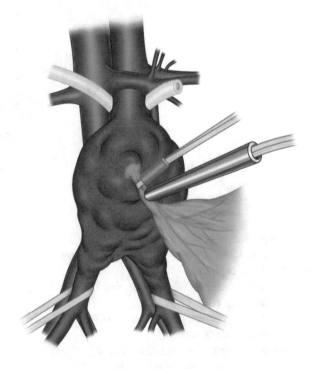

- **Step 8.** After adequate exposure has been achieved, give systemic heparin in a dose of 0.6–1.0 mg/kg of body weight.
- **Step 9.** Clamp the iliac arteries, then the infrarenal aorta.
- **Step 10.** Incise the aortic wall vertically (Fig. 17.13).
- **Step 11.** Remove loose, laminated thrombus.
- **Step 12.** If lumbar arteries are back-bleeding into the aneurysm, ligate with interrupted figure-of-eight sutures (Fig. 17.14).
- **Step 13.** Cut to length a bifurcated, collagen-impregnated polyester graft (18 to 22 mm in size) and suture it end-to-end to the proximal aortic stump with

Fig. 17.13 Incision of the aortic wall and common iliac arteries, facilitating removal of thrombus

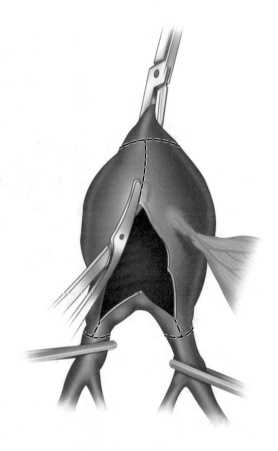

Fig. 17.14 Ligation of
back-bleeding lumbar
arteries with figure-of-
eight sutures

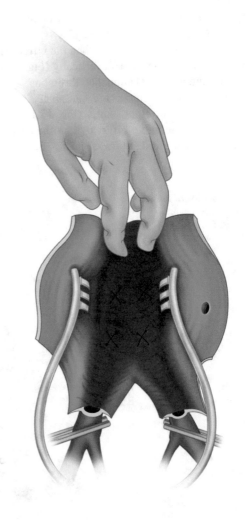

running continuous 3–0 polypropylene suture (Fig. 17.15). This suture-line
should be started on the back wall and carried anteriorly around the aorta from
each side.

- **Step 14.** Distally, make an anastomosis to each iliac artery in end-to-end fashion
using 4–0 continuous suture (Fig. 17.16). Exercise caution in the circumferential
dissection of the iliac arteries to avoid injuring the iliac veins or ureters.
- **Step 15.** Prior to completing the final anastomosis, flush the aorta and graft.
- **Step 16.** Remove occlusion clamps stepwise and ascertain hemostasis at the
suture lines.

Fig. 17.15 The proximal suture line is started on the back wall and brought anteriorly from each side with a continuous running suture

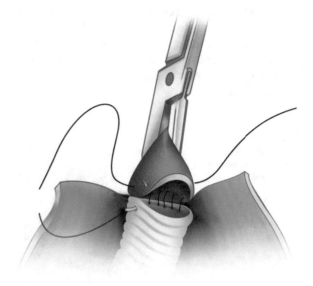

Fig. 17.16 End-to-side anastomosis is fashioned to each iliac artery using a continuous running suture

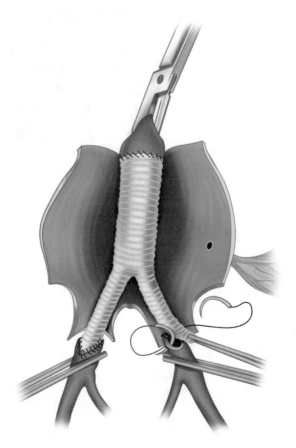

- **Step 17.** If the inferior mesenteric artery shows minimal back-bleeding, reimplant its orifice onto the aortic graft (Fig. 17.17). A side-biting vascular clamp allows for flow through the graft during reimplantation.
- **Step 18.** After heparin reversal, inspect the field for hemostasis and close the aneurysm sac around the prosthesis with a single layer of running suture (Fig. 17.18).

Fig. 17.17
Reimplantation of the
inferior mesenteric artery
onto the aortic graft

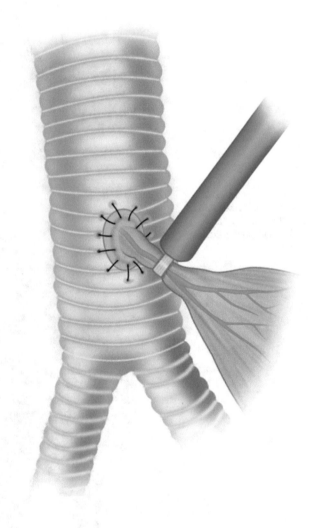

Fig. 17.18 Closure of the
aneurysm sac around the
prosthesis

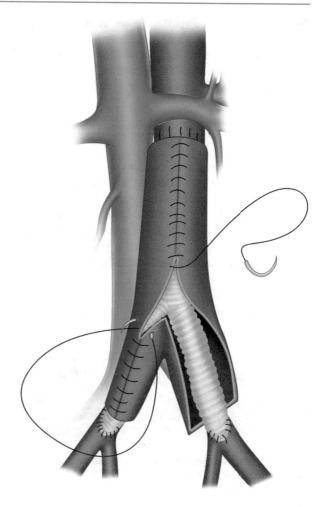

- **Step 19.** Suture the posterior parietal peritoneum to prevent adherence of the
  small bowel to exposed graft material.

Remember
- During dissection it is possible to dislodge thrombus material from the
  aneurysm sac, which may embolize distally. Thus, it is important to demonstrate good back-bleeding intraoperatively and to confirm the presence
  of distal pulses immediately postoperatively.
- In 5% of the population, there exists a retroaortic renal vein. Therefore, the
  course of the left renal vein should be demonstrated to prevent injury during cross-clamping.
- If preoperative imaging suggests that the inferior mesenteric artery is an
  important visceral collateral, or if intraoperative Doppler interrogation
  shows inadequate blood flow, the vessel should be reimplanted.

Femoropopliteal Bypass, Below Knee, with Saphenous Vein

PRIOR TO SURGERY: Imaging studies (angiogram, MRA, arterial duplex ultra-sound mapping) are vitally important to proper preoperative planning. Preoperative duplex ultrasound vein mapping will assist in identifying the presence (or absence) of adequate venous conduit.

POSITION: Supine.

ANESTHESIA: General or spinal.

- **Step 1.** Make a vertical incision overlying the femoral pulse.
- **Step 2.** Identify the saphenous vein and dissect it out. Follow it down the medial aspect of the leg with either one incision or skip incisions along its course (Fig. 17.19). The vein can also be harvested endoscopically.
- **Step 3.** With 4–0 silk ligate venous tributaries 1–2 mm from the main trunk to allow for expansion with arterial pressure. Their distal aspect may be either clipped or tied off in a similar manner (Fig. 17.20).

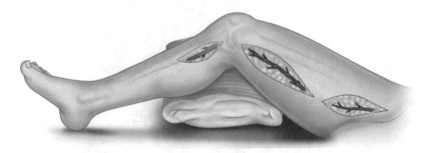

Fig. 17.19 Incisions along the medial aspect of the leg facilitating dissection of the femoral and popliteal arteries, as well as harvest of the saphenous vein

Fig. 17.20 Venous tributaries are ligated with 4–0 silk 1–2 mm way from the vessel. The distal aspect may be clipped or tied off in a similar manner

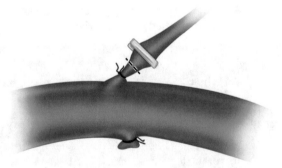

- **Step 4.** Gently irrigate the saphenous vein with saline solution containing heparin.
- **Step 5.** Ligate missed tributaries with silk sutures. The harvested vein can then be stored in a similar heparin solution, until ready for use.
- **Step 6.** Expose the below-knee popliteal artery through an incision 2 cm behind the tibia on the medial aspect of the leg.
- **Step 7.** Reflect the gastrocnemius muscle posteriorly and incise the fascia overlying the popliteal artery and vein.
- **Step 8.** The origin of the soleus muscle that arches across the below-knee popliteal artery may have to be incised to allow for exposure.
- **Step 9.** Dissect the distal popliteal artery away from its accompanying vein. Proximal and distal control of the vessel is obtained via vessel loops around the proximal popliteal, tibioperoneal, and anterior tibial arteries (Fig. 17.21).
- **Step 10.** Expose the common femoral artery through the original femoral incision. Obtain proximal and distal control via vessel loops around the proximal common femoral, superficial femoral, and profunda femoral arteries, respectively.
- **Step 11.** Create a tunnel from the below-knee popliteal space passing directly behind the knee joint and then medially through the subcutaneous tissue to the groin inflow site.
- **Step 12.** Anticoagulate the patient systemically with heparin.
- **Step 13.** Perform an end-to-side anastomosis by suturing the spatulated, reversed saphenous vein to an arteriotomy in the below-knee popliteal artery with continuous 6–0 monofilament polypropylene suture (for calcified vessels, 5–0 suture material is more suitable) (Fig. 17.22).

Fig. 17.21 The below-knee popliteal artery exposure showing branching of the anterior tibial artery

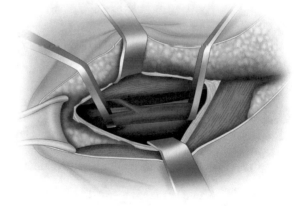

Fig. 17.22 End-to-side anastomosis of spatulated vein to below-knee popliteal artery

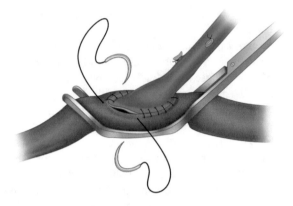

Fig. 17.23 End-to-side femoral anastomosis

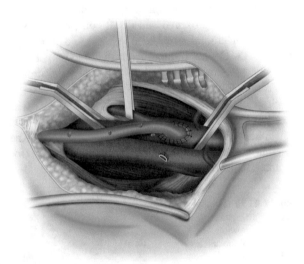

- **Step 14.** Draw the saphenous conduit through the prepared tunnel to the groin, taking care to avoid kinking or twisting of the vein graft.
- **Step 15.** Perform the femoral anastomosis in an end-to-side manner (Fig. 17.23).
- **Step 16.** Close incisions in layers.
- **Step 17.** Use of closed suction drainage is optional.

Remember
- Good arterial inflow, suitable outflow, and an adequate conduit are the three requirements for a successful bypass.
- Complete hemostasis and avoidance of tissue desiccation are essential.

Arteriovenous Fistula (AVF)

Preoperative assessment must include evaluation of patient's history with regard to previous catheters, superficial venous thrombosis (SVT), and deep vein thrombosis (DVT) in the upper extremities. Determine the patient's dominant arm and, if possible, use the nondominant arm first.

Examine the patient's veins with a tourniquet in place. Examine arterial pulses from the axillary distally and verify a brisk Allen's test (assessment of collateral circulation).

Obtain ultrasound vein mapping of the upper extremities. Consider obtaining a venogram in cases where the patient has had multiple prior access procedures and/or central vein catheters that may impede a successful access.

If the patient in question is already on hemodialysis, consideration should be given to performing the procedure on a "non-dialysis" day. Immediately prior to a dialysis, the patient may experience volume overload and electrolyte imbalance. In addition, the patient may be hypovolemic immediately after dialysis and tend toward hypotension while under sedation during the procedure.

Generally, dialysis access operations can be performed under local anesthesia with mild sedation, although this decision must be modified individually based on the anticipated length and complexity of the procedure.

Radiocephalic AVF

- **Step 1.** Prep the entire arm circumferentially from the shoulder to the hand. Cover the hand itself with a sterile towel and use adhesive bandage or a towel clamp to affix the towel in place.
- **Step 2.** Make a short incision axially along the radial artery just proximal to the wrist.
- **Step 3.** Initially identify the cephalic vein by undermining toward the dorsal surface of the wrist. Dissect the cephalic vein distally and proximally; free a sufficient length to allow the vein to reach the radial artery easily without tension. Ligate and divide branches with 4–0 silk.
- **Step 4.** Ligate the cephalic vein distally and spatulate its open end. Flush the vein with heparinized saline. Inflate the vein gently.
- **Step 5.** Proceed to expose the radial artery. Take great care to avoid injury to the adjoining structures. Encircle the radial artery proximally and distally with vessel loops.
- **Step 6.** At this time you may heparinize the patient. Some operators choose not to administer systemic heparin and instead locally flush the artery with a heparinized saline solution. Both approaches are acceptable.
- **Step 7.** Clamp the artery with vessel clamps such as angled Debakey clamps or Heifetz clips, or control with vessel loops.
- **Step 8.** Create an arteriotomy with an 11 blade and extend it with Potts scissors.

- **Step 9.** Sew the vein to the radial artery with standard vascular anastomosis technique 7–0 Prolene suture.
- **Step 10.** Once the anastomosis is completed, release the clamp on the proximal radial artery and the cephalic vein first so as not to flush any inadvertently retained debris to the hand. Finally, release the clamp on the distal radial artery. Examine the pulse in the fistula. You should feel a thrill and hear a bruit with Doppler. Examine the fistula where it is visible in your operative field. Make sure that there are no kinks in the AVF and that the fistula is not tethered in any way. Release any tethering bands of soft tissue.
- **Step 11.** Approximate the subcutaneous fascia over the fistula. Close the skin with a subcuticular suture.

Note
- Consider using ultrasound intraoperatively to mark the course of the cephalic vein and its major tributaries.

Brachiocephalic AVF
Step 1. Make a transverse incision just distal to the antecubital crease.
Step 2. In the subcutaneous fat, identify the medial cubital vein and the cephalic vein to which it drains.
Step 3. Mobilize the cephalic vein sufficiently so that it will reach the brachial artery without tension.
Step 4. Divide the bicep aponeurosis axially. Identify the underlying brachial artery. The brachial vein generally lies over the artery. Take great care not to injure the vein and the adjacent median nerve.
Step 5. Encircle the brachial artery proximally and distally.
Step 6. Heparinize the patient.
Step 7. Create a short arteriotomy in the brachial artery.
Step 8. Assess the correct length of cephalic vein needed to reach the artery and proceed to spatulate the vein.
Step 9. Sew the anastomosis with 6.0 Prolene suture.
Step 10. Flush the anastomosis with heparinized saline and complete it.
Step 11. Examine the portion of the fistula visible in your incision and small skin flap. The vein should lie tension-free. Release any restrictive soft tissue bands.
Step 12. Close the incision with 3.0 Vicryl for the subcutaneous fascia and 4.0 Monocryl for the skin.

Note
- Reestablish flow first to the fistula and then to the distal brachial artery. Expect an easily palpable thrill.

Brachio-axillary Arterial Venous Graft

- **Step 1.** Make a short axially oriented incision just proximal to the antecubital crease over the brachial artery pulse.
- **Step 2.** Sharply dissect the artery proximally and distally and encircle with vessel loops.
- **Step 3.** Make another short axially oriented incision in the proximal upper arm in the axilla. Identify the axillary vein. Dissect the vein free; avoid injury to neighboring structures. Encircle the vein proximally and distally.
- **Step 4.** Use a large clamp or curved tunneler to create a subcutaneous tunnel between the two incisions. Do not make the tunnel any wider that it needs to be in order to pass the graft through it snuggly. Orient the tunnel in an arched course and make sure that the majority of the graft will lie over the anterior portion of the bicep muscle.
- **Step 5.** Pass a 4–7 mm tapered polytetrafluoroethylene (PTFE) graft in the tunnel with the 4 mm end toward the artery. Do not trim the 4 mm segment, because it provides resistance to flow and thereby reduces the risk of steal syndrome.
- **Step 6.** Heparinize the patient.
- **Step 7.** Clamp the brachial artery and create an arteriotomy.
- **Step 8.** Sew the PTFE graft to the open brachial artery in an end-to-side fashion.
- **Step 9.** Clamp the graft and reestablish flow in the brachial artery.
- **Step 10.** Clamp the axillary vein.
- **Step 11.** Make a venotomy in the vein.
- **Step 12.** Trim the graft to length for a tension-free anastomosis.
- **Step 13.** Sew the graft to the open vein in an end-to-side fashion with a 6–0 Prolene.
- **Step 14.** Flush the graft and vein prior to completion of the anastomosis.
- **Step 15.** Complete the anastomosis and establish flow in the graft. You should expect a palpable thrill in the graft.
- **Step 16.** Close the incisions. Use 3.0 Vicryl suture for the subcutaneous fascia and 4.0 Monocryl for the skin.

Anatomic Complications in Vascular Surgery

Anatomical complications in vascular surgery are divided into local non-vascular and vascular complications. The most common non-vascular complications are failure of wound healing, wound infection, and lymphatic fistula. Inguinal incisions are common in vascular surgery and are often complicated by poor wound healing due to subcutaneous lymphatic vessels or infection related to proximity of the anogenital region. Transverse incisions are sometimes preferred to longitudinal incisions to decrease tension on closure of skin at the inguinal area with the risk of more limited proximal and distal exposure. Asepsis, atraumatic tissue handling and antibiotic prophylaxis are also important in reducing infection and delayed healing.

The most common vascular complications are failing grafts or infection. Early graft failure is often the result of inappropriate tissue handling, size mismatch, graft kink, or stenosis of the vascular anastomosis. Long-term graft failures can be the result of the graft material itself or progression of inflow and outflow lesions. Autogenous veins are superior to synthetic grafts in maintaining patency and are more resistant to infection. Infected synthetic grafts must be removed and replaced with in situ autogenous graft or homograft or with extra-anatomic bypass grafts.

Uterus, Tubes, and Ovaries

18

Ramon A. Suarez

Anatomy

Relations and Positions of the Uterus, Tubes, and Ovaries

The uterus lies in the pelvis between the bladder and rectum. The normal position of the uterus—whether anteverted, midplane, or retroverted—is maintained by the round ligaments. The ligaments insert laterally, anterior to the fallopian tubes, and then plunge into the pelvic sidewall. The round ligaments may be viewed as the roof of the broad ligament. The broad ligament contains the blood supply, lymphatic channels, and nerves of the corpus uteri.

The ureter courses just below the insertion of the uterine artery into the lower uterine segment, and it should be identified clearly to avoid injuring it. The lower uterine segment and cervix are bordered anteriorly by the bladder and posteriorly by the rectum. Moving downward, the surgeon encounters the uterosacral ligaments, which provide critical support to the uterus. Laterally and downward the broad ligament joins the cardinal ligament until the cervical/vaginal junction is reached.

The fallopian tubes emerge from the fundus and are in close proximity to the ovaries. The mesosalpinx descends from the tubes. The ovaries are joined to the uterus via the utero-ovarian ligament and to the pelvic sidewall by the infundibulo-pelvic ligament. The infundibulopelvic ligament contains the ovarian vessels.

R. A. Suarez (✉)
Department of Gynecology and Obstetrics, Emory University School of Medicine, Atlanta, GA, USA

Gynecology – Obstetrics, Piedmont Hospital, Atlanta, GA, USA

© Springer Nature Switzerland AG 2021
L. J. Skandalakis (ed.), *Surgical Anatomy and Technique*,
https://doi.org/10.1007/978-3-030-51313-9_18

Vascular System of the Uterus, Tubes, and Ovaries

Arterial Supply
The uterine artery arises from the internal iliac artery, as do the cervical, vaginal, and other collateral vessels.

Venous Supply
The veins follow a course analogous to the internal iliac vein. The ovarian artery and vein course in a cephalad direction and have no pelvic origin.

Lymphatic Drainage
Coursing parallel to the internal iliac vessels, the drainage from the corpus uteri and cervix ends in the deep pelvic lymph nodes. The drainage from the ovaries is in a cephalad and midline direction, coursing to the periaortic nodes, adjacent to the inferior vena cava and aorta.

Technique

Abdominal Hysterectomy and Bilateral Salpingo-oophorectomy

In addition to understanding the surgical technique of hysterectomy, the surgeon should realize the significance of the procedure to the patient. Removal of the uterus will, under usual circumstances, sterilize the patient. Removal of the ovaries will result in castration of the patient. The possible need for estrogen replacement therapy, with all its attendant controversies, might then develop. It is beyond the scope of this chapter to consider these issues, but the surgeon is encouraged, when possible, to clearly understand the patient's wishes and perspective.

The incision for hysterectomy is often determined by the indications for the procedure. When cancer is suspected, a midline incision is performed from the umbilicus to the symphysis pubis. For large fibroids or extensive endometriosis, a Maylard incision (muscle-cutting transverse incision) might be performed. A tubo-ovarian abscess can be approached with either a Maylard or a midline skin incision. For benign disease of limited dimension, a Pfannenstiel incision (low transverse muscle-spreading incision) is often performed.

The following general technique of hysterectomy is suitable when there is no significant disruption of the normal anatomy; modifications are needed according to disease processes encountered.

Preoperative: Prepare the vagina carefully with a Betadine solution; administer antibiotics.

- **Step 1.** Make incision. Generally a transverse muscle-splitting or muscle-cutting incision is performed. This choice of incision is associated with less postoperative pain and a more desirable cosmetic result. For a transverse incision, the skin is cut approximately 2 cm above the symphysis pubis and 3–4 cm to each side of the midline.

- **Step 2.** Incise the rectus abdominis fascia and extend this incision laterally. Grasp the superior edge and sharply dissect the underlying muscle away from the fascia with Metzenbaum scissors. Bleeding from perforated vessels can be controlled with electrocautery.
- **Step 3.** Take a Kelly clamp and identify the midline of the muscle. Gently separate the bellies and extend the incision superiorly and inferiorly, reaching the limits of your previous dissection.
- **Step 4.** Grasp a peritoneal fold. Enter cautiously to avoid injury to underlying bowel. Extend the peritoneal incision superiorly and inferiorly.
- **Step 5.** If a neoplasm is suspected, take pelvic washings and submit for cytology. If an infectious process is apparent, take fluid for culture.
- **Step 6.** Place Kelly clamps on each corner of the uterus encompassing the round ligaments, utero-ovarian ligaments, and fallopian tubes.
- **Step 7.** Place gentle traction on the clamps. With a curved Heaney, Zeppelin, or Masterson pelvic clamp, clamp the round ligament approximately 2 cm lateral to its uterine insertion. Cut the round ligament with a scalpel, leaving a pedicle approximately 3 mm distal to the clamp. Secure the pedicle with a 0 or 2–0 Vicryl suture ligature. All subsequent sutures are the same unless otherwise indicated (Fig. 18.1).

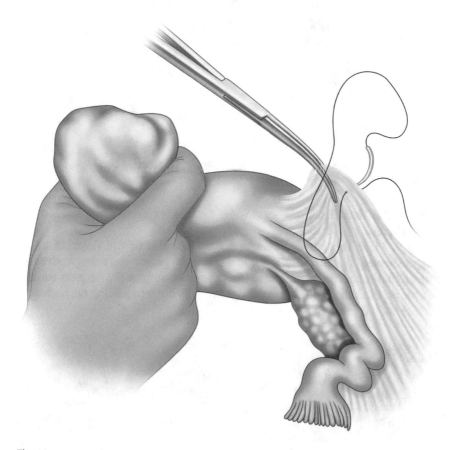

Fig. 18.1 Round ligament is clamped, ligated, and cut. Broad ligament is opened

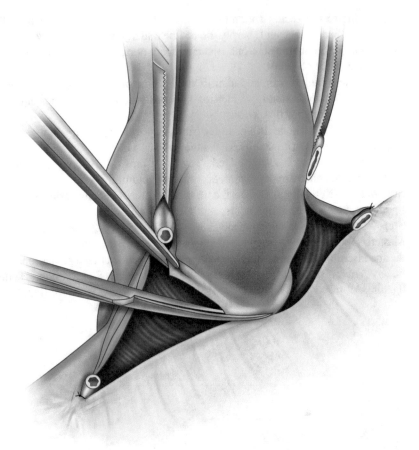

Fig. 18.2 Leaves of the broad ligament are incised. To avoid unnecessary blood loss, the bladder is not dissected away from the uterus at this point

- **Step 8.** Use Metzenbaum scissors to open the anterior and posterior leaves of the broad ligament (Fig. 18.2).
- **Step 9.** Place two curved clamps on the utero-ovarian and fallopian tubes, approximately 1–2 cm lateral to the uterus. Cut the pedicle and secure with a free tie around the most lateral clamp. Remove the clamp as the surgeon stitches down on the knot. Place a second ligature below the remaining clamp before removing it (Fig. 18.3).

Note
- If performing bilateral salpingo-oophorectomy (BSO): Place two clamps across the infundibulopelvic ligament 1–2 cm from the ovary. Secure the pedicles as above. Therefore, the placement of the clamp either in front of or behind the ovary will determine whether the adnexa are removed or preserved.

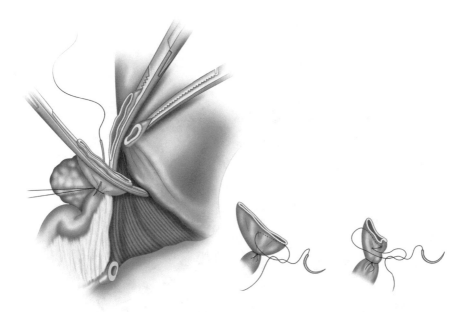

Fig. 18.3 Double clamping. The lateral clamp is replaced with a free tie that surrounds the pedicle and occludes the vessels (inset: *left*). The middle clamp is replaced by a transfixion suture ligature (inset: *right*)

- **Step 10.** Use the Metzenbaum scissors to open the broad ligament until the uterine vessels are viewed and skeletonized. With the scissors pointing away from the bladder and toward the cervix, carefully dissect the bladder away from the cervix and lower uterine segment (Fig. 18.4).
- **Step 11.** At the level of the internal cervical os, perpendicular to the cervix, place the first clamp. Place the second clamp immediately above it, and the third clamp above that, leaving enough of a gap to cut an adequate pedicle. Use the scalpel to cut to the tip of the clamp. Place a suture ligature at the tip of the bottom clamp and secure the bottom of the pedicle. Remove the bottom clamp. Place a second suture at the tip of the remaining bottom clamp. When the suture is secure, remove the pedicle. The third clamp is used to control any resultant back bleeding (Fig. 18.5).
- **Step 12.** Between the uterus and the vascular pedicle above, advance straight clamps approximately 1 cm. It is important that the heel of this clamp be in direct contact with the secured previous pedicle. If it is not, tissue will be cut that is not encompassed by a ligature. Later attempts to arrest resultant bleeding are associated with an increased risk of injury to the ureter. Cut the pedicle and secure with a suture ligature (Fig. 18.6).
- **Step 13.** Sequentially advance straight clamps: clamp, cut, and suture ligate until the uterosacral ligaments are encountered.
- **Step 14.** With a straight clamp, clamp the uterosacral ligament 1 cm from the cervix. Cut and secure with a ligature.

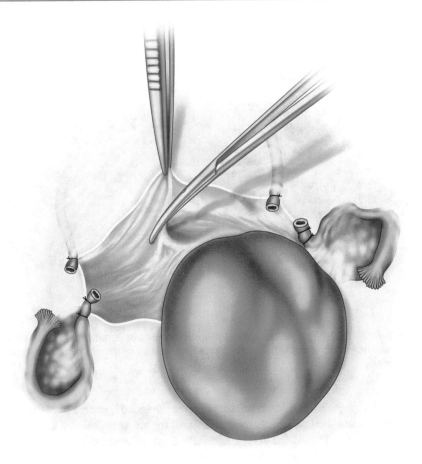

Fig. 18.4 Mobilization of bladder

- **Step 15.** Using a scalpel, make a superficial incision between the uterosacral ligaments; usually 1–2 mm must be cut. Try to ensure that the entirety of the cervix is felt between the fingers and then apply a curved clamp at the cervical-vaginal junction. Cut the pedicle, and the vagina is entered. Suture ligate the pedicle and secure it with a Kelly clamp.
- **Step 16.** On the opposite side, repeat all these steps sequentially.
- **Step 17.** Using Jorgensen scissors or a scalpel, cut the entire cervix away while removing as little vagina as possible (Fig. 18.7).
- **Step 18.** Following a hysterectomy, the most common site for postoperative bleeding is the vaginal cuff. Carefully close the vagina in an anterior-to-posterior fashion with figure-of-eight stitches. If too much tissue is incorporated into a ligature, the risk of cellulitis increases.

Fig. 18.5 Skeletonization of uterine vessels and placement of suture ligatures

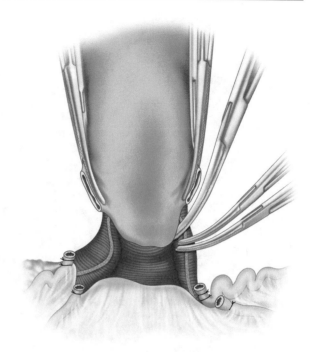

Fig. 18.6 Line of incision

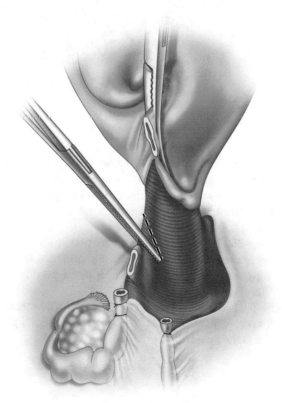

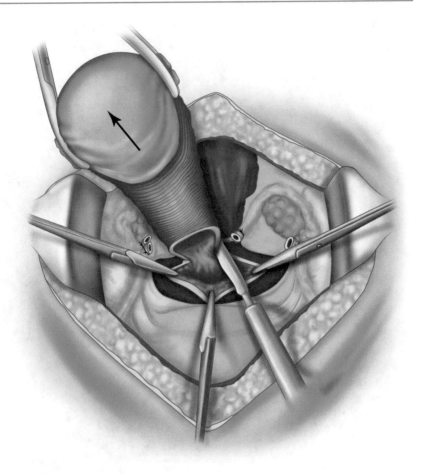

Fig. 18.7 Cervix is removed

- **Step 19.** Carefully place a suture through the uterosacral pedicle close to the previous ligature, the posterior wall of the vagina, and the opposite uterosacral ligament. Caution is required to avoid injury to the ureters. This suture diminishes the likelihood that enterocele or vaginal vault prolapse will develop (Fig. 18.8).
- **Step 20.** If there is evidence of pelvic infection, the vagina is not closed. Secure the vaginal edges with a continuous interlocking stitch. Before closing the retroperitoneal space, a drain may be placed with a running 3–0 Vicryl suture.
- **Step 21.** Carefully irrigate the pelvis with normal saline and inspect all pedicles for complete hemostasis. The visceral or parietal peritoneum may be closed, but this is not mandatory.

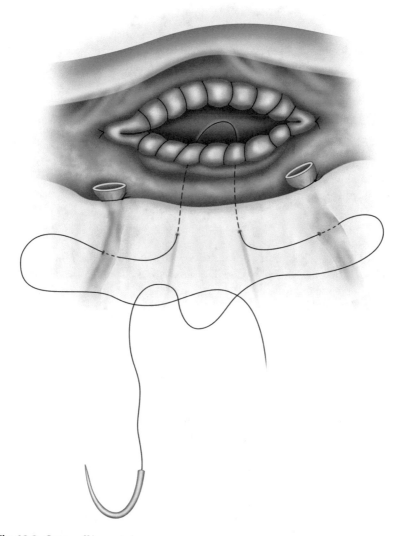

Fig. 18.8 Open cuff is created

- **Step 22.** If the muscles have not been cut, typically they fall back together. After placing one interrupted 2–0 Vicryl suture at the midline, close the fascia with a 2–0 Vicryl running suture.
- **Step 23.** Carefully irrigate the subcutaneous tissues and observe for hemostasis. The skin may be closed with a 3–0 or 4–0 subcuticular closure. Standard bandages may be applied.

Remember

- Postoperative infection is a common complication following hysterectomy. Incidence can be reduced with the use of preoperative antibiotics; first-generation cephalosporins are usually used and should be administered before the incision is made.
- The wise surgical technique of limiting pedicle size will minimize the necrotic tissue left behind.
- Injury to the ureter is a rare but serious mishap. The surgeon performing a hysterectomy must know the course of the pelvic ureter. Once the broad ligament has been opened, careful dissection will reveal the presence of the ureter below the uterine vessels.
- Postoperative ileus is not always preventable, but the likelihood of its development can be reduced by avoiding irritation to the bowel. In particular, avoid packing away the intestines unless absolutely necessary and then always use moistened lap pads.
- Use of cautery and other newer energy-dependent devices should be avoided when the vascular pedicle is reached. Collateral thermal injury may put the ureter at risk.

Ovarian Cystectomy

In this era of extensive use of imaging, it would be unlikely for a surgeon to be surprised by the presence of an ovarian cyst (Fig. 18.9a). Nevertheless, the surgical management of these entities is relevant to all who enter the abdomen.

The ovary has the capacity to produce many benign and malignant tumors. In general, maximal effort should be focused on the preservation of useful function when the presumed histology is benign (Fig. 18.9a). When a ruptured, bleeding cyst is encountered, the surgeon should perform careful dissection with Metzenbaum scissors to excise the cyst from the surrounding ovarian parenchyma (Fig. 18.9b). The dissection plane becomes obvious as the cyst wall is peeled away from the residual ovarian tissue (Fig. 18.9c). The ovary may be stabilized with a Babcock clamp and the cyst pulled away with smooth forceps. Deep stitches of 3–0 or 4–0 Vicryl are used cautiously to close the inner ovarian stroma. The ovarian cortex is then closed with interrupted 4–0 Vicryl (Fig. 18.9d) or a continuous baseball stitch (Fig. 18.10).

Care should be taken to remove as little ovarian stroma or cortex as possible. Hemostasis is improved by cautious use of the needlepoint Bovie prior to closure on obvious bleeding sites. Care should be taken not to compromise the ovarian blood supply by overly zealous cautery use. Copious irrigation with lactated Ringer's solution will diminish adhesion formation. Adhesion barriers on the repaired ovary have not conclusively demonstrated benefit and are not recommended.

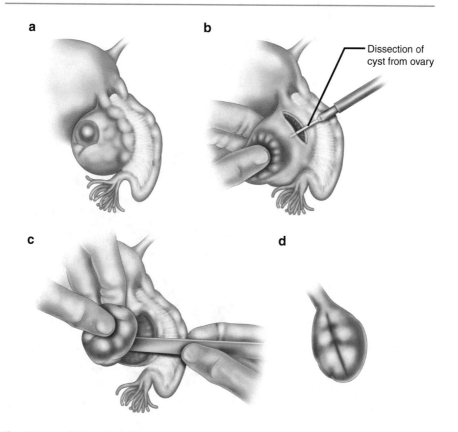

Fig. 18.9 (**a–d**) Resection of benign cyst

When an unruptured cyst is encountered in a premenopausal patient, size will suggest management. In general, cysts less than 7 cm should be left undisturbed. Larger cysts can be removed using the procedure for ruptured cysts. Care should be taken to avoid rupturing an intact cyst. If the surgeon encounters an asymptomatic cyst, it is best left undisturbed; most asymptomatic cysts are functional and will resolve spontaneously.

The presence of an ovarian cyst in a postmenopausal patient has a higher association with malignancy. If the cyst must be removed, peritoneal washings and omental biopsies should be obtained before oophorectomy. The infundibulopelvic ligament is isolated 1–2 cm next to the ovary, clamped, cut, and secured with 2–0 Vicryl sutures. The utero-ovarian ligament and fallopian tube are similarly clamped, cut, and ligated. If frozen section analysis confirms malignancy, a full staging operation of total abdominal hysterectomy, BSO, and pelvic and aortic lymphadenectomy should be performed by an appropriately trained surgeon.

Fig. 18.10 Closure of the
ovary with a baseball stitch

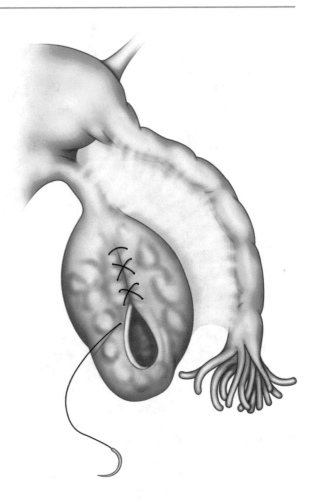

Remember
- Be careful to avoid injury to the ureter when clamping the infundibulopel-
  vic ligament.
- Always adhere to the "golden rule" of gynecologic surgery—preservation
  of useful function. Never remove an ovary unless it is absolutely necessary.
- Careful attention to hemostasis decreases adhesion formation.
- Ovarian surgery is associated with a significant risk of infertility. Often the
  best approach is not to disturb the ovary.

Carpal Tunnel Release

19

John Gray Seiler

Anatomy

The surgical anatomy and anatomical entities related to the carpal tunnel syndrome are presented through illustrations and tables (Figs. 19.1, 19.2, 19.3, 19.4, 19.5 and Tables 19.1, 19.2, 19.3).

Technique

Surgical Treatment of Carpal Tunnel Syndrome

Patients with chronic carpal tunnel syndrome may benefit from a number of different nonsurgical and surgical treatments. Often surgical release of the carpal canal is necessary to help alleviate patient's symptoms. Surgical decompression of the nerve works by increasing the space available for the median nerve, giving the nerve better opportunity to conduct impulses more normally.

While multiple surgical variations have been reported, none has been shown to be superior to a traditional open carpal tunnel release. The purpose of the chapter is

J. G. Seiler (✉)
Department of Orthopaedic Surgery, Emory University, Atlanta, GA, USA

Piedmont Hospital, Atlanta, GA, USA
e-mail: jgseiler@gahand.org

© Springer Nature Switzerland AG 2021
L. J. Skandalakis (ed.), *Surgical Anatomy and Technique*,
https://doi.org/10.1007/978-3-030-51313-9_19

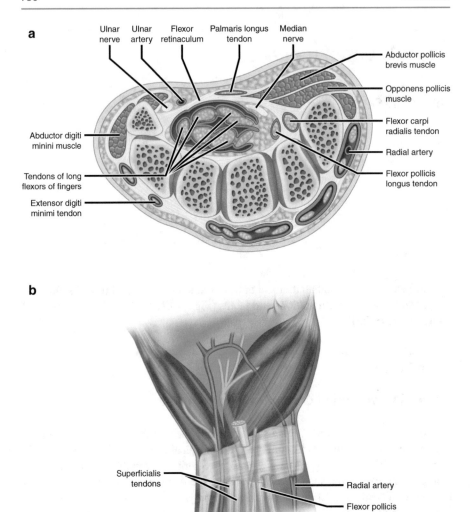

Fig. 19.1 (**a**) Cross section of the wrist. (**b**) The tunnel and its relations

to present a method of open carpal tunnel release for the purpose of treating chronic carpal tunnel syndrome. Because the surgical anatomy of the palm is complex, thorough knowledge of the local anatomy is important to optimize the outcome. Surgical complications can be related to anatomic variants that go unrecognized at the time of the procedure.

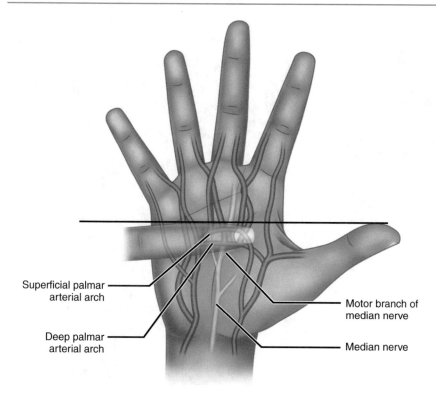

Fig. 19.2 The superficial and deep palmar arches and the topography of the motor branches of the median nerve

Surgery is usually performed on an outpatient basis using a regional or local anesthetic block, a sterile facility, and an optical magnification. Routine prophylactic antibiotics are not necessary to perform a surgical timeout with the patient.

- **Step 1.** Tourniquet management. The procedure can be performed with the use of a well-padded brachial or antebrachial tourniquet, which is inflated to a pressure 100 mm/hg over the patient's systolic blood pressure (but not to exceed 250 mm/hg).
- **Step 2.** Generate anesthesia for the procedure. For OR procedures done under local anesthesia, I use 0.5% plain Marcaine. Perform a proximal median and ulnar nerve block with 10 cc and then infiltrate the line of the incision. The block is best done approximately 30 min prior to incision time.

Fig. 19.3 Superficial
relations of the flexor
retinaculum. (*1*) Radial
artery, (*2*) flexor carpi
radialis tendons, (*3*)
palmaris longus tendon, (*4*)
ulnar artery and nerve, (*5*)
flexor carpi ulnaris tendon,
(*6*) palmar cutaneous
branch of median nerve,
(*7*) palmar branch of radial
artery, (*8*) three thenar
muscles, (*9*) palmar
cutaneous branch of ulnar
nerve, and (*10*) three
hypothenar muscles

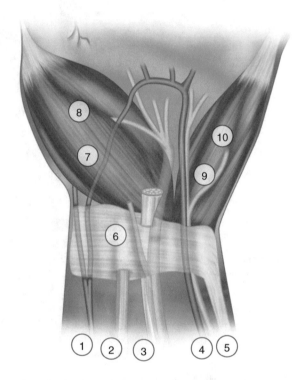

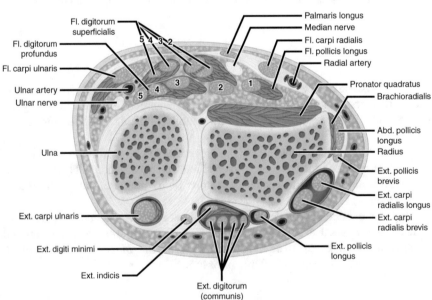

Fig. 19.4 The proximal surgical zone

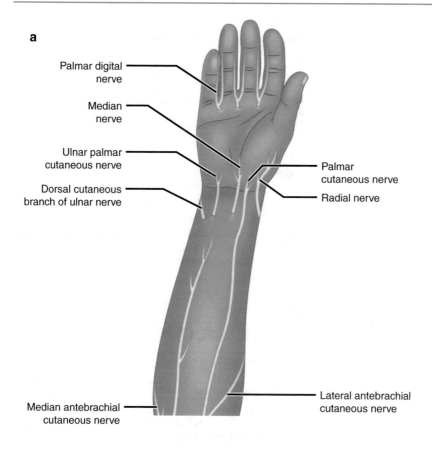

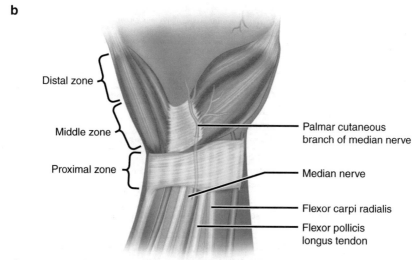

Fig. 19.5 (**a**) Palmar cutaneous branches of the ulnar, musculocutaneous, radial, and median nerves. (**b**) Palmar cutaneous branch of the median nerve

Table 19.1 Upper proximal zone divisions

Ulnar side		
Ulnar trio	Flexor carpi ulnaris	
	Ulnar nerve	
	Ulnar artery	
Central (median) area		
Ulnar bursae with flexor digitorum superficialis and profundus tendons		
Median duo	Palmaris longus	
	Median nerve	
Radial side		
Radial trio	Radial artery	
	Flexor carpi radialis	
	Flexor pollicis longus within the radial bursa	

From JE Skandalakis, GL Colborn, PN Skandalakis, et al. The carpal tunnel syndrome: Part II. *Am Surg* 58(2):77–81, 1992. Reprinted with permission from American Surgeon

Table 19.2 Central zone (carpal tunnel) divisions

Ulnar side
Ulnar bursa: Eight tendons (sublimis and profundus)
Central area
Median nerve and its branches (with possible variations)
Radial side
Radial bursa and flexor pollicis

From JE Skandalakis, GL Colborn, PN Skandalakis, et al. The carpal tunnel syndrome: Part II. *Am Surg* 58(2):77–81, 1992. Reprinted with permission from American Surgeon

Table 19.3 Distal zone divisions

Ulnar side
Ulnar nerve branches
Ulnar artery and superficial arch
Ulnar bursa: four profundus tendons
Ulnar bursa: four superficialis tendons
Central (median) side
Median nerve branches
Recurrent branch thenar muscles
One or two digital nerves for thumb
Four or five digital nerves for index, middle, and radial side of ring finger
Radial side
Flexor pollicis longus with radial bursa
Median nerve palmar cutaneous branch

From JE Skandalakis, GL Colborn, PN Skandalakis, et al. The carpal tunnel syndrome: Part II. *Am Surg* 58(2):77–81, 1992. Reprinted with permission from American Surgeon

Fig. 19.6 Preferred skin incision to avoid underlying neurovascular structures

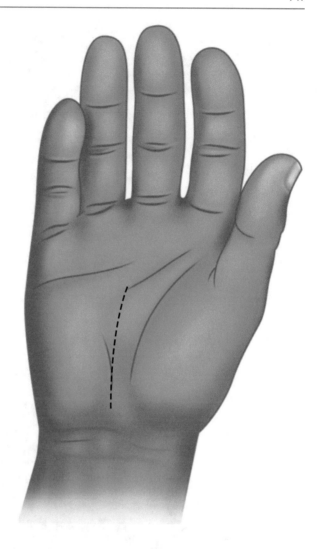

- **Step 3.** Make a curving incision that is in line with the ring finger metacarpal (Fig. 19.6).
- **Step 4.** Blunt subcutaneous dissection allows for identification and preservation of the crossing cutaneous nerves. These nerves may originate from either the palmar cutaneous branch of the median nerve or the palmar cutaneous branch of the ulnar nerve (Fig. 19.7). Longitudinally incise the longitudinal fibers of the palmar aponeurosis.
- **Step 5.** Identify the transverse carpal ligament. The ligament is thick, and the fibers are transverse. The origin of the thenar muscles is found on the radial margin; the hook of the hamate can be palpated on the ulnar aspect (Fig. 19.8). The ulnar artery and nerve are housed beneath the thick fibers of the palmar carpal ligament, just

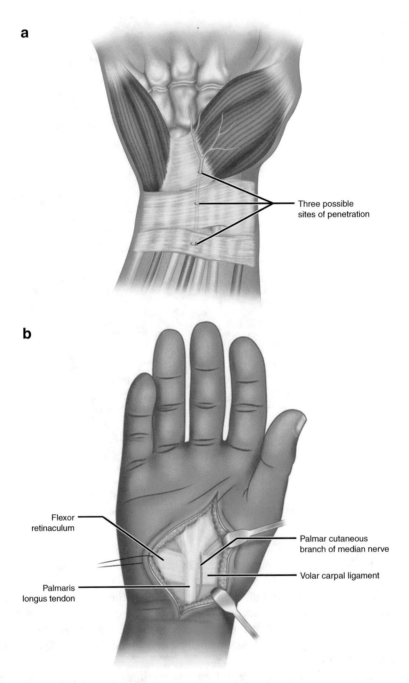

Fig. 19.7 Superficial dissection to identify the distal palmaris longus tendon insertion into the palmar fascia and the distal palmar fat pad. (**a**) Three possible sites of penetration of the palmar cutaneous nerve. (**b**) Note the palmar cutaneous branch of the median nerve that parallels the palmaris longus tendon

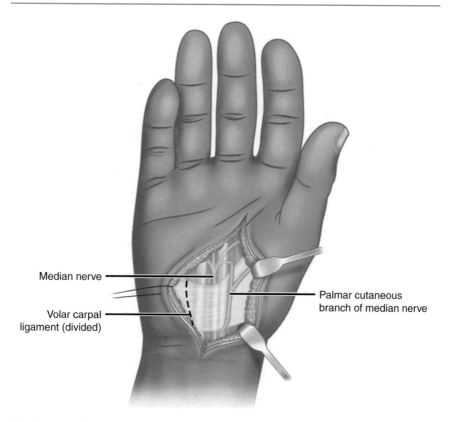

Median nerve

Palmar cutaneous
branch of median nerve

Volar carpal
ligament (divided)

Fig. 19.8 Identification of the transverse carpal ligament. Release of the ligament near its ulnar insertion limits risk to variant branches of the recurrent motor branch of the median nerve

ulnar and palmar to the transverse carpal ligament. Distally, the palmar fat pad will mark the distal extent of the transverse carpal ligament. Proximally, the ligament will become confluent with the thinner, distal antebrachial fascia.

- **Step 6.** Use a 15 blade to sharply release the transverse carpal ligament along the line of the ring finger metacarpal. Release along this line should be just ulnar to the position of the median nerve.
- **Step 7.** Under direct vision, release the distal antebrachial fascia in the proximal end of the incision.
- **Step 8.** Inspect the cut edge of the ligament to ensure that the entire ligament is released. Inspect the carpal tunnel contents for anatomical abnormality, degenerative elements, and/or inflammatory conditions that may require additional treatment (Fig. 19.9). Make note of the condition of the median nerve (Fig. 19.10).
- **Step 9.** Irrigate. Close the wound with a subcuticular absorbable suture. Close the wound with interrupted 4–0 or 5–0 nylon or with a subcuticular absorbable suture. For uncomplicated cases, a comfortable, soft dressing is used. For complicated cases, a volar plaster splint is applied for 2 weeks.
- **Step 10.** Ensure that the sterile soft dressing allows for full finger range of motion.

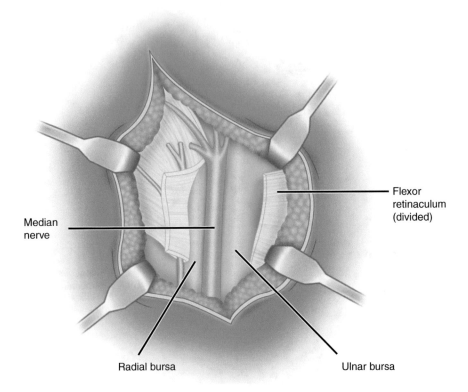

Fig. 19.9 Division of the flexor retinaculum. Inspect the carpal tunnel contents

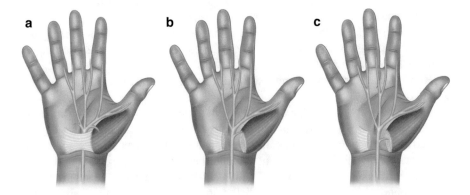

Fig. 19.10 Anatomical variations of the median nerve in the carpal tunnel. (**a**) Regular branching of the median nerve, 55 percent. (**b**) Thenar branch leaving the median nerve within the carpal tunnel (subligamentous), 31 percent. (**c**) Transligamentous course of the thenar branch, 14 percent

Anatomical Complications

- Wound sensitivity
- Wound infection
- Median nerve injury
- Recurrent motor branch of median nerve injury
- Palmar cutaneous branch of median nerve injury
- Ulnar nerve injury
- Ulnar artery injury
- Superficial palmar arch injury

Microsurgical Procedures

20

John Gray Seiler

Introduction

The era of microsurgery, which followed the introduction of ultrafine, nonreactive sutures, precision surgical instrumentation, and improved optical magnification, led to digital replantation, free tissue transfer, vascularized bone grafting, and other procedures. This chapter provides basic information about microsurgical procedures, techniques, and the equipment needed to perform them.

Microsurgical Instrumentation

Because of the exacting requirements of microsurgical procedures, high-quality instrumentation is crucial. Microsurgical tools require specialized storage conditions and individual cleaning, as well as regular inspections, repair, and replacement to ensure that they are ready for use by the surgical team. To ensure readiness for cases, all instrumentation should be inspected by a qualified technician at least quarterly.

A basic set of instruments should include microsurgical forceps (4, 5A), vessel dilating forceps, curved scissors, straight scissors, and vascular clamps (single and double for both arteries and veins). For more advanced procedures, surgical background with color contrast, microsutures, and micro-irrigation syringes are needed. Some complex cases may be facilitated by custom instruments.

J. G. Seiler (✉)
Department of Orthopaedic Surgery, Emory University, Atlanta, GA, USA

Piedmont Hospital, Atlanta, GA, USA
e-mail: jgseiler@gahand.org

Methods of Magnification

Operating loupes—easily used and customized to each surgeon—work well for procedures in which lower levels of optical magnification (2.5–6.5×) are sufficient. The disadvantage of loupes is that magnification and depth of field are fixed.

An operating microscope is necessary for surgeries that require higher levels of magnification. This larger instrument provides exceptional image clarity and vibrant light. The operating microscope can be set up for use by a single operator or two surgeons. Newer microscopes have the capability for in-room televised display and recording of the operation. However, operating microscopes are more cumbersome to use than loupes, are expensive, and require significant maintenance.

Procedures often done with loupe magnification include:

- Pediatric hernia repair
- Hypospadias
- Discectomy
- Coronary artery bypass graft
- Arterial bypass graft using reversed saphenous vein interpositional graft
- Larger nerve repair
- Blepharoplasty
- Tendon repair
- Arterial repair
- Larger vein repair

Procedures often done with use of the operating microscope include:

- Replantation
- Free tissue transfer
- Hand aneurysm resection and repair
- Smaller vessel repair (digital artery)
- Smaller nerve repair (digital nerve)
- Vascular repair

Psychomotor Skills Training

Like most surgical skills, precision techniques for microsurgery are best taught in a laboratory setting; standardized instruction is available in a number of centers. Typically, students begin with simple methods for arterial repair. As their skills improve, they advance to more difficult procedures, such as interpositional vein grafting. Because live animals are used, surgeons obtain direct feedback on the outcome. The significant learning benefit from this method is that students know their success rate for various procedures prior to taking them to a clinical setting.

Surgical Setup

The setup for each case varies, but planning the procedure is time well spent. For most orthopedic and hand surgeries, the microscope should be set up for "opposing" use, i.e., surgeon and assistant across from one another. For some ENT procedures, the surgeon and assistant may be oriented at right angles.

Suture Materials

Surgeons generally prefer 7–0 to 11–0 monofilament, nonabsorbable sutures for vascular repair and for nerve repair. Our preferences are for nylon and prolene.

Procedure for Vascular Repair

Dissection/Preparation

For arterial repair in the limbs, regional or general anesthesia can be administered. The initial dissection should allow both proximal and distal control of the vessel. Usually this dissection is done with a broad pneumatic tourniquet inflated to a pressure that is 100 mmHg above the patient's systolic blood pressure.

End-to-End Arterial and Venous Repair

The segment for repair (Fig. 20.1) is dissected free, and the arterial ends are sharply trimmed using optical magnification. Using straight, sharp scissors, cut the vessel at right angles to the long axis of the artery. Gently dilate the artery, clean the artery's interior of clot, and irrigate with a heparinized saline solution. With the tourniquet deflated, confirm satisfactory inflow and then apply a vascular occlusion clamp to the proximal artery. The two arterial ends are then positioned within the double clamp, leaving a small gap. For visual contrast, place a colored plastic background or suction mat behind the artery.

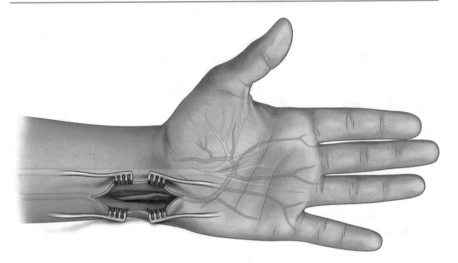

Fig. 20.1 Vascular segment is dissected free

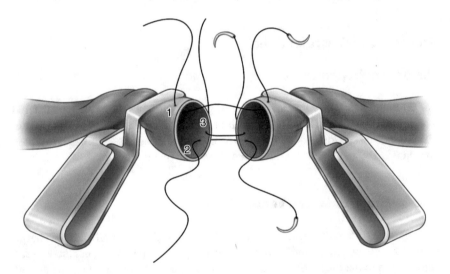

Fig. 20.2 Interrupted suture technique

Suture the artery using an interrupted technique, everting the vessel edges. Place the initial two sutures 180° apart and then place the third suture halfway between them (Fig. 20.2). Each subsequent suture should again be placed halfway between the adjacent sutures until the vessel repair is complete (Figs. 20.3 and 20.4).

Turn the vessel over (180°) in the clamp. By opening the back wall with forceps, the surgeon can inspect the first half of the repair for accuracy. Again irrigate the vessel with a heparinized saline solution.

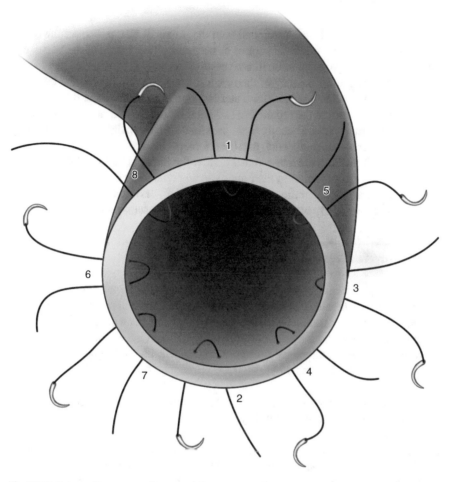

Fig. 20.3 Intermediate suture placement

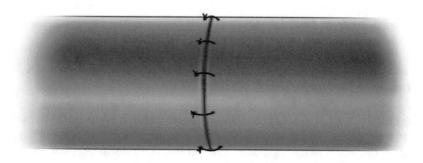

Fig. 20.4 Back wall of sutured vessel

Assessing Patency

Next, remove first the distal clamp and then the proximal clamp. Inspect the repair for leakage and insert additional sutures as necessary. The surface of the vessel can be irrigated with Xylocaine to facilitate vessel dilation.

Begin assessment of patency of the repair. Inspect the distal color and capillary refill and feel for a distal pulse. Use a sterile Doppler to listen to the flow and perform a "milking test" of the repair: use two smooth forceps and place them side by side over the artery several centimeters proximal to the repair; occlude the artery with both forceps; and gently slide the distal forceps distally across the repair site to a position well distal to the anastomosis so that the artery is "milked" flat. Release the arterial forceps proximal to the repair site and document anterograde flow that crosses the anastomosis in the artery. When possible, design a wound closure that places normal (or nearly normal) skin over the site of vascular repairs.

Procedure for Nerve Repair

For nerve repair, clamps and positioning devices are usually not needed. Primary peripheral nerve repair is commonly done using an interrupted epineural suture method. For repair of traumatic injury, the proximal and distal ends of the artery are carefully identified and then mobilized by longitudinal dissection. When the nerve ends are mobilized sufficiently for end-to-end repair, the nerve must be oriented. Orientation will be facilitated by:

- A general working knowledge of the internal topography of the nerve
- Epineurial surface vessels that may be aligned in the repair
- Inspection of the internal fascicular array of the nerve

With the nerve oriented, the surgeon begins the repair by placing two sutures 180° apart in the external epineurium. Additional sutures are placed to bisect the distance between adjacent sutures until the repair is complete (Figs. 20.5 and 20.6).

Recommended suture gauges for specific nerves are as follows:

- Median, ulnar, and radial nerves: 7–0 to 10–0
- Common digital and proper digital nerves: 9–0 to 10–0

Procedure for Neuroentubulation

Neuroentubulation is an alternate method of nerve repair. It positions the transected nerve ends within 2–3 mm of each other and then allows repair to occur in the protected environment of the nerve tube. Previously, neuroentubulation was done with

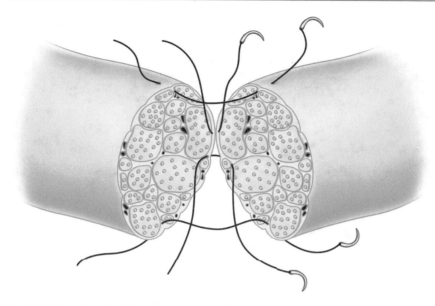

Fig. 20.5 Nerve is oriented, and first sutures are placed

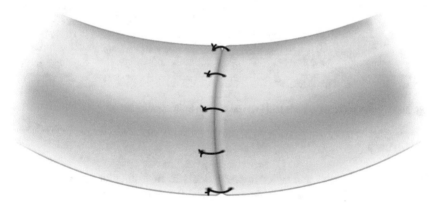

Fig. 20.6 Intermediate sutures are placed

autogenous vein. There are now a number of commercially available devices for nerve entubulation. Initial dissection mobilizes the cut nerve ends. The cut ends are freshened with a sharp, straight scissors. With a suture method, the ends are advanced into the tube (Fig. 20.7).

Alternatively, the tube may be split, the nerve ends are laid into the tube (Fig. 20.8), and the tube is sutured closed with a running suture. The tube diameter should be slightly larger than the nerve to allow for postoperative edema in the nerve.

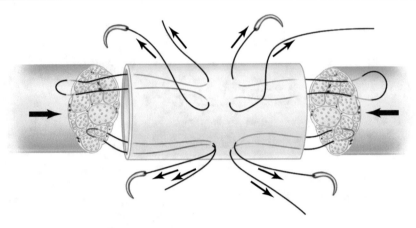

Fig. 20.7 Neuroentubulation

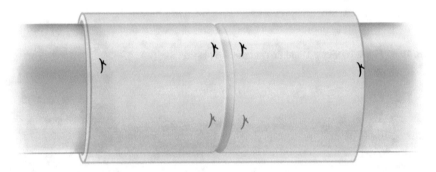

Fig. 20.8 Tube split, nerve ends laid in, tube closure with running suture

Summary

Optical magnification and other improvements in instrumentation have expanded the surgeon's ability to treat a wide variety of difficult conditions. Appropriate tools and training enable the surgeon to repair vessels of less than 1 mm satisfactorily.

Miscellaneous Procedures

21

Lee J. Skandalakis

Technique

Device Insertion

Subclavian Vein Catheter Insertion

- **Step 1.** Place the patient in Trendelenburg position.
- **Step 2.** Prep and drape the subclavian area. Make sure that the sternal notch is visible.
- **Step 3.** Infiltrate the skin with a local anesthetic just underneath the clavicle at a point approximately halfway to two-thirds out from the sternal notch. While doing this, make sure that the needle gently touches the clavicle. Then, step down the injection so that the position of the needle is underneath the clavicle. Do not go deep enough to access the subclavian vein.
- **Step 4.** Use the Seldinger technique to access the subclavian vein. Access is accomplished by using the needle that has been provided in the kit. The needle punctures the skin and is directed underneath the clavicle and aimed toward the sternal notch. As the needle is advanced, gentle back pressure is placed on the syringe. As the needle is advanced when the vein is accessed, the syringe will easily fill with the blood. If on the way the vein is not accessed, slowly withdraw the syringe, keeping gentle negative pressure. Quite often the vein will be accessed as the needle is withdrawn.
- **Step 5.** Once the vein is accessed, insert the guide wire through the needle and advance into the vein. Remove the needle and continue advancing the guide wire (15 cm should be adequate).
- **Step 6.** Place the introducer sheath over the guide wire and advance.

L. J. Skandalakis (✉)
Department of Surgery, Piedmont Hospital, Atlanta, GA, USA

© Springer Nature Switzerland AG 2021
L. J. Skandalakis (ed.), *Surgical Anatomy and Technique*,
https://doi.org/10.1007/978-3-030-51313-9_21

- **Step 7.** Remove the inner rigid portion leaving the peel-away introducer sheath and insert the catheter into the introducer. Advance approximately 15 cm and then peel away the introducer sheath, leaving the catheter in place.
- **Step 8.** Identify and isolate the superior thyroid artery. Flush all ports and secure the catheter to the skin with a 20 silk suture.

Remember
- It is important not to change the orientation of the needle during insertion. Whatever angle you choose to insert, the needle should be maintained until the needle is removed. Changing that angle when the needle is underneath the clavicle could injure the vein or artery.
- If the patient is being monitored, make sure that there are no premature ventricular contractions during insertion of the guide wire, which could be in too far and stimulating the heart. If the patient feels pain in the ear during insertion of the guide wire, the guide wire has likely traveled up the internal jugular vein.
- Avoid damage to cranial nerves during dissection by properly placing retractors or vascular clamps and by precise use of electrocoagulation current. If you are unable to access the vein with this technique, then try changing the angle of the needle insertion. I would suggest insertion so that the needle is aimed toward the sternoclavicular joint and aimed down approximately 30° to 45°.
- Make sure chest X-ray is obtained after this procedure to check placement of the line and to ensure that a pneumothorax has not occurred.

Chest Tube Insertion
- **Step 1.** Place patient in a semi-decubitus position.
- **Step 2.** Prep and drape chest at the level of the fourth intercostal space at the anterior axillary line.
- **Step 3.** Infiltrate the skin with a local anesthetic of your choice approximately 2 cm distal to the fourth intercostal space. Infiltrate the tissue around and over the fifth rib. Step the needle up the fifth rib into the fourth intercostal space just above the rib.
- **Step 4.** Make your incision through the skin with scalpel. Extend into the subcutaneous tissue.
- **Step 5.** Using either a 6 or 8 in. Kelly clamp, begin blunt dissection, spreading with the clamp up toward the fourth intercostal space.
- **Step 6.** Spread the tissue just above the fifth rib. With the clamp closed, push into the chest; once in, spread the clamp. At this point the index finger is inserted.
- **Step 7.** Choose an appropriately sized chest tube depending on indications: larger for blood evacuation and smaller for pneumothorax or thin fluid. Using the Kelly clamp, grasp the end of the chest tube with the clamp so that the end of the clamp is even with the end of the tube.

- **Step 8.** Insert the chest tube through the incision and direct posteriorly toward the apex of the thorax.
- **Step 9.** Secure the chest tube to the skin using a 0 silk suture. It may be necessary to approximate the skin edges at one end or the other to get a good seal and prevent air from being sucked in.

Remember
- The incision is made a little distal to the fourth intercostal space so that when the tube is eventually pulled, there will be a good seal and less chance for pneumothorax. It will also help to prevent air from being sucked around the tube when it is connected to the suction.
- The intercostal neurovascular bundle travels just inferior to each rib. It is for this reason that the tube is inserted over the rib and not under the rib.

Biopsy

Sural Nerve Biopsy
Indications: Sural nerve biopsy is a well-established diagnostic procedure for peripheral neuropathies.

- **Step 1.** Prep and drape the area of the lateral malleolus.
- **Step 2.** Infiltrate the skin with a local anesthetic of your choice between the lateral malleolus and the Achilles tendon. This incision should be approximately 4 cm in length. If necessary extend the incision distally, following the curvature of the lateral malleolus and approximately 1 cm distal to the lateral malleolus.
- **Step 3.** Commence blunt dissection when you have entered through the skin. The nerve, a glistening white structure approximately 3 mm in diameter, will be easily found.
- **Step 4.** Infiltrate the nerve proximally and distally with a local anesthetic. Using scissors, transect the nerve proximally and distally. Try to obtain at least a 2 cm segment.
- **Step 5.** Close the wound in layers. Use a 30 Vicryl for the subcutaneous tissue and a 40 nylon for the skin.

Muscle Biopsy
Indications: Muscle biopsies can be useful to help diagnose patients who present with symptoms such as weakness, muscle pain, cramps, and fatigue with activity. These symptoms in the presence of a neuropathy would also suggest a nerve biopsy. The muscle with pain or weakness is the one to biopsy.

- **Step 1.** Prep and drape the anterolateral thigh.
- **Step 2.** Infiltrate an area approximately 4 cm in length with a local anesthetic of your choice. This area will likely be over the rectus femoris. Infiltrate the local anesthetic into the subcutaneous tissue and muscle.

- **Step 3.** Using Metzenbaum scissors, perform blunt dissection down to the muscle investing sheath.
- **Step 4.** Score the investing sheath with a 15 blade.
- **Step 5.** Grasp the underlying muscle with an Allis clamp.
- **Step 6.** Remove a segment of muscle measuring approximately 3 × 2 cm. This is usually sent to pathology as a fresh specimen on ice.
- **Step 7.** Close the wound in layers with 30 and 40 Vicryl.

Remember
- Prior to removing the specimen, the Bovie is not to be used because it can destroy and alter the histology of the specimen.

Bariatric Surgery

22

Charles D. Procter

General Description of Gastric Bypass

The Roux-en-Y gastric bypass has taken on many forms over the last five decades. While it is still performed as an open procedure across much of the country, the laparoscopic variant has enjoyed increasing popularity among bariatric surgeons and patients since Clark and Wittgrove first described their technique in 1994. The advancement of the Roux limb may be performed in an antecolic/antegastric, retro-colic/antegastric, or retrocolic/retrogastric fashion. While each of these techniques has its own merits, it is advantageous for the practitioner to understand and be facile with each one; variations in patient anatomy as the situation presents may require the surgeon to diverge from his or her preferred approach.

What is described below is our technique for a laparoscopic retrocolic Roux-en-Y gastric bypass. We recognize that there are many ways to "skin a cat," with each resulting in an excellent outcome. While not described in this manuscript, we will often employ an antecolic approach based on the patient's body habitus. We recognize, as well, that the use of a circular stapler placed transabdominally in order to create a stapled gastrojejunostomy is perfectly acceptable. However, this technique is not used in our practice. Furthermore, we now employ the DaVinci surgical robot for this procedure with the added advantage of enhanced visualization and intracorporeal dexterity. The technique of the procedure as described below, however, is the same regardless of the surgical approach.

C. D. Procter (✉)
Department of Surgery, Piedmont Atlanta Hospital, Atlanta, GA, USA
e-mail: cproctermd@bbsg.life

© Springer Nature Switzerland AG 2021
L. J. Skandalakis (ed.), *Surgical Anatomy and Technique*,
https://doi.org/10.1007/978-3-030-51313-9_22

Anatomy

Gastric anatomy is presented in Chap. 7, stomach.

Technique

Retrocolic Roux-En-Y Gastric Bypass

Diet prior to surgery	We employ a 2-week modified protein liquid diet in order to reduce the size of the liver, which aids in the visualization of the gastroesophageal junction.
Tests prior to surgery	*H. pylori* testing is mandatory. Postoperative gastric ulcers in the remnant stomach are not only quite morbid but also can be a diagnostic and treatment dilemma. We have not found bowel prep to be beneficial preoperatively.
Endoscopy	Routine preoperative upper endoscopy to rule out gastroduodenal lesions which will not be approachable endoscopically once the remnant stomach has been bypassed. Preoperative endoscopy also will help to define posterior herniation of the fundus that may not be evident at the time of the operation and which can lead to suboptimal pouch construction.

- **Step 1.** The surgeon stands on the patient's right side with an assistant on the left.
- **Step 2.** Prep and drape patient widely in anticipation of conversion to an open procedure if necessary.
- **Step 3.** Establish pneumoperitoneum in the normal manner. We prefer introduction of a Veress needle just below the left subcostal margin.
- **Step 4.** Enter the abdomen using a 5- or 10-mm optical viewing trocar 15–18 cm below the xiphoid and just to the left of the midline.
- **Step 5.** Place two ports on the patient's right side: one just below the tip of the right lobe of the liver and the other in a line midway between the first port and the umbilicus. The second port should be a 12-mm port in order to accommodate a linear stapler.
- **Step 6.** Place one or two more assistant ports in the left upper quadrant.
- **Step 7.** Retract the left lobe of the liver anteriorly, using a Nathanson liver retractor placed through a small incision just below the xiphoid process.
- **Step 8.** Inspect the entire abdomen. Any adhesions should be carefully taken down.
- **Step 9.** Creation of Roux loop prior to the creation of the gastric pouch.
- **Step 10.** Identify the ligament of Treitz by retracting the greater omentum and transverse colon cephalad.

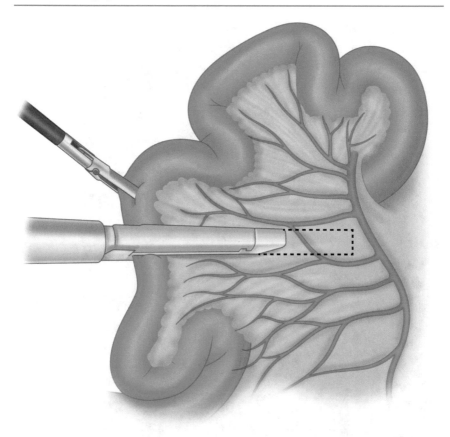

Fig. 22.1 The small bowel is divided using a linear stapler. Two more firings of the stapler are used to divide the mesentery. This provides additional mobility for the Roux limb

- **Step 11.** Using a linear stapling device, divide the small bowel 40 cm distal to the ligament of Treitz. A vascular load is preferred when stapling the small bowel in order to reduce the incidence of staple line bleeding.
- **Step 12.** To avoid ischemia of the two stapled ends, divide the mesentery for 4–5 cm in a direction perpendicular to the bowel (Fig. 22.1).
- **Step 13.** Create the Roux limb from the distal stapled bowel. We prefer a 120-cm Roux limb for patients with a BMI less than 50 and a 150-cm Roux limb for patients with a BMI greater than 50 kg/m^2 (Fig. 22.2).
- **Step 14.** An energy device is used to create an enterotomy on the antimesenteric border of the base of the Roux limb and near the stapled end of the proximal biliopancreatic limb.

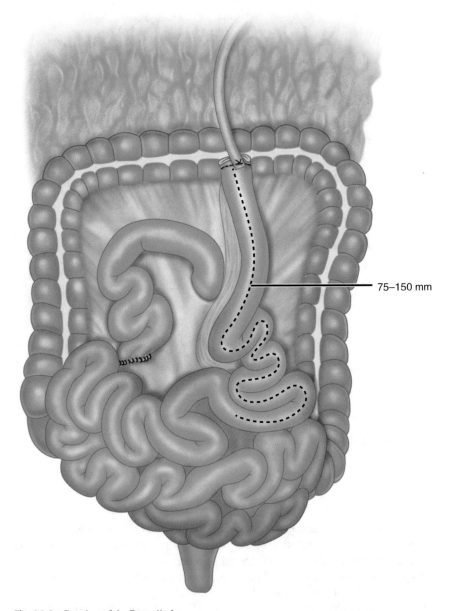

75–150 mm

Fig. 22.2 Creation of the Roux limb

- **Step 15.** Create a side-by-side isoperistaltic anastomosis by placing a linear stapler into these enterotomies. After deploying the stapler, it is wise to slightly close it while it is being removed from the bowel lumen to avoid unnecessarily widening the common defect (Fig. 22.3).

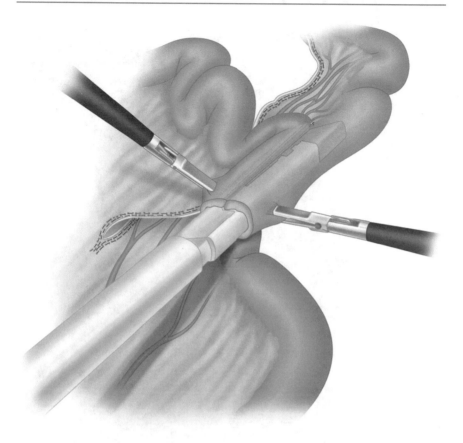

Fig. 22.3 After the Roux limb is measured, it is approximated to the biliopancreatic limb. Enterotomies are made. A linear stapler is used to create the anastomosis

- **Step 16.** Close the common defect by aligning the edges of the bowel and deploying another staple load externally or by oversewing the defect with a single layer of running 2–0 absorbable suture.
- **Step 17.** The mesenteric defect must then be closed in order to prevent internal bowel herniation, which can be catastrophic. Close with a single running layer of nonabsorbable suture from the base of the mesenteric defect to the bowel. Care should be taken to avoid ligation of the small arterioles which may cause ischemia of the anastomosis (Fig. 22.4).
- **Step 18.** For a retrocolic Roux limb, the transverse mesocolon is held upright. A dimple can usually be seen just to the left of the middle colic vessels anterior to the ligament of Treitz. An energy device is used to open the mesocolon for about 2.5 cm and to create a window into the lesser sac.
- **Step 19.** Place the Roux limb into the lesser sac, with care taken to avoid twisting. This is best achieved by keeping the divided end of the mesentery oriented to the left.

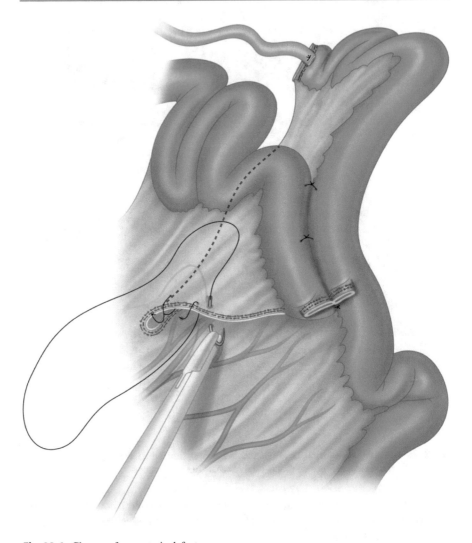

Fig. 22.4 Closure of mesenteric defect

- **Step 20.** Place the greater omentum and transverse mesocolon back into anatomic position.
- **Step 21.** Inspect the gastroesophageal junction. Excise the anterior fat pad with an energy device so that the angle of His can be dissected.
- **Step 22.** If a hiatal hernia exists, it is wise to dissect out the entire GE junction and repair it in the standard manner.
- **Step 23.** Construct the pouch by creating a defect in the lesser omentum 6 cm distal to the GE junction. Enter the lesser sac from the lesser curvature of the stomach (Fig. 22.5).

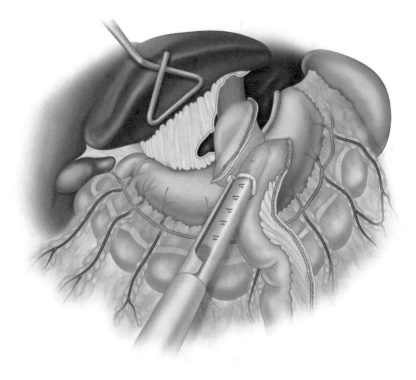

Fig. 22.5 Creation of gastric pouch

- **Step 24.** After ensuring that all transoral intragastric devices have been removed by the anesthesia team, create a horizontal staple line with a 45-mm standard GI load linear stapler 6 cm distal to the GE junction.
- **Step 25.** Inspect the posterior stomach. Take down any adhesions to the posterior lesser sac.
- **Step 26.** The anesthesia team places a 36-French bougie transorally to the level of the staple line. It will be used to protect the esophagus and to calibrate the size of the gastric pouch.
- **Step 27.** Carry the staple line cephalad through the angle of His. A complete division of the stomach must be ensured, because a gastrogastric fistula can lead to weight regain.
- **Step 28.** The Roux limb is brought out through an opening in the gastrocolic ligament in an antegastric fashion or brought out from behind the divided remnant stomach in a retrogastric fashion. Approximate the antimesenteric border near the stapled tip to the lower end of the gastric pouch

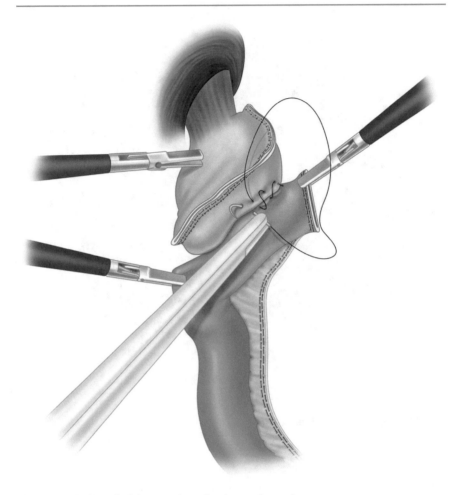

Fig. 22.6 The Roux limb is approximated to the gastric pouch

- **Step 29.** Use a single layer of running 2–0 absorbable suture to approximate the base of the pouch to the antimesenteric border of the Roux limb (Fig. 22.6).
- **Step 30.** Use an energy device to create 1-cm mirroring defects in the lower edge of the gastric pouch and the Roux limb anterior to the suture line.
- **Step 31.** Run a posterior layer of running 2–0 absorbable suture to approximate the posterior edges of the gastrojejunostomy.
- **Step 32.** Run the anterior inner layer of the gastrojejunostomy with a second 2–0 absorbable suture. Advance the 36-French bougie across the anastomosis into the small bowel in order to calibrate the size of the stoma (Fig. 22.7).
- **Step 33.** Finally, a second anterior layer of running 2–0 absorbable suture is run in a Lembert fashion to complete the two-layer anastomosis.
- **Step 34.** Test the integrity of the anastomosis. Clamp the Roux limb just distal to the anastomosis. With the anastomosis submerged in saline, either infuse methy-

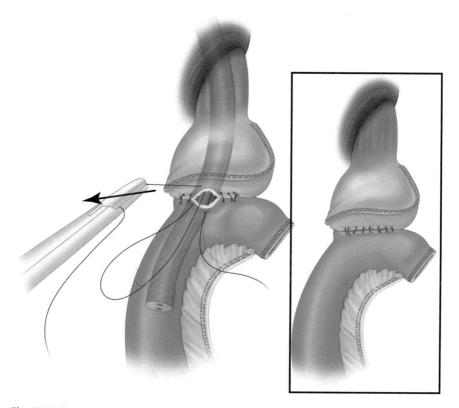

Fig. 22.7 Completing the anastomosis. *Inset*: Common opening is closed

lene blue through an orogastric tube or perform upper endoscopy to insufflate the pouch. The latter technique allows the surgeon to rule out an intraluminal anastomotic bleed, which can be immediately controlled by oversewing.

- **Step 35.** With a competent anastomosis, surgical drains are typically not left in place unless there is a concern with the tissue's ability to heal.
- **Step 36.** In the case of a retrocolic Roux limb, the underside of the transverse mesocolon is again inspected. In order to prevent problems with poor emptying, gently reduce any redundant bowel back below the mesocolic defect. Close the defect by running a 2-0 permanent suture to approximate the cut edges of the transverse mesocolon, the bowel. Take care to include the entire Peterson defect, which can be found on the patient's right side just below the site of entrance of the bowel through the mesocolic defect.
- **Step 37.** The greater omentum and transverse mesocolon are again placed back in anatomic position. In order to prevent injury to the spleen or the newly formed gastrojejunostomy, carefully remove the liver retractor under direct visualization
- **Step 38.** Remove the trocars. The carbon dioxide is completely expelled from the abdominal cavity (Fig. 22.8).

Fig. 22.8 Completed
Roux-en-Y gastric bypass

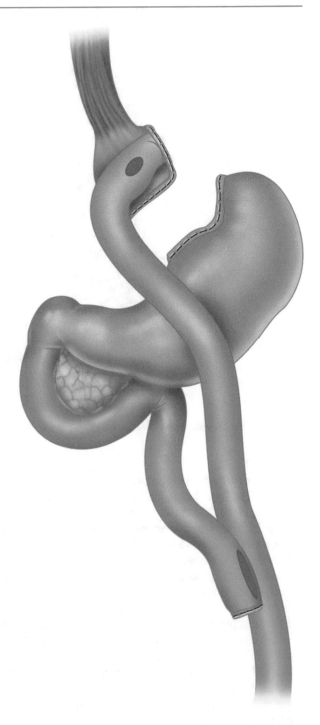

Postoperative

- Pain control is generally not an issue postoperatively. Pain is generally well controlled with a PCA (patient-controlled analgesia) device that can be removed the morning following surgery and replaced with a liquid narcotic for a few days.
- A Foley catheter, placed after induction of anesthesia, is left overnight to monitor urine output. It is removed the morning following surgery.
- Unless there is concern about the anastomosis, patients are allowed ice chips on the night of surgery and started on a sugar-free clear liquid diet on the morning of post-op day 1.
- We do not employ swallow studies routinely. There is a well-published 50% false-negative rate for these studies. Intraoperative testing of the anastomosis should be all that is needed to ensure a competent suture line.
- Patients should ambulate as early as the night of surgery and be kept on subcutaneous DVT (deep vein thrombosis) prophylaxis throughout the hospital stay.
- In our practice, any patient with a history of DVT, pulmonary embolism, or with a BMI of 50 kg/m^2 or greater is sent home on subcutaneous anticoagulation for 1 week.
- Patients who are tolerating liquids without nausea and ambulating may be discharged home on postoperative day 1 or 2.
- Patients are kept on a liquid diet for 1 to 2 weeks post-op. This diet consists of liquid protein supplementation, sugar-free fluids, and chewable vitamins.

Laparoscopic Vertical Sleeve Gastrectomy

Anesthesia: General

Patient Positioning
1. Patient in the supine position with both arms out.
2. Footboard secured to bed.
3. Care is taken to ensure that the patient's heels are on the footboard with toes out, to minimize the risk of ankle subluxation when in the standing position.
4. Surgeon stands on the patient's right with assistant on the left.
   Other: Foley catheter, orogastric tube, and sequential compression devices

- **Step 1.** Prep and drape in standard fashion for either open or laparoscopic access.
- **Step 2.** Administer perioperative cephalosporin and low-molecular-weight heparin in the pre-op holding area.
- **Step 3.** Establish carbon dioxide pneumoperitoneum to 15-mm Hg with a Veress needle inserted in the left subcostal margin.
- **Step 4.** Enter abdomen with a 12-mm optical viewing trocar just left and superior to the umbilicus.
- **Step 5.** Port position as shown: Assistant 5-mm port in the left mid-abdomen, 15-mm port in the right mid-abdomen, and 5-mm port in the right upper quadrant. Subxiphoid incision for the hook liver retractor.

- **Step 6.** Once trocars are in position, patient is placed in slight reverse Trendelenburg. The liver retractor is fixed to the bed with a mechanical arm.
- **Step 7.** Dissection begins on the greater curve of the stomach 5 cm proximal to the pylorus. This is usually in the area of the insertion of the right gastroepiploic artery.
- **Step 8.** All of the gastrocolic, gastrosplenic (short gastric vessels), and gastro-phrenic attachments are divided using a harmonic scalpel, ligasure, or enseal device depending upon surgeon preference. The most cephalad aspect of the dis-section on the greater curve is complete when the left crus is identified.
- **Step 9.** Inspect the hiatus for a hiatal hernia.
- **Step 10.** If a hiatal hernia is encountered, the hiatus is circumferentially mobi-lized, and a posterior cruroplasty is performed with interrupted 0-Ethibond sutures. Use a 60-Fr bougie to calibrate the posterior cruroplasty (if performed).
- **Step 11.** A 36-Fr round, non-tapered tip bougie is advanced and situated along the lesser curve of the stomach. Take care to ensure that there is no orogastric tube or esophageal temperature probe in the patient's mouth at this time to elimi-nate the risk of accidental division of these tubes when the stomach is divided.
- **Step 12.** Starting 5 cm proximal to the pylorus on the greater curve of the stomach, use a surgical stapler to begin the vertical gastrectomy. We routinely start with the 4.1-mm-thick tissue loads and transition to the 3.8- or 3.5-mm tissue loads. Often, we also use tissue reinforcement (although this is still debatable) (Fig. 22.9).
- **Step 13.** The vertical gastrectomy continues, using the bougie as a guide. Care is taken to avoid narrowing the gastric pouch at the incisura. Care is also taken at the most cephalad aspect approaching the gastroesophageal junction to not hug the bougie, in order to avoid an inadvertent side bite on the distal esophagus.
- **Step 14.** Perform an on-table leak test. Options include an air leak test using an endoscope, a saline submersion leak test, or a dye leak test. If the leak test is negative, we do not routinely perform a post-op day 1 upper GI series, unless it is clinically indicated.
- **Step 15.** The portion of the stomach to be removed is placed in an endocatch bag and removed via the 15-mm trocar site.
- **Step 16.** Remove all trocars under direct vision. Close the 15-mm fascial inci-sion with 0 vicryl (Fig. 22.10).

Postoperative

- Patients begin ambulating the evening of surgery.
- Ice chips are allowed immediately following surgery.
- The patient is advanced to a liquid diet postoperative day 1. Patients are dis-charged home if they are able to tolerate at least 4 ounces of liquids per hour.

Biliopancreatic Diversion with Duodenal Switch

This section outlines our technique for performing the biliopancreatic diversion with duodenal switch (BPD-DS). This is a procedure we offer patients with a body mass index in the range of 55 to 70 kg/m2. We feel that patients with a BMI below that range will find success with a less aggressive procedure and patients with a

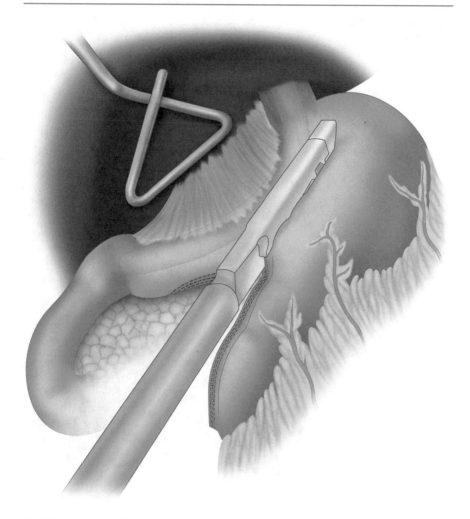

Fig. 22.9 The stapler is fired successively from the antrum to the angle of His adjacent to an intragastric bougie

BMI above 70 will be counseled to undergo a staged procedure beginning with a sleeve gastrectomy with a later conversion to either the BPD-DS or gastric bypass once they have lost down to a weight that will reduce their operative risk. Recognizing that this operation is widely performed in both the open and minimally invasive techniques. We have described the procedure as it may be performed by either method. Our technique begins very deliberately with the sleeve gastrectomy. With this portion safely completed, we then move to the distal enteroenterostomy. We leave division of the duodenum with the duodeno-enterostomy as a final step.

It is important that patients understand, prior to choosing this procedure, that it will necessarily entail lifelong vitamin supplementation. Patients who forgo the prescribed supplements will most certainly find themselves with significant nutrient deficiencies. We prescribe three bariatric multivitamins, calcium, vitamin D, iron, and B12. Nutritional

Fig. 22.10 Completed
laparoscopic sleeve
gastrectomy

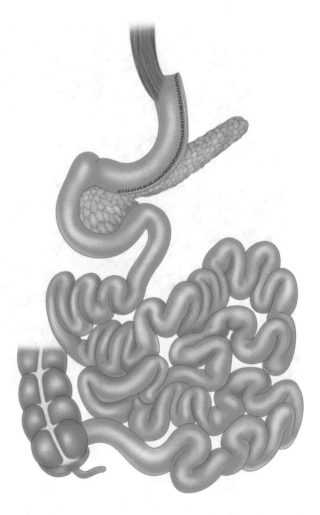

labs are checked twice a year, and the patients are seen by our dietician every 6 months. When managed conscientiously by the patient, physician, and weight loss team, this operation can yield an excellent result in larger patients who might otherwise find more moderate results with the sleeve gastrectomy or gastric bypass procedures.

- Of the commonly performed bariatric procedures today, the biliopancreatic diversion with duodenal switch stands as the most aggressive procedure with regard to weight loss and the resolution of comorbid, metabolic conditions. This operation has been shown to result in the most significant weight loss and the least amount of weight regain when compared to the gastric bypass or sleeve gastrectomy. It is important to note that the anatomy of this operation will decrease the patient's ability to absorb dietary fats as well as fat-soluble vitamins. This will necessitate a very stringent lifelong course of vitamin supplementation, and the patient should be well aware that lifelong nutritional monitoring will be required. Below is our technique for performing this procedure. Please note that the common approaches to performing this procedure are

(1) through the standard open technique, (2) laparoscopically, or (3) robotically. Whatever route is chosen for surgical access, the procedure performed remains the same. Some of the most salient points to remember in this brief description are the lengths of the common and alimentary channels as well as the technique for creating the sleeve gastrectomy, which may very somewhat from a standard vertical sleeve gastrectomy when performed alone. Our preference is to perform a hybrid laparoscopic/robotic technique as described below.

- The patient is placed in the supine position with the arms out.
- All pressure points are padded. A Foley catheter is placed following induction of general anesthesia.
- The abdomen is prepped and draped to allow wide access to the entire abdominal cavity from the xiphoid to well below the umbilicus.

- **Step 1.** Initial access is gained about 25 cm below the xiphoid just to the left of center using an optical viewing trocar.
    - Upon gaining access, the abdomen is insufflated, and general inspection was undertaken to ensure that there are no gross, visual abnormalities, or significant adhesive disease.
    - Significant adhesive disease from prior surgery may require prolonged lysis, conversion to an open technique, or transition to performing a sleeve gastrectomy only.
- **Step 2.** Placement of trocars (Fig. 22.11)

Trocars are then placed under direct visualization in the right upper quadrant just below the tip of the right lobe of the liver. A "stapling" trocar is then placed between this right upper quadrant trocar and the umbilicus. A fourth port is then placed in the left upper quadrant.

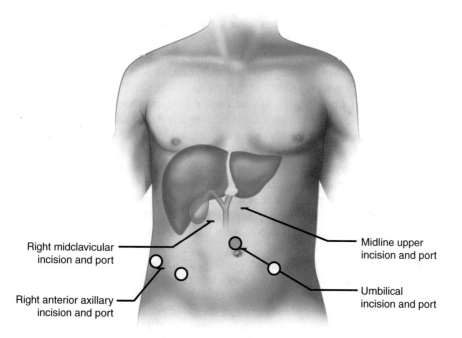

Fig. 22.11 Sites of incisions and ports

- **Step 3.** A liver retractor is placed through a stab incision just below the xiphoid in order to retract the left lobe of the liver anteriorly.
- **Step 4.** Sleeve gastrectomy is performed. Refer to technique earlier in this chapter.
- Our procedure begins with the creation of the sleeve gastrectomy.
    - This is typically done by using either an ultrasonic dissector or monopolar device to dissect the omentum from the greater curvature of the stomach.
    - As in the case of a typical sleeve gastrectomy, care should be taken to perform this dissection as close to the stomach as possible in order to avoid injury to the gastroepiploic epiploic vessels.
        Injury to these vessels could cause bleeding or, possibly, thrombosis of the portal vein.
    - The dissection is carried up to the level of the left crus of the diaphragm.
        If a hiatal hernia is noted. We recommend repairing it in the typical standard fashion.
    - With the greater curvature now fully mobilized, a bougie is placed transorally down to the level of the pylorus in order to calibrate the size of the sleeve. We will typically use a larger bougie, than we would with a standard sleeve gastrectomy. Either a 56- or 60-French bougie are commonly used when performing the BPD-DS.
    - A staple line is started on the greater curvature, 6 cm proximal to the pylorus, and a linear stapler is used to divide the stomach along the bougie up through the cardiac angle of the stomach.
    - The bougie is then removed. A leak test will be performed at the conclusion of the procedure.
- **Step 5.** Duodenal dissection
- With the sleeve gastrectomy now completed, attention is turned to the duodenal dissection.
    - The duodenum is dissected from its retroperitoneal position using an energy device. Care must be taken to do this slowly and deliberately as there is a complex of small vessels just below the first portion of the duodenum which could easily bleed, obscuring the field and making the dissection more precarious. If needed, the pylorus can be marked prior to this dissection with a single stitch as it is sometimes somewhat more difficult to identify after the dissection has been completed. During this portion of the dissection, extra care must be taken to avoid injury to the gastroduodenal artery and common bile duct which lie just posterior to the first and second portions of the duodenum.
    - Once these structures have been identified, a window can be made through the fat overlying the cephalad portion of D1 so that a stapler can be placed across. We generally reserved this portion of the case until after we have made our enteroenterostomy.
- **Step 6.** Creation of enteroenterostomy (Fig. 22.12)
    - We find it helpful to place a 12-mm trocar just to the left of midline below the umbilicus. The camera is now placed in the left upper quadrant trocar, and instruments are placed through the prior camera port and infraumbilical trocar.

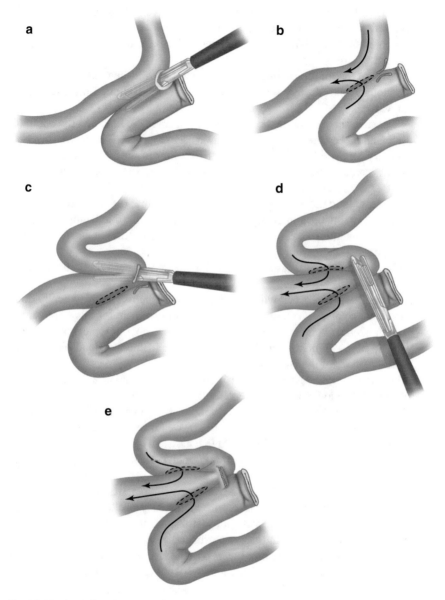

Fig. 22.12 (**a–e**) Creation of duodena-duodenostomy

- The terminal ileum is identified, and the ileum is measured proximally 100 cm. This will be the common limb and is marked with clips.

  We placed two clips proximally and one distally to mark the direction of "downhill" flow.

- From this point, we measure another 150 cm proximally where the small bowel is divided with a vascular linear stapler.

- We mark the tip of the alimentary limb with several clips in order to avoid confusion when making our anastomosis.
- The mesentery is divided using an energy device to decrease tension on the alimentary limb.
- The tip of the more proximal, biliopancreatic limb is then placed next to our previously placed clips on the common channel 100 cm from the ileocecal valve.
- We place a stay suture on the tip of the biliopancreatic limb and the common limb and make enterotomies on the antimesenteric side of each. We then perform a side-by-side anastomosis with two firings of the 60-mm vascular load linear stapler. The common defect can then be oversewn or closed with another staple fire.
- The mesenteric defect is then closed with a running 2-0 silk suture.
    At this point, the alimentary limb is brought up to the duodenum. If needed, the omentum can be divided to create less tension on the duodeno-enterostomy.
- **Step 7.** Division of duodenum and creation of duodeno-enterostomy (Figs. 22.13, 22.14, and 22.15)
- At this point, we'll proceed with dividing the duodenum. This is typically done with a linear stapler. We choose to use staple reinforcement for this staple fire.
    - The duodenal stump may be oversewn, but this is not our typical practice.
    - The tip of the alimentary limb is then placed in an end to side fashion next to the stapled tip of the duodenum.
    - These two structures are then approximated with a running 2-0 silk suture.
    - An anterior duodenotomy and enterotomy are then made. We tend to try to make these enterotomies as wide as possible to avoid a stenosis of the entero-enterostomy. Because the pylorus is intact, we do not try to keep this anastomosis, narrow as we typically would in a gastric bypass.
    - We then hand sew the posterior and anterior layers using a running 3-0 absorbable suture.
    - Until you have developed a lot of experience with this, we recommend sewing this anastomosis over a stent to ensure the patency of the anastomosis. This can easily be done using the standard gastroscope which will facilitate in testing the anastomosis and the sleeve postoperatively.
    - Once the posterior and anterior layers have been sewn together, we run a final layer in a Lembert fashion using another 3-0 absorbable suture.

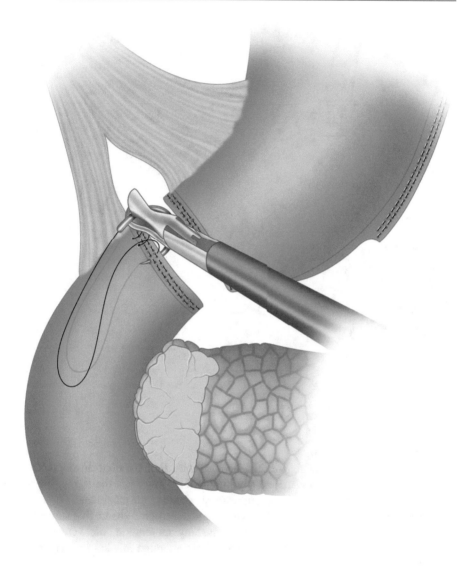

Fig. 22.13 Division of duodenum

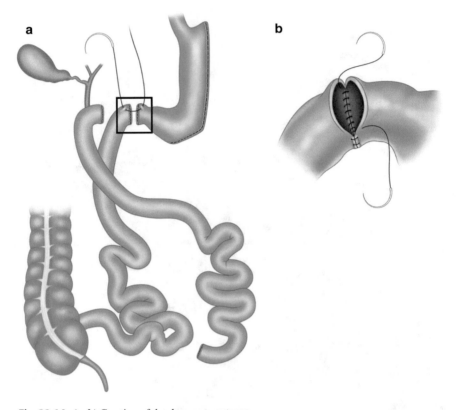

Fig. 22.14 (**a**, **b**) Creation of duodeno-enterostomy

- **Step 8.** Testing for a leak
- The sleeve and anastomosis are then stressed with air from a gastroscope. The gastroscope allows us to visualize any internal bleeding from the staple line or leaks that may be occurring at the anastomosis or along the staple line.
    - Leaks can generally be managed with single interrupted absorbable sutures.
    - It is sometimes recommended to close the large mesenteric defect created by the antecolic passage of the alimentary limb, although this has not typically been our practice.
    - Following a negative leak test, a 10-French flat JP drain is placed so that it is in proximity to the staple line, the duodeno-enterostomy, and the duodenal stump.
    - This may be removed the next day, if the patient is tolerating liquids and no bilious effluent is seen in the drain.
- **Step 9.** Remove gastric remnant and trocars.
- Remove the resected portion of the stomach using a retrieval bag.
    - The liver retractor should be removed under direct visualization.
    - The abdomen is deflated, the trocars are removed, and the sites are closed in standard fashion.

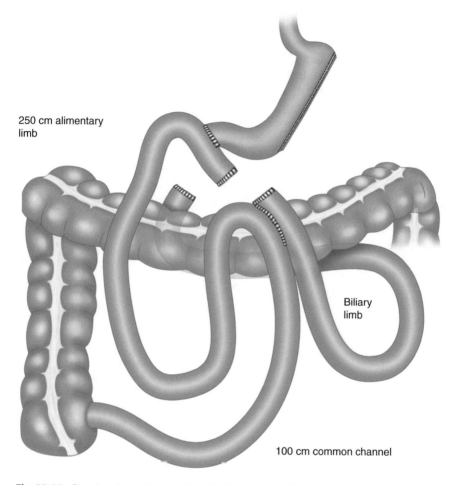

250 cm alimentary
limb

Biliary
limb

100 cm common channel

Fig. 22.15 Completed operation showing the duodenal switch and all anastomoses

Post-op

Our patients will generally stay one to two nights on the bariatric floor of the hospital.

- We began feeding them clear liquids the next morning.
- We do not routinely perform fluoroscopic swallow studies unless the patient is having significant nausea lasting more than 48 h or there is concern for a leak.
- Any bilious material that is seen in the drain on postoperative day 1 should be treated as a leak from the duodenal stump and should necessitate a diagnostic laparoscopy.
- The patients are sent home on a full liquid diet for 2 weeks and then advanced over the course of the next few weeks to a regular diet.

- We will generally check nutritional laboratories often in the first year at 3 months, 6 months, and in 12 months.
- Nutrition should also be checked annually or semiannually to ensure that proper supplementation is being maintained.
- It is very important that the patient take a vitamin that has the adequate amount of vitamins A, D, E, and K, as these are difficult for the patient to absorb following this procedure.

Sports Hernia

23

Jeffrey S. Hoadley

Anatomical and Physiologic Considerations

The diagnosis of sports hernia, aka athletic pubalgia or core muscle injury, has always been shrouded in some mystery. Hopefully, with the understanding of pathophysiology and anatomy, the diagnosis and treatment will become much clearer. Awareness of this injury is important because 0.5–6.2% of patients presenting to a sports injury clinic complain of groin pain. Of patients suffering a groin injury, 46% participate in soccer followed by hockey at 17% and football 13%. The reality is that just about any recreational activity can lead to this type of injury. As in any disease process, an understanding of the mechanism of injury followed by the differential diagnosis allows a complex decision process to be much more simplistic.

The mechanism of injury is based on the forces in and around the anterior pelvis. Torquing or twisting of the pelvis leaves the pubic tubercle as a fulcrum for the generated forces. The rectus abdominis and the oblique muscles pull and rotate opposite the directional forces of the adductor longus. The resulting injury is based on the theory that the anterior core muscles are relatively weaker than the legs. This mechanism is why adductor-dominant athletes such as soccer and hockey players are more prone to this injury. Athletic loading of the pubic tubercle or symphysis leads to shearing forces and symphyseal instability. If the majority of shear load is across the pubic bone, then the patient is prone to osteitis pubis or stress fracture of the pubis. If the majority of shear load is across the tendon, then the patient can develop adductor tendinitis or sports hernia with the rectus abdominis/conjoined tendon or floor of the inguinal canal bearing the brunt of the forces. This describes the pathophysiology of core and boney injuries across the pubis, but patients presenting with groin pain have a much broader differential. Understanding the full differential will allow the treating physician to properly select those with a core muscle injury.

J. S. Hoadley (✉)
Department of Surgery, North Atlanta Surgical Associates, Atlanta, GA, USA

© Springer Nature Switzerland AG 2021
L. J. Skandalakis (ed.), *Surgical Anatomy and Technique*,
https://doi.org/10.1007/978-3-030-51313-9_23

Despite the emerging recognition of core muscle injuries, true inguinal hernias are the most common cause of groin pain. Perhaps the second most common cause would be neuralgia or scar disruption from previous hernia repairs. As previously discussed, osteitis pubis or stress fracture of the pubic bone can manifest as groin pain. Because the rectus abdominis-adductor aponeurosis shares connection across the front of the pubic bone, adductor tendinitis can have an inguinal pain component as well. If the diruption occurs at the insertion of the conjoined tendon at the pubic tubercle or the floor of the inguinal canal is dirupted without classic herniation, then a sports hernia injury has resulted. But perhaps the most insidious presentation of groin pain involves primary hip pathology. Hip flexor tendinitis, labral tears, and bursitis can all present with groin pain due to the medial location of the acetabular socket. While imaging can be helpful, physical exam should allow the diagnosis to emerge from the differential.

While the patient can usually describe the specifics of the injury, many have an insidious onset especially during cooldown or the day after activity. Specific questioning will rule out any intra-abdominal pathology such as appendicitis or nephrolithiasis which can occasionally present as groin pain. Physical exam starts with the patient standing. A true inguinal hernia, especially small indirect hernias, needs to be ruled out. Patients with a core muscle injury may have discomfort at the external ring, along the floor of the inguinal canal and especially at the insertion of the conjoined tendon at the pubic tubercle exacerbated with Valsalva maneuver. Palpation of the adductor insertion will elicit adductor tendinitis. Palpation of the mid-pubic bone allows for osteitis pubis or stress fracture to be diagnosed. Secondly, the patient is examined supine and dynamic. Patients with core muscle injury will have pain performing an in-line sit-up especially with palpation throughout the inguinal ligament and the insertion of the conjoined tendon at the pubic tubercle. Adductor palpation should be done with resisted adduction. Most importantly, hip pathology must be ruled out. If the patient has pain with internal/external rotation with both knee and hip flexed as well as pain with medial loading of the hip, then hip pathology must be ruled out with imaging or assessment by hip specialist prior to any inguinal intervention.

Ultrasound, CT, and MRI can assist in working through the differential. Ultrasound can allow the patient to be dynamic and can demonstrate convex bulging of the inguinal floor. Unfortunately, ultrasound is user dependent. CT is best to rule out intra-abdominal pathology. The gold standard is pelvic MRI which does a very good job of assessing the muscle, tendon, and bone. MR arthrogram is able to adequately assess for hip pathology. In regard to athletic pubalgia, unfortunately the most common MRI finding is "normal." So physical exam and patient complaints reign supreme with imaging complimenting clinical assessment. In addition, adductor-dominant athletes often have multiple findings on MRI which represent old injuries and not of current clinical significance.

Treatment is obviously driven by diagnosis. Osteitis pubis responds well to cortisone injection. Stress fracture of the pubis requires long rest and perhaps non-weight bearing. Hip pathology is dependent on the hip specialist. In regard to core muscle injury, prolonged rest followed by physical therapy is the first mainstay. A

2015 article in the *British Journal of Medicine* reported on a retrospective study that physical therapy was equal to operation. This strengthens the argument for physical therapy but was not a prospective randomized trial and did not address those athletes who fail physical therapy. Physical therapy can take 4–6 weeks to complete, complimented by dry needling, deep tissue massage, and core short support. 10–15% of patients do not respond adequately to nonoperative modalities. Those patients require platelet-rich plasma (PRP) injection and/or operative intervention.

Patients with adductor tendinitis who cannot return to sport-specific activity with PT require PRP injection. The theory is that the adductor tendon does not have sufficient blood supply to recover and PRP injection brings a bolus of growth factors to the injury. The discrete insertion of the adductor tendon allows for this technique. For the rare athlete who does not respond to PRP injection, then adductor operative release should be contemplated. Unfortunately, the broad insertion of the rectus/conjoined tendon and associated injuries does not allow PRP injection to be adequate for the abdominal component of core muscle injury aka sports hernia. This requires operative intervention.

Operating Room Strategies, Considerations, and Technique

Operative findings include a spectrum of injuries in and around the inguinal canal. These include longitudinal tears in the external oblique especially along nerve exit sites, splaying of the external ring, laxity of the inguinal floor, and palpable step-off at the conjoined tendon suggesting a tear in this structure. Operative technique centers on the pain at the insertion of the conjoined tendon at the pubic tubercle. The conjoined tendon is plicated first to the pubic tubercle and then the medial aspect of Cooper's ligament.

- **Step 1.** An oblique incision is made just medial and parallel, to the inguinal ligament.
- **Step 2.** The external oblique aponeurosis is identified. This structure is then opened from the external ring extending beyond the internal ring.
- **Step 3.** The spermatic cord is mobilized and elevated off the tubercle, dividing cremasteric fibers to rule out an indirect defect. The conjoined tendon is plicated as described above. Lightweight mesh is placed over the repair and extends 1–2 cm over the tubercle. The mesh is allowed to extend laterally beyond the internal ring fashioning a keyhole around the cord structures.
- **Step 4.** The mesh is sutured to the transversalis fascia medially and Poupart's ligament laterally. This supports both the conjoined tendon repair and the floor of the inguinal canal. In addition, the iliohypogastric nerve may play a role in the pain syndrome. For this reason and the possibility of post-op neuralgia, the iliohypogastric nerve is excised.
- **Step 5.** The splayed external ring and tears in the external oblique are repaired during wound closure.

- **Step 6.** In patients who have significant adductor symptoms, an adductor release is performed. This is a partial release consisting of making 2–3 cm incisions over the upper adductor tendon near the groin crease. Five to seven of these incisions are made.

Postoperative Course

After 2 weeks of recovery, physical therapy is again initiated. Full recovery can be expected in a 6–8 week time frame. If properly selected, nearly 100% of athletes should return to sport-specific activity. If not, give consideration to a concomitant secondary injury such as hip pathology.

Ablative Techniques for Management of Symptomatic Superficial Venous Disease

Charles B. Ross, Veer Chahwala, and Garnet Roy Craddock Jr.

Patient Selection

Treatment of patients with venous disease begins with a detailed history and physical examination. Venous disease affects all ages and both genders. Heaviness, aching, swelling, throbbing, itching, (HASTI) are common symptoms [1]. Specific factors to be considered include a history of venous thrombosis, extremity trauma, extremity swelling, spontaneous bleeding, personal and/or family history of thrombophilia, duration of symptoms, and physical findings. In women, parity is contributory, and reproductive history is always recorded. Atherosclerotic cardiovascular disease frequently co-exists in older patients with chronic venous insufficiency and should be identified. Patients should be scrutinized for confounding disorders including suprainguinal venous disease such as nonthrombotic iliac venous compression, lymphedema, arterial insufficiency, and lumbosacral spine disease which may change one's therapeutic approach. The focused physical examination should include documentation of all pulses, documentation of location and estimated size of varicose veins as well as spider and reticular venous complexes. In the calf, pruritis, dermatitis, induration, edema, hyperpigmentation, scarring from healed ulcers, and active ulcers should be documented. It is helpful to document physical findings

C. B. Ross (✉)
Vascular and Endovascular Services, Piedmont Heart Institute, Piedmont Atlanta Vein Center, Piedmont Atlanta Hospital, Atlanta, GA, USA
e-mail: Charles.ross@piedmont.org

V. Chahwala
Vascular and Endovascular Surgery, Piedmont Atlanta Vein Center, Piedmont Atlanta Hospital, Atlanta, GA, USA

G. R. Craddock Jr.
Southern Vein Care, The Piedmont Clinic, Piedmont Newnan Hospital, Newnan, GA, USA

© Springer Nature Switzerland AG 2021
L. J. Skandalakis (ed.), *Surgical Anatomy and Technique*,
https://doi.org/10.1007/978-3-030-51313-9_24

by photography. Maximal circumference of each ankle, calf, and thigh is recorded as well. It is considered good practice to classify patients' venous disease using the CEAP classification system [2]. Clinical scoring of symptoms and findings is also important. In our practice, we use the Venous Clinical Severity Score (VCSS) [3].

The next step in patient evaluation is a detailed duplex venous ultrasound [4]. This study uses gray scale imaging with/without compression and Doppler assessment of flow to document superficial and deep vein patency and valvular incompetency. Signs of venous outflow obstruction including continuous flow and reduced phasicity are documented and considered for further investigation. Below the inguinal ligament, venous reflux of 500 milliseconds or longer is considered pathologic, but treatment is always clinically driven, generally with much longer reflux duration. Sources of reflux from the deep to superficial system are mapped. The subcutaneous course of the saphenous veins is mapped including duplicated segments, accessory saphenous vein, and locations where the vein courses outside its fascial envelope. Highest and lowest points of reflux are noted. Finally, the diameter of the great and small saphenous veins should be documented at regular intervals along their entire length.

Patients whose clinical histories and physical findings suggest symptomatic venous insufficiency are initially managed with compression hose (20–30 mmHg), periodic limb elevation, regular walking, and variable topical agents. Venous ulceration requires more advanced wound therapy and must be provided. Pain is managed with nonsteroidal anti-inflammatory agents or with other nonnarcotic alternatives. Some patients will improve with symptomatic therapy. Many others will reach a point of maximal benefit and still have symptoms for which they desire definitive therapy. Once third-party payer and/or departmental standards have been met, appropriate patients may be considered candidates for ablative therapy. In March 2020, at the 32nd annual meeting of the American Venous Forum, appropriate use criteria guiding management of chronic lower extremity venous disease, formulated by multidisciplinary working group headed by Masuda and colleagues, were presented [5]. When considering a patient for intervention and/or when discussing coverage of services for a patient in an insurance denial appeal, this document may provide clarity and guidance.

Options for Axial Vein Ablation

Endovenous thermal ablation with tumescence (TT) is a minimally invasive technique which produces excellent cosmesis and quick recovery for patients. It is equally efficacious compared to surgical stripping and may result is less recurrent neovascularity than stripping plus high ligation [6–8]. The basic principle is local direct application of thermal energy to the vein wall resulting in vein wall injury, contraction, and intraluminal thrombosis – with acute injury evolving to chronic closure of the vein. Thermal energy may be applied by radiofrequency or laser. Multiple catheters and systems are available. The basic technique is to insert the RFA or laser catheter into the greater saphenous vein just above the level of the tibial plateau or distal thigh, advance the catheter to a position 2 to 3 cm below the saphenofemoral junction, infiltrate tumescent anesthesia along the entire course of the target vein, recheck position of the catheter tip, and then treat either segmentally or with slow, continuous

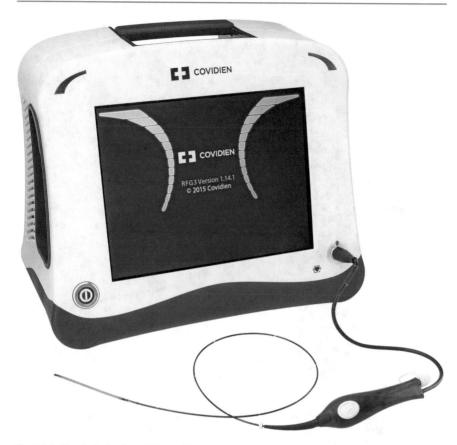

Fig. 24.1 Vendor's display of ClosureFast™ catheter and generator. (©2019 Medtronic. All rights reserved. Used with the permission of Medtronic)

withdrawal depending on the catheter system used. Operators should work with vendors and mentors to carefully study the nuances of the specific catheter and technique available in their center. In this chapter, we describe use of the ClosureFast™ radiofrequency ablation system (Medtronic, Plymouth, MN, USA) (Fig. 24.1).

Nonthermal, nontumescent ablation (NTNT) may be accomplished using multiple techniques [9]. The procedures are performed with ultrasound guidance. Catheter tips are positioned 3 to 5 cm below the junction of the saphenous vein with deep vein. Treatment is administered as the catheter is pulled back. Again, operators should take required training modules and courses provided by the vendor and take advantage of mentors as early experiences are accumulated.

MOCA, mechanical occlusion chemically assisted ablation (Clarivein ™, Merit Medical Systems, Inc., South Jordan, UT, USA), is an NTNT ablation technique that uses a small diameter steerable catheter with spinning wire-tip. The tip rotates at 3500 rpm causing endothelial damage and wall spasm. Sclerosant (1.5% sodium tetradecyl sulfate) is injected while the tip spins and the catheter is slowly pulled back (1 cm/7 seconds). This results in minimal discomfort, is efficient, and is well-tolerated. Another NTNT ablative technique relies on tissue adhesion. CAE,

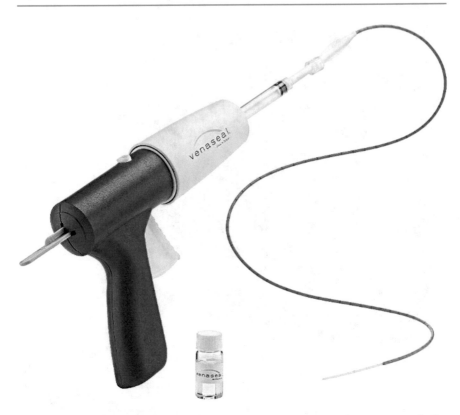

Fig. 24.2 Vendor's display of Venaseal™ system showing gun, coaxial catheter system, and adhesive. (©2019 Medtronic. All rights reserved. Used with the permission of Medtronic)

cyanoacrylate embolization (Venaseal ™), uses a 5F catheter inserted via a 7F sheath through which cyanoacrylate (CA) adhesive is injected into the vein. Once exposed to blood, the adhesive rapidly sets and occludes the vein. An inflammatory reaction results and further assists in scarring and permanent closure. Other NTNT techniques include foam sclerotherapy, including Varithena™ which is a proprietary, polidocanol microfoam (Boston Scientific, Inc., Natick, MA, USA) and VBAS (V-block assisted sclerotherapy) which involves endovenous placement of an occlusive plug behind which foamed sclerosant is injected (proprietary technique available in Europe). All the abovementioned techniques result in minimal discomfort, are efficient, and are well-tolerated [9]. In this chapter, we describe use of the CAE Venaseal™ system (Fig. 24.2).

Considering TT and NTNT techniques, the field is rapidly evolving. Meta-analyses of clinical trials comparing TT and NTNT techniques have shown no significant differences in closure rates but a tendency toward less pain with NTNT procedures [10]. Selection of one technique over another depends on multiple factors such as ultrasound and patient characteristics including vein diameter, length of vein to be treated, tortuosity, course in relation to depth and fascia, above versus below knee position, concerns about neighboring structures such as nerves and skin, and presence or absence of advanced tissue changes in the region of treatment. In general, larger veins located above the knee are most commonly treated by TT whereas veins below the knee where nerves and skin are at risk, tortuous suprafascial veins at any level, and veins in regions of advanced tissue changes are best treated with NTNT techniques. These decisions are covered in a recent review by Elias [11].

Ultrasound Guidance for Venous Ablative Procedures

Percutaneous ultrasound (US) guidance is fundamentally important to the safe conduct of ablation procedures. Venous access to initiate ablative procedures is easily mastered. The basic steps of US-guided intervention are as follows:

Step 1. After sterilely prepping and draping the extremity, the US transducer is placed in a sterile sleeve with generous conductive jelly. The skin is also lubricated, and the target vein is identified and surveyed.

Step 2. The target location for entry is selected. Local anesthesia is then injected with US guidance using a 25-gauge needle. It is helpful to observe the infiltration of local solution because one can develop an understanding of the trajectory of needle that will be necessary for successful vein puncture.

Step 3. Next, a 22-gauge micropuncture needle is used to puncture the target vein. One may use either the US short-axis view with the transducer placed perpendicular to the target or the long-axis view. The long-axis view allows better visualization of the needle as it enters the vein (Fig. 24.3).

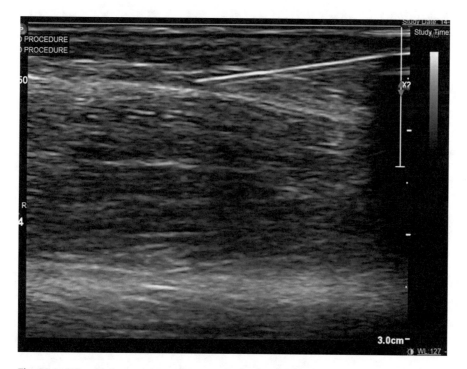

Fig. 24.3 US-guided percutaneous venous access, long-axis view

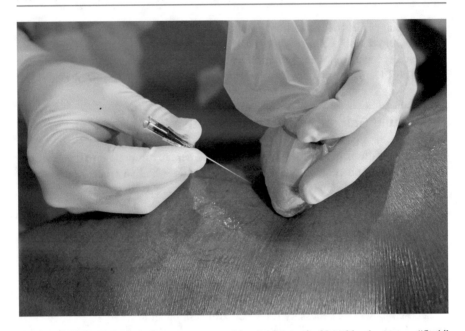

Fig. 24.4 US-guided percutaneous access, working in short axis. Note blood return or "flash" with successful puncture

Step 4. While the physician is concentrating on the puncture, the physician and the assistant must watch for a flash with egress of blood (Fig. 24.4). When the flash is noted, a 0.018 Nitinol guidewire is placed, and it is followed in the vein by US (Figs. 24.5 and 24.6). All movements with the needle and the wire should be steady and fine.

Step 5. When satisfactory wire placement is achieved, the tip of an 11-blade scalpel is used to make a small nick at the wire entry point in the skin. Then, the dilator and the sheath are placed (Fig. 24.7). It is our practice to aspirate blood from the sheath and then to flush with injectable normal saline.

Step 6. After access, US guidance is necessary for safe positioning of the ablation device or catheter within the target vein distal to the saphenofemoral junction (SFJ) and deep system. A long-axis view is obtained which demonstrates the tip of the ablation device and SFJ. The distance between SFJ and the tip of the radio-frequency ablation device should be no less than 2.0 cm. We prefer 2.5 to 3 cm (Fig. 24.8). When performing ablation using the Venaseal™ technique, the tip of the injection catheter must be 5 cm from the SFJ.

Step 7. The position of the device/catheter relative to the SFJ is documented with a saved or hard copy image with distance annotated in the image.

Step 8. At the completion of an ablation procedure, US is used to document the proximal extent of vein closure as well as unimpaired common femoral venous flow and normal compressibility.

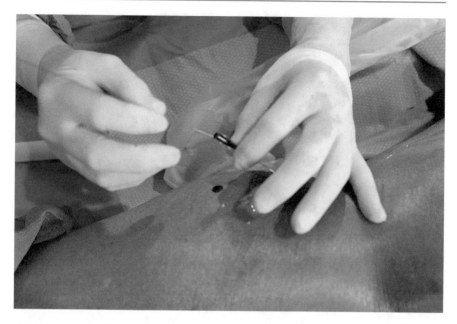

Fig. 24.5 Detailed view of nitinol wire advance into the vein

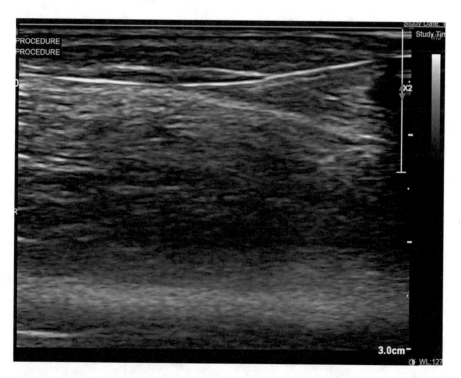

Fig. 24.6 Detailed US view of nitinol wire entering vein lumen

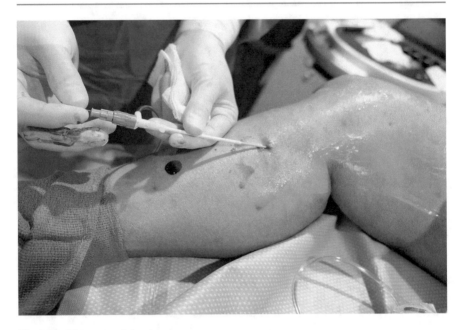

Fig. 24.7 Placement of sheath

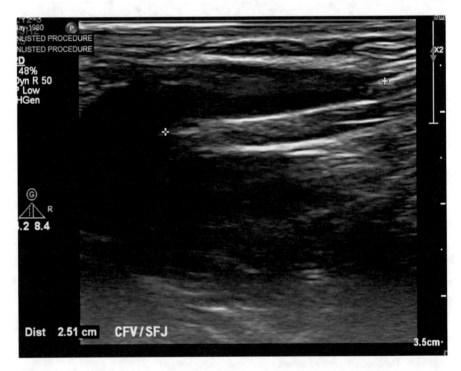

Fig. 24.8 US documentation of distance between saphenofemoral junction and RFA catheter tip

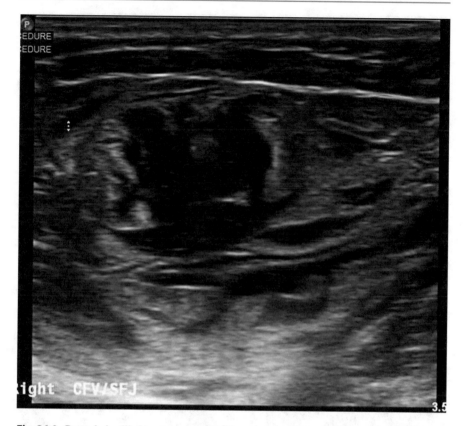

Fig. 24.9 Properly instilled tumescence with vein and catheter appearance as a "bullseye"

In the course of a TT procedure, US guidance is used to direct instillation of tumescent anesthesia fluid into the perivenous space. This may be done with a syringe or foot pump depending on surgeon preference. Tumescence is important. It provides anesthesia. It compresses the vein around the tip of the ablation device. It also serves as a heat sink and thus protects against injury to the overlying skin and adjacent soft tissue and nerves. Care should be taken to instill fluid both posterior and anterior to the vein. With proper tumescence, the catheter within the target vein ideally should appear as a "bullseye" within the fluid-filled saphenous sheath (Fig. 24.9). Inadvertent puncture of the target vein should also be avoided in order to minimize bleeding and ecchymosis. When using tumescence with an extra-fascial vein, care should be taken to elevate the dermis at least 1 cm from the RAF catheter.

Radiofrequency Ablation Technique

Radiofrequency ablation using the ClosureFast™ catheter precisely heats a 7 cm (also available in 3 cm length) vein segment in one 20-second interval to shrink and collapse the target veins to achieve a fibrotic seal and occlude the refluxing vein

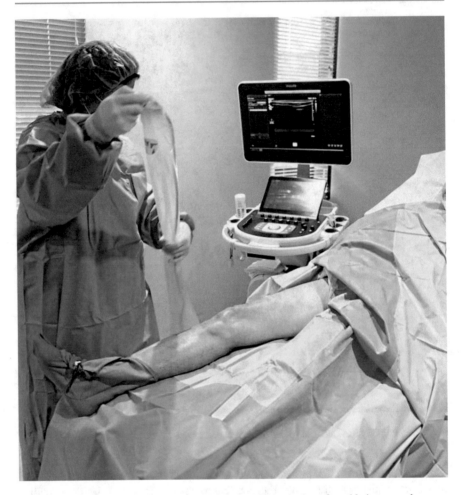

Fig. 24.10 A properly prepped and draped patient at the beginning of an ablation procedure

segment. The temperature is kept at a stable 120 degrees Celsius during the 20-second treatment cycle. The catheter delivers radiofrequency (RF) energy which uses ohmic heating to cause collagen contraction, which leads to obliteration of the lumen through endothelial destruction, inflammatory response, fibrosis, and permanent occlusion.

Step 1: Positioning

The patient is prepped and draped circumferentially from the groin crease to the ipsilateral toes (Fig. 24.10). The patient is placed in reverse Trendelenburg position to allow maximal vein distention in the early stages of the procedure.

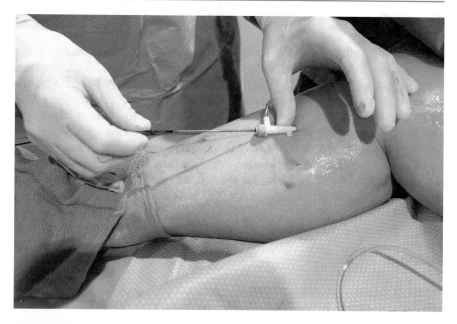

Fig. 24.11 Detailed view of insertion of the 7 cm RFA catheter. Note, an RFA catheter with 3 cm treatment zone is also available for use when treating short vein segments such as an accessory saphenous vein

Step 2: Access

As previously described, ultrasound-guided access of the great saphenous vein is obtained using a 21-gauge micropuncture needle and .018-inch wire at the level of the distal thigh or just below the knee. The tapered 7-Fr sheath is placed over the wire. The ClosureFast™ catheter is then placed through the 7-Fr sheath (Fig. 24.11) and advanced to the level of the SFJ. The distance between SFJ and the tip of the radiofrequency ablation device should be no less than 2.0 cm (see Fig. 24.8). We prefer 2.5 to 3 cm. Occasionally, a 0.25inch guidewire may be required to help guide the catheter if the vein is particularly tortuous.

Step 3: Tumescence

The entire treatment length of the vein must be circumferentially anesthetized with dilute 0.1% lidocaine tumescent solution prior to beginning ablation. The superficial fascia anterior to the vein and the muscular fascia posterior the vein create the saphenous canal. Using ultrasound guidance, the tumescent solution (445 ml of 0.9% saline, 50 ml of 1% Lidocaine with 1:100,000 epinephrine and 5 ml of 8.4% sodium bicarbonate) is injected circumferentially around the vein in the saphenous canal and to have at least 1 cm separation from the dermis.

Step 4: RFA Treatment

RFA may begin after appropriate instillation of tumescent solution along the entire treatment length of the vein and final positioning of the RF catheter is rechecked and confirmed to be 2–3 cm from the saphenofemoral junction (SFJ). Importantly, two cycles of RF energy (20 seconds each) are delivered for the first treatment zone adjacent to the SFJ. This helps ensure adequate closure of the vein at this critical location. Next, the catheter is retracted in 6.5 cm segments, and each vein segment is treated with a single 20 second cycle. Venous segments >10 mm in diameter may be treated with an additional RF cycle. After the final segment of vein has been treated, the catheter and the sheath are removed and manual pressure is applied at the sheath insertion to achieve hemostasis. An elastic stocking or bandage is applied for 24–48 hours postoperatively.

Follow-Up

A venous duplex is performed within 72 hours to confirm venous ablation and to rule out deep venous thrombosis.

Endovenous Laser Ablation (EVLA)

The technique for EVLA is very similar to that of RFA, with some notable differences.

After access to the GSV, the endovenous sheath is inserted. The endovenous sheath for EVLA must be long enough to reach the saphenofemoral junction (SFJ) (either 25-,35-,45-, or 65-cm lengths). The sheath is tracked over the wire to the SFJ. Anesthetic tumescence is given in the saphenous sheath. The laser fiber is advanced to the sheath tip, and then the sheath is retracted 1 cm to expose the laser fiber tip. Once exposed, the laser fiber tip should be positioned at least 2 cm distal to the SFJ. Finally, the patient is treated as the laser fiber is pulled back such that 60–80 J/cm is delivered. Manual pressure is held during the pull back as well. At the termination of the laser pull back, the laser is deactivated and laser and sheath are removed together. Manual pressure is held at the access site for hemostasis, and the leg is wrapped with a compression bandage.

Complications of Thermal Ablation with Tumescence

Several (usually minor) complications may arise after an ablative procedure. The patient may experience bruising and local discomfort for the first 24–48 hours, but this is usually self-limiting. Potential complications also include paresthesias, thrombophlebitis, deep vein thrombosis, hematoma, infection, staining, skin dimpling, and skin burns. Major nerve injuries are rare but possible, especially when treating the small saphenous vein. Paresthesias, numbness, and skin injury may be avoided by proper perivenous tumescence – elevating the skin at least 1 cm away from any point of ablation and filling the sheath fully to protect the saphenous nerve. If the vein resides extra-fascially and less than 1 cm beneath the dermis, staining and dimpling may still occur even with copious tumescence and may be avoided by selection of an alternative NTNT technique or stab phlebectomy.

Proper positioning of the RFA device tip from the SFJ and its superficial epigastric branch is essential in preventing propagation of thrombus into the common femoral vein. With modern devices, this phenomenon, endovenous heat-induced thrombosis (EHIT), occurs in less than 2% of cases [12]. But it is considered standard-of-care to bring all patients back to the vein center 72 hours after RFA procedures for venous ultrasound examination to rule out EHIT. Patients with large vein diameters (> than 8 mm) are at higher risk for EHIT [12]. Classification and management of EHIT is shown in Table 24.1. Guidelines for management of EHIT have been recently updated [13]. These guidelines recommend no extra treatment or surveillance for EHIT I. For EHIT II, the guidelines suggest surveillance only versus either aspirin or oral anticoagulation with surveillance. Our preference is use of a direct oral anticoagulant. We have the patient return in 2 weeks for repeat venous ultrasound and discontinue therapy as the thrombus retracts into the treated superficial vein. Rarely do we find it necessary to continue therapy more than 2 to 4 weeks. Anticoagulation is definitely recommended for class III and IV EHIT. Management of EHIT IV follows standard DVT practices.

Table 24.1 Endovenous heat-induced thrombosis [13]

Class	Description and management
1	Thrombus extends to the superficial-deep junction but does not extend into the deep vein lumen (Fig. 24.12) Observation with repeat ultrasound in 1 week
2	Nonocclusive thrombus extends into the lumen of the deep vein but causes less than 50% reduction in cross-sectional area of the vein Surveillance until thrombus retracts into the treated SFJ or SPJ and no longer occupies the deep vein; adjunctive aspirin or anticoagulation may be considered
3	Nonocclusive thrombus extends into the lumen of the deep vein and causes > than 50% reduction in cross-sectional area of the vein Anticoagulation with LMWH or DOAC until thrombus retracts and no longer occupies the lumen of the deep vein
4	Thrombus extends into the deep vein and results in a completely occlusive deep vein thrombosis Anticoagulation with LMWH or DOAC per standard DVT practice

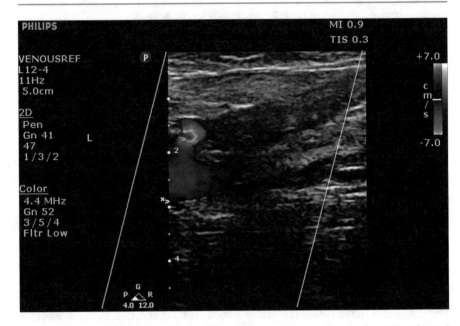

Fig. 24.12 US appearance of EHIT Class 1. Note thrombus extending to the saphenofemoral junction

Brief Note Regarding Adjunctive Stab Phlebectomy

It is optional to add stab phlebectomy to ablative procedures targeting the greater or lesser saphenous veins. It is our general practice to add phlebectomy to treat bulging, unsightly or symptomatic tributary varices. As noted, varices are marked preprocedurally with the patient standing (Fig. 24.13). After ablation, we use ultrasound to confirm our markings. One percent Lidocaine is injected in the dermis and subcutaneous tissues around the vein. A 2 to 3 mm incision is made with the tip of an 11-blade scalpel, phlebectomy device, 15 degree ophthalmic scalpel, or 16 g needle tip (surgeon's choice). The vein is engaged either with a crochet-hook phlebectomy device or mosquito hemostat. Tumescence is often infiltrated along the course of the vein, and the vein is removed through push–pull technique. Skin may be closed with 4-0 or 5-0 Nylon sutures using plastic technique or with skin glue and adhesive strips. We prefer to use tapered as opposed to cutting needles to further minimize trauma. Complications include local paresthesias, infection, and hematoma. Nerve injury, however, is possible, and great caution should be exercised if phlebectomy is performed in the posterior thigh, popliteal fossa, or region of the fibular head. In rare cases, sciatic and or peroneal–tibial nerve injuries with permanent foot drop have been litigated [14].

Fig. 24.13 Preprocedural marking of varices to be treated with RFA plus adjunctive stab phlebectomies

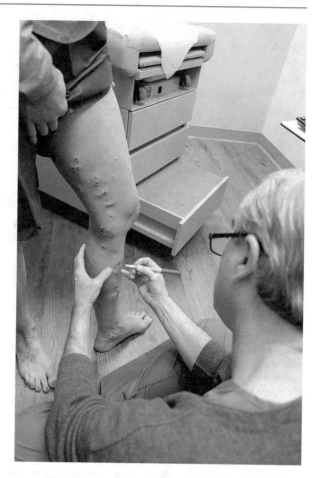

Nonthermal, Nontumesence (NTNT) Ablation Technique

The Venaseal™ system comes with a 5 ml vial of cyanoacrylate, co-axial sheath/catheter system, and delivery gun. Steps for the Venaseal closure procedure are as follows:

Step 1. US-guided access is obtained, and a 7F sheath is placed.

Step 2. A 0.035 guidewire is advanced from entry to the deep system across the SFJ. The system's long 7F sheath is advanced over the wire and positioned 5 cm distal to the SFJ.

Step 3. Next, a 5F delivery catheter with loaded injection gun is advanced into the sheath. The delivery catheter has a laser mark 5 cm from its hub. When that mark reaches the

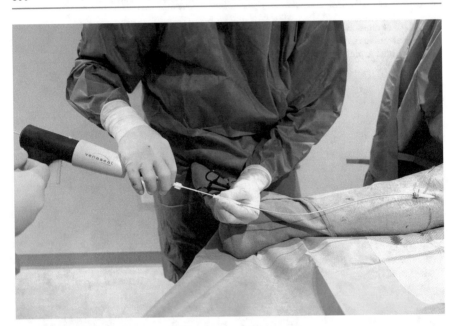

Fig. 24.14 Demonstration of proper final positioning of the Venaseal catheter before first injection of adhesive. The tip of the (blue) introducer has been localized by US 5 cm distal to the saphenofemoral junction. The (white) delivery catheter is inserted into the introducer to the laser mark. The delivery catheter is then held steady while the introducer is pulled back to the hub and locked. US is then used again to verify that the delivery catheter tip is no less than 5 cm from the saphenofemoral junction. Once verified, the transducer is used to firmly compress the saphenous vein between the catheter tip and the junction. Then, the trigger is depressed and procedure initiated

hub of the sheath, the delivery catheter is steadied and the sheath is pulled back and married to the hub of the delivery catheter – thus exposing the tip of the delivery catheter 5 cm from the SFJ (Fig. 24.14). US is used to confirm tip position.

Step 4. To begin, proper delivery catheter position is confirmed by US measurement. The catheter is easily visualized in its short access as a star pattern (Fig. 24.15).

Step 5. Then, the transducer is used to compress the GSV approximately 2.5 cm from the SFJ. The trigger is squeezed, and the first aliquot of CA is delivered.

Step 6. The delivery catheter is immediately pulled back 1 cm and a second injection is made. The catheter is immediately pulled back 3 cm. Transducer compression is maintained during this entire sequence and the subsequent 3 minutes. The Venaseal™ delivery gun has an audible click. With each squeeze and click, 0.1 cc of CA is deposited. The substance is viscous, so the trigger should be held for 3 seconds per injection. External hand pressure over the area of the vein where the adhesive was delivered is applied for 3 minutes.

Step 7. After 3 minutes, an injection is made, and the catheter is pulled back 3 cm. External pressure (Fig. 24.16) is again applied and maintained for 30 seconds over the deposited adhesive just proximal to the catheter tip. This sequence is repeated until the catheter has treated within 3 cm of the entry point.

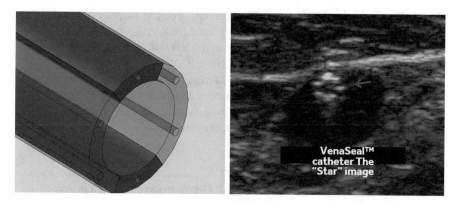

Fig. 24.15 Diagram of the delivery catheter and its "star" appearance under US inspection. (Source: Courtesy of Medtronic AVE, Santa Rosa, CA.)

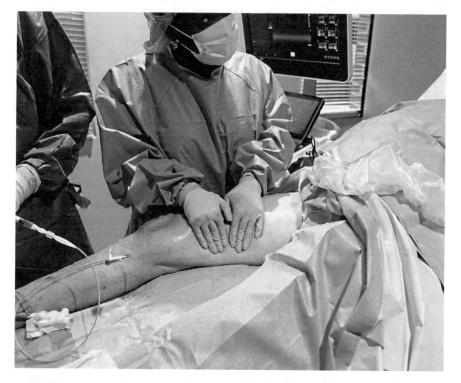

Fig. 24.16 Demonstration of manual compression over a venous segment which has just been injected with adhesive

Step 8. The last injection is made, pressure applied, and catheter removed. Care should be taken to be sure CA is only placed intravenously, as it may elicit an inflammatory reaction in soft tissues or at the level of the skin (this is not a dermal closure adhesive).

Step 9. After treatment, the vein should be surveyed by US, and patency of the common femoral vein and SFJ should be confirmed and documented. In our experience, 1.2 to 1.5 mls of CAC is usually used. It is our practice to have the patient return to the vein center in 3 to 5 days to reassess the vein closure and to rule out potential deep vein thrombosis.

Complications of CAE Nonthermal, Nontumescent Ablation

Complications of CAE include an inflammatory phlebitis in up to 18% of patients in early experience [15]. This may be managed with nonsteroidal anti-inflammatory agents. Because of this inflammation, some authorities have advised against use of the Venaseal procedure in extra-fascial veins located near the skin surface. Also, as noted, care should be taken to prevent CA from entering soft tissues at the point of catheter entry. With these modifications, the mild inflammatory reactions are lessening. Deep vein thrombosis is exceedingly rare, but care should be taken when treating venous segments in communication with large perforating veins. Importantly, nerve injury has not been associated with CAE.

Treatment of the Small Saphenous Vein

Both TT and NTNT techniques may be used to treat the small saphenous vein. In the region of the saphenopopliteal junction, injury to the peroneal or tibial nerves is possible. When using TT techniques, it is our habit not to advance to tip of the RFA catheter beyond the level in the proximal calf at which it turns deep. Given our heightened concern for the rare but possible occurrence of a nerve injury and also considering less distance from skin to vein within the calf, our preference for ablation of the small saphenous vein leans toward NTNT techniques.

Expected Primary Outcome   Durable Venous Closure

Radiofrequency Ablation with ClosureFast™ System

Successful vein closure using the ClosureFast™ system has been documented between 90 and 100% in multiple registries. In a longitudinal prospective study, Kaplan–Meier analysis showed GSV occlusion rates of 91.9% and freedom from reflux of 94.9% [16]. Compared to surgical stripping, closure by RFA has been associated with less pain, faster recovery, and better cosmetic results [6].

Cyanoacrylate Embolization with Venaseal™ System

CAE results in successful vein closure in 92 to 99% of cases producing results equal to those obtained by RFA [11, 17, 18]. All measures of patient comfort, pain during and after procedures, and quality of life equal or exceed the results obtained by RFA in early trials.

Acknowledgment The authors express appreciation to Joseph A. Zygmunt, Jr, RVT, RPhS of Medtronic APV, Endovenous Division, for his critique of our discussion of the ClosureFast and Venaseal procedures.

References

1. Rabe E, Pannier F. Epidemiology of chronic venous disorders. Chapter 10, pages 121–127. In: Gloviczki P, Dalsing MC, Ecklof B, Lurie F, Wakefield TW, editors. Handbook of venous and lymphatic disorders. 4th ed. Boca Raton: Guidelines of the American Venous Forum. CRC Press; 2017.
2. Lurie F, Passman M, Meisner M, Dalsing M, Masuda E, et al. The 2020 update of the CEAP classification system and reporting standards. J Vasc Surg: Venous Lym Dis. 2020;8:342–52.
3. Vasquez MA, Harris L. Outcomes assessment for chronic venous disease. Chapter 67, pages 771-782. In: Gloviczki P, Dalsing MC, Ecklof B, Lurie F, Wakefield TW, editors. Handbook of venous and lymphatic disorders. 4th ed. Boca Raton: Guidelines of the American Venous Forum. CRC Press; 2017.
4. Zygmunt JA. Duplex ultrasound for chronic venous insufficiency. J Invasive Cardiol 2014 E149–55. Accessed December 2, 2018: https://www.invasivecardiology.com/articles/duplex-ultrasound-chronic-venous-insufficiency.
5. Masuda E, Ozsvath K, Vossler J, Woo K, Kistner R, et al. The 2020 appropriate use criteria for chronic lower extremity venous disease of the American Venous Forum, the Society for Vascular Surgery, the American Vein and Lymphatic Society, and The Society for Interventional Radiology. J Vasc Surg: Venous and Lym Dis. 2020;8:505–25.
6. Dietzek AM, Blackwood S. Radiofrequency treatment of the incompetent saphenous vein, Chapter 37, pages 443-454. In: Gloviczki P, Dalsing MC, Ecklof B, Lurie F, Wakefield TW, editors. Handbook of venous and lymphatic disorders. 4th ed. Boca Raton: Guidelines of the American Venous Forum. CRC Press; 2017.
7. Morrison N. Laser treatment of the incompetent saphenous vein. Chapter 38, pages 455-463. In: Gloviczki P, Dalsing MC, Ecklof B, Lurie F, Wakefield TW, editors. Handbook of venous and lymphatic disorders. 4th ed. Boca Raton: Guidelines of the American Venous Forum. CRC Press; 2017.
8. Kheirelseid EAH, Crowe G, Sehgal R, Liakopoulos D, Mulkern E, et al. Systematic review and meta-analysis of randomized controlled trials evaluating long-term outcomes of endovenous management of lower extremity varicose veins. J Vasc Surg: Venous Lym Dis. 2018;6:256–70.
9. Elias S. Emerging endovenous technology for chronic venous disease: mechanical occlusion chemically assisted ablation (MOCA), cyanoacrylate embolization (CAE), and V block-assisted sclerotherapy (VBAS). Chapter 39, pages 465-474. In: Gloviczki P, Dalsing MC, Ecklof B, Lurie F, Wakefield TW, editors. Handbook of venous and lymphatic disorders. 4th ed. Boca Raton: Guidelines of the American Venous Forum. CRC Press; 2017.
10. Harlock JA, Elias F, Qadura M, Dubois L. Meta-analysis of nontumescent-based versus tumescent-based endovenous therapies for patients with great saphenous insufficiency and varicose veins. J Vasc Surg: Venous Lym Dis. 2018;6:779–87.

11. Elias S. Evaluating options to treat superficial venous disease in 2018. Endovascular Today. 2018;17:92–7. Accessed 2 Dec 2018: https://evtoday.com/2018/07/evaluating-options-to-treat-superficial-venous-disease-in-2018/.

12. Sufian S, Arnez A, Labropoulos N, Lakhanpal S. Incidence, progression, and risk factors for endovenous heat-induced thrombosis after radiofrequency ablation. J Vasc Surg: Venous Lym Dis. 2013;1:159–64.

13. Kabnick LS, Sadek M, Bjarnason H, Colman DM, Dillavou ED, et al. Classification and treatment of endothermal heat-induced thrombosis: recommendations from the American venous Forum and the Society for Vascular Surgery. J Vasc Surg: Venous Lym Dis. 2021;9:6–22.

14. Giannas J, Bayat A, Watson SJ. Common peroneal nerve injury during varicose vein operation. Eur J Vasc Endovasc Surg. 2006;31:443–5.

15. Vos CG, Unlu C, Bosma J, van Vlijmen CJ, Jorianne de Nie A, et al. A systematic review and meta-analysis of two novel techniques of nonthermal endovenous ablation of the great saphenous vein. J Vasc Surg: Venous Lym Dis. 2017;5:880–96.

16. Proebstle TM, Alm BJ, Gockeritz O, Wenzel C, Noppeney T, et al. Five-year results from the prospective European multicenter cohort study on radiofrequency segmental thermal ablation for incompetent great saphenous veins. BJS. 2015;102:212–8.

17. Gibson K, Morrison N, Kolluri R, Vasquez M, Weiss R, et al. Twenty-four month results from a randomized trial of cyanoacrylate closure versus radiofrequency ablation for treatment of incompetent great saphenous veins. J Vasc Surg: Venous Lym Dis. 2018;6:606–13.

18. Morrison N, Kolluri R, Vasquez M, Madsen N, Jones A, Gibson K. Comparison of cyanoacrylate closure and radiofrequency ablation for the treatment of incompetent great saphenous veins: 36-month outcomes of the VeClose randomized controlled trial. Phlebology. 2019;34:380–90.

Kidney and Ureter

25

Nikhil L. Shah and M. Fred Muhletaler

Kidney and Ureter

Kidney

Anatomy

The kidneys are located in the retroperitoneum. The projected area where the kidneys lay has four sides, and its boundaries are the 12th rib, the iliac crest, the vertebral column, and a longitudinal line starting at the ipsilateral anterior superior iliac line. The right kidney is usually lower than the left kidney because of the right hepatic lobe.

The muscles of the back around the kidney can be divided into three layers (Fig. 25.1):

(a) Superficial: latissimus dorsi and external oblique muscle
(b) Middle: posteroinferior serratus, sacrospinalis, and internal oblique muscle
(c) Deep: quadratus lumborum muscle, psoas major, and transverse abdominis muscle

The right kidney is related anteriorly to the liver superiorly, to the duodenum (close to the renal hilum) and the ascending colon inferiorly (Fig. 25.2).

The left kidney is adjacent to the stomach, the spleen, and the tail of the pancreas superiorly and medially and the descending colon anteriorly (Fig. 25.3).

N. L. Shah (✉)
Minimally Invasive, Minimal Access & Robotic Surgery, Department of Surgery, Piedmont Health Care, Atlanta, GA, USA

M. Fred Muhletaler
Robotic and Minimally Invasive Surgery, Department of Surgery, Palms West Hospital and Palm Beach Urology, Wellington, FL, USA

© Springer Nature Switzerland AG 2021
L. J. Skandalakis (ed.), *Surgical Anatomy and Technique*,
https://doi.org/10.1007/978-3-030-51313-9_25

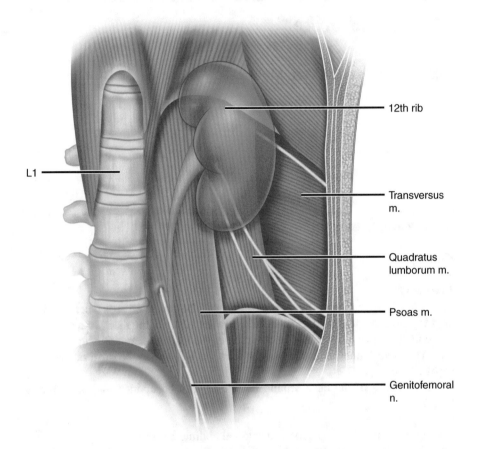

Fig. 25.1 Depiction of the musculature and spine relating to normal anatomic relationships of the kidney

The transversalis fascia splits into posterior and anterior perirenal fascial layers that for Gerota's fascia. The kidneys, adrenal glands, ureters, and renal hilar structures are enclosed in Gerota's fascia. This fascia is typically well closed superiorly to the kidney, but not so well fused inferiorly and medially. Within Gerota's the kidney is slightly movable.

Gross Structure

The kidney is a bean-shaped, soft, and brown-colored structure. It is covered by a fibrous capsule that can be easily stripped.

An adult kidney measures 9–12 cm in the longitudinal axis, 4.5–6.5 wide, and 3–4 cm thick. An average adult kidney weighs 100–140 gr.

The kidney parenchyma can be divided into cortex and medulla. The cortex is the thinner that the medulla, and it contains the glomeruli and the convolute tubules (4–5 mm). The medulla is composed of 8–15 conical masses called pyramids. The bases of the pyramids are continuous with the cortex and the apices project into the

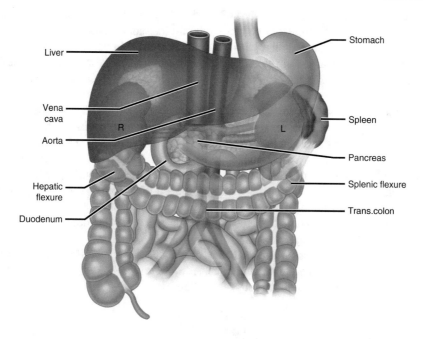

Fig. 25.2 The right kidney's anterior surface in relation to the abdominal viscera

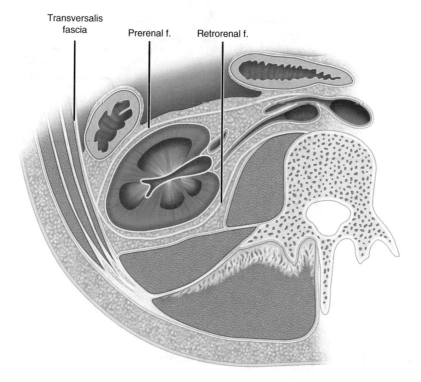

Fig. 25.3 A cross section of the mid-left kidney, revealing anatomic relationships

renal minor calices of the renal pelvis (Fig. 25.4). The minor calices join to form the 2–3 major calices. These major calices open into the renal pelvis. The renal pelvis is a funnel-shaped structure that joins the ureter at the ureteropelvic junction.

The renal arteries arise from the lateral abdominal aorta below the superior mesenteric artery. Both arteries reach the kidneys medially at the hilum. The right renal artery usually courses behind the vena cava. and it is longer than the left renal artery. Renal arteries can branch into several smaller arteries before entering the kidney. It has been well described that a lower pole segmental renal artery branch can cause ureteral obstructions. These branches can cause significant bleeding if not well recognized during renal surgery.

The renal veins lie typically anterior to the arteries, and the left renal vein can be found in front of the aorta, and it is longer than the right renal vein (Fig. 25.5).

Of importance, the left gonadal vein joins the left renal vein on the left side, and the right gonadal vein joins the cava directly on the right side.

Renal lymphatics emerge from the hilum via larger trunks that drain into retrocaval trunks behind the major vessels.

The kidneys have sympathetic and parasympathetic nerve supplies. The majority of nerve fibers run along the renal arteries. A few nerve fibers are received directly from the solar plexus into the kidney and its capsule.

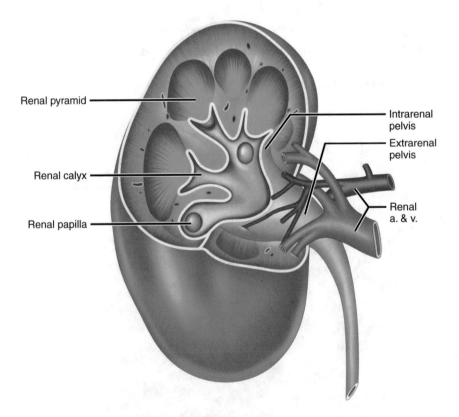

Fig. 25.4 Gross structure of kidney: the hilum, vasculature, and the renal pelvis

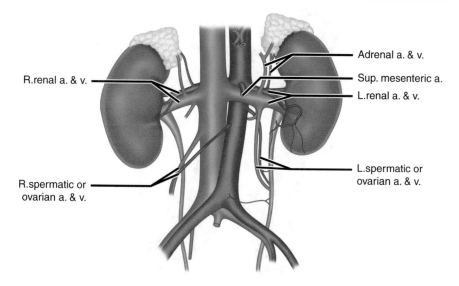

Fig. 25.5 Vascular supply to (and from) the kidney

Incision Techniques

Lumbar/Flank Approach

- **Step 1.** After indication of general anesthesia, the patient is positioned on the side with the appropriate kidney exposed (Fig. 25.6a). Adhesive tape can be used to keep the position at the hip and shoulder. The arm should be kept horizontally, and the knees and legs should be protected.
- **Step 2.** The incision line can be made below the 12th rib or over the distal half of the 12th rib (Fig. 25.6b). The incision is carried through the skin into the subcutaneous tissues exposing the external oblique muscle. If the rib needs to be resected, the incision has to be extended into the body of the 12th rib. Additionally, a lumbar incision can be used as alternative incisions (Fig. 25.6c).
- **Step 3.** Once the external oblique muscle was reached and incised, the internal oblique muscle will be seen. This muscle can be easily recognized for its classic is fan-shape (Fig. 25.7a).
- **Step 4.** Once the internal oblique muscle has been incised, the transversus abdominis fascia and the lumbodorsal fascia will be identified (Fig. 25.7b). The transversus abdominis muscle is the deepest muscular layer of the three lateral abdominal muscles.
- **Step 5.** At this point of the incision time, care should be taken to not injure the 12th thoracic and first lumbar nerves. These nerves can be found between the internal oblique and the transversus abdominis muscles.
- **Step 6.** The next layer of the dissection is Gerota's fascia, which contains the kidney and other structures as described above.

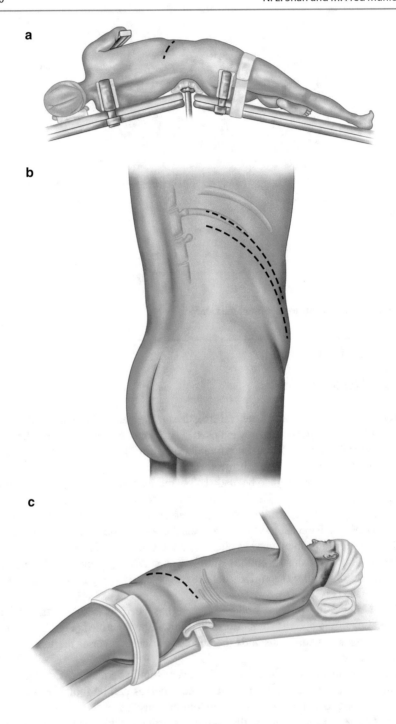

Fig. 25.6 (**a**) Patient in left lateral recumbent positioning with the table flexed, kidney rest fully engaged and the table in slight Trendelenburg. (**b**) Demarcation of a right subcostal incision from flank to the anterior abdomen. (**c**) Depiction of a lumbar incision, left anterior oblique approach

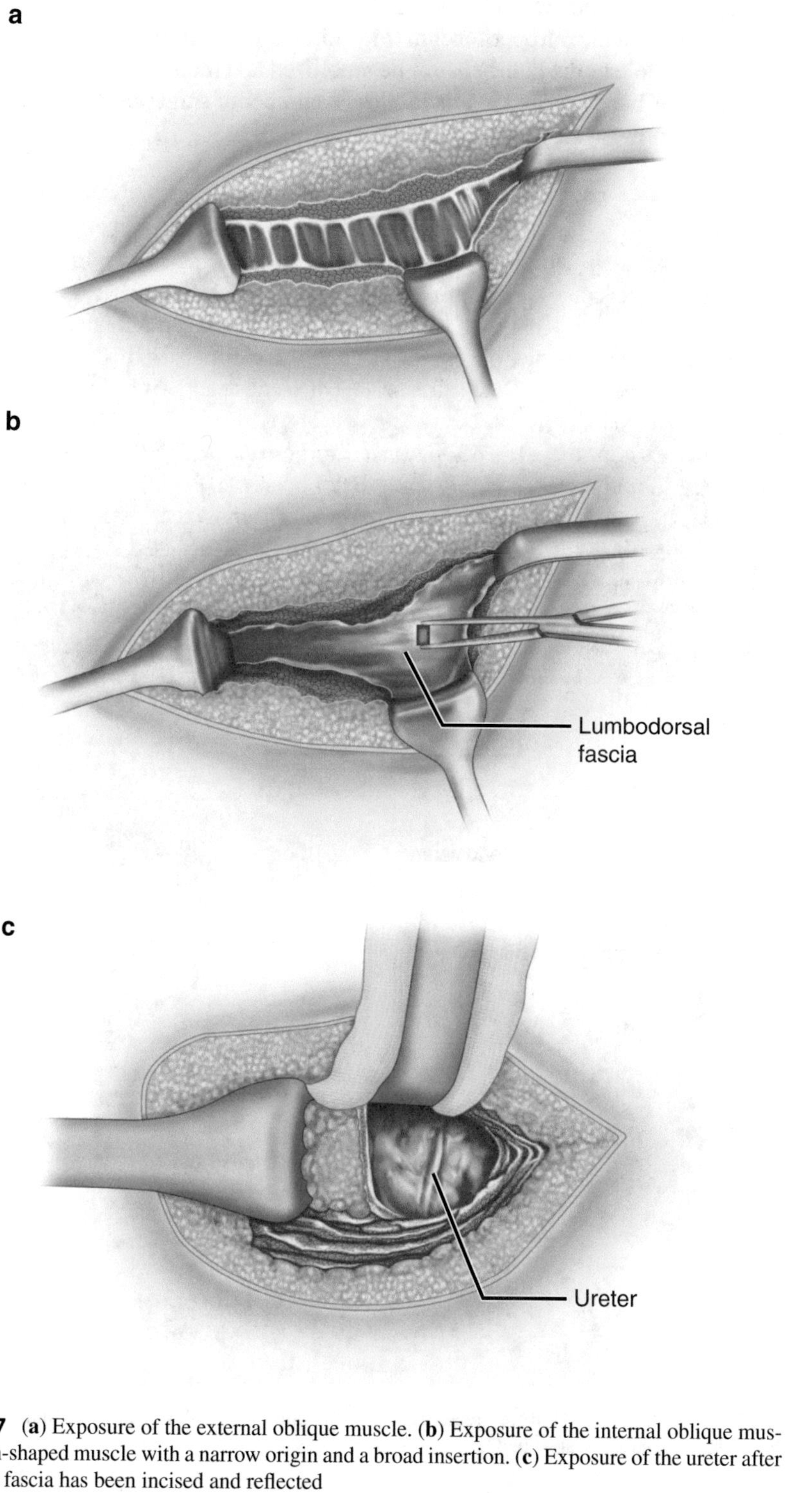

Fig. 25.7 (a) Exposure of the external oblique muscle. (b) Exposure of the internal oblique muscle, a fan-shaped muscle with a narrow origin and a broad insertion. (c) Exposure of the ureter after Gerota's fascia has been incised and reflected

- **Step 7.** The ureter will be identified as a structure with very clear peristaltic movements in the retroperitoneum (Fig. 25.7C). In order to see the ureter clearly, the lower pole of the kidney has to be mobilized and retracted medially. Once the kidney has been exposed in this fashion, a number of surgeries can be done (ureterolithotomy, pyeloplasty, pyelolithotomy, etc.).

Note
- If a bigger exposure is needed, the 12th rib could be resected (Fig. 25.8). For this, the incision has to be extended over the body of the 12th rib. For this dissection, the following muscles have to be divided: external oblique, internal oblique, and latissimus dorsi. Using a periosteal elevator, the rib can be elevated and cut (see images below) after incising the periosteum. After the rib is cut, the lateral abdominal muscles can be incised, and the exposure greatly improved.
- On occasion, the 11th rib may need to be removed in the same manner. Care should be taken at this point to not open the pleural space.
- An alternative technique can be used after removing the rib to enter the retroperitoneum. The distal periosteal bed can be used as a handle to develop an avascular plane underneath it. This maneuver will allow the surgeon to keep the peritoneum medially and, using blunt dissection, enter the retroperitoneum using this avascular plane.

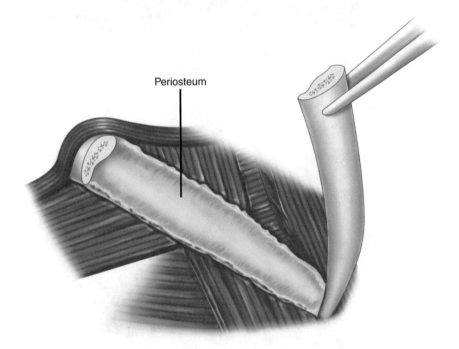

Periosteum

Fig. 25.8 12th rib resection for greater access to the kidney: the rib is transected and lifted from the underlying subperiosteal bed

Fig. 25.9 Midline transperitoneal incision encompassing the umbilicus

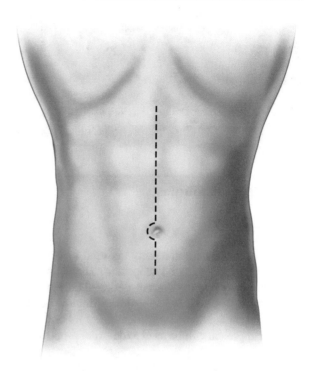

Anterior Abdominal/Transperitoneal Approach

Some cases may require a wider exposure then the one offered by the flank incision Such is the case of a very large renal mass or a trauma situation where rapid control of the renal hilum is needed. Furthermore, in a patient with severe pulmonary insufficiency, the position needed for a retroperitoneal approach may not be adequate. For these situations, a transperitoneal approach should be used.

- **Step 1.** A vertical, midline incision is made (Fig. 25.9). A subcostal oblique incision can be done to facilitate the lateral renal dissection.
- **Step 2.** Upon entry into the peritoneum, inspection and palpation of the abdominal contents is done.
- **Step 3.** The following structures have to be mobilized to expose the kidneys:
  - Right kidney: ascending colon, duodenum (which will be kocherized from the lateral border) and hepatic attachments
  - Left kidney: descending colon, tail of pancreas, splenic attachments, and sometimes the stomach (laterally)
- **Step 4.** At this point, the vascular structures will be seen after some careful dissection: vena cava with the gonadal vein insertion into it and the right renal vein or, contra laterally, the left renal vein with the gonadal vein inserting into it.

Note
- The renal arteries will not be seen well anteriorly, since the renal veins will be usually covering them in the anterior approach.
- There are other incision techniques, for example, the thoracoabdominal approach (for very large upper pole masses), the anterior L-type incision or the subcostal incisions. These are mostly for very specific purposes and are beyond the purpose of this chapter.

Operative Techniques

Nephrectomy

The term "radical nephrectomy" is used to describe an oncologic procedure for renal masses and potential neoplasms. The perirenal structures should be removed with the kidney (Gerota's fascia, perirenal fat, etc.). The term "simple (sub capsular) nephrectomy" is used in the context of removal of a kidney for nonneoplastic reasons (nonfunctioning kidney, trauma, etc.). For the following description, the right anterior approach will be used to describe surgical steps.

- **Step 1.** After the steps mentioned above (incision and entering into the peritoneum, medialization of the ascending colon, and kocherization of the duodenum), the ureter should be dissected and traced up into the renal hilum. This should be done with care to leave the right gonadal vein intact if possible.
- **Step 2.** The renal vessels should be dissected (artery and vein) using split and roll techniques. There are many ways to control and cut the renal hilar structures. The two techniques more frequently used are double-clamp technique (trying to isolate the artery and the vein and tie them off separately) and the use of manual or mechanical staplers. If ligated, the renal vessels should be doubly ligated on the stay side. The renal artery should be ligated and cut first and then the renal vein. Use nonabsorbable material for this purpose. With the use of the newer mechanical stapling devices, an en bloc staple and division of the vessels can be attempted.
- **Step 3.** During a radical nephrectomy, adrenal sparing techniques can be used. In this case, to dissect the adrenal gland off the kidney, care has to be taken to control smaller vessels to the upper pole of the kidney. Hemostatic tools like a harmonic scalpel of a vessel sealer can be helpful.
- **Step 4.** Upon closure, a drain is not needed if the surgical bed is dry and clean.

- **Step 5.** The incision should be closed in layers using absorbable suture.

The discussion of other renal surgical procedures (simple and partial nephrectomy, nephropexy, pyelolithotomy, etc.) is beyond the scope of this chapter.

Ureter

Anatomy

The ureters are bilateral fibromuscular structures that transport urine from the renal pelvis to the urinary bladder. The ureters are 24–35 cm long, and the left ureter is slightly longer than the right one.

From the ureteropelvic junction to the bifurcation of the iliac vessels, the ureters lie on the anterior surface of the psoas major muscles. The gonadal vessels run medially to the ureters for the superior half of the course, and then they cross over more lateral location.

The best way to identify a ureter is to observe its peristaltic activity, which can be also elicited by softly holding it with atraumatic graspers or forceps.

The pelvic ureter crossed the bifurcation of the iliac artery, passes along the lower border of the internal iliac artery, and crosses its anterior branches.

The distal ureter is surrounded by a plexus of veins and small arteries. Finally, as the ureter enters the bladder, there is a segment called the intramural ureter (2 cm).

In the male, the terminal ureter is crossed by the vas deferens just above the ureterovesical junction (Fig. 25.10a, c).

In the female, the distal ureter is in close proximity to the supravaginal portion of the cervix, and it is covered by the uterine artery and veins (Fig. 25.10b). Here is where the ureteral injuries most commonly happen during gynecologic surgery.

Anatomically, the ureter has three narrow areas: the ureteropelvic junction, the area over the iliac vessels, and the ureterovesical junction (which is the tightest of the three). Here is where the passage of kidney stones gets impeded.

The vascular supply to the ureter comes from several sources. The upper third of the ureter is supplied by renal artery and aorta. The mid ureter gets its vascular supply from branches derived from the gonadal artery, colic artery, and internal iliac artery. The distal ureter, in turn, gets irrigation from the superior and inferior vesical artery branches.

These details about the vascular supply to the ureters have to be taken into consideration when ureteral dissection is undertaken. Potential ureteral ischemia will potentially lead to long-segment ureteral strictures.

Most of the open surgical techniques for ureteral surgery have been replaced by endo-urological procedures, which are less invasive.

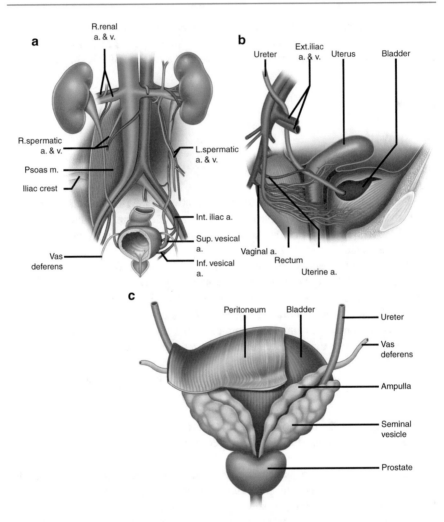

Fig. 25.10 (**a**) The anatomy and relationships of the ureter and vascular supply in the male. (**b**) Deep pelvic part of ureter in the female, lateral view. (**c**) Posterior view of the prostate, seminal vesicles, and vasa

Operative Techniques

Most ureteral surgeries are reconstructive in nature in the current clinical practice. These surgeries should be undertaken by an experienced urologist. In this chapter, we will describe and end-to-end ureteroureterostomy. This procedure could restore continuity of the ureter if it gets accidentally transected during a surgical procedure.

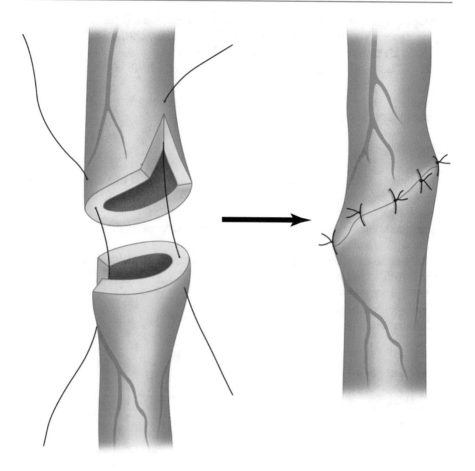

Fig. 25.11 Spatulated, end-to-end anastomosis of the ureter using interrupted absorbable, synthetic suture

End-to-End Ureteroureterostomy

If a ureteral injury occurs (secondary to surgical injury or trauma), this structure can be anastomosed primarily in an end-to-end fashion. This technique works best if the ureter was transected or if the damaged segment is no longer than 2 cm.

The steps to this procedure are as follows:

- **Step 1.** Make sure that the edges of the ureters are viable (with bleeding and with no thermal injury).
- **Step 2.** Spatulate the ureter ends on opposite sites (180° apart). This is done by cutting the ureteral wall longitudinally approximate 7 mm (Fig. 25.11).

- **Step 3.** Suture the ends with interrupted or running stitches (hemi-circular) using fine absorbable suture (e.g., 5–0 PDS). During this point, a Double JJ (e.g., 6 × 24 JJ) ureteral stent should be left in place.
- **Step 4.** Leave a drain at the end of this surgery for 24-m 48 hours.

Anatomical Complications

Renal Surgery

- Diaphragmatic injury – occasionally the posterior lamina of the road is fascia which is fixed to the diaphragm. So when traction is applied to the kidney, the diaphragm can tear.
- Pneumothorax – this can occur with a diaphragmatic injury or with a flank incision with or without rib resection.
- Bleeding from injury to the adrenal gland, spleen, pancreas, and liver.
- Pancreatitis from pancreatic injury.
- Bile leak secondary to liver injury.
- Duodenal injury/perforation.
- Colonic injury/perforation.

Ureter Surgery

- Bleeding
- Ligation
- Laceration or division
- Stripping
- Stenosis
- Fistula
- The most common sites of ureter injury are as follows:
    1. The pelvic wall lateral to the uterine vessels
    2. At the ureterovesical junction
    3. Base of the infundibulopelvic ligament

Index

© Springer Nature Switzerland AG 2021
L. J. Skandalakis (ed.), *Surgical Anatomy and Technique*,
https://doi.org/10.1007/978-3-030-51313-9

Printed in the United States
by Baker & Taylor Publisher Services